Biomedical Platforms

Inside Technology
edited by Wiebe E. Bijker, W. Bernard Carlson, and Trevor Pinch

Janet Abbate, *Inventing the Internet*

Charles Bazerman, *The Languages of Edison's Light*

Marc Berg, *Rationalizing Medical Work: Decision Support Techniques and Medical Practices*

Wiebe E. Bijker, *Of Bicycles, Bakelites, and Bulbs: Toward a Theory of Sociotechnical Change*

Wiebe E. Bijker and John Law, editors, *Shaping Technology/Building Society: Studies in Sociotechnical Change*

Stuart S. Blume, *Insight and Industry: On the Dynamics of Technological Change in Medicine*

Geoffrey C. Bowker, *Science on the Run: Information Management and Industrial Geophysics at Schlumberger, 1920–1940*

Geoffrey C. Bowker and Susan Leigh Star, *Sorting Things Out: Classification and Its Consequences*

Louis L. Bucciarelli, *Designing Engineers*

H. M. Collins, *Artificial Experts: Social Knowledge and Intelligent Machines*

Paul N. Edwards, *The Closed World: Computers and the Politics of Discourse in Cold War America*

Herbert Gottweis, *Governing Molecules: The Discursive Politics of Genetic Engineering in Europe and the United States*

Gabrielle Hecht, *The Radiance of France: Nuclear Power and National Identity after World War II*

Kathryn Henderson, *On Line and On Paper: Visual Representations, Visual Culture, and Computer Graphics in Design Engineering*

Peter Keating and Alberto Cambrosio, *Biomedical Platforms: Realigning the Normal and the Pathological in Late-Twentieth-Century Medicine*

Eda Kranakis, *Constructing a Bridge: An Exploration of Engineering Culture, Design, and Research in Nineteenth-Century France and America*

Pamela E. Mack, *Viewing the Earth: The Social Construction of the Landsat Satellite System*

Donald MacKenzie, *Inventing Accuracy: A Historical Sociology of Nuclear Missile Guidance*

Donald MacKenzie, *Knowing Machines: Essays on Technical Change*

Donald MacKenzie, *Mechanizing Proof: Computing, Risk, and Trust*

Maggie Mort, *Building the Trident Network: A Study of the Enrolment of People, Knowledge, and Machines*

Paul Rosen, *Framing Production: Technology, Culture, and Change in the British Bicycle Industry*

Susanne K. Schmidt and Raymund Werle, *Coordinating Technology: Studies in the International Standardization of Telecommunications*

Dominque Vinck, editor, *Everyday Engineering: An Ethnography of Design and Innovation*

Biomedical Platforms

Realigning the Normal and the Pathological in Late-Twentieth-Century Medicine

Peter Keating and Alberto Cambrosio

The MIT Press
Cambridge, Massachusetts
London, England

This book was set in New Baskerville by SNP Best-set Typesetter Ltd., Hong Kong and printed and bound in the United States of America.

Library of Congress Cataloging-in-Publication Data

Keating, Peter, 1953–
Biomedical platforms: realigning the normal and the pathological in late-twentieth-century medicine / Peter Keating and Alberto Cambrosio.
p. ; cm. — (Inside technology)
Includes bibliographical references and index.
ISBN 0-262-11276-0 (hc : alk. paper)
1. Social medicine. 2. Biotechnology. I. Cambrosio, Alberto, 1950– II. Title. III. Series.
[DNLM: 1. Sociology, Medical. 2. Biological Markers. 3. Biotechnology. 4. Immunophenotyping. WA 31 K25b 2003]
RA418.K39 2003
306.4′61–dc21

2002044414

10 9 8 7 6 5 4 3 2 1

To our parents:
Douglas and Phyllis Keating
Athos and Flora Cambrosio

Contents

Preface

According to an Italian saying, "Il mondo è fatto a scale, c'è chi scende e c'è chi sale," or, in English translation: "The world is made like stairs: there are those who walk down and those who walk up." While the proverb is meant to provide a fatalistic account of individual destinies, it can also be applied to innovations, medical or otherwise: some meet with success, others end in failure and are quickly forgotten. The saying, however, glosses over an important point: stairs do not generally consist solely of steps, they are regularly interrupted by landings or platforms marking each floor. Without these platforms, stairs would have no purpose nor would they exist qua stairs. In turn, platforms are not simply convenient resting places between steps; rather, they give access to apartments and living rooms. This book is about platforms and the rooms to which they give access.

Stairs and platforms in general follow simple paths. We prefer to think of them as in one of the famous Escher drawings where a number of stairs and platforms lead into each other without a clear sense of vertical hierarchy. In other words, we are not interested in linear paths, with well-established beginnings and ends, for we recognize the retrospective existence of multiple paths. In fact, we are not even interested in paths per se but, rather, in the materials and conventions that have been used to design them. We are interested in scattered platforms that interrupt paths and, often, launch them in new directions, providing for both continuities and discontinuities.

Our book analyzes *biomedical* platforms. For reasons that should become clear to readers, we do not think that there are social science platforms. This does not mean that we were able to complete this book without material and conceptual contributions from a number of social science sources. Let us start with financial support. Research for this book has been made possible by several grants. The Social Sciences and

Humanities Research Council of Canada awarded us two successive grants, on "Standards, Instruments and Techniques in the Biological and Biomedical Sciences" (1994–97) and on "Scientific Instrumentalities and the Transformation of Medical Judgment after World War II" (1997–2000). Since 1994, Quebec's Fonds FCAR (now FQRSC) has provided ongoing support for our research program on the regulation of biomedical practices entitled "Techno-scientific Innovations, Biomedical Research and Clinical Interventions." Between 1994 and 1997, the Hannah Institute for the History of Medicine of Associate Medical Services, Inc. (Toronto) provided funds for a more restricted project on visualization in the biomedical sciences, traces of whose results can be seen in chapter 8. The Burroughs Wellcome Fund also contributed decisively to this book by granting to one of the coauthors (P.K.) an award to spend a year at the National Humanities Center, Research Triangle Park, in North Carolina and to the other coauthor (A.C.) a 40th Anniversary Award in the History of Medicine to spend a year in a place of his choice. Additional travel funds were provided to A.C. in 1999 by the Wellcome Institute for the History of Medicine (London) and the Max Planck Institute for the History of Science (Berlin). During 2001, the French Institut National pour la Santé et la Recherche Médicale awarded A.C. a one-year position as a Senior Invited Researcher in the Unit 379 Épidémiologie et sciences sociales appliquées à l'innovation médicale, in Marseilles. Last but not least, both our universities have granted us a sabbatical year during the preparation of this book: P.K. spent it in part at the Mario Negri Institute in Santa Maria Imbaro, Italy (1997–98) and A.C. at the Centre de Sociologie de l'Innovation of the École des Mines in Paris (1996–97).

In addition to funding, good research assistants are an active ingredient of a research project. We would like to single out for special thanks Jean-François Auger, Élaine Gauthier, Anne-Julie Houle, Claudio Interdonato, Martha Poon, and Gavin Svensson. Michael Rutherford and Janalyn Prest cleaned up the mess we had left in the unformatted footnotes of our manuscript. Our students Zlatko Anguelov, Eric Francoeur, Yoshio Nukaga, Sébastien Piché, and Andrew Scyner, and postdoctoral fellows Kenton Kroker and Eve Seguin, while not directly involved in research for this book, stimulated our thinking about technology and biomedicine in contemporary and historical perspectives. Carole Smith and Guy L'Heureux of McGill's Biology Image Centre did a marvelous job scanning and reworking the illustrations used in this book.

Archival collections were a rich source of empirical material for our project and our work there was greatly facilitated by the professional help provided by many archivists. In France, we would like to mention Hélène Chambefort of the INSERM archives in Le Vésinet, Louis Cosnier of the CNRS archives in Paris, Michelle Sabourin of the CNRS archives in Gif-sur Yvette, Sylvain Riquier of the Assistance Publique–Hôpitaux de Paris archives in Paris, and Denise Ogilvie of the Institut Pasteur archives in Paris. In the United Kingdom, we would like to thank for their invaluable help Philip Toms, Records Manager of the Medical Research Council, Dr. David Grant, Scientific Director of the Leukemia Research Fund (LRF) who gave us access to documents held at the LRF headquarters, Miss Frederika A. Phillips, Clerk to the Council of the Imperial Cancer Research Fund (ICRF) (Lincoln's Inn Fields), Julia Chester, Head of Library and Information Services at the ICRF, Robert J. Moore, Librarian at the National Institute for Medical Research (Mill Hill), and Lesley A. Hall of the Contemporary Medical Archives Centre of the Wellcome Library for the History and Understanding of Medicine, all in London. In the United States, Charles Freiman of the Engineering Institute (New York) graciously opened the doors to the corporate archives. Victoria Harden at the National Institutes of Health (NIH) and Judy Grosberg at the National Cancer Institute (NCI) were instrumental in guiding us to the relevant library and archival material in that enormous biomedical complex. Finally, Mike Rhode of the Army Institute of Pathology (Washington, D.C.) was equally generous with his time.

In addition to archival work, interviews with more than eighty scientists, clinicians, and company officials in the United States, Canada, United Kingdom, France, Germany, the Netherlands, and Italy provided a rich documentary basis for this book. Many of these individuals went out of their way to provide unpublished material, correspondence, advice, and close readings of preliminary chapters. They are, in an important sense, less social science "subjects" than valued collaborators. An appendix at the end of this book, giving the list of those who accepted to be interviewed (a few, repeatedly) for this project, is our way of thanking each of them by name. Without their help and understanding, we could simply not have written this book. We see their collaboration as further proof that the history and sociology of science and medicine need not result in "science wars," which are more the product of the disgruntled imagination of a few philosophers or scientists turned ideologues.

Earlier versions of "platform sociology" were presented at a number of meetings, namely the 1997 (Tucson) and 1998 (Halifax) meetings of the Society for Social Studies of Science (4S), the 1998 Lisbon conference of the European Association for the Study of Science and Technology (EASST), the 1998 International Conference on Science, Technology and Society (Tokyo, Hiroshima, and Kyoto), and the 2000 meeting of the American Association for the History of Medicine (Bethesda, Md.). Additional presentations of our ideas on platforms as they were taking shape were presented at several invited talks, including those at the Center for the Sociology of Innovation (École des Mines, Paris, 1996 and 2001), the INSERM Unit 158 (Paris, 1996), Centre for Research into Innovation, Culture and Technology (CRICT) Brunel University (Uxbridge, Middlesex, 1999), the Max Planck Institute for the History of Science (Berlin, 1999), the University of Freiburg (1999), the University of Lausanne (2001), the École des Hautes Études en Sciences Sociales (Paris, 2001), the University of Perugia (2001), and the INSERM Unit 379 (Marseilles, 2001). On each of these occasions we profited from the comments and criticisms of the participants.

We would like to single out, for special thanks, the following friends and colleagues: in France, Madeleine Akrich, Isabelle Baszanger, Pascale Bourret, Michel Callon, Nicolas Dodier, Jean-Paul Gaudillière, Daniel Jacobi, Claire Julian-Reynier, Anne Lovell, Ilana Löwy, Cécile Méadel, Jean-Paul Moatti, Andrei Mogoutov, Anne Marie Moulin, Philippe Mustar, Pierre Lascoumes, Jean-François Picard, and Vololona Rabeharisoa; in Germany, Hans-Jörg Rheinberger and Thomas Schlich (who has now joined us in Montreal); in Portugal, Joao Arriscado Nunes; in the United Kingdom, Harmke Kamminga, Michael Lynch (who has now moved to the United States), Soraya de Chadarevian, and Tilly Tansey; in the United States, Jim Bono, Geof Bowker, Adele Clarke, Angela Creager, Joan Fujimura, Thomas Gieryn, Sheila Jasanoff, Harry Marks, Paul Rabinow, Arthur Silverstein, Susan Leigh Star, and Fred Tauber; in the Netherlands, Marc Berg, Annmarie Mol, and Bernike Pasveer; in Italy, Gilberto Corbellini, Maria Benedetta Donati, Giovanni de Gaetano, and Pino Schirripa; in Switzerland, Marc Audétat and Alain Kaufmann; and, of course, our Canadian colleagues at the Département d'Histoire of the Université du Québec à Montréal, the Centre Interuniversitaire de Recherche sur la Science et la Technologie (CIRST), and the Department of Social Studies of Medicine at McGill University, especially Margaret Lock, Allan Young, and George Weisz.

Although the material used in this book has been entirely rewritten and refocused around the notion of a biomedical platform, several chapters draw from previous publications. An initial, general overview of our argument was presented in:

Keating, Peter, and Alberto Cambrosio. "Biomedical Platforms." *Configurations* 8 (2000), 337–87. Material reproduced with permission by Johns Hopkins University Press.

Scattered components of our argument, not yet connected by the notion of a platform, were included in the following texts:

Cambrosio, Alberto, and Peter Keating. "Of Lymphocytes and Pixels: The Techno-visual Production of Cell Populations." *Studies in History and Philosophy of Biological and Biomedical Sciences* 31 (2000), 233–70. Material reproduced with permission from Elsevier Science.

Keating, Peter, and Alberto Cambrosio. "Real Compared to What?: Diagnosing Leukemias and Lymphomas." In *Living and Working with the New Medical Technologies. Intersections of Inquiry,* ed. Margaret Lock, Allan Young, and Alberto Cambrosio, 103–34. Cambridge, UK: Cambridge University Press, 2000. Material reproduced with permission from Cambridge University Press.

Keating, Peter, Camille Limoges, and Alberto Cambrosio. "The Automated Laboratory: The Generation and Replication of Work in Molecular Genetics." In *The Practices of Human Genetics,* ed. Michael Fortun and Everett Mendelsohn, 125–42. Dordrecht, Netherlands: Kluwer, 1999. Material reproduced with kind permission of Kluwer Academic Publishers.

Keating, Peter, and Alberto Cambrosio. "Interlaboratory Life: Regulating Flow Cytometry." In *The Invisible Industrialist: Manufacturers and the Construction of Scientific Knowledge,* ed. Jean-Paul Gaudillière and Ilana Löwy, 250–95. London: Macmillan/New York: St. Martin's Press, 1998. Material reproduced with permission of Palgrave Macmillan.

Cambrosio, Alberto, Peter Keating, and Ronald D. Guttmann. "New Medical Technologies and Clinical Practice: A Survey of Lymphocyte Subset Monitoring." *Clinical Transplantation* 8 (1994), 532–40. Material reproduced with permission of Blackwell Science Ltd.

Keating, Peter, and Alberto Cambrosio. "'Ours Is an Engineering Approach': Flow Cytometry and the Constitution of Human T-Cell Subsets." *Journal of the History of Biology* 27 (1994), 449–79. Material reproduced with kind permission of Kluwer Academic Publishers.

Cambrosio, Alberto, and Peter Keating. "A Matter of FACS: Constituting Novel Entities in Immunology." *Medical Anthropology Quarterly* 6 (1992), 362–84. Material reproduced with permission of the American Anthropology and Association.

Finally, we would like to thank Kisho Kurokawa for sending us a photograph of one of the buildings he designed and granting us permission to use it for the cover picture of this book.

Biomedical Platforms

1

An Introduction to Platforms

Michel Foucault, discussing the work of conductor and composer Pierre Boulez, once said that the most passionate Western intellectual debates were about form, not content.[1] And indeed, if one looks back at the twentieth century, questions of form—in literature, music, the visual arts—have consistently overridden issues of content. As far as literature goes, just think of the (no longer so "nouveau") *nouveau roman* and its strategy of systematically disrupting traditional narrative conventions. Yet, in spite of limited and not entirely convincing attempts to import "new literary forms" into the field of science and technology studies,[2] history and the social sciences have resisted attempts to subvert the standard scholarly rules of presentation. This book is no exception, except for a modest attempt, in its opening chapters, to introduce its subject matter progressively, through the accretion of several layers of examples. A few colleagues (and, most important, referees!), fearing that such an approach would put off hurried readers, urged us to capture their attention immediately by beginning with a somewhat more traditional summary of the argument. We comply.

The Argument Summarized

In this book, we introduce the notion of *biomedical platform* and use it to analyze the development of innovations and routines in postwar biomedicine. Our analysis entails the articulation of three well-known dichotomies: biology/medicine, science/technology, and innovation/routine. Concerning the first, we claim that, since World War II, biology and medicine have come together, both institutionally and intellectually, in a hybrid practice that is neither syncretic nor synthetic. We show, through example, that a new way of conducting research in biology and medicine has emerged and that this modality aligns normal and pathological phenomena and their representation in a novel way. Within this problematic space of scientific representation, truly biomedical entities—e.g., cell-surface markers, oncogenes, DNA profiles, etc.—exist as both normal biological entities and as pathological signs, i.e., as *biomedical* substances with regard to their origins, their uses, and their meanings. We argue that these entities are constitutive of biomedical platforms and their products.

Figure 1.1 is a 1991 representation of a hierarchical set of procedures used to diagnose blood cancers. As the figure suggests, a patient expressing the relevant clinical signs will generally undergo a biopsy. The tissue sample will then be investigated with the help of histochemical dyes using different techniques beginning with morphological diagnosis to examine the architectural arrangement and the shape and size of the cells in the sample. A form of diagnosis called immunophenotyping follows this initial investigation. Here, panels of standardized antibodies that are often combined with the use of computerized, laser-based equipment detect distinctive molecules at the surface of the malignant cells. Molecular genetics analysis is the last step. Suspicious cells are examined for culpable RNA, DNA fragments, and genes using molecular biologi-

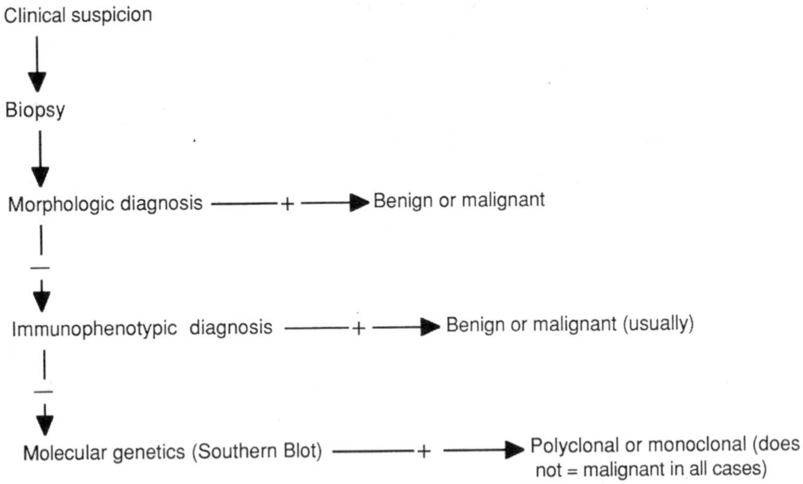

Figure 1.1
A diagnostic algorithm for lymphoid tumors showing platform hierarchies. (From: Whittaker and Willman. "A Practical Guide to the Use of Molecular Genetic Techniques in the Diagnosis of Lymphoid Malignancies," 124. © United States and Canadian Academy of Pathology. Reprinted by permission.)

cal techniques. We believe that each of these steps mobilizes a distinctive biomedical platform. We will thus speak of the morphological platform, the immunophenotyping platform, and so on.

Our subsequent analysis of biomedical platforms focuses on the interlaboratory level of scientific and medical research. Unlike laboratory research, research at this level concerns less the production of local and unprecedented "epistemic things"[3] than the constitution and circulation of protocols, instruments, and substances between laboratories and the establishment of conventions that allow them to be used in the generation of biomedical facts. Usually neglected as a field of mundane regulatory activity, here, accepted divisions between science and technology and innovation and routine break down. We show, thus, how modern biomedicine requires a description of scientific practice that offers a distinctive place for technology and its development other than that of a simple tool for the furtherance of intellectual goals. In particular, we show that biomedical research programs are embedded in technology in the form of substances produced on biomedical platforms and that regulatory activities conducted at all levels of research are constitutive of platforms and their effective functioning as agents of change within the biomedical sciences.

We have chosen a specific biomedical platform known as "immunophenotyping" and describe its emergence as an experimental system with roots in biology (immunology) and pathology (oncology). We then show how this experimental system was transformed into a biomedical platform, initially for the diagnosis of leukemia, at first in one, then in many laboratories. Our description does not resort to the diffusion of ideas or instruments but details the interlaboratory constitution of conventional substances—in our case cell-surface markers—and the equipment, procedures, and clinical and scientific categories required for the conduct of interchangeable activities on a global level. By targeting this level of practice, we avoid two pitfalls commonly associated with the description of scientific activities. First, by concentrating on the platforms that link laboratories, we avoid the action-at-a-distance causality that underlies descriptions of science as a paradigm-ordered or theory-driven activity. Second, although we occasionally describe experiments in individual laboratories, our analysis of activities that seek to stabilize existing practices and the entities they produce allows us to outline conditions for the production of novelty and routine within a single laboratory.

Our analysis of the immunophenotyping platform draws together a range of activities in contemporary biomedicine running from laboratory research to clinical trials and routine diagnosis. This enables us to describe biomedical platforms as specific combinations of techniques, instruments, reagents, skills, constituent entities (morphologies, cell-surface markers, genes), spaces of representations, diagnostic, prognostic, and therapeutic indications, and related etiologic accounts. More specifically and more abstractly, our study enables us to define biomedical platforms as material and discursive arrangements that act as the bench upon which conventions concerning the biological or normal are connected with conventions concerning the medical or pathological.

Finally, through comparison of different clinical instantiations of the immunophenotyping platform, we observe that while platforms form the locus of biomedical innovation and routine, the development of a new platform does not necessarily result in the replacement of the previous platform. Rather, new platforms are often articulated and aligned in complex ways with existing ones, and thus integrated into an expanding set of clinical-biological strategies.

Readers will find below a short chapter-by-chapter overview of the book. For the moment, we ask them to accompany us through the doors of a hospital.

A Visit to a Hospital

The tertiary hospital provided specialized care to patients afflicted with rare or deadly diseases such as leukemia and lymphoma, cancers affecting the cells and organs of the hemopoietic (blood cell–forming) system. The large American flag in front of the massive building reminded us that we were in the United States. Overhead, emergency helicopters flew patients in from the tristate catchment basin on an around-the-clock basis. Upon entering the premises, we were struck by a giant quilt on the walls of the entrance hall (figure 1.2a). Although the "quilt" turned out to be made of ceramic tiles, the recent revival of the American tradition of quilting in response to the AIDS crisis had immediately brought the term to mind.[4] Cancer patients had designed the individual tiles that featured childlike drawings of cartoon characters and that consequently reminded onlookers of the emotional lives of children with leukemia.[5] Short texts, in adult handwriting, occasionally accompanied the tiles and expressed heartfelt gratitude—sometimes to God, sometimes to a doctor—for successful therapy (figure 1.2b).

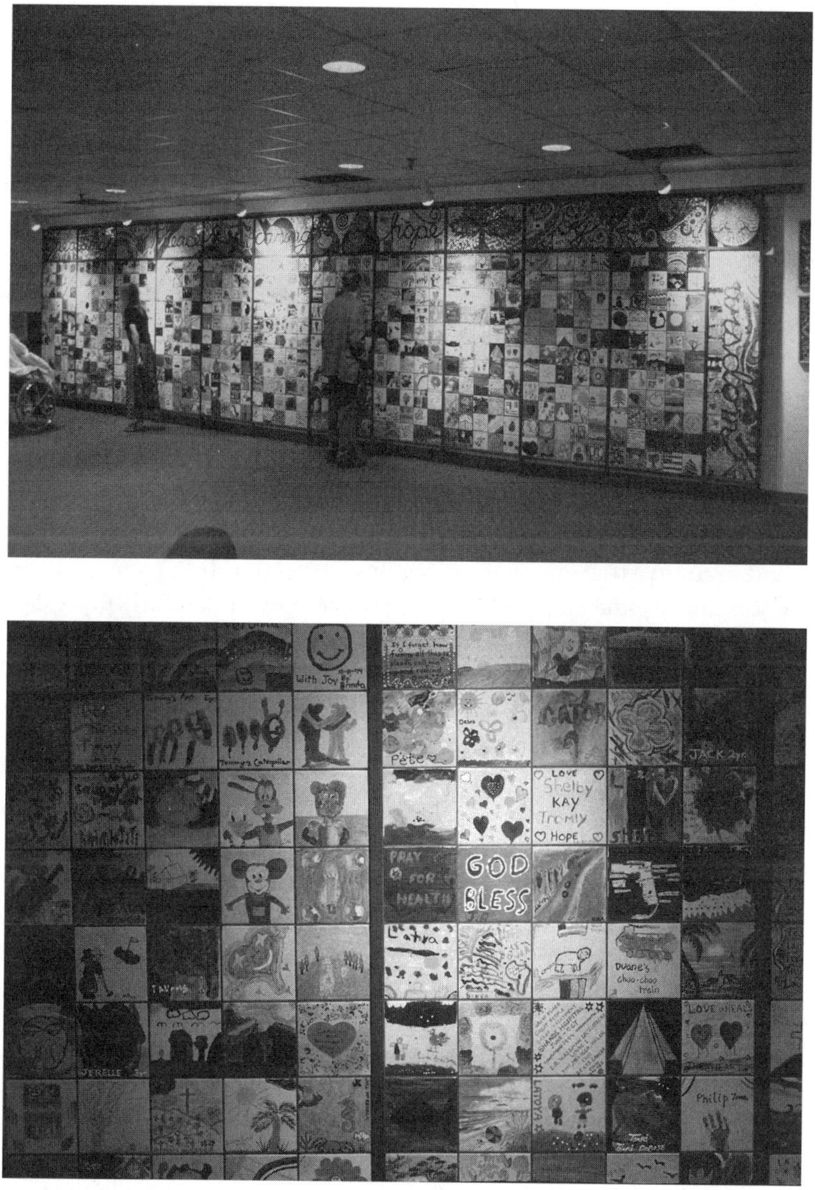

(*a*)

(*b*)

Figure 1.2
Overview (*a*) and close-up (*b*) of the "quilt" on the walls of an American cancer hospital. (Photographs: A.C.)

The quilt interwove numerous narratives of personal despair and suffering and of hope.

We had come to the hospital to visit an important laboratory medicine team and to learn about recent developments in the diagnosis and prognosis of cancer. We hoped to gain firsthand knowledge of old and new procedures and to gather oral-historical information from the head of the local hematopathology (blood pathology) unit. The tile "quilt" confronted us with the patient's view of the medical developments we had come to investigate. Was this the voice of the "lifeworld," i.e., the subjective experience of disease, as opposed to the voice of medicine, i.e., the objectifying language of medical diagnosis, as expressed in numbers and esoteric terminology?[6]

Past the entrance hall, several flights up, we followed a sign reading Hematopathology to a large laboratory. Hospital policy excluded patients, in the ordinary sense of the term, from these rooms. We nonetheless encountered a number of "patients" in the form of blood and bone marrow samples undergoing inspection by a team of pathologists and technicians. Although these patients were clearly metaphorical, it was not our metaphor. Having taken us out to lunch, the chief laboratory pathologist had told us somewhat nervously partway through the meal that he had to "rush back to his patients." We had assumed that he had planned to visit patients in the wards—an unusual move for a pathologist—but as soon as we reentered the laboratory he pointed to a set of blood and marrow slides (figure 1.3), saying, "Here are my patients." Is this further evidence of the divorce between the voice of the lifeworld, where it only makes sense to speak of patients as whole persons, and the voice of medicine, where patients can be reduced to body samples exposed to the objectifying gaze of healthcare professionals and automated laboratory equipment?

As we soon learned, to construe the pathologist's utterance—"Here are my patients"—as evidence of the narrow, reductionist nature of "the biomedical model,"[7] overlooked the fact that clinicians generally initiate chemotherapeutic treatment of patients presenting the clinical signs of acute leukemia after the diagnosis has been confirmed by laboratory analysis. It can literally be a matter of hours before it is too late to reverse the course of the disease. This is why the laboratory we visited was staffed on a 24-hour basis and this is why the microscope slides, ultimately integrated with "whole" patients waiting in the wards for lifesaving or, at least, life-prolonging therapy, were of crucial importance to their treating physicians.[8] In other words, there was, despite appearances, no deep

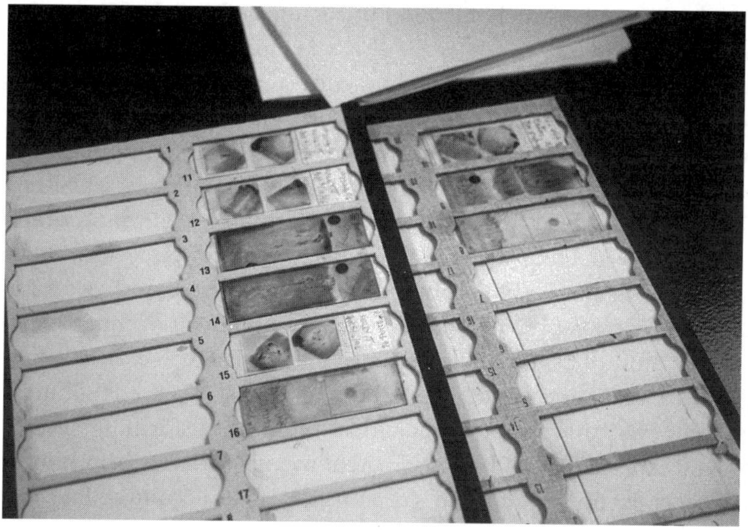

Figure 1.3
"Here are my patients": blood and bone marrow slides in a pathology laboratory. (Photograph: A.C.)

division between the patient and the laboratory. Indeed, in contemporary hospitals all sorts of body samples leave the patient to travel routinely and frequently to diagnostic laboratories. But they also return to the patient in the form of results that acquire meaning as part of the therapeutic relationship that exists between patients and increasingly complex teams of healthcare professionals. Traces of this process can easily be found in the material and organizational structure of hospitals that have been redesigned to take into account the large flow of samples (see chapter 2).

In this book, we examine the social and historical conditions for the establishment of both discursive and material relations between bodies and samples. Commonly referred to as links between the clinic and the laboratory, these relations are defined by the intersection of distinctive arrangements of instruments and programs that seek to articulate biological and population data with diagnostic and prognostic singularities. We call such configurations of people and equipment, several of which have been developed during the second half of the twentieth century, "biomedical platforms." We will show that the latter are a critical site of biomedical innovation and that new biomedical entities, produced, managed, and regulated on the platform, become defining elements of patients' bodies and, as such, channel the actions of the physicians who deal with them.

Scientific and clinical research and practice create and reproduce new entities, new actors.[9] Initially confined to the esoteric space of the laboratory, they (or, at least, some of them) subsequently redefine not only the patient's clinical identity but also our daily lives. Indeed, as Silverman has noted, medical discourse "has entered into our own accounts of ourselves, thus making the distinction between 'lifeworld' and 'medicine' itself problematic."[10] Microorganisms are a case in point[11]: we wash our hands and take care to prevent the deleterious effects of "microbes," entities that most of us have never seen or manipulated.[12] As Porter suggests, in the case of germs, medicine has migrated "from the laboratory to the lavatory," infiltrating our imagination and transforming "everyday beliefs, experiences and habits."[13] Actions and behaviors, both individual and collective, have been (re)constituted to accommodate the new entities produced by modern biomedicine.

While the case of bacteriology is particularly well documented, the argument applies just as well to the entities generated more recently by other medical specialties such as hematology and immunology, or, more precisely, by the development of the biomedical platforms used by those specialties. T4 cells, also known as CD4 cells, the white blood cells attacked by the virus human immunodeficiency (HIV) and whose sharp decline signals the passage from HIV-positive status to AIDS, provide a significant contemporary example. Less than thirty years ago, T4 cells did not exist in laboratories or medical textbooks. Chapters 4 and 5 reconstruct the complex chain of events that, independently of the impending AIDS pandemic, resulted in the production of the biomedical platform that lies behind the existence of T4 cells. For the moment, let us simply note that they are now taken for granted in both medicine and everyday life. Anyone strolling through downtown Paris in 1997, for instance, saw the magnified pictures of T4 cells hanging from the city walls (figure 1.4). For AIDS patients, T4 cells had by then become a daily reality. Counting the T4 cells contained in a cubic millimeter of blood produced a number that, following initial diagnosis, continuously mediated their subjective bodily experience and narratives. Consider the following AIDS patient who experienced a dramatic recovery after the initiation of triple therapy:

> Look at me now!—says a young HIV positive patient while executing a *pas de deux* in the corridors of the Cochin hospital—Six months ago I could feel death taking over, I was at zero T4, I was skinny, I had one infection after another, I was witnessing my own passing away. Since the beginning of triple-therapy, I have 180 T4s, my viral load is undetectable, I have put on 3 kilos, I will start working again, and I am even asking myself whether or not I should have a child.[14]

No longer confined to the hospital or to the bodies of individual patients, T4 cells have entered the political arena, further reinforcing their status in medical settings.[15] A case in point is the decision by the U.S. Centers for Disease Control and Prevention (CDC) to modify the definition and staging of AIDS. The latter had initially been based solely on clinical criteria (a list of opportunistic diseases and clinical conditions). In 1985, following the identification of HIV, the CDC added the results of the HIV antibody test. Then, in 1993, the CDC ruled that a cell count of less than 200 CD4 (T4) cells/mm^3 combined with an HIV-positive status defined AIDS. The switch from a clinical to a laboratory-based definition generated considerable controversy, for it immediately produced a major increase in the prevalence of official AIDS cases and created the possibility of diagnosing patients with AIDS before the expression of symptoms.[16] Prior to the 1993 decision, the CDC had organized an extremely adversarial meeting with lay activist groups.[17] The transcripts of the meeting on the implications of the change in the definition of AIDS contain many angry personal narratives from HIV-positive patients who contrasted their lived experiences with the objectifying nature of laboratory-generated values purveyed by the CDC's medical experts.

Yet, as chronicled in Steven Epstein's detailed analysis of AIDS activism, when lay groups such as ACT UP confronted the medical establishment, contesting, for instance, the design of clinical trials, they turned themselves into "lay experts" making full use of the biomedical entities that inhabit clinical discourse.[18] Challenging, for example, the use of a patient's death as an appropriate endpoint for clinical trials, AIDS activists promoted, instead, CD4 counts as "surrogate markers."[19] CD4 counts, as we have seen, had become routine components of the therapeutic management of AIDS both from the medical and the patient's point of view. By accepting the clinical significance of CD4 cells, patients and activists operate on the biomedical platform that has generated and reproduced those entities. In other words, while medical and lay actors position themselves vis-à-vis a given platform, contributing, for instance, as in the present case, to its further entrenchment, they cannot

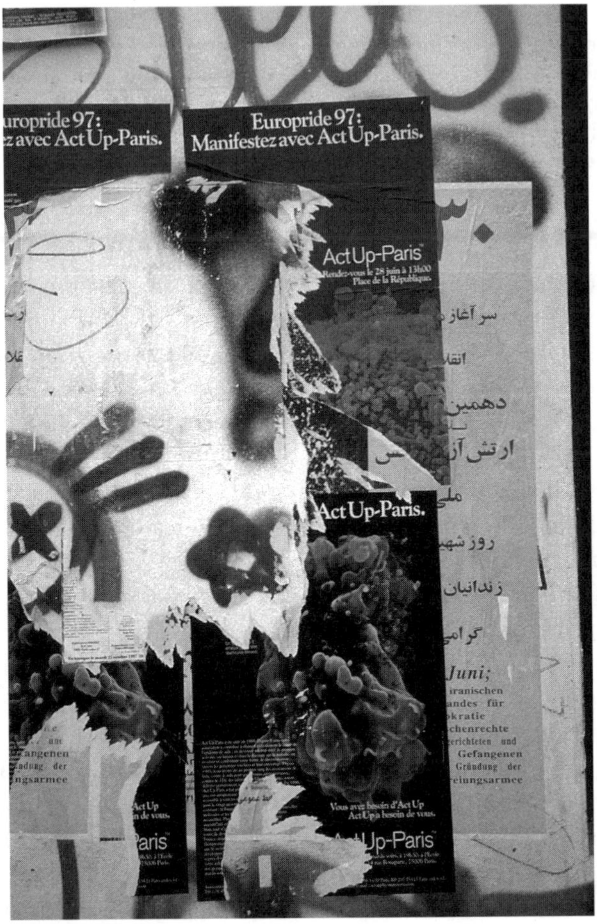

(*a*)

Figure 1.4
ACT UP posters displaying CD4 cells on the walls of buildings in downtown Paris (*a*), and a clean version (*b*) of one of the posters. (Photographs: A.C.)

operate "off" the platform, unless, of course, they decide to opt out entirely from Western medicine by embracing alternative medical cosmologies.

The situation we just described can be analyzed as part of the long-term historical trend whereby physicians no longer rely on narratives of symptoms offered by patients during a medical encounter, but turn instead to an expanding collection of diagnostic signs.[20] Yet, as we argue in chapter 3, the post–World War II period, rather than simply corresponding to a quantitative extension of this process, has led to a quali-

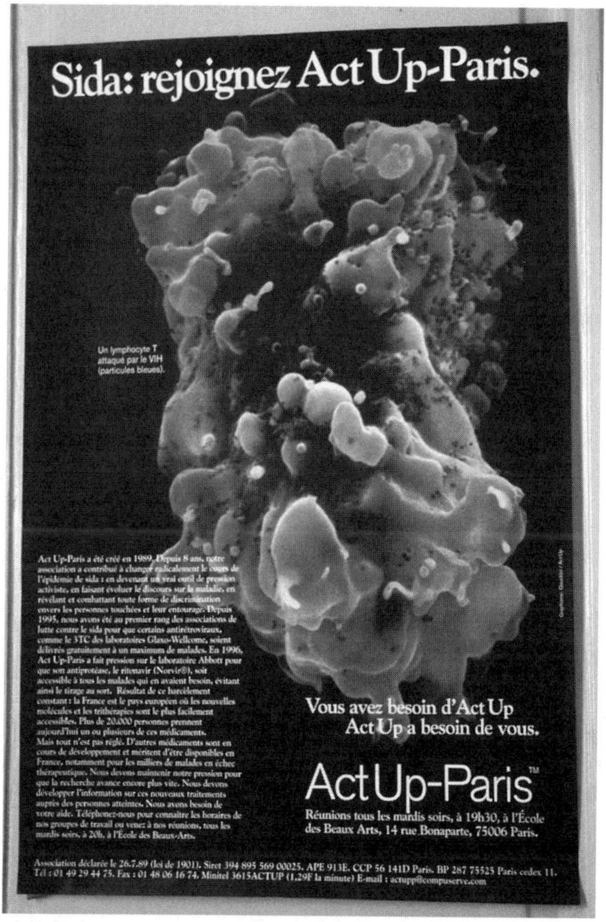

(*b*)

Figure 1.4
(continued)

tative transition aptly captured by the neologism "biomedicine." If then, in an important sense, being a patient now is quite different from being a patient several decades ago, this is not simply because a growing number of the entities, such as CD4 cells or, say, cancer susceptibility genes, that are constitutive of those diagnostic signs are of recent origin. Rather, it is because the understanding of these entities resides at the intersection of medicine and biology or, in other words, is linked to the emergence of a new configuration of the relations (conceptual, material, and institutional) between the normal and the pathological. We conceived of this book as a contribution to the study of this profound transformation of modern medicine, which we will track through the analysis of the development of biomedical platforms. Before going any further, then, we must outline, by way of a concrete example, the notion of "biomedical platform."

Platforms: An Example

Here is an excerpt of a message posted to a clinical electronic discussion forum used by cancer pathologists seeking help in difficult diagnoses:

> I have a bone marrow biopsy on a 63 yr. old male with severe peripheral pancytopenia. Biopsy is atypical lymphoid infiltrate consistent with [non-Hodgkin's lymphoma] small cleaved cell. . . . The phenotype . . . seems to fit best with follicular lymphoma except for the CD10 negativity. I wonder what others of you may think about this phenotype?[21]

For the moment, ignore the compressed nature of the message,[22] and consider the description of a biopsy featuring simultaneously an "atypical lymphoid infiltrate," "small cleaved cell," and a "phenotype" with "CD10 negativity." What do these terms mean?

"Lymphoid infiltrates" and "small cleaved cells" belong to the richly descriptive language of pathological morphology. Typically, pathologists examine blood samples, as well as bone marrow and tissue specimens surgically obtained from patients (biopsies), under a microscope to detect cells and tissues that have pathognomonic value, i.e., that are characteristic of a given disease or subclass thereof. The term "infiltrate," in this context, designates unusual cell growth patterns or the migration of cells to tissues other than those of origin, both signs of cancer. In this same context, "small cleaved cells" refer to a particular kind of white blood cell (lymphocyte) presenting a characteristic deformation: their nuclei display infoldings or deep indentations. Figure 1.5 shows three pathologists examining the same slide under a multiocular microscope. The chief pathologist controls the settings of the microscope, exploring different parts of the slide and increasing or decreasing magnification to observe individual cells or the overall cell pattern. While doing so, he solicits the opinion of his colleagues, and, together, they reach a diagnosis before moving to the next slide/patient.[23]

"Phenotypes" (or "immunophenotypes," as they are also called) arise in a significantly different practice. Here, sophisticated equipment

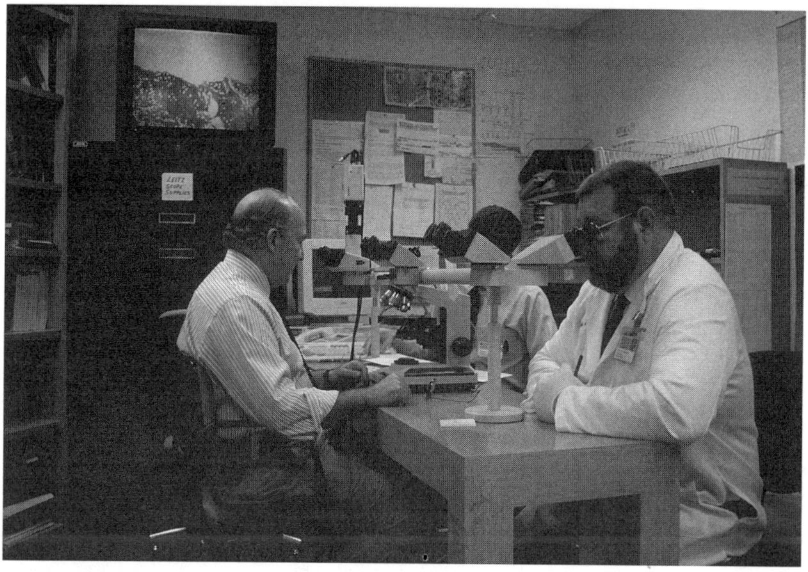

Figure 1.5
The collective production of morphological diagnosis: pathologists looking into a multiocular microscope. The chief pathologist (on the left) operates the microscope. One of the oculars is connected to a camera, allowing additional observers to follow the diagnostic session on the television screen. (Photograph: A.C.)

(known as flow cytometers) and exquisitely specific immunological reagents (antibodies), classified according to an internationally accepted CD nomenclature (see chapters 6 and 7 for a detailed discussion of flow cytometry and the CD system), conspire to produce a quantitative analysis of the cell populations found in normal and pathological blood and bone marrow specimens. The CD reagents bind to molecularly distinct yet visually indistinguishable structures (so-called markers; see chapters 4 and 6) on the surface of cells, and fluorescent substances linked to the reagents allow the cytometer's laser beam, optical detectors, and photomultipliers to detect a given set of markers. Figure 1.6 shows a pathologist sitting in front of a flow cytometer looking at results on the equipment's computer screen. We discuss the distinctive imagery produced by the cytometer in chapters 7 and 8. For now, suffice it to say that, as shown in figure 1.7 (see also figures 7.7 and 9.1), it bears no resemblance to the morphological shapes pathologists have painstakingly learned to recognize and name.

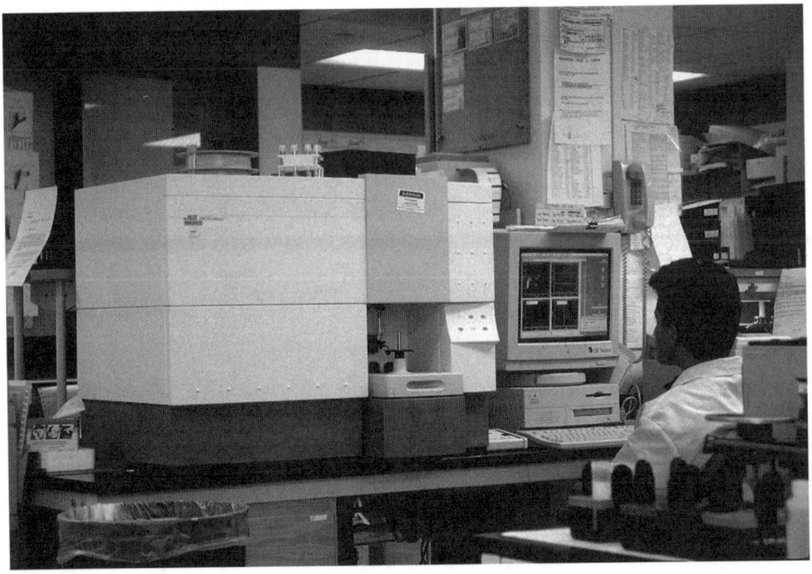

Figure 1.6
A pathologist sitting in front of a flow cytometer, inspecting phenotypic imagery on the computer screen. (Photograph: A.C.)

Let us return to our electronic message. The patient mentioned in the excerpt had a marked reduction in the number of cells normally present in the blood (pancytopenia). The author of the message interpreted this symptom as indicating a type of cancer known as lymphoma. He wondered how to further classify the disease since the two *platforms* on which he routinely relied—morphological analysis and phenotyping—provided contradictory answers. Morphology pointed to one of the most common subtypes of lymphoma in the United States, follicular (itself a morphological term)[24] lymphoma, but, were this so, then the cells should have been CD10 positive.

Reactions to the message varied. Some respondents favored exclusive reliance on the morphological platform: "the actual pattern of the lymphoid infiltrate would be more helpful in suggesting follicular lymphoma."[25] Others favored a hierarchical ordering of both platforms, with morphology as "the gold standard."[26] Yet others gave precedence to phenotyping over morphology:

I think that we are all gratified that the continual evolution in lymphoma classification has begun to utilize immunophenotypic descriptions more and

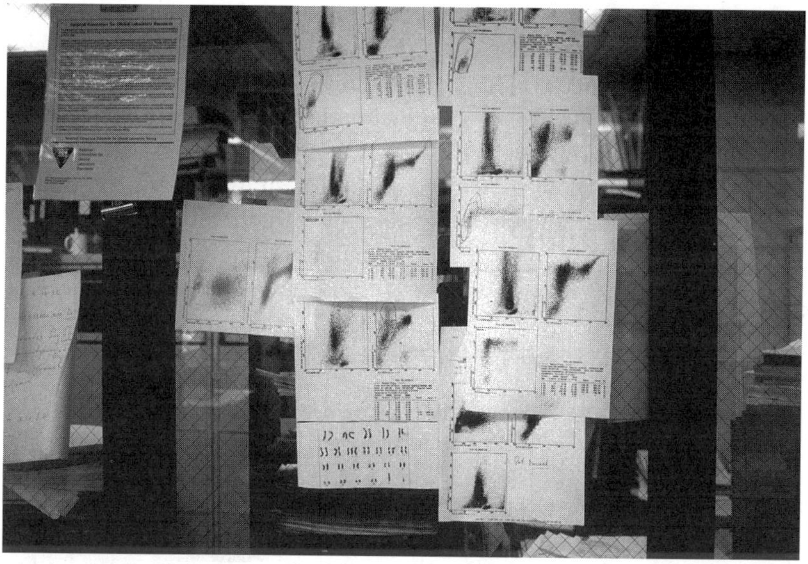

Figure 1.7
Printed samples of phenotypic images posted on a glass partition in a diagnostic laboratory. (Photograph: A.C.)

more—this is long overdue. However, we must remember that all of the historical classifications, especially those including such terms as "follicular," "mantle," etc. are based on (highly subjective in my view) morphology.[27]

Some perceived this last opinion as a threat not simply to the morphological platform, but, more important, to the biological and clinical reality of the disease entities defined on the basis of that platform. While admitting that there were "those gray cases which are not typical for anything and the state of the art is such that we can't give an accurate diagnosis and must give a best guess," the author of the following message maintained that

Mantle cell lymphoma has a characteristic morphology, immunophenotype and [genotype]. It also has a clinical prognosis that is distinct from other [related kinds of cancer]. It is not a subjective morphological diagnosis. Any good hematopathologist can diagnose a typical mantle cell lymphoma. Follicular lymphoma is even easier and again not only has morphologic, immunophenotypic and genotypic criteria but there is also an associated clinical prognosis. Follicular lymphoma is a disease that we know a lot about, not a subjective morphological classification.[28]

The previous message implicitly acknowledged the existence of multiple platforms that somehow converged to lead to the differential diagnosis of distinct (and "real")[29] disease entities. And indeed, the issue of how the different platforms should be aligned became the focus of subsequent discussion, for, as is obvious, as soon as clinical laboratories routinely produce data generated by different platforms, alignment becomes a practical and pressing necessity. Alignment, however, does not necessarily mean overlap or triangulation[30] insofar as it entails hierarchies (e.g., "gold standards"), choices, and the production of unexpected events. It is itself a controversial procedure, as shown by the juxtaposition of the following three excerpts:

> We are asking for a lot of confusion, and we are doing ourselves a disservice, if we keep trying to align morphologic descriptions with specific immunophenotypes.[31]

> Modern classification of lymphoma combines [morphologic, immunologic, and genetic] features, and in most cases the morphologic features fit very well with the immunophenotype. . . . Adding these other methods allows us to further define entities, but should not entirely replace the significance of the morphologic features. When immunologic features do not fit the morphologic features, I go back and review the morphology again.[32]

> I would suggest that it is in the process of "trying to align morphologic descriptions with specific immunophenotypes" that we make progress in sorting out which morphologies and which immunophenotypes actually define true pathological entities. . . . The efforts to correlate these various criteria (morphologic, immunologic, genetic, and clinical) clearly result in the recognition and better understanding of specific disease entities.[33]

The electronic exchange just reported concerned the diagnosis of lymphoma, i.e., the determination of the type or category of lymphoma from which the patient suffered. A similar discussion occurred a year later concerning "staging," i.e., the determination of the specific extent of spread of the disease following diagnosis. Typically, in a procedure known as a bone marrow aspiration, the surgeon inserts a needle into the patient's hip bone and extracts liquid bone marrow, which is then examined morphologically under a microscope and phenotypically with flow cytometry. The opening message of this exchange read, in part:

> If the pathologist did not see any abnormal cells, and the immunophenotyping showed a small clearly monoclonal population of, say, 1–2% of the nucleated cells, how would this information get used, in terms of patient management and treatment? To me it seems that the gray area between when the pathologist cannot see abnormal cells and the flow ability to detect them is in the 1–5% range.[34]

A first reply came from a pathologist who represented the situation as follows:

> In my experience, what happens when you detect a small population of malignant cells that the pathologist (myself included) can't see depends on the clinician. Some clinicians here understand the power of flow and will accept .01% malignant cells. Another won't accept anything but morphology (therefore making flow almost a waste for staging).[35]

After noting that the question had been "addressed (although not totally resolved)" by a recently published consensus statement (we discuss the production of consensus recommendations in chapter 9), a second contributor, while averring that "immunophenotypic analysis of bone marrow with morphologically obvious lymphoma . . . is generally considered redundant," nonetheless conceded that

> Detection of minimal disease does at times create a therapeutic dilemma. . . . However, it does provide what most consider useful, objective information and can increase the rate of detection by another 10–20% . . . I believe a good practice is to perform flow if there is any doubt. At the very least, the combination of morphology and flow immunophenotyping will reduce the frequency of staging procedures with the final interpretation of "atypical lymphoid infiltrate, suspicious for lymphoma," which is of little value to the treating clinician.[36]

Once again, alignment between different platforms, a practical necessity derived from their coexistence under the same medical roof, turned out to be the critical issue.

Platforms: Initial Theoretical Musings

The situation depicted in this example is relevant to anyone interested in biomedical practices and, more specifically, in biomedical innovation, for we have here an instance of an older, established practice—morphological pathology—being challenged (but not superseded) by a newcomer, immunophenotyping. But who or what is challenging whom or what? In other words, how should one describe the participants in this debate, analyze its development, and, more generally, describe biomedical routines and innovation?

A traditional sociological answer to this question and one often implicitly adopted by historians treats the debate as the result of a collision or confrontation of different "social worlds," i.e., professional groups or subgroups, each characterized by a distinctive shared identity. These conflicting identities were held to have a variety of sources. In their classic papers on "professions in process," for instance, Bucher and Strauss argued that the identity of a given group would vary according to the tasks performed by its members, the methodology and techniques they used, the clients they served, the colleagues with whom they interacted, and the interests and values they shared.[37] In spite of the recognition that shifts in methodology might lead to redefinitions of the field and give rise to debating segments, Bucher and Strauss concluded that social relations among and between members of the various segments would ultimately determine the definition of a given segment. The conflicts between groups would thus be ultimately social conflicts prompted by threatened identities. There are no things in this world: just words.

According to Bucher and Strauss, human actors make up groups and these actors just happen to "take up" techniques and instruments in the course of their professional life. More recent work in this tradition has replaced these groups or "segments" with "social worlds."[38] But a change of words does not entail a change in perspective. The expansion from group or segment to world is entirely discursive. Sociologists who use the "social worlds" perspective to examine technical, scientific, and medical issues—i.e., fields saturated with tools and techniques—focus first and foremost on human collectives, their words and deeds.[39] Although techniques, instruments, and research materials (organic or otherwise) do occasionally figure in their accounts, their appearance and status is entirely secondary. They are either black-boxed and construed as rhetorical tools mobilized in the turf struggles between competing camps, reduced to social variables, or dissolved into an increasingly vague, all-encompassing notion of practice(s). In contrast to these sociological accounts, we wish to treat objects as mediators and coordinators of biomedical activities.[40] To this end, borrowing in part from language used in the healthcare sector (see chapter 2), we have devised the notion of biomedical platforms to draw together within a single category biomedical instruments and programs and related patterns of cooperation between biologists, clinicians, and companies that produce reagents and equipment.

To explain why we have done so, it is useful to return to the debate featured in the previous section. It should be obvious to most readers that a narrow focus on human collectives and professional rivalries can hardly account for the confrontation between the morphological and the immunophenotyping platforms. True enough, a clever sociologist could always identify each of the opinions concerning a given platform as the product of a distinct group or social world, either by multiplying the number of ad hoc distinctions between groups or by tailoring opinions to fit a predetermined group. But such divisions would be at odds with the participants' views. The researchers and clinicians who posted the conflicting messages are clearly engaged in what they perceive as the same kind of activity and thus, in some sense, belong to a single group. In other words, taken on their own terms, the actors we quoted inhabit a single world in addition to a single electronic discussion forum. This common world also houses many platforms, whose role in that world, judging from the debate we have just summarized, is far from marginal. Why, then, should the sociologists' view, according to which participants inhabit different "worlds" or partake in different "groups," take precedence over the participants' view? Clearly, there is no compelling reason to do so.

This is not to say that patterns of segmentation between different occupational groups are absent from the biomedical enterprise. Professional and specialty divisions are common features of the latter. Indeed, some authors have characterized the proliferation of medical specialties as the hallmark of the development of modern medicine.[41] But how should one describe these segmentation processes or, to use a related term from yet another sociological tradition, this ever-evolving division of labor? Studies of the organization of craft and industrial activities have tended to define the division of labor as a division of laborers, furthermore assuming that the latter always precedes the division of the objects upon which people work: first you divide the workers, then you divide the work. This approach was, in large part, a reaction against attempts to "naturalize" the division of labor by assuming the presence of a stable, predefined division of the world into a number of discrete objects or kinds, around which different occupations would establish themselves. This latter approach makes little sense, especially in the case of modern occupations, but the former approach also raises major problems.

Reverting to our central concern, we can easily see that biomedicine does not have a stable division of labor corresponding to an unproblematic partition of the object of work, namely the human body. New specialties are created around different, overlapping organizing principles: organ systems (e.g., cardiology, ophthalmology), regions (e.g., internal medicine), gender-specific functions (e.g., obstetrics and gynecology), life stages (e.g., pediatrics, gerontology), occupational criteria (e.g., sports medicine, industrial medicine), and so on. The heterogeneity of principles does not mean, however, that biomedical practitioners can arbitrarily establish divisions within medicine and biology in order to create distinct and independent domains of professional expertise. The independence of a biomedical specialty is inevitably relative: hematologists, for example, cannot ignore pathology reports when it comes to treating patients. In medicine, this mutual dependency is stronger than in most other modern professions, such as engineering, since the object of medicine is not the body per se, as previously suggested, but, rather, models of the body.

Not all sociologists would agree with our analysis. Some, taking their cue from historians such as Michel Foucault, have described a dispersion of "the clinical gaze" through a fragmentation of the patient's body, whereby the latter "is no longer localized in the discrete, integral body of the actual patient," but, rather, is distributed (figuratively speaking) among a number of different specialties, and (in a literal sense) simultaneously present as a set of samples in different sections of a hospital.[42] As just noted, this fragmentation of the body is, moreover, held to mimic social fragmentation, as instantiated in the increasingly complex division of labor. Yet, to speak of a fragmentation of the patient is to lose sight of all the work that goes into keeping everything together, into making sure that, for instance, the sample that has left the body will rejoin it in terms of meaningful (for the task-at-hand) results.[43] The apparent body fragments are, in fact, body *samples*, which in turn are always samples of some-thing or some-body. Of some-body because they come from a given patient (to whom, for instance, a medical record containing the various laboratory reports is attached),[44] and of some-thing because sampling operates less on the actual body than on the body as construed through *models* of the body, such as those that decompose the latter into various bodily "systems."

The twin practices of modeling and sampling correspond to sequential patterns of representation and intervention.[45] Samples and test results, be they numbers or images, circulate between the laboratory performing the tests, the general practitioner who ordered them, the specialist to whom the patient and his or her double, the medical record, have been referred, and so on. They thus both presuppose and give rise to patterns of cooperation that cannot be dissociated from the tools used to produce representations of body parts and, ultimately, to intervene upon the patient's body. The dominant pattern is not one of diverging, competing segments (although this is also part of the story) but, rather, as we have noted, one of consult and mutual dependency.[46] Since, as we will see in chapters 8 and 9, individual tools acquire consistency and meaning only through the regulatory activities generated by a given platform, such interdependency patterns are, in a strong sense, platform dependent. This also means that platforms (such as immunophenotyping) cannot be reduced to human collectives such as medical specialties or defined in terms of the social ties that keep those specialties together. Without platforms and the pattern of activities they generate, human collectives would fall apart. By choosing platforms as a unit of analysis of contemporary biomedical activities, we do not wish, of course, to promote a new sort of technological determinism. To the contrary, we provide ample room for social and cultural contingencies. The latter, however, cannot be dissociated from the configuration of material components and symbolic activities we call a platform.

The notion of platform that we advance in this book is intended to question the rigid dichotomy between the social and the technical that lies behind both technological and social determinist accounts of scientific and medical activities.[47] Readers may nonetheless suspect that the conflicts and debates that permeate contemporary biomedicine are most fruitfully approached by focusing primarily on human activities rather than on the techniques and technologies that make them possible. One could, for instance, examine how actors position themselves vis-à-vis a specific platform and argue, for example, in favor of morphology over immunophenotyping rather than examine how those platforms came to be.[48] From this perspective, platforms do not determine the actors' position; actors situate themselves vis-à-vis a platform. We would like to offer a contrasting perspective wherein, rather than caught up in a narrow dialectic of debate, biomedical platforms define new domains of clinical and scientific action. Within these domains, a variety of stances and attitudes are possible and they range from controversy to peaceful coexistence and cooperation. These positions (either individual or collective) are not grafted onto the platform, dividing it up according to exogenous criteria. Rather, they correspond to differences within platforms and between different, overlapping platforms.[49] In the rest of this book, we provide ample evidence supporting this analytical stance.

One final reservation: our argument in this book is specific to biomedicine and its empirical support is drawn exclusively from this field. Our aim, in other words, is to define and analyze *biomedical* platforms as prominent features of late-twentieth-century medicine, and not to offer some generic theoretical construct—"platforms"—that accounts for or enters into any and all social action. This specificity, we believe, strengthens our proposal. Indeed, we maintain that a study of biomedical platforms, built on historical investigation, highlights biomedical events and processes overlooked by other analytical frameworks. In particular, and this theme runs through the book, the notion of biomedical platforms sheds new light on the articulation and the regulation of the practices focused on the normal and the pathological that characterize contemporary biomedicine.

Plan of the Book

This short introductory chapter sought to provide readers with an initial sense of the issues and topics that cluster around the notion of platform. It also sought to introduce readers to the medical domains from which we have extracted the material for this book. We designed the final discussion of social theoretical issues as an initial positioning within the social sciences. All three of these goals have been attained with the sketchiest of means.

After a short examination of the etymology and semantic field of the notion of platform, chapter 2 analyzes the recent evolution of hospital architecture, and relates it to the rise of medical biology and the post–World War II institutional and epistemological program of combining biology with medicine. We are thus led to reexamine, in chapter 3, the problem of the relation between the normal and the pathological, as initially defined by historical epistemology, in the light of more recent events, such as the rise of automated biomedical instrumentation. Chapter 3 thus details our understanding of "biomedicine" as a distinctive postwar configuration of medical work, and, in so doing, investigates the increasing importance of diagnostic examinations and the automation of laboratory tasks. As we do not intend to pursue the themes just mentioned in isolation, these two chapters provide a map of their changing relations and of the polarities (biology and medicine, the laboratory and the clinic, etc.) through which they are expressed. Thus, they take a broad view.

In contrast to chapters 2 and 3, which create the framework for our study, the subsequent four chapters describe the development of a specific platform, the immunophenotyping platform. Chapters 4 and 5 draw on a rich infrastructure of interviews, archival material, and content analysis of the published literature to examine the rise of a new field of biomedical investigations focused on the study of the cell surface. Begun in the 1950s, work on the cell surface became a dominant trend in immunology (in conjunction with the rise of cellular immunology) in the 1970s. Cell surface studies also figured prominently in cancer research where the former came to be seen as a key to unlocking the mysteries of the transformation of normal into pathological cells. We show that two different versions of these historical events can be elaborated: the dominant biological story and a counterstory that focuses on contributions from pathology and the clinic. We furthermore show how these two lines of work converged in clinics and laboratories on both sides of the Atlantic to constitute the notion of cell or tumor marker (as both a notion and a set of reagents) and the related immunophenotyping platform. This allows us to specify how the diagnosis and prognosis of leukemia and the conduct of clinical trials for leukemia were profoundly transformed by these events.

Chapters 6 and 7, although based on numerous historical sources, are, in a way, the sociological counterpart to the two previous chapters. We argue that the immunophenotyping platform consists of core and peripheral elements and that, accordingly, there are various instantiations of the platform. This allows us to show that the platform is more than an instrument or device, but is a specific configuration of instruments and individuals that share common routines and activities, held together by standard reagents. These chapters accordingly examine the different kinds of coordination inscribed in platform components and describe the industrial contribution to their production and management. In particular, we analyze the commercial production of core components—"markers"—and the correlative constitution of an international nomenclature of reagents that established equivalences between locally produced antibodies. With regard to the peripheral components, we look at the two principal instantiations of the immunophenotyping platform, namely microscope-based slide techniques (immunocytochemistry) and the more technologically sophisticated development of laser and computer-based instrumentation. Discussion of the latter leads us into a technological underground where computer companies mingle with atomic energy facilities, space exploration agencies, academic biology laboratories, and hospital clinics.

Finally, chapters 8 and 9 bring to the surface an undercurrent of the previous chapters, the problem of regulation. We show that in order to understand how regulation enters into the production and maintenance of biomedical platforms, one has to take the larger view and go beyond the narrow sense of regulation as a form of government intervention through regulatory agencies. We will see how regulations—formal and informal, explicit and implicit—invade all practices related to platform stabilization and maintenance. Chapter 8 analyzes the historical development of regulatory activities on both sides of the Atlantic and then goes on to examine the practices, instruments, reagents, and images that need to be managed by regulators. Regulation of these interacting components of a platform makes possible the production of meaningful results and interlaboratory and interclinical comparisons. Chapter 9 centers on the development of a key regulatory instrument of clinical work, disease classification. In this chapter, we examine the transformation of classifications through the use of new platforms and the consequent use of consensus development techniques to align different platforms.

Chapter 10 draws together the different strands of our story and shows how the notion of a biomedical platform offered in this book allows one to describe and examine events and processes that are overlooked by alternative approaches. In addition to discussing possible objections to our approach, this concluding chapter also suggests further inquiries made possible by the notion of a biomedical platform.

2

Hospital Platforms

In the opening chapter, we discussed a medical debate implicating two different "biomedical platforms" without explaining the meaning of the latter. The time has come to take a closer look at the central concept of our study and show why this notion is useful for the understanding of the conduct and organization of work in the biomedical sciences.

When we first used the term in oral presentations, it often provoked puzzlement. Audience members typically queried, "Biomedical platforms? I have heard of oil platforms and train platforms, but I've never heard of *biomedical* platforms!" Indeed, while each word—biomedical and platform—is commonly used in ordinary language, together they make an unusual combination. In this chapter, we explore the meaning of the expression by first focusing on the etymology of "platform." This linguistic excursion is followed by an analysis of its use in hospital settings which, in turn, leads to a discussion, in the following chapter, of the transformation of postwar medicine through the establishment of new relations between biology and medicine. Here again, we undertake an etymological inquiry, this time of the neologism "biomedicine."

Note that while "biomedicine" generally refers to modern, Western medicine—a body of knowledge and practices often assumed to originate in the bacteriological laboratory in the second half of the nineteenth century—casual use of the term disguises two important facts. First, the term itself is of recent coinage (c. 1923) and its widespread use postdates World War II. Second, the relations between biology and the clinic are, even today, far from seamless and unproblematic; it is difficult to reduce pathology to biology and attempts to do so often meet with stubborn social and material resistance. We do not hereby suggest that biomedicine is an epistemological "monster," as the French would say, or a practical impossibility. Rather, we suggest that the relationship between biology and pathology should not be taken for granted, but, instead, analyzed in terms of the articulation of material and discursive practices. Replacing normative epistemology with analytical description, in other words, will enable us to pinpoint the distinctive *biomedical* dimension of biomedical platforms.

In this chapter and the next we examine mundane uses of "platform" and "biomedical." We do so for a reason but the reason is not the one normally given. In the social science literature, methodological prescriptions often contrast native terminology—normally equated with mundane use—with scholarly, analytical notions. In the present case, however, we eschew the alternative consisting in *either* going native and contenting ourselves with a description of the actors' language *or* in developing an analytical metalanguage divorced from the actors' own meaning and practices.[1] Rather, we seek intersections between the questions actors ask and the questions we raise, between the practical answers they provide and the theoretical framing we offer, thus focusing on what a group of sociologists known as ethnomethodologists call "perspicuous phenomena," i.e., "topics or themes which preoccupy particular groups and which resonate with social science issues."[2]

So, let the etymologies begin.

Etymologies I: Platforms

Et comme le nom est joli, dis-je, on aimerait savoir l'origine de ces noms-là.[3]

"Platform" has an interesting etymology.[4] It originated in fifteenth-century France where *platte-fourme* referred to a flat form, a plane, elevated surface, be it natural (the flat top of a small hill) or artificial (the top of a flat building). Although the natural referent still occurs in geology (a continental platform or plateau), the artificial referent has dominated subsequent extensions of the term. The latter, the product of metonymy, has seen the term spread to the military (the surface on which artillery pieces are mounted), street paving, and, following the industrial revolution, to other instances of flat, supporting surfaces in transportation (the surface on which rails are fixed, the open portion at the end of a railway car, the raised walk at which trains arrive and depart), the oil industry (the surface on which sea drilling equipment rests), and, more recently, space travel (an orbiting, fully equipped station) and navigational equipment (an "inertial platform" is the rigid structure on which gyroscopes are fixed for the guidance of ships, airplanes, or missiles).

The idea of a horizontal surface serving as a support for something leads easily to metaphor, such as when present society is described as a ready-made platform, built by and inherited from previous generations.[5] Today's main metaphorical use of the term is as a set of ideas, objectives, and principles supporting a common course of action and upheld by a political party, a union, or any other organized group. One finds a similar use of the term in late-sixteenth-century English to refer to a scheme of church government and discipline.[6] The modern figurative meaning—a declaration of principles and policy—however, did not arise until the 1840s when it developed in the United States in reference to the tribune (or speaker's platform) used for electoral speeches.[7] From the United States, it traveled back to Europe, appearing, for instance, in France in 1855.

The shift from the material to the figurative entailed a shift in connotation from platforms as passive supports to platforms as springboards for future action. In this process, technical and political meanings became inextricably linked. For instance, in scientific articles on AIDS, the term platform sometimes refers to *both* the equipment and technologies used to measure the number of white blood cells targeted by HIV (the CD4 cells) and the implementation and coordination of AIDS control activities.[8] This is not simply a case of using the same word for different purposes. Surveillance policies critically depend on the definition of the nature and evolution of AIDS, a task that requires dependable (available and regulated) CD4 measurements. In turn, as mentioned in chapter 1, the heated controversies surrounding the decisions to include these laboratory measurements in the definition of AIDS (rather than follow a list of clinical conditions as before)[9] or to use them as an alternative endpoint of clinical trials,[10] highlight the political dimension of CD4 counts.

"Platform's" semantic reach thus embraces natural and artificial entities, material artifacts and their blueprints, and technical, political, material, and symbolic referents. At one end of the semantic spectrum lies the engineering/physics idea of a simple bench or surface onto which other devices are fixed in a definite but not definitive way. At the other end of the spectrum lies the political platform, an arrangement of statements and positions with respect to particular issues. A platform, then, is less a thing than a way of arranging things in both a material and discursive sense. In both senses (as an instrument or a project), the platform creates the basis for the organization of activities. In neither sense does it offer a foundation for these activities, insofar as its adoption and the comparative advantages it confers require no criterion of truth or any other criterion of correspondence to a specific order of things. Platforms furnish pragmatic criteria: what works best for a given purpose, given a necessarily limited amount of information, opportunities, and resources.[11]

Far from having a fixed meaning, the term platform has recently undergone further development. It has entered high-tech domains such as the computer and the biotech industry where it presents itself as a basis for change and innovation, thus retaining some of its original connotation while extending its technical use. In the early electronic industry, for example, engineers spoke of a computer platform as a way of abstracting or black-boxing different hardware configurations sharing a capability of running the same software; in other words, they spoke of bracketing technical differences that, for a given practical purpose, did not make any difference.[12] In the contemporary computer industry, the term platform usually refers to the hardware system and the system software used by a computer program (e.g., a Macintosh and a MacOS platform).[13] Economists of industrial innovation have expanded this notion by defining it as an interface standard that allows for the clustering of knowledge, physical capital (system software, applications, and peripherals), and human capital (programmers and end users). So defined, computer platforms cut across social institutions such as firms. Platforms, not firms, account for the dynamics of technological competition in the sector: "Existing [economic] theory emphasizes competition among firms. The dynamic part of technological competition in computing, by contrast, is competition between platforms."[14]

Given the obvious connections between computing and modern biomedical instrumentation, readers should not be surprised to learn that the latter often employs the term platform. For example, in the course of our research, an employee of Immunotech, a wholly owned subsidiary of a vertically integrated biomedical instrumentation company, described the parent company's activities to us. These included the design and production of interacting hardware, software, and diagnostic reagents. According to the employee, each subsidiary produced components as a relatively autonomous *platform*—an organizational unit smaller than the whole firm, yet larger than a single laboratory—that organized activities such as design, quality control, and so on.[15] In the broader field of biotechnology, the term signifies the link between technical singularities and generic applications. For instance, a large Canadian biotech investment firm issued an advisory to its clients that divided "the risk reward spectrum" of therapeutics into "platform technologies, early stage clinical trials, late stage clinical trials and companies with approved products."[16] From the investment examples given, readers learned that the notion of platform referred to a therapeutic technique or technology that potentially could be applied to a large number of diseases. Generality, however, was not the only criterion for the classification. As suggested above, the platform category stood at the research end of the R&D spectrum. In the world of biotechnology venture capital, then, a platform constituted a high-risk generality.

This use of the term platform has gained widespread recognition among financial specialists: Ernst & Young and Pricewaterhouse Coopers, major firms in the field, routinely distinguish between the more recent platform technology–based biotech companies that sell services (e.g., in the genomics field), and traditional biotechnology firms that focus on long-term product development, the former offering a higher degree of capital valuation.[17] In turn, as shown by a recent sampling of article titles, molecular biologists increasingly use the term platform to describe technological developments.[18] Perhaps spurred by such developments, the general director of the French Medical Research Institute (INSERM), called upon to define his organization's strategy, singled out the development of "technological platforms" throughout France (a map was included) as his first priority.[19]

Organizational scientists have gone one step further and advanced the notion of a platform organization, which they describe as a flexible unit with fuzzy contours that replicates the structure and functioning of a computer platform in its capacity to be configured for many different uses.[20] Traditional notions of industrial platforms had focused on their role in providing different users with a shared set of tools and systems, an arrangement implying both standardization (to establish links with different users) and flexibility (to cater to their specific needs). From this point of view, and insofar as they function as production units rather than as mere dispatching sites, platforms represent the active nodes of a network.[21] The notion of a platform organization reverses the subordination of platforms to networks. In high-tech companies, a platform organization typically rests on a pool of schemes, arrangements, and resources that enable it to cope with "sudden events [that] can tilt established patterns of identity, organization, culture, routines and capabilities."[22] Platforms, so described, share some of the properties of networks: they are flexible and subject to distributed, as opposed to centrally planned, forms of coordination. Yet, although descriptions of particular networks remain part of the overall picture, the notion of a platform organization shifts our attention from effects to causes. Networks become ex post accounts of the configurations generated by a platform.[23]

We can conclude from this literature that it is possible to account for both innovation and routines in terms of a unit of analysis, the platform, that, by providing a new topography of the field under consideration—i.e., by making descriptions of a given field in terms of either its constitutive social units (e.g., professions or firms) or its defining technologies obsolete—escapes both social and technical reductionism. In addition to avoiding these forms of reductionism, the notion of platform allows for historical contingency. For example, whereas the platform forms the basis for political or technical projects, participants recognize it as a timely construct. The platform holds the party or the devices together only for the time being. We can also conclude that, unlike, say, Kuhnian paradigms,[24] in order to operate, a platform does not need shared understandings. The order created by a platform, in the simplest sense, results from consistency between the various parts, be it consistency of purpose, consistently measurable distances, or consistent interfaces as, for example, in the case of the components of an optical or electronic device.

So much for platforms. What about *biomedical* platforms? Here again, inspection of native usage provides us with a good empirical starting point for exploring the intricacies of the notion. In particular, although the term biomedical platform is yet to be found in dictionaries, a close equivalent—*plateau médico-technique*—has recently become common in French hospital circles, both in everyday language and as an academic construct to which numerous meetings and publications have been devoted.

Platform Hospitals and Hospital Platforms

The Saint-Louis Hospital entrance on Claude-Vellefaux Avenue in Paris confronts visitors with a sharp contrast. On the left lies the old Saint-Louis, a collection of low-rise buildings that includes the original Quadrilateral, built in 1607 in response to recurring plague epidemics, as well as several other pavilions added in the following centuries. On the right lies the new Saint-Louis, a building inaugurated in 1984 and consisting of a podium or platform supporting six small towers[25] (see figures 2.1 and 2.2). The clinical wards, and thus the patients, are located

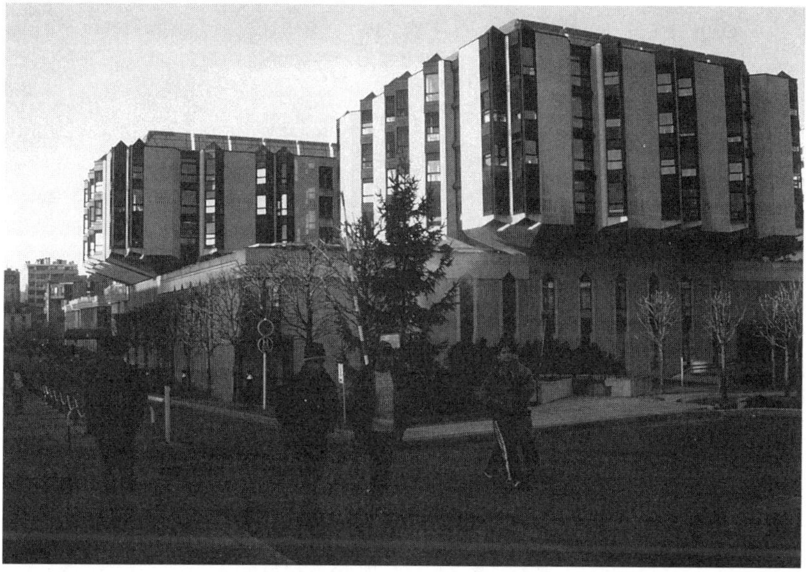

Figure 2.1
The new Saint-Louis Hospital in Paris. (Photograph: A.C.)

in the towers. The platform houses the operating theatres and several laboratories (bacteriology, virology, parasitology, biochemistry, hematology, etc.) that, taken together, form what hospital plans and administrative documents refer to as the "plateau médico-technique," a term we can freely translate as medical-technical platform.[26] The services and laboratories housed on the platform share a common technical and administrative infrastructure. Patients and various body samples move freely between the rooms in the towers and the platform.

Particularly striking because of the juxtaposition of the old and the new, Saint-Louis is not, however, an isolated example. A common denominator of Western postwar hospital architecture in general, and, since the 1960s, of French architecture in particular, has been the increased space devoted to the hospital platform at the expense of space devoted to patient beds. In Marseille hospitals, for instance, platform space rose from 7% of overall surface area in 1945, to 20% in 1965 and 35% in 1985. The project of building platforms and, consequently, of replacing a collection of laboratories isolated in various parts of the hospital with a specific construct harboring complex, expensive instruments, and a logistic infrastructure has become common.[27] The introduction of new diagnostic equipment has accompanied a profound

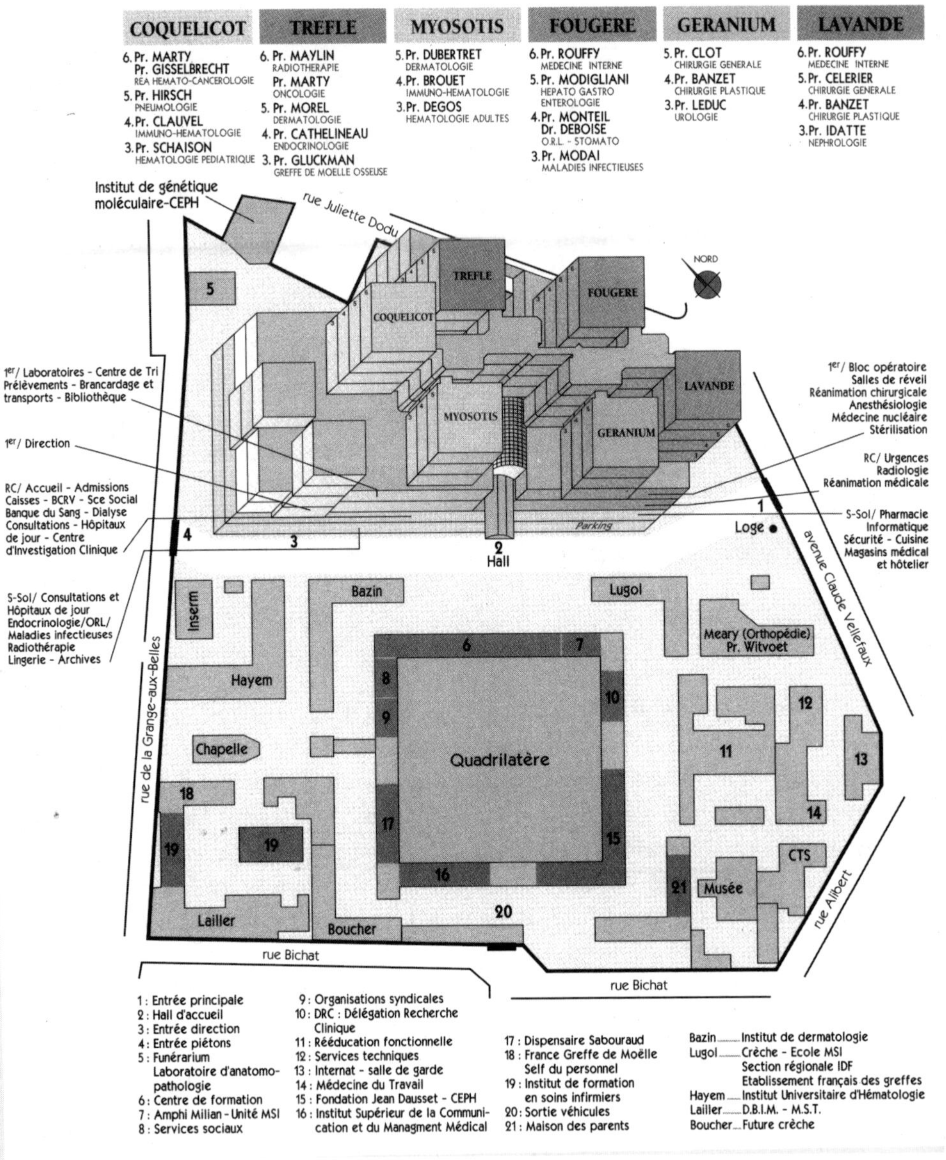

Figure 2.2

Plan of the Saint-Louis Hospital, showing the old and the new Saint-Louis. (Source: CHU Saint-Louis/AP-HP Paris: undated [c. 1996] brochure. Reprinted with kind permission of CHU Saint-Louis, AP-HP Paris.)

transformation of hospital architecture, the daily functioning of hospitals, and the medical pathways that patients are required to follow.[28] As a consequence, the very center of gravity of the hospital has moved from hospitalization to the "medico-technical" department where a greater range of increasingly sophisticated means of diagnosis and treatment come together.[29] Unsurprisingly, given the circumstances, hospital planners since the 1960s have shown an explicit interest in the topographical relations between clinical wards and technical platforms, two components of the hospital that have come to be seen as distinct.[30] French architects now believe that since the "modern hospital" has been redefined as the "locus" of equipment and tools for diagnosis, treatment, teaching, and research, laboratory and diagnostic medicine should be recognized as a discrete entity to which "architectural dignity" could and should be granted.[31]

Architects have applied the platform approach to both old and new hospital buildings. Refurbished buildings include the Paris-based Lariboisière Hospital. Dating back to 1853, the latter is widely acknowledged as a paradigmatic example of nineteenth-century pavilion architecture, according to which doctors distributed patients by specific disease in separate buildings under the control of different clinical specialties.[32] Today's visitor to Lariboisière is initially exposed to the old pavilion plan: a central courtyard surrounded by a rectangular building, from which a series of pavilions project outward[33] (see figure 2.3). One soon learns, however, that under the courtyard lies a technical platform built in the 1970s. Thus, as with recent hospitals, and even though the construction sequence has been inverted, the clinical wards, rest on a platform.

A particularly noteworthy example of a new platform building is the Caen hospital. Officially opened in 1975, it was the first to be explicitly conceived as an architectural expression of the 1957 Debré healthcare reform aimed at unifying clinical, research, and teaching activities within the hospital and that resulted in the establishment of the institution known as the Hospital-University Center (CHU, Centre Hospitalo-Universitaire).[34] The Caen hospital consists of a large platform housing the faculty of medicine and the hospital laboratories as well as other medical-technical services, and an H-shaped tower (an obvious metaphorical gesture),[35] containing clinical wards[36] (see figure 2.4).

Examples could be multiplied, but readers are by now entitled to ask whether these developments are unique to France or whether, to the contrary, they correspond to an international or, at least, Western trend. It so happens that the latter is the case.[37] According to historians of archi-

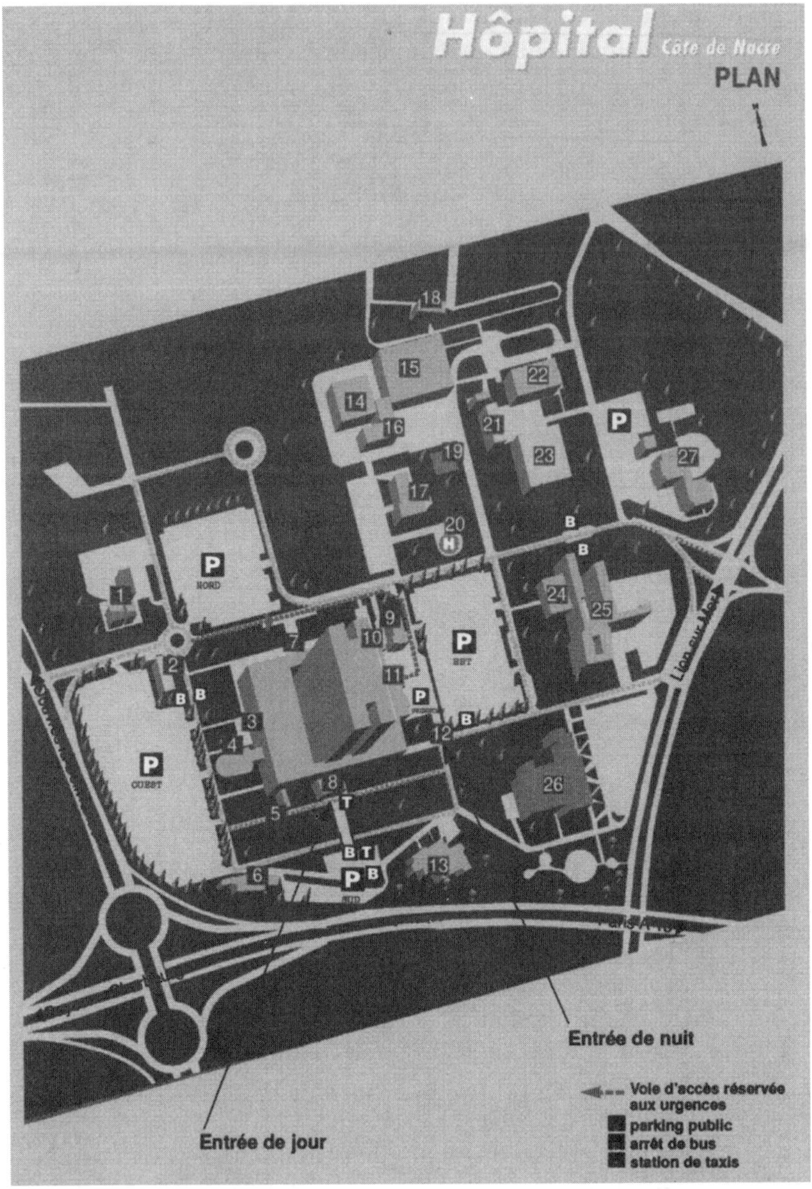

Figure 2.3
Plan of the Caen University Hospital. (Source: Caen University Hospital. Reprinted with kind permission of CHU Caen.)

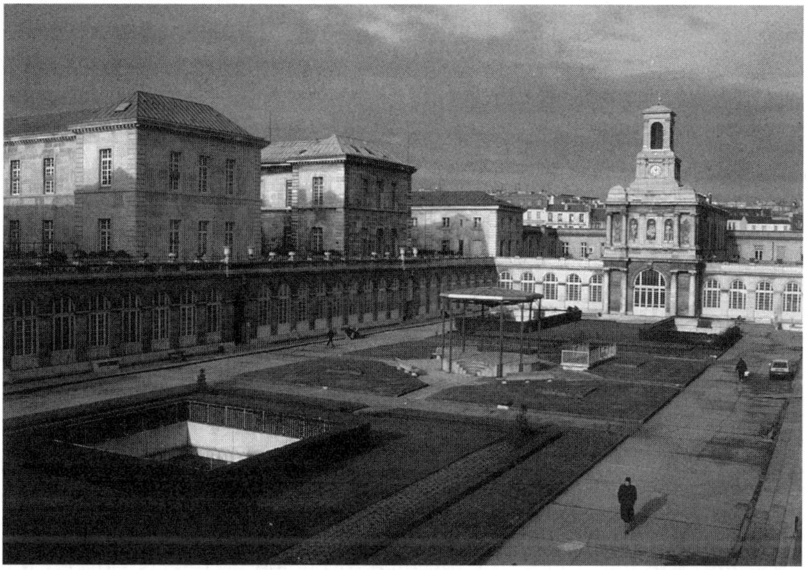

Figure 2.4
The Lariboisière Hospital in Paris: central courtyard and the original pavilion buildings. (Photograph: A.C.)

tecture, the modernist International Style that grew out of the Bauhaus school of the 1920s dominated hospital design by the 1960s. Platform architecture participates in this general trend that is characterized by "a tripartite structure of below-grade service base, an administrative base at grade level, and a patient tower on top."[38] Hardly monolithic, the International Style integrated national idiosyncrasies, such as differences in the organization of the healthcare system or the pace of renewal of the hospital network in the aftermath of Warld War II. This, in turn, has separated the United States from Europe. In the United States, following the Hospital Construction Act of 1946, the construction of thousands of facilities extended over many decades.[39] As a result, although 80% of the projects financed by the act in 1948 targeted new constructions, by 1971 96.5% of the projects involved modernization and renovation of existing structures. In the United States, then, a modern hospital network has been in existence for some time, and present-day hospitals are often the result of incremental additions.[40] In contrast, Europeans (especially the French, German, and British) have constructed new hospitals from scratch during a relatively short period of time under the centralized control of government planners.

The striking transformation of the hospital landscape in Europe has been described as the advent of the "European urban platform hospital," a term that obviously resonates with our own terminology and that is meant to highlight "the role of high technology as a determinant of form." In other words, for example, "technology drove the need to place autonomous nursing units above a high-tech platform or base," and "[t]his use of a monolithic base with patient towers above might best be termed 'platform.'"[41] This trend has followed different national paths within Europe. In the United Kingdom, following the establishment of the National Health Service in 1948, a group of modernist architects designed a series of hospitals in the late 1950s and early 1960s characterized by the tower-on-podium form, also known as matchbox-on-a-muffin. In architectural circles, the United Kingdom subsequently became known as the land of "brutalist hospitals."[42] In France, a flourish of architectural activity followed a postwar period dominated by the construction of standardized, faceless hospital buildings. Between 1980 and the mid-1990s, for instance, over 300 architects worked for the "Assistance Publique–Hôpitaux de Paris" (AP-HP), the agency in charge of hospitals in the French capital, designing hospitals such as the new Saint-Louis.[43] In Germany, university central clinics (*Zentralkliniken*) became exemplars of platform hospitals. Completed in the late 1960s, the health center of the Free University of Berlin (referred to as a "self-contained urban machine"), soon to be followed by similar buildings in Hannover, Munich, Cologne, Göttingen, and Münster, is often cited as the first in a series of hospitals that embodied the new high-tech credo of German medicine[44] (see figure 2.5).

So as not to overstate our case, let us admit that many different elements enter into the production and widespread adoption of a given architectural form. Consider, for instance, the tower-on-podium scheme. Its connection to the International Style movement as well as the fact that its prototypical example was not a hospital, but a 1952 New York landmark office building known as Lever House, clearly demonstrates the explicit involvement of hospital architects with the symbolic and practical expression of modernity. Notions of modernity have also been translated into a rhetoric of efficacy and rationality and the search for architectural forms leading to a better flow of patients, records, and samples throughout the hospital. Keywords such as "flexibility," "adaptability," and "expansion" have been routinely used to justify a particular hospital design. The advent of paying patients and hospitalization insur-

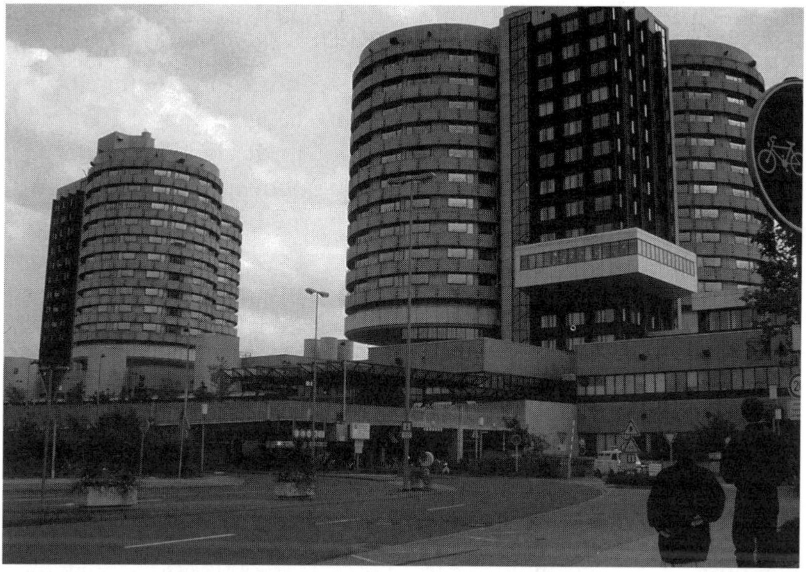

Figure 2.5
The university hospital in Münster. (Photograph: A.C.)

ance plans has resulted in a demand for smaller wards, each needing a window, that could be placed in the tower. Similarly, with its absence of natural light or air, the podium has provided a response to the development of and demand for climate and light control for spaces such as operating rooms.[45] In short, an architectural scheme such as the tower-on-podium is clearly overdetermined and cannot thus be accounted for in terms of a single cause.

We are interested, however, in exploring only a particular aspect of this complex process, namely the connections between new architectural forms and the transformation of medical knowledge and practices. Following Foucault's innovative analysis of hospital architecture,[46] other authors have looked for such connections. Among them, Lindsay Prior has traced the development of hospital architecture from pavilion hospitals, linked to a miasmatic understanding of disease, to the installation of isolation cubicles following the rise of the germ theory of disease, to the modern development of the dispensary as the embodiment of social medicine.[47] By focusing exclusively on the wards, Prior has, however, neglected the more decisive transformation in spatial relations between the wards and other sectors of the hospital.[48] Similarly, those analysts that do recognize the emergence of platform hospitals as a key development of the postwar period unfortunately devote most of their attention to ward design as an indicator of both the tensions and countercurrents within the modernist movement, and of changing medical attitudes toward the patient (e.g., from the "machine for healing" metaphor to a patient-centered approach).[49] While we do not deny the interest in such analyses, we maintain that much can be learned by looking at the hospital platforms themselves.

In France, the development of hospital platforms as distinct architectural spaces is clearly reflected in the increasing use of the notion in healthcare management publications.[50] Moreover, several hospitals now have a "medical-technical platform committee" and a "technical platform coordinator." Professional organizations of hospital biologists and laboratory and clinical technicians regularly organize seminars and meetings on hospital platforms. When questioned about these activities, interviewees usually reply with an evolutionary narrative describing how, in the beginning, early postwar laboratories, staffed by a versatile technician, were first added to each clinical ward; how, subsequently, diagnostic tests in a single field (e.g., biochemistry or hematology) were centralized in laboratories staffed by specialized technicians; and how, finally, different central laboratories came together on a hospital platform.[51]

Clearly, this reallocation of personnel and material entailed an investment in form that enabled previously heterogeneous equipment (in the largest sense of the term) to function together as a new sociotechnical unit. Indeed, in using Laurent Thévenot's suggestive notion of investments in form, we would remind readers that the establishment of hospital platforms involved more than the stroke of an architect's pen. Platform organizers (architects included) had to establish some sort of equivalency between "cognitive categories, classificatory tools, social beings, customs, social representations, collective persons, juridical or institutional entities, rules, conventions and technical objects," in order to create new collective identities and to produce standards and other tools of simplification.[52]

Platform committees, coordinators, and meetings are all expressions of platform-related investments in form. So are legal instruments such as the 1985 ministerial order that created a nomenclature for the diagnostic tests to be reimbursed by the French Medicare system (the *Nomenclature des Actes de Biologie Médicale*). Frequently revised by a special government committee, the *Nomenclature* has expanded beyond its original nine to fifteen considerably larger sections.[53] The *Nomenclature* establishes equivalencies by assigning a number (preceded by the letter *B* for biology) to each test it features, according to the relative value of the test. For example, a simple test such as a urine sugar measurement is categorized as B2; a more cumbersome, yet routine test such as a Pap smear as B60; and a sophisticated, relatively rare test such as leukemia or lymphoma immunophenotyping as B300. B units thus allow one to compare across diagnostic tests not only for Medicare purposes (e.g., during the periodic revision of the monetary value of a B unit) but also for the assessment and monitoring of hospital technology.

The organizational flow chart of a French platform hospital offers a vivid illustration of the connection between platform activities and clinical practices. A promotional brochure of Saint-Louis Hospital depicts two piles of smaller boxes lying on a larger, rectangular box—the platform (see figure 2.6). Inscribed on the boxes on the left, corresponding to "Medical-surgical activities by pathological discipline," are the names of a traditional specialty (hematology, dermatology, nephrology, etc.), while the boxes on the right, collectively designated "Transversal activities," are named according to more recent domains of clinical intervention: genetics, oncology, and molecular biology. According to the diagram, the platform, far from merely supporting the other activities, has become the obligatory passage point through which the specialty-based activities on the left are connected to the transversal activities on the right.[54] In other words, today's hospital is not simply organized *around* the technical platform.[55] Platforms redefine clinical practices, and they do so by embodying the "fabulous and irresistible rise" of medical biology.[56] We return to medical biology later in this chapter. For now, let us simply note that to the question of whether hospital platforms are a solution to a technical problem (insofar as they allow patients to move easily between their beds and the central diagnostic facilities), an economic problem (insofar as centralization allows for economies of scale), or an epistemological problem (insofar as the isolated specialists of the old pavilion medicine are replaced by "synthetic" multidisciplinary teams), the answer is: all of the above.

To develop our argument further, we need to take a closer look at the content of hospital platforms. For purposes of illustration, we have chosen the platform of the University Hospital Center in Nantes, inaugurated in October 1990 and widely cited as a successful, innovative example of platform architecture and practice.[57] The external design, a typical platform shape—albeit surrounded by, instead of supporting, the

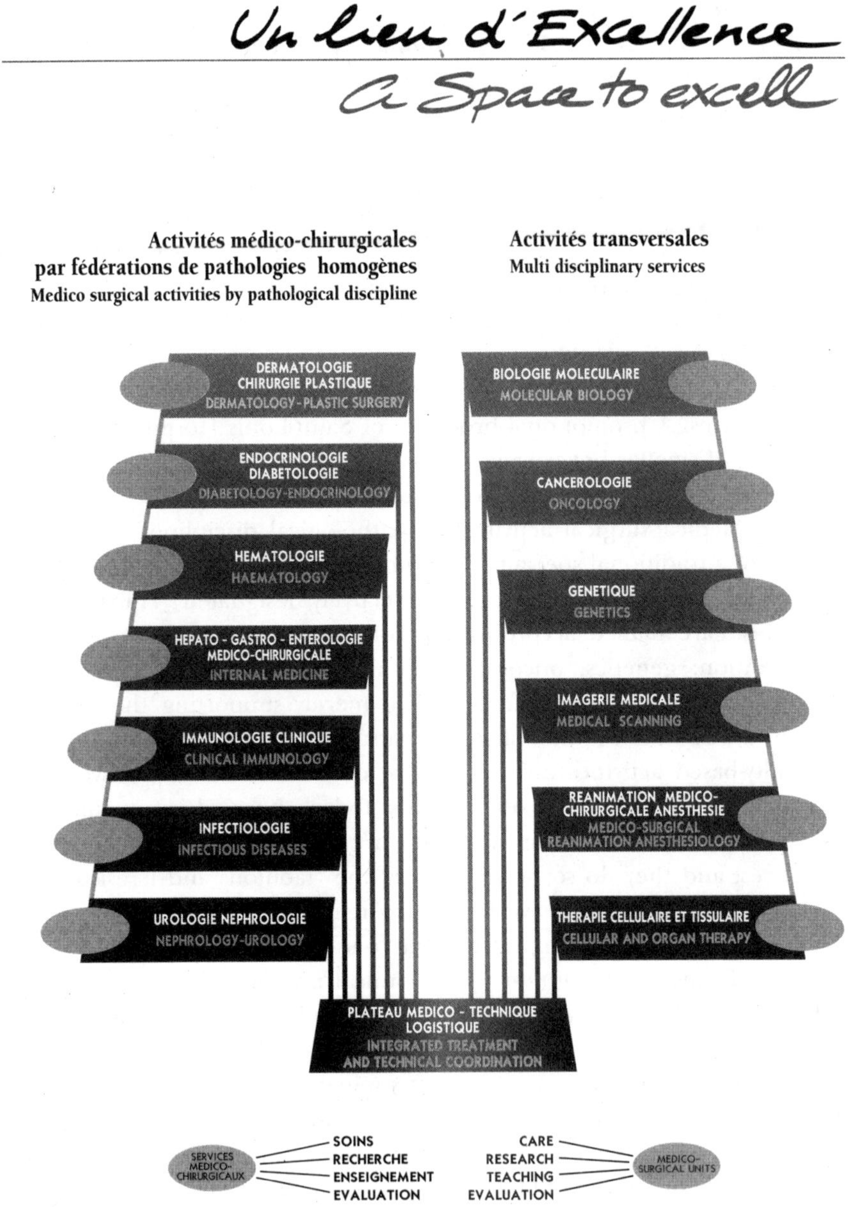

Figure 2.6
Organizational flow chart of the Saint-Louis Hospital. (Source: CHU Saint-Louis/AP-HP Paris: undated [c. 1996] brochure. Reprinted with kind permission of CHU Saint-Louis, AP-HP Paris.)

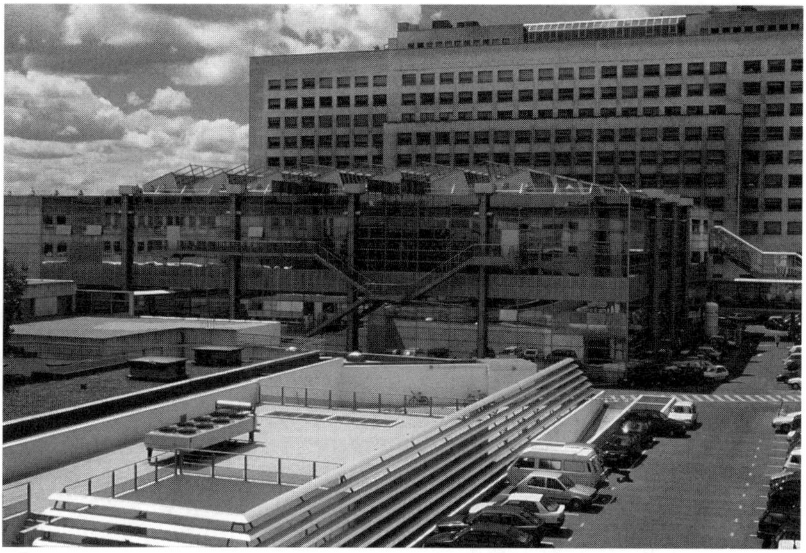

Figure 2.7
Exterior of the Nantes hospital platform. (Photograph: A.C.)

hospital towers—while eye-catching because of walls of glittering glass, is hardly a major architectural achievement (see figure 2.7). More interesting is the internal structure: an open space of 6000 m^2 that can be easily reorganized by shifting removable panels and thus modifying the spaces devoted to the various biomedical specialties housed on the platform, namely biochemistry, hematology, immunology, microbiology (bacteriology, virology, and parasitology), cytogenetics, pharmacology, and molecular biology (see figure 2.8). Platform creators justify this flexible, open design by the need to break down barriers and increase coordination among specialties, as well as to continuously adapt internal spatial arrangements to new developments and innovations. Following spatial readjustments, tissue and fluid samples can be rerouted to their new destination via a system of automated, computer-controlled wagons running from the ceiling. Some of the high-tech equipment, namely the cell-sorting equipment used for immunophenotyping (see chapter 4), occupies a special place insofar as it overlaps several specialties.

Readers may have noted that pathology, the prototypical discipline of laboratory medicine, does not appear in the list of specialties represented on the Nantes platform. There is a reason for this. Being physicians and thus legitimately qualified to interpret diagnostic findings,

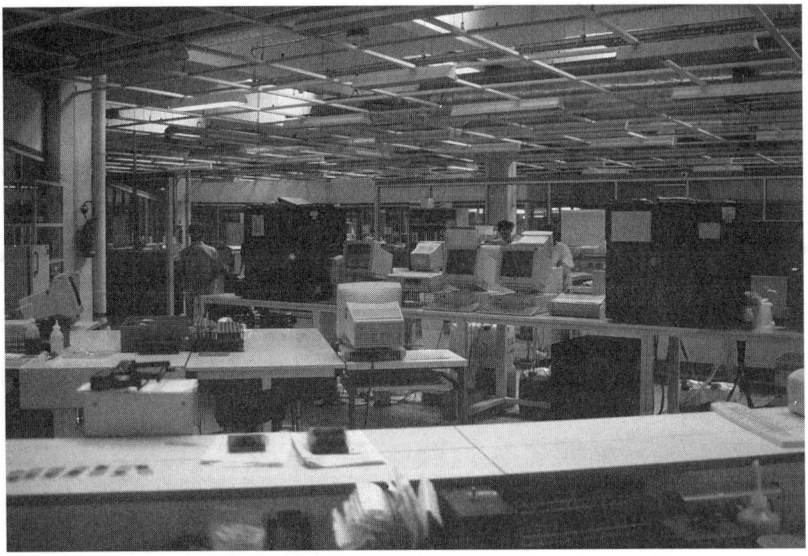

(*a*)

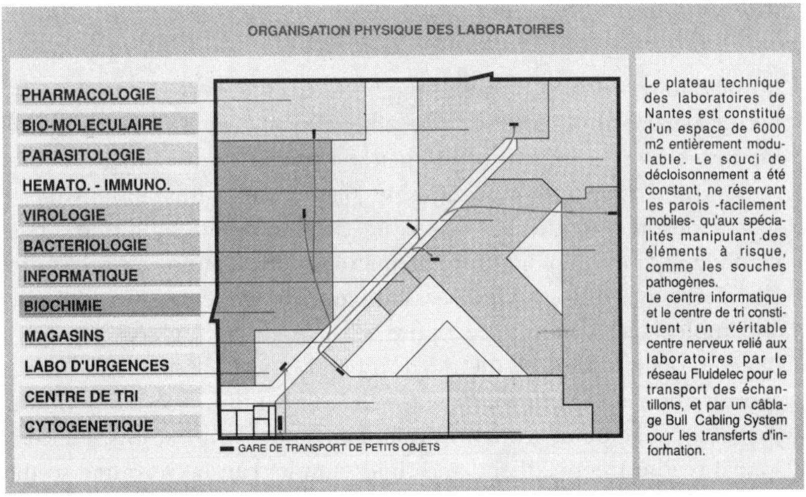

(*b*)

Figure 2.8

Interior (*a*) and plan (*b*) of the Nantes platform. (Photograph: A.C. Plan: undated [c. 1996] CHU Nantes brochure.) Reprinted with kind permission of CHU Nantes.

pathologists have set themselves apart from medical biologists and have obtained different codes for Medicare reimbursement purposes.[58] Yet, things are changing. Younger pathologists work on the platform and pathology will be officially represented on the new platforms that have been established for other hospitals, such as the University Hospital Center in Toulouse and the brand-new Georges Pompidou European Hospital in Paris.[59] We are aware that the turf struggle between pathologists and medical biologists could be used to argue that, contrary to what we maintained in chapter 1, professional segments are the key to an understanding of the situation. We would disagree. The professional categories in this case are the epiphenomena. Medical biologists are defined by the hospital platform. Pathologists, in turn, had to choose whether or not to embark. In other words, the professional issue is derivative of the problems imposed by the platform. Moreover, while professional identities are not rigidly dependent on the changing content of professional activities, they do not in any way act as an independent variable. Rather, we increasingly observe a conflation of social and technical aspects of professional activities, as when it is claimed, for example, that the direct modification of the core of pathological phenomena made possible by molecular biology also affects professional identities. In this case, not only does the change in technical content modify the substance of diagnostic findings, it subverts horizontal and vertical relations between various hospital sectors (which is precisely the idea that the flow chart of Saint-Louis Hospital tried to convey).[60]

Turning now to platform equipment, according to a spokesperson of the Nantes team, the purpose of the sophisticated scopes, meters, and hybrids of the two that one finds on a hospital platform is not simply automation, understood as a faster, cheaper, and large-volume alternative to manual laboratory activities. Rather, it is a question of doing *different* things by doing the same things differently.[61] Platform equipment embodies the transformation of the relation between biology and the clinic that allows medical biologists to increasingly intervene in the clinical realm and thus reshape the organization and content of medicine.[62]

A sense of why this is so can be gained by looking at the recent history of medical diagnostics. Recall that, in his classic account of the rise of medical technology, Reiser described a rapid postwar increase in the number of diagnostic tests being performed in American hospitals: from a 100% increase between 1938 and 1958, to a doubling every five years from the mid-1950s through the 1960s, and an even faster increase rate in the 1970s, a trend which included the automation of laboratory analysis. French data show an estimated 237% increase in the number of diagnostic tests performed between 1970 and 1980.[63] These numbers, as well as similar ones for Canada and Great Britain, translate what Reiser ironically calls "a marvelous faith in laboratory tests" and they have left their mark on both hospital building plans and patient care in the wards. Yet, again according to Reiser, because of their many shortcomings in terms of medical decision-making (overdependence on technology, loss of tacit clinical skills), and in spite of their significant advantages, we should view laboratory tests as mixed blessings or, at the very least, treat them with caution.[64] A recent French contribution to the history of medical diagnosis adopts an even more critical stance vis-à-vis laboratory diagnosis. In a section significantly entitled "diagnosis without the clinic," the author notes that in the 1950s, following the British and American lead, French hospitals adopted the diagnostic laboratory as a relatively autonomous component of "paraclinical" activities.[65] Formerly subordinated to clinical goals and arrangements, these activities now threaten to displace if not replace the former. Having become the first step of any clinical investigation, they now take precedence over patient complaints and clinical examinations.[66]

The same electronic discussion forum that provided the example used in chapter 1 offers an illustration of how this is so. The discussion began with a message claiming that all cases of B-chronic lymphocytic leukemia (CLL) were CD23 positive.[67] When researchers at the National Cancer Institute countered that "Although almost all CLL is CD23 positive, we have seen CLL that is negative for CD23. Never say always or never in [cancer],"[68] the original writer retorted: "Of course there is no absolute 100% in biology . . . BUT . . . if we make some diagnostic criteria . . . why not stick to them."[69] This comment provoked a rather blunt reply from a defender of the primacy of clinical data over laboratory data: "Clinical criteria dictate clinical syndromes, not immunophenotypic patterns, correct? Correlative laboratory data are confirmatory rather than 'diagnostic.'"[70] The equally blunt rejoinder cautioned: "Yes, clinical findings describe clinical syndromes and when the immunophenotype is not the expected, one of the options is to rethink the clinical syndrome. In my experience neither [has] 100% specificity and sensitivity."[71]

Ostensibly a confrontation between data provided by immunophenotyping and clinical findings, this confrontation shows how the former, by generating biological entities, calls into question the status of preexisting clinical entities. While immunophenotyping challenged, or, better, reshaped clinical primacy, it did so in complex, open-ended ways.

These confrontations will not be limited to diagnostics and prognostics, as therapeutics will likely face similar challenges on the platform in the near future.[72] Part and parcel of the challenge is the transfer of medical judgment from the individual clinician to the companies that design automated equipment, the development of a thick layer of regulations to ensure the validity of automated diagnostic results (see chapter 5), a redefinition of the notion of normality, a transformation of the medical division of labor, the introduction of new practices such as the screening of asymptomatic "patients," and so on and so forth. Our point in raising these issues is not to support or dismiss these claims and complaints but, rather, to show how platform activities do indeed embody an essential tension within biomedical practices.

Allow us one final remark concerning hospital platforms. According to their promoters, some confusion surrounds their exact referent, so that the best definition of a hospital platform may very well be: "what each hospital describes as such." In practice, definitions of hospital platforms always include a prototypical core consisting of the diagnostic laboratories and imaging services. Other units, such as operating theaters and anesthesia services, are generally, but not always, excluded, depending on architectural, organizational, political, and professional arrangements.[73] Even this loose definition falls apart, however, if we stretch the notion of a hospital platform to include those found in institutions such as the Albert Bonniot Institute (IAB) in Grenoble. Established in 1994 to take advantage of the many high-tech computing firms in the region and built on a site close to the university hospital, the IAB was conceived from the outset as a *bioclinical* (their term) research center operating at the interfaces of biology, medicine, and computing in fields related to cellular pathology and cancer.[74] In addition to the research teams, its noteworthy architectural structure[75] houses three medical pilot units (surgery, pathology, and cytogenetics) where the methods and technologies developed in the institute can be tested on real patients (see figure 2.9). Thus, while the Nantes hospital platform has been built within the hospital, in Grenoble the hospital (or, at least, a sample of it) has been built within the platform. Rather than contrasting configurations, however, the Nantes and Grenoble platforms represent different points along a continuum. In both cases, they can be described as "ecological niches" that promote associations between hospital practitioners and researchers, make the confrontation between laboratory results and clinical data possible, and link the development of diagnostic expertise to the development of routine and specialized bioclinical interfaces.[76]

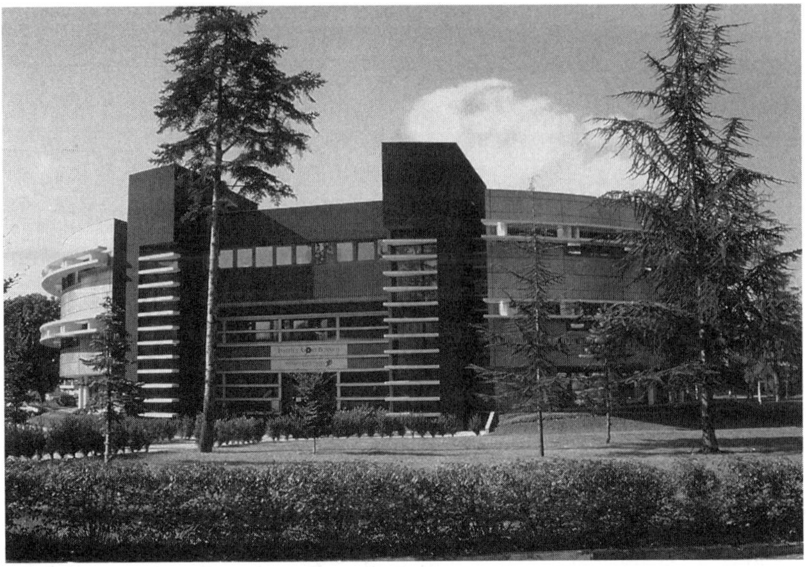

Figure 2.9
The Albert Bonniot Institute in Grenoble, France. (Photograph: A.C.)

These interfaces are not established after the fact, i.e., after each side—the biological and the clinical—has independently developed its own tools and practices. Rather, as shown in the case of the IAB and similar institutions, they are the fruit of constant interaction.

To define the work done at these interfaces, biomedical administrators have invented yet another neologism—translational research. Practical usage of the term, although restricted mostly to the United States,[77] is consistent with the larger trends just described. Current definitions of the term can be found, for example, in a recent newsletter of an American agency that funds translational research. Translational research is defined here as "the two-way transfer between basic research and the treatment of patients," with the further specification that the "awards will enable recipients to explore important scientific questions, to apply the resulting knowledge at the bedside, and to bring insights from the clinical setting back to the laboratory for further exploration."[78] This definition suggests the existence or necessity or both of a mutual link between laboratory work and clinical work. In spite of interpretations that imply a more traditional unidirectional model,[79] most authors seem to favor the bidirectional approach: "The link between the basic laboratory and the clinic has been termed translational research, and this bridge must be crossed in both directions, bringing concepts from the laboratory into the clinic and taking observations from the clinic to the laboratory."[80]

While some authors employ the metaphor of a new space situated somewhere between the laboratory and the clinic ("The term 'translational research' refers to investigations at the interface between the laboratory and the clinic"[81]), others, as in the above quotation and in the following one, indulge in the notion of a bridge connecting two different worlds: "Basic science and clinical medicine have long existed within separate worlds that only occasionally meet in an uneasy partnership. . . . The bridge between these two worlds is difficult but necessary to build."[82] In the rest of the book, we look more closely at the issues and problems raised by these claims and, more generally, by the term "biomedicine." If, as some advocates of translational research maintain, biology and medicine are separate worlds characterized by distinctive sets of issues and entities, then their successful hybridization must involve the creation of a new epistemological, institutional, and material configuration, one that is no longer biological or clinical but biomedical and, as such, irreducible to both medicine and biology. As we show in chapter 3, the emergence of such a configuration did not have to await the invention of the term "translational research."

To sum up, what should we make of hospital platforms and how do they relate to our notion of biomedical platforms? Our preceding remarks point in one direction: to account for the development of hospital platforms one has to examine the changing relations between biology and medicine. This means that one has to go beyond the analysis of hospital platforms as architectural, organizational, or logistic units, and develop a notion of *biomedical* platforms, as distinct from hospital platforms. To do so means that we must take apart the collection of equipment and devices housed on the hospital platform and show that only some of these qualify as components of biomedical platforms. As a first step in this direction, the next chapter inspects the ramifications, etymological and otherwise, of the terms "biomedical" and "biomedicine."

3

Biomedicine and Platforms

Since World War II, the relations between biology and medicine have taken on a new form in the Western world. The exponential rise in public funds made available to university and parapublic research since 1945 has put a lot of biology on the market and has generated numerous public and private schemes to translate that knowledge into clinically useful practices. In the same vein, the wave of reform that ran through the Western world in the postwar period vastly expanded the notion of public health to include funding for basic medical research. In Britain, for example, the creation of the National Health Service (NHS) in 1948 gave the health ministry the power to fund and conduct research. Together with the Medical Research Council (MRC), the NHS set up over forty-six clinical research units throughout the country both in universities and hospitals in the period 1950–70.[1] In the United States, the National Institutes of Health (NIH), founded in 1948, quickly became the leading source of continuous federal funding for medical research, supplying 70% of all funds by 1975.[2] In the twenty-five years after the war, total federal support of biomedical research rose from $27 million to 1.7 billion.[3] The rise in funds accompanied a concomitant rise in clinical personnel in university departments of medicine. In 1950, there were perhaps 1000 academic clinicians in the United States.[4] In 1980 there were twelve times that number. As clinical departments became more academic, medical schools became increasingly research-oriented, to the extent that by 1980 they awarded 42% of all PhDs given in the biological sciences.[5]

But maybe there is nothing new under the sun. After all, have not historical variations of biology and medicine interacted since the ancient Hippocratic authors first ascribed disease to a mere excess or lack of the four physiological humors? Has not pathology attempted to model itself on biology since the seventeenth century when Sydenham invented the former by proposing that diseases be treated as autonomous entities, like plants and animals, and be subjected to similar schemes of description and classification?[6] In a more modest time frame, could one not still claim, as is often the case, that contemporary biomedicine goes back at least to the bacteriological and laboratory revolution of the second half of the nineteenth century,[7] or to Virchow's establishment of a cellular pathology by applying cell biology to the understanding of pathological processes?[8] On the contrary, we maintain that modern "biomedicine" constitutes a novel institutional and scientific activity that is incommensurable with the practices of, say, a Louis Pasteur, a Robert Koch, or a Rudolf Virchow. We claim, in particular, that unlike previous efforts to combine biology and medicine, present efforts have succeeded in a way that the others did not: biology and medicine are now tightly intertwined research enterprises. As we will see further on, unlike the nineteenth century, it is now no longer a question of *attempts* to apply biology to medicine. Biology now "applies" to medicine in the sense that practitioners of the activity known as biomedicine can no longer say beforehand whether a particular research project, clinical investigation, or even clinical intervention will result in the production of biological or medical facts. Somewhat like the distance between pure and applied research, the distance separating biology and medicine has collapsed without, albeit, erasing the distinction between the two activities.

Etymologies II: Biomedical/Biomedicine

The appearance of the neologism biomedicine (and its adjectival form, biomedical) acts as a linguistic marker of this event.[9] As we noted at the outset of chapter 2, the notion of biomedicine is both common and controversial. As late as 1968, the famous French hematologist Jean Bernard declared the term a smokescreen that hid the fact that clinical observations often stimulated biological investigations.[10] More than thirty years later, the issue remains. In a 1999 *Nature* commentary, for example, the president of the U.S. Biophysical Society, Ken Dill, defined the biomedical enterprise as a tendency that had emerged in the course of the last century to "reduce the problems of disease to problems of molecular science: to identify the relevant molecules, to purify them, to determine their three-dimensional structures at atomic resolution, and then to create drugs to bind to them, atom by atom."[11] This definition did not stand unchallenged. In a subsequent issue, Alan Schechter, a clinical researcher at the NIH criticized Dill for naïve reductionism and accused him of having conflated "biology and medicine into an ill-defined hybrid 'biomedicine.'"[12] Schechter did not so much deny the existence of biomedicine as object to the one-way street proposed by Dill leading from the basic sciences to biology and medicine. According to Schechter, the "unidirectional model" belied the fact that "advances in biology and medicine feed back into and stimulate what he [Dill] terms the 'basic sciences,' and may lead to whole new research paradigms."[13] While our sympathies may lie with Schechter in this dispute, the point is not to decide who is right or wrong but to note that the very idea of biomedicine presupposes some idea of how innovations are produced in the gray zone that lies between biology and other "basic sciences" and medicine.

Notwithstanding one commentator's insinuation according to which the NIH introduced the term "biomedical science" in the 1960s in order to justify its "diversion of funds" from "the study of human health and disease, into basic molecular biology," we suggest that there is more to the term than vested interests and inflated rhetoric.[14] Let us return to the dictionaries. Webster's 2nd edition (1970) of its *New World Dictionary* defines *biomedicine* as "a branch of medicine that is combined with research in biology."[15] This sounds harmless enough. The "social etymology" of the word, however, reveals a somewhat more tortuous history. Indeed, to avoid unnecessary misunderstandings, allow us to immediately distance ourselves from one widespread negative connotation of "biomedicine" used in many medical sociology and medical anthropology publications. Here, in contrast to mass media usages where "biomedicine" evokes high-tech, heroic medicine, the term is more often than not accompanied by a ritual exorcism of the "mechanistic" and "reductionist" nature of contemporary medical practice. The latter are unfavorably contrasted with the allegedly "holistic" or "broader" work on the social determinants of health and illness often carried out by social scientists.[16] Although these narcissistic skirmishes form part of the history of the term, we eschew further investigation as our interest lies in the contrasting positive definitions of the term and, especially, the context of its postwar diffusion.

The *Barnhart Dictionary of New English Since 1963* traces "biomedicine" back to 1970.[17] One finds similarly recent origins in French dictionaries, such as the *Dictionnaire historique de la langue française* (1970) and the *Dictionnaire des mots nouveaux* (1965).[18] Obviously, these dates do not indicate the earliest use of the word. Rather, they record the approximate date at which the term entered general use. For earlier usage, we must turn to other dictionaries that describe a more specialized use of "biomedicine." The *Merriam Webster Collegiate Dictionary* (10th edition) dates the term back to a 1947 Rockefeller Foundation report,[19] and the *Random House Unabridged Dictionary* to 1945–50.[20] The earliest, prewar dating for biomedicine is found in the *Oxford English Dictionary Additions Series,* which mentions a 1923 occurrence in the 12th edition of *Dorland's Medical Dictionary.*[21] We are here confronted with a case of self-reference whereby one dictionary (*Dorland's*) serves as a citational authority for another dictionary (the *OED*). The self-reference becomes entire when we realize that the source of the *Dorland's* definition remains unknown since, owing to computerization, the publisher has kept no citational evidence prior to 1974. We do, however, know that Dr. W. A. Newman Dorland, a U.S. Army lieutenant colonel, was a member of the American Medical Association committee on the nomenclature and classification of diseases, and that he worked on his eponymous dictionary in collaboration with a professor of bacteriology and biochemistry at the Virginia Medical College. These two circumstances may explain why *Dorland's* listed "biomedicine" at such an early date, in spite of the fact that we can find only isolated instances of the word prior to World War II.

True, the composite term biochemistry, constructed on a similar basis, entered general circulation in the 1920s. Both *Random House* and the *OED* date early use of that word to 1880–85, while historians point to Hoppe-Seyler's introduction of the term in 1877 and Hofmeister's firm establishment of it in 1901.[22] However, in the early twentieth century it still had an aura of novelty prompting the surprised reaction, in 1912, of an English physician: "I struck a hybrid the other day, a bio-chemist!"[23] Biophysics appeared toward the end of the nineteenth century and was soon followed by other composite terms, such as biomechanics, biodynamics, and bioengineering, which refer to topics ranging from the physical aspects of cellular biology to engineering and rehabilitation.[24] Several of these terms appear as keywords in the third and fourth series of the *Index Catalogue of the Surgeon General's Library* (the precursor of today's MEDLINE) published between the two world wars. No mention, however, of biomedicine. So, while one may stumble across isolated interwar examples of the use of "biomedicine" or its adjectival form—a Chicago psychiatrist writing in 1931 speaks of the "psychological and strictly bio-medical aspects of mental disorders"[25]—it is not until the second half of the twentieth century that the word entered routine discussions of medical matters and even then in initially highly unusual situations. Indeed, as we will see below, the composite term's first official use emerged in the late 1940s in connection with research on the biological and medical consequences of atom bomb testing. It then spread, in the early 1960s, to descriptions of NASA space travel programs, emerging in the late 1960s–early 1970s as a standard category of healthcare policy and administration.

Enough about dating. What about definitions? While the prize for originality certainly goes to a 1994 French dictionary defining *biomedicine* as that "part of medicine investigating treatments designed to conserve life and vital functions,"[26] most definitions found in English dictionaries offer two related, yet distinct meanings. They describe, on the one hand, the *epistemological* idea of a cross-fertilization of medicine and biology. On the other hand, they define biomedicine as a *substantive area*, namely the study of environmental stresses on the human body. *Dorland's* 1923 definition ("Clinical medicine based on the principles of physiology and biochemistry") remained unchanged until the 1940s and is an example of the first meaning, as are more recent definitions such as *Random House's* ("The application of the natural sciences, esp. the biological and physiological sciences, to clinical medicine") or *Webster's* ("Medicine based on the application of the principles of the natural sciences and especially biology and biochemistry").[27]

The *OED* also adopts the epistemological approach, although in its definition the hybridization of biology and medicine seems to have reached the stage of fusion: "Biology and medicine collectively, the biomedical sciences."[28] Examples of the second meaning are provided by *Random House* ("The science concerned with the effects of the environment on the human body, esp. environments associated with space travel"), *Barnhart* ("The biological and medical study of man's tolerance to environmental stresses, specially in space travel"), and another medical dictionary, *Stedman's* ("A discipline concerned with analyzing human tolerances to different environments and with methods of protecting against the effects of exceeding these tolerances").[29] The two definitions of biomedicine—the epistemological and the substantive—are mirror images. The former refers to the investigation of pathological situations using biological theories and methods: the laws of the normal applied to pathological bodies. The latter focuses on normal bodies challenged, so to speak, by pathological environments.

An early institutional juxtaposition of biology and medicine occurred in 1948 when the Atomic Energy Commission (AEC) formed its Division of Biology and Medicine.[30] The division had been preceded in

1943 by the formation of a small health group at Los Alamos to monitor and protect the personnel involved in the Manhattan Project from the adverse effects of radioactivity. Obviously, the situation had called for more than routine medicine, since the potential patients confronted previously unknown environmental threats created by the presence of novel substances such as plutonium. The AEC subsequently established a small biochemistry section so that, by 1948, when the health group evolved into a health division, the biochemistry section became the Biomedical Research Group (H-4) of that division.[31]

The group acquired a unique expertise in the study of the biological and medical effects of nuclear radiation and the physiology of radioactive elements and developed a whole array of new instruments and related techniques for which they actively sought biomedical applications in the emerging field of nuclear medicine.[32] Following the discovery in the mid-1950s that radioactive elements from fallout due to the testing of nuclear devices were deposited in organic material, the group initiated a screening program for milk, hamburger meat, and humans.[33] The 1960s saw an increased emphasis on fundamental research, particularly in the fields of molecular and cellular biology that, once again, prompted the development of instrumentation, and in particular high-speed electronic cell counting, sizing, and sorting. Los Alamos authorities disbanded the Biomedical Research Group in 1973 and reorganized it into four new groups, namely mammalian radiobiology, cellular and molecular radiobiology, biophysics and instrumentation, and organic and biosynthesis.[34] We return to Los Alamos in chapter 7, when we have an opportunity to discuss some of the instrumentation produced in that setting and that ended up as a component of the immunophenotyping platform.

A radioactive world is one pathological environment; outer space is another. In 1958, following the October 1957 launch of *Sputnik* by the Soviet Union, U.S. Congress established the National Aeronautics and Space Administration (NASA), with the mandate of placing a man into orbit.[35] American space operations, however, did not begin with NASA. In addition to NACA (National Advisory Committee for Aeronautics), NASA's predecessor agency, the military, and in particular the Air Force, had already developed extensive expertise in this field. The Air Force maintained leadership in the medical aspects of space flight due, in part, to the contribution of German scientists who had been brought to the United States after the war. The Air Force established the world's first department of space medicine in 1950 at the Air Force School of

Aviation Medicine.[36] Interestingly enough, there was no talk at that time of biomedicine, but, rather, of space (or aerospace) medicine and of space biology. In 1958, however, immediately after the establishment of NASA, a letter from NASA to the Pentagon mentioned "three biomedical flights involving primates,"[37] and a January 1959 internal memo, entitled "Bio-medical Interests of NASA" recommended the creation of a "biomedical unit" and of "a small biomedical research laboratory."[38]

The selection and training of astronauts and the development of ways of monitoring the astronauts' physiological functions on earth and during flight featured among the major "biomedical" tasks faced by NASA in 1958. Astronaut selection involved the prior establishment of the clinical norms to be expected of successful candidates and the development of means to test body performance in extreme situations. Monitoring procedures necessitated the development of bioinstrumentation; yet, given the uncharted environment in which the operations had to be performed, researchers admitted that "the principal value of bioinstrumentation [as initially designed] would be to test the instruments and monitoring procedures themselves and thereby contribute to the design and development of reliable devices for use in subsequent flight programs."[39] The connection between these programs and Earth-based medicine lay in the fact that postwar practices, such as the advent of continuous monitoring of patients' physiological variables, were

> appreciably advanced by the invention of sophisticated equipment to observe physiological changes in animals and astronauts during the space exploration program that grew during the 1960s. As one enthusiast commented, "If monkeys 100 miles in the air can be monitored, there is no reason why patients cannot be monitored."[40]

And indeed, in parallel with the performance of biomedical experiments on the Skylab station, a landmark 1970 report that reoriented NASA activities toward unmanned planetary explorations and exobiological investigations (the search for extraterrestrial life forms) singled out the transfer of biomedical knowledge and technology from the space program to Earth-based medicine as an explicit goal.[41] As we will see in chapter 7, one of the instruments eventually integrated into the immunophenotyping platform was initially developed at Stanford University as part of work on automated equipment for NASA's exobiology program.[42]

We have discussed in some detail the early use of the terms *biomedicine* and *biomedical* by NASA and the Los Alamos laboratories not simply because these institutions played a key role in their circulation but also because of the connotations of these neologisms. Two are of particular interest in the present context: first, the location of biomedical activities at the interface between the normal and pathological, and, second, their relation to the development of instrumentation. These two meanings are, in an important sense, coextensive, insofar as biological variables, by definition, vary continuously and thus apply to populations. They consequently open the door to screening and automation in medicine, as carried out, for instance, by the instruments that measure biological variables on a hospital platform. Screening and automation, in turn, draw pathology and biology into a single domain of description.

We return to these questions later, but first let us add that early uses of "biomedicine" also have a political and administrative dimension. In this respect, the 1960s ushered in the first official reports on biomedicine[43] and the organization of international meetings such as the Symposium on National Policies for Biomedical Research organized by the NIH in Williamsburg, Virginia in 1965, or the Science Policy and Biomedical Research meeting sponsored in Paris in 1968 by the International Council of Biomedical Sciences, with the support of UNESCO and the World Health Organization.[44] Several of these meetings included attempts to establish distinctions between the various kinds of research (basic, clinical, public health, technological, and so on) covered by the umbrella term biomedicine. As a result, the term itself lost its distinctiveness (either substantive or epistemological) and became somewhat of a catchall, as exemplified in this 1992 definition of *biomedical* as the "inclusive word . . . for the many kinds of research funded by the NIH and performed in our medical schools and medical research institutes by MDs, MD-PhDs, PhDs, and others, and whose content runs the gamut from strictly biological to strictly clinical."[45]

A short 1972 address to the Institute of Medicine by Lewis Thomas, a leading reformer of American medicine and chairman of the President's Biomedical Research Panel, stood out, however, as an exception to this trend and thus merits further attention.[46] In an attempt to present a coherent conceptual account of the idea of biomedicine, Thomas distinguished two types of medical technology. First were the so-called high technologies such as those involved in chemotherapy, radiotherapy, and transplantation. Thomas argued that such technologies were misleadingly described as medical high technologies as they did not require an understanding of the pathological mechanisms at work in disease. Physicians called upon these technologies only after the disease had done its damage. Thomas contrasted the former with the "real high technology of medicine," consisting of antibiotics, antibodies, hormone treatments for endocrinological disorders, or treatments for nutritional disorders (and, one could add with hindsight, tools such as cells, enzymes, and genes). Based in part on an understanding of pathological mechanisms, these technologies could be used to prevent the emergence of disease or to return affected cells and tissues to their normal state, thus making the cruder forms of intervention unnecessary. Thomas located the origin of medical high technologies in advances of biology and thus in the improved comprehension of the basic functions *and* dysfunctions of biological mechanisms. Although Thomas did not say so explicitly, biomedicine corresponded to this collapse of the boundaries between the normal and the pathological. As we will see in chapter 3, Thomas's position, typical of advanced American "biomedicine," resonated closely with similar programs advanced at roughly the same time in the United Kingdom by reformers who gained control of key institutions such as the Imperial Cancer Research Fund.

To sum up: our etymological detour has revealed an inversion of the relationship of biology to medicine. Once a handmaiden to pathology, biology now counts as the ultimate description and account of disease origins and mechanisms. It is true that the qualitative, synthetic judgment that the pathologist or clinician uses when identifying a specific disease in an individual has not been eliminated. Yet, while biology has yet to substitute itself, in the reductionist sense, for pathology, it has to a certain extent encircled medicine. As prediagnostic biological tests for individuals and screens for groups or as therapeutic monitoring procedures, the investigation of quantifiable, biological variables pervades the practice of medicine. We will have occasion in the following section to distinguish between devices dedicated to the measurement of a single item of medical interest and biomedical instruments that measure a biological variable and attempt (not always successfully) to bring pathology and biology together within a single space of representation.

Biomedicine as Instrumentation and Automation

The development of machines and devices dedicated to the measurement of biological variables is one way of integrating biology and medicine. As previously mentioned, automation is not simply the process of doing the same thing more quickly or efficiently. Practitioners know this. Here is an example from hematology. In 1978 and 1980 two hematology journals—the *Nouvelle Revue Française d'Hématologie* and *Blood Cells*—published special issues devoted to automation.[47] The transformation of hospital work and architecture through the injection of massive amounts of equipment and devices had prompted a growing preoccupation with automation. In turn, contributors to the journals felt that automation had affected the conditions and content of medical practice and judgment. Summing up the *Blood Cells* symposium, Jean Bernard declared that automation had engendered competing points of view based on four fundamental divisions. He described these divisions as those that opposed "numbers or quantities, and a unique quality or specificity," "the subjective and objective viewpoints," "morphology and physiology, or . . . appearance and function," and, finally, different representations of the world of blood diseases as, for instance, cells (under a microscope) or "clouds of particles" (on the screen of a computerized instrument).[48] In this respect, "the future of hematology" depended on automation insofar as it obviously entailed far more than the acceleration of laboratory tasks.

Bernard's concerns reflected a process initiated in the 1920s with the introduction of devices dedicated to the measurement of red blood cells.[49] As argued in the previously mentioned address by Lewis Thomas, however, with the substitution or addition of biological technologies (enzymes, proteins, and, subsequently, stretches of DNA) for the strictly physicochemical counting devices that had preceded them, hospital technologies underwent a marked transformation in the 1960s and 1970s. Biomedical technology could now be used at an explanatory cellular and molecular level. In contrast, the measurement of pathological phenomena whose existence depended upon the expert judgment of a pathologist remained singularly resistant to automation. Herein lay part of the reward of reducing the pathological to a quantitative extension of the biological: biological variables could be measured, making possible gains in "mechanical objectivity"[50] (the epistemological edge) and labor time (the operational edge).

Note, here, that in order to automate in the field of biomedicine, problems of pathology had to be reduced to problems of biology; pathological singularities had to be translated into expressions of biological function. In other words, measuring devices had to operate on quantitative differences before transforming these differences into qualitative distinctions. In an important sense, biomedicine and the multiple institutional and scientific investments of the postwar period presupposed that just such a reduction was possible. In the next section we discuss the problems raised by the attempt to construe pathology as operating according to the same laws or along the same lines as biology. For the moment, we will take a closer look at automation, for considerable confusion surrounds the meaning of this term.

What happens, for instance, when scientists and engineers attempt to automate something like "diagnosing cancer?" Common sense would tell us that someone invents a machine capable of carrying out such an activity. In reality, however, just as diagnosis requires some sort of mechanical mediation—even in the absence of tools or equipment, a "hands-on" diagnosis requires disciplined gestures and draws upon the mechanical or statistical treatment of previous encounters—there is no machine judgment that substitutes for human judgment. Rather, researchers rearrange the process of producing that judgment. The process of diagnosis and the very nature of the disease in question are consequently redefined. Nonetheless, if one were to turn to the sociology of work,[51] where automation has been a central topic of study since the 1940s, one would conclude that human judgment and the skills needed to exercise such judgment are indeed automated. Sociologists commonly describe automation as a process of deskilling wherein labor and laborers are divided until their skills can be incorporated into the physical design of, and their actions mimicked by, nonhuman devices. As Stephen Barley has pointed out, however, most studies in this tradition are somewhat misleading, as empirical studies have shown repeatedly that to deskill a task does not necessarily entail deskilling a worker.[52]

Harry Collins agrees with Barley when he tells us that automation is simply the ability of a machine to substitute for human action and not humans.[53] That substitution is, moreover, not an identical substitution but a functional substitution based on mimicry. According to Collins, a successful substitution depends upon not only a social consensus as to what counts as the same thing or action but also upon the ability of humans to make good the deficiencies that inevitably result from mimicry. Collins thus claims that when machines "replace" humans, they do so only in the special sense that they rarely do the same thing the humans did; they often appear to do so only because humans make good the deficiencies in the performance; and that when the replacement appears to work, it appears so because the human performance is itself modeled upon or mimics a mechanical or machine-like performance.[54] Nonetheless, underlying this careful functionalism and its "social" stipulations remains the idea that technology substitutes for human activity whether it be the activity of a group or an individual. Indeed,

Collins contends that when it comes to automation, we are dealing with a "social prosthesis."[55]

In so doing and despite his rejection of the commonsense notion of substitution, Collins's position results in an implicit refusal to recognize a division of labor even though he is conscious of divisions among workers. Collins would no doubt recognize that humans at work perform work routines and that these, per se, are not reducible to isolated human actions or behaviors, as they do not occur in the absence of tools.[56] Moreover, work routines take place within a division of labor that transcends the simple sum of an individual's actions. Work and its routines thus entail a variety of interactions between the living and the dead and the human and the nonhuman. What is replaced through automation or by a machine is not some fragment of the human body or some ultimately indescribable series of physical or mental gestures, but a way of *making* something. Successful automation is thus not an automated mimicking of human operations by a more efficient machine, but a *substitution* of one process (involving more than humans) by another. Automation is not a deskilling of humans and the replacement of human judgment by machines by embedding human skills in an automaton, but the creation of a new field of operations that redistributes actions between humans and machines and among the humans themselves.

Practitioners implicitly acknowledge these differences in their ad hoc typologies of equipment. Automators in the biomedical sciences, for example, generally recognize two kinds of equipment: devices and instruments. The terms of the division are not ours. Reviewing, in the early 1990s, all the instruments produced in the course of 30 years of attempts to automate the Pap test, a British research group described the technology developed in Europe, the United States, and Japan as falling into just these two categories. The first and oldest category included all those *devices* that "have been designed to emulate the human screening process." These devices were bound together by the fact that "the features selected [for automated processing] have a direct relation to the conventional criteria: morphology, optical density, texture, etc." The second category of technology, following the "current trend in biomedical science," described *instruments* that "complement, or perhaps replace, conventional morphological criteria by measurements of signals derived from cell chemistry and immunocytochemistry, nuclear DNA characteristics and newer markers."[57] While *devices* involved the attempt to recognize some pathological entity, then, biomedical *instruments* move the problems of automation out of the sphere of pathology and human judgment into the sphere of biology and quantification. So far, according to the actors themselves, products developed under the first heading have been less successful than those developed under the second.

In fact, continued attempts to automate the Pap test since World War II clearly illustrate the limits of automating devices and the difficulties of reducing a pathological singularity, in this case cervical cancer, to a biological continuum.[58] In order to explore these problems further, we will briefly analyze the history of the devices, instruments, and programs set up to automate the Pap test. The history will show an ambivalence in the relationship between devices and instruments, one that is, moreover, consistent with the more general rise of biomedicine that we have been describing. Let us begin with one of the high points of this history, the inauguration of the Cytology Automation Program by the National Cancer Institute (NCI) of the United States in July of 1972.[59] Designed to fund applied research destined to automate the Pap test and run by a committee on cytology automation, the program was fueled by funds from the recently announced "war on cancer."[60] Although the program's funding went as often to "pure technology" and "general biomedical applications" as it did to "clinical applications,"[61] the resulting instruments were intended to be transformed into devices dedicated to the automatic detection of cervical cancer cells.[62] This did not happen. In 1978, administrative reorganizations within the NCI reduced the cytology automation committee to a purely advisory capacity.[63] Two years later, the NCI abolished the committee and the program ended, somewhat acrimoniously, having failed to achieve its objectives.[64]

The NCI program had capped a movement that had emerged in the wake of the first conference on "Automatic Cytology" organized by the Engineering Foundation, a private research foundation of modest means, and held in Henniker, New Hampshire in 1971. Many members of the future NCI committee met for the first time at this conference. Drawing participants from seven countries, the conference generated a growing sense of an international research effort. Conference organizers boasted that the "field" of cytology automation had grown from "less than a dozen in 1966 into a body of well over 100 workers."[65] Far from being a homogeneous field with a common project or purpose, however, meeting participants came from strikingly different disciplines and institutions. Attendees included George Wied from the University of Chicago's Department of Pathology and an expert in the Pap smear and developers of various instruments from the Los Alamos Scientific

Laboratory, the Lawrence Livermore National Laboratory, and the Stanford University Department of Genetics (these latter institutions return in chapter 7).

Why did the NCI think they could automate a medical activity—namely the diagnosis of cervical cancer—by funding instrument development? To answer this question, we must return to the original Pap test. First developed by George Papanicolaou in the 1920s, the Pap test was not, strictly speaking, a diagnostic test. It was a method of classifying cells taken from the cervix and placed on a microscope slide. Sometimes those cells were perfectly normal, in which case the slide fell into class I. Sometimes the cells appeared to indicate cancer. In this case, the slide fell into classes IV and V. Classes II and III, as can be imagined, lay somewhere in between. At no point in the classification procedure could one be said to have diagnosed cancer. The classification thus represented an early attempt at a "biology of cancer" with its assumption that there was a visible continuum between normal cells and pathological cells.[66]

Papanicolaou encountered two obstacles to the acceptance of his test. First was the widespread observation among pathologists that, under a microscope, nothing in particular distinguished cancer cells from normal cells.[67] Second, pathologists marginalized Papanicolaou's work by noting that he was neither a pathologist nor a clinician, but an anatomist. Papanicolaou had foreseen the problem and had used the biological terminology of classes to avoid conflict with pathologists. Nonetheless, although entirely dependent on traditional microscopic techniques of cell identification, it took a veritable campaign conducted by the American Cancer Society and the NCI before the Pap smear and its interpretation finally entered clinical medicine in the United States and subsequently in Europe in the postwar era.[68]

The continuum between the normal and the pathological created by Papanicolaou's classification raised the question: at what point did the biology of cervical cells slide into disease? In other words, although "hailed as the ultimate tool in cancer detection and prevention,"[69] it was not always clear in the 1940s and 1950s how pathologists should read the findings of a positive Pap smear (i.e., the presence of cancerous cells). In particular, some pathologists doubted that cancerous changes detected on the outermost tissue of the cervix (the epithelium) and referred to as carcinoma in situ, would inevitably lead to a genuine cancer of the cervix, referred to as invasive cancer. An early practitioner of the Pap smear, Dr. Lewis Robbins, recalled the kind of disputes the test generated in the 1940s:

> The Pap smear isn't diagnosing cancer, it's diagnosing a precursor. Why do they call it cancer then? Because nobody would pay any attention if they called it dysplasia (abnormal tissue). If you call it carcinoma in situ, then they will examine it, do something with it. I remember a battle at Roswell Park in 1946, the pathologist was saying that the Pap smear is no good. One physician said carcinoma in situ is not cancer, but we have to call it cancer. The pathologist said we can't call it cancer if it doesn't metastasize or if it hasn't already metastasized. But we did.[70]

These problems persisted well into the 1950s. To answer these and other questions, such as the age at which women were most in danger of developing cervical cancer, the NCI undertook experimental mass screening programs for cervical cancer beginning in the late 1940s in Arkansas.[71] Expanded in 1951 to Tennessee,[72] by the late 1950s the NCI funded six separate experimental screening projects.[73] Preliminary results showed that "vaginal cytology readily lends itself to use as a mass screening device."[74] The massive nature of the undertaking, however, created a demand for a new kind of instrument, a device devoted to the analysis of the Pap test. Note here the emergence of a new kind of diagnostic activity that is decidedly not diagnostic. As defined in the 1950s, "Screening tests sort out apparently well persons who have a disease from those who probably do not. A screening test is not intended to be diagnostic."[75] This novel activity—screening—formed the bridge between biology and medicine.

The NCI announced its intentions to produce such an instrument in 1955 with a press release bearing the headline: "Can a Machine Distinguish between Cancer and Normal Cells? The Government and the American Cancer Society Are Betting $100,000 That It Can."[76] Consequently, in 1955, Airborne Instruments Limited received a grant to develop what came to be known as the cytoanalyzer. Founded as a division of Cutler-Hammer Inc. in 1945 to develop electronic components for the Air Force and air traffic control, in the early 1960s Airborne Instruments employed over 3000 people, twenty of whom were assigned to the Department of Medical and Biological Physics. The latter, opened in 1955, operated under the belief that the "physical sciences are the key to many hoped-for areas of biological research and to many desirable programs in mass diagnosis and prognosis."[77] Walter Tolles, a physicist at the Airborne Instruments laboratory developed the prototype.[78] Moving back and forth over a microscope slide, the cytoanalyzer measured the area and density of cells on the slide by transforming the variation in light passing through the sample on the slide into an electric current. The electric current could then be run through a computer supplied with rules to distinguish a normal from an abnormal current, thus translating the cells into electric currents.[79]

Between 1955 and 1961, Tolles and Airborne Instruments produced a number of instruments field-tested by the NCI and outside collaborators. In its first controlled clinical trial, the cytoanalyzer managed to eliminate 40% of the negative (normal) slides and missed none of the positive (classes III–V in the Pap classification) slides. The field testers concluded that the cytoanalyzer was a "workable device."[80] A second clinical trial held in 1959 analyzed samples from over 11,000 vaginal smears from the Columbus Ohio Cancer Survey Project and from patients treated in the gynecology service of the Walter Reed Army Hospital. Results showed the machine capable of eliminating approximately 37% of all negative smears.[81] Shortly thereafter, Tolles and his coworkers announced greatly improved results. In 1961, they reported a trial showing no false negatives and a mere 15% false positives, which, in their terms, constituted "a very effective screening level."

It would be, however, the last time anybody achieved a false-negative rate of 0%, a rate that is today considered next to impossible, for, despite these promising numbers, the cytoanalyzer subsequently disappeared.[82] Several reasons for its demise have been offered. Leo Koss tells us that "the entire Cytoanalyzer effort was soon abandoned for lack of fiscal support."[83] The story within the NCI, the source of the fiscal support, is substantially different. Reviewing the situation in 1965, the director of the Diagnostics Research Division of the NCI concluded that although the cytoanalyzer "performed its purpose well," the "biological programming" did not work.[84] Specifically, further work on the instrument suggested that clumps of white blood cells (leukocytes) had "fooled" the machine into thinking that they were cancerous cells. The leukocytes present in the smears were indeed signs of incipient cancer so the instrument got the right answer for the wrong reason. But incipient was not early enough as the machine "therefore misses early lesions in which leucocytic infiltration and exudation are lacking."[85] Since the whole point of the program was early detection, the machine was self-defeating. Following the failure of the cytoanalyzer, company officers at Airborne Instruments "gained a profound respect for the [unspecified] philosophies of the life sciences."[86]

Rather than abandon the whole project, the NCI turned to its chief contractor for yet another device with greater computing capacity. Developed during the period 1961–63,[87] CYDAC grew directly out of the cytoanalyzer program. Not only were components of the cytoanalyzer transferred directly to CYDAC, but the Diagnostics Research Division of the NCI, the original sponsors of the cytoanalyzer, provided funding.[88] Despite the continuity of program, CYDAC differed from the cytoanalyzer in one major respect. Rather than scanning hundreds of cells looking for normal and abnormal cells, it scanned hundreds of cells and reconstituted a digitized image of a normal cell. In a sense, it could be argued that in developing CYDAC, the NCI had abandoned clinical medicine and devices for the wider field of biological instrumentation; automating the pathological was now to be pursued through the digitization of the normal. Indeed, the express purpose of the instrument was to digitize microscope images of cells and thus transform what was essentially a classification of normal cells based on morphological appearances to one based on measures of those same images. In spite of this difference, CYDAC measured the same variable as the cytoanalyzer, namely the ability of different cells to absorb different amounts of light. CYDAC, however, was field-tested in an entirely different field, namely chromosome analysis, where it ended up being outflanked by immunocytochemical analytical techniques.[89]

The idea that a machine could automate the Pap test did not go away. In 1963, Lovis Kamentsky, an IBM engineer, and Myron Melamed at New York's most prominent cancer research facility, the Memorial Sloan-Kettering Cancer Center,[90] began research on the automation of the Pap test, instituting a collaboration that would last for more than a decade.[91] In the absence of a specific pathological criterion distinguishing cancer cells from normal cells, Kamentsky and Melamed needed a biological variable. To do so, Kamentsky created a spectrophotometer that exploited the ability of the nucleus of the cell and its constituent nucleic acids to absorb light at a specific wavelength. Measurements of the amount of ultraviolet light absorbed by cells in the apparatus showed that "some" cancer cells absorbed more light than normal cells.[92]

A double-blind test comparing human cytologists and the spectrophotometer also showed the device capable of detecting "at least 95% of the cervical cancers."[93] A large-scale clinical trial carried out in conjunction with the NCI brought this number down to 85%. However, while these results may have been sufficient back in the 1950s, the field had changed considerably in the interim and the false-negative rate (the percentage of undetected abnormal cells) had become the number to consider. No longer the strict purview of the NCI and the American Cancer Society, the Pap test had become a relatively common procedure and over 120 government-supported schools of cytotechnology had produced an abundance of cytotechnologists.[94] Moreover, since 1966, the Pap test had been a reimbursable procedure under Social Security only if a pathologist or an individual certified by the American Society of Cytology provided the service. Run by George Wied at the University of Chicago, the American Society of Cytology acted as a form of unofficial quality control in the field of the Pap test. If they did not like the device, then it would not fly.

Shortly after the announcement of the results of the NCI clinical trial, Wied announced what were to become the unofficial rules of the game as far as Pap test automation was concerned. Essentially, they boiled down to 0% false negatives or, in other words, 100% success in cancer detection. The idea that the machine could not miss any cancer cells even though cytotechnicians and pathologists sometimes did set up the following Catch-22: the machine must do as a pathologist, but if it did, then it was inadequate. The only way out of the paradox was to make the machine judgment-proof, hence through the reduction of false negatives to zero. As Wied put it in 1968, "Naturally, it would be folly to say that if a technician misses so many cancer cells in 10,000 the projected machine would be adequate if it missed the same percentage. A machine which misses tumor cells and registers the cancer case as 'normal' is an instrument of automatic malpractice for this particular patient who is possibly dying of cancer because of an ill-designed machine."[95] In this comparison with cytopathologists, Kamentsky's apparatus fared even worse. According to Wied, the use of cellular criteria like the absorption of light was no substitute for what cytopathologists really do. In reality, cytopathologists never evaluated single cells. Rather, they looked at "cell patterns," and "associations of cells." Consequently "[a]ny method that removes cells from their 'pattern' tends to decrease diagnostic accuracy."[96]

As can be seen, according to the American Society of Cytology, the ideal machine became not one that merely takes over a human task, but one that replaced human judgment. On these grounds, Kamentsky's spectrophotometer was destined to fail and fail it did. Nonetheless, the initial confusion was now dissipated: there would be no machine to replace human judgment. This did not, of course, preclude automation if the machines could do something that humans simply could not do. Rather than automating morphology, the time had come to circumvent it through the redefinition of the biologically normal cell on the basis of new instruments.

Kamentsky and Melamed articulated this movement from the automation of clinical tasks to biological automation in the late 1960s. Presenting their machine in a special issue of the IEEE journal organized in 1969,[97] they pointed out that, despite the origin of the demand for such equipment, the primary use for an automated instrument was not to identify pathological cells: it was to identify "specimens that are entirely normal." They drew this lesson explicitly from the attempt to automate the Pap test. Once the initial identification had been achieved, then it would be possible to think of "separating, concentrating or marking abnormal cells in a specimen."[98] But even in this case, the apparatus would not necessarily serve as a substitute for human judgment. Rather, it would function in the absence of human judgment insofar as it provided heretofore unknown or "unique methods to characterize cells." In this sense, paradoxically, there was no automation in the classic sense of the term as there was no prior human action to be automated.

Although it had been developed to automate the Pap test, the fact that Kamentsky's apparatus measured and separated cells on a biological basis meant that it had a much wider use than originally intended. Even though he described the invention in his 1965 patent as "a separation apparatus which is fast, accurate and amenable to use in the mass screening area,"[99] the screening of abnormal cells from the cervix in the hopes of isolating a cancerous cell was simply a case in point. The "detection of abnormal biological [as opposed to pathological] cells in samples of body fluids" defined the more general purpose of the project. The patent described, in other words, a biological instrument that would "selectively separate the components or constituents of a biological sample according to type or condition." Consequently, the project to automate the Pap test had resulted, once again, in the production of an apparatus that identified—scanned and separated—different biological entities without actually diagnosing anything. In a sense, it was adequate to the task as the Pap test did not actually diagnose anything either. Kamentsky's apparatus, however, made no attempt to imitate the human eye or its powers of discrimination. Rather than search out the abnormal cell or digitize the normal cell, Kamentsky's instrument isolated normal and abnormal populations on the basis of parameters invisible to the human eye.

As American initiatives in Pap test automation wound down, interest in Europe and Japan heated up. Between 1975 and 1981, the Europeans developed eleven different systems[100] and between 1983 and 1987, four of these went into limited clinical trials funded by the European

Community as part of a larger program entitled "Concerted Action Automated Analytical Cytology" (CAAC). Although designed for limited use, an interesting feature of the prototypes is how much the Pap test itself had been transformed in the effort to automate it. To begin with, the stains used in the prototypes were not always the original Pap stain. Moreover, the devices rarely read a slide prepared by a human. In some systems, a centrifuge that deposited cells on a specially coated slide prepared the specimen. Others prepared the slide using a series of fine meshes to reduce the sample to a single layer of cells that were then spread on a slide. Note that in neither case can we speak of a smear.[101] In addition, the machines rarely read the slides alone but as part of an interactive process. The Dutch system, for example, selected positive images for evaluation by a cytologist. The machine screened the tests and presented images on a TV monitor for humans to determine whether a test was positive.[102]

Despite these and many other ingenious inventions, in their final report to the European Community the cytology automation researchers admitted that "the early hopes and expectations of the CAAC have not been fulfilled."[103] Research continues as many believe that the reasons for the commercial "failure" of the devices were more economic than technical.[104] In particular, enthusiasts suggest that the fragmented European market composed of many small test laboratories could not shoulder the high cost of the systems. As for the U.S. market, although centralized into seven "Pap test mills" handling tens of thousands of tests a year, the International Academy of Cytology had erected a formidable barrier to entry by imposing the aforementioned "almost impossible accuracy requirement" of 0% false negatives.[105] Based partly on the assumption that this was potentially the accuracy of human analysts and thus the only level of acceptable risk from the actuarial and litigation point of view, a series of articles critical of the "Pap mills" and their elevated levels of false negatives in the *Wall Street Journal* in 1987 laid that myth to rest and rekindled interest in automation in the United States.[106]

In 1992, the author of a review on the field of cytopathology automation claimed that since 1987 the field had been dramatically transformed.[107] "Dramatic" is certainly overblown, since the transformation amounted to little more than the appearance of several commercial systems with preliminary positive results. And indeed, despite the optimism, by 1998 none of the systems mentioned in the 1992 review had found broad clinical use.[108] A 2001 report from a French medical technology assessment team, citing similar findings from a 1998 Australian study and a 2000 New Zealand study, concluded that the automated systems had failed to show any superior value when compared to manual techniques.[109] We have suggested that the history of attempts to automate the Pap test have been beset by the ambiguous relationship between medical devices and biological instrumentation. As we have just seen, the project to create a medical device to automate the Pap test has been a relative failure despite the fact that it did succeed in generating biological instrumentation in more than one instance. The persistent ambiguity and the failure can be partly understood within the larger framework of the relations between the normal and the pathological and, in particular, between the quantitative measurement of the normal and the qualitative definition of the pathological.

Biomedicine: The Normal and the Pathological Revisited

Quelqu'un emploie-t-il à tout propos le mot "vie"?—sachez que c'est un malade.[110]

The relationship between biological knowledge and medical practice should be relatively straightforward. Since disease and death are consequences of life, knowledge of pathological processes must necessarily be a subset of the laws of life. Nonetheless, in an influential book published over fifty years ago, the French historian and philosopher of medicine Georges Canguilhem argued that the application of biology to the understanding of disease had been more verbal than real. Canguilhem's much-translated and oft-cited *On the Normal and the Pathological* claimed that the definition of pathological processes as simply quantitative extensions of normal physiology was, in fact, more wishful thinking or "scientific ideology," as he later termed it, than common scientific or medical practice. Far from being a normative stance, Canguilhem based his contention on the historical argument that the numerous attempts since the end of the eighteenth century to define disease as a mere continuation of physiological processes had always failed insofar as they had invariably been shown to be mistaken.

To gain some idea of what Canguilhem observed as a recurrent form of reasoning within modern medicine, consider one of the central examples of his thesis, the analysis by Claude Bernard, the great nineteenth-century physiologist, of the symptoms and cause of diabetes. According to Bernard, each of the major symptoms of diabetes could be understood as merely a quantitative extension of a normal physiological process. Thus, he claimed that different degrees of the intense thirst, frequent urination, weight loss, and sugar in the urine found in diabetes patients could all be found in a normal human being. While varying intensities of the first three symptoms can be commonly observed in humans under normal conditions, Bernard had particular difficulty demonstrating the presence of the last and, indeed, cardinal symptom, glycosurea, in normal subjects. Failing to make the required demonstration, Bernard simply asserted that there must be something wrong with the measuring equipment used to measure glucose in urine (i.e., that it was not sensitive enough).[111] Yet, as Canguilhem remarked, that particular symptom of diabetes could not and cannot be described as simply too much sugar in the urine; normal people do not have any sugar in their urine. It was not and is not a question of quantity; it is a question of quality.

As far as the underlying cause of the symptoms was concerned, Bernard took glycosurea to be simply a consequence of increased sugar production in the body. Following upon his celebrated discovery of the glycogenic function of the liver, Bernard postulated that the liver had put too much sugar into the blood and that the kidney was flooded; the consequent overflow then leaked into the urine. Canguilhem's criticism in this case centered on what Bernard could not have known, namely that the sugar in the blood is not the result of a mere quantitative increase in glycogenesis but, as was shown in the 1920s, the result of an absolute (qualitative) lack of insulin. Now, Canguilhem did not criticize Bernard for not knowing what he could not have known. Rather, he sought to show that Bernard persisted, almost perversely, throughout his career, in believing, despite considerable clinical evidence to the contrary, that pathological processes such as diabetes must be little more than biological processes such as glycogenesis "writ large," so to speak.[112]

Canguilhem raised a second objection to the identification of the normal and the pathological, namely, that such an identification presupposes an objective definition of the normal.[113] Without an objective definition of normal, there is no starting point for the quantitative extension of the normal to the pathological. Such numbers do not, according to Canguilhem, exist and the argument is as follows. In physiology, the norm is generally taken to be the mean of a series of observations. It is assumed that these numbers do not vary according to the environment but are specific to the organism under observation. This leaves out, however, the fact that the number—the mean—is not itself the norm but the numerical expression of the norm. It is not an objective number in the sense that it is the result of a prior process of selection by an environment.

More specifically, Canguilhem points out that the investigation of any physiological process is necessarily the investigation of a process that has a positive (qualitative) value prior to having a quantitative expression. The positive value derives from the fact that, assuming that there are no useless (neutral) physiological processes, then any process must contribute in some way to the maintenance of the life of the organism and must have been the result of natural selection. In other words, all physiological processes had at some point, and retain so far, some positive selective value. Similarly, negative physiological values, like the body temperature of a dinosaur, must already be extinct (and presumably cannot be measured anyway).[114] Given natural selection then, physiological norms are ultimately dependent on the environment and thus cannot be taken as stand-alone, external standards. And indeed, physiological norms can be shown to vary, sometimes quite spectacularly, according to the environment.

If the pathological is not reducible to the normal, then it might be asked, what, besides "nature," gives pathology its autonomous status vis-à-vis physiology? The answer, according to Canguilhem, is that pathology has access to an independent body of observations that emerge in the clinic in the contact between doctor and patient. Clinical facts are not physiological facts even though they are often the basis for such facts. Indeed, the history of medicine shows that despite textbook descriptions, the initial impetus for most physiological research lies in the clinic as opposed to the physiological laboratory. The discovery of the normal function of the islets of Langerhans, for example, was the product of research on diabetes. As Canguilhem puts it, "Almost every time it is said in human physiology, 'We now know that . . . ,' one will find, if one looks hard enough—and without reducing the role of experimentation—that the problem was raised and the solution outlined in the clinic and through therapeutic intervention, and often at the expense, biologically that is, of the patient." In other words, the claim is clear: not only is pathology independent of physiology, it almost always precedes it.[115] Pathology, in turn, is dependent upon a clinical encounter.

Canguilhem explains the primacy of the patient in pathology in a fictitious example. Suppose a murder victim is discovered to have cancer that had not been diagnosed and had not even been suspected by the victim who had remained symptom-free until his or her untimely death.

Did the murder victim have cancer? According to Canguilhem, the answer is no if the question is interpreted to mean: is it possible for a pathologist to diagnose cancer without some sort of clinical encounter? In the case at hand, it is possible to say that the individual had cancer only if he or she had cancerous cells or a tumor. In turn, it is possible to say that only because similar cells or tissue had been seen in some other person who indeed expressed the symptoms of cancer to a physician. In other words, even though clinical scientists use laboratory techniques to detect diseases that individuals may not be aware of, these techniques, in the final assizes, derive their meaning from previous clinical encounters. As Canguilhem puts it, "If today a physician's knowledge of disease allows him to foresee the experience of the disease by the patient, it is because in the past the patient called upon the physician." In history, then, pathology precedes physiology. "Cells of the renal, pulmonary or splenic parenchyma can only be said to be sick, and sick from some disease, today, by an anatomo-pathologist who never sets foot in a hospital or clinic because they were removed or resemble those that were removed yesterday or one hundred years ago, it does not matter which, by a practicing clinician from the body or amputated organ of a man whose behavior he had observed."[116]

How does Canguilhem's analysis relate to our present discussion? Let us clarify what we mean when we say that biomedicine constitutes a new alignment of the normal and the pathological in the postwar era. To begin with, and as previously mentioned, we are not claiming that there has been no discussion of how the normal relates to the pathological or more generally how biology is related to medicine prior to this period. As previously pointed out, we are aware that, since the seventeenth century, part of clinical medicine has tended to describe itself as a form of natural history.[117] Nor do we ignore the fact that since the middle of the nineteenth century an understanding of the basic sciences, such as physiology and chemistry, has been considered the backbone of scientific medicine. Our claim concerns, rather, the articulation of the normal and the pathological in such a way that research in one is immediately available to research in the other. While there are several ways of depicting this relation, we contend that, with minor exceptions, it is only in the second half of the twentieth century that the term "biomedicine" readily applies to a hybrid form of research and therapy that combines the normal and the pathological.

A number of objections spring immediately to mind. Two of the most important advances in modern medicine, cellular pathology and the germ theory of disease, would seem to fit our description of biological research that is immediately applicable to pathology. Consider the first example. Cell theory and tumor theory were elaborated at the same time and in the same laboratory. Schwann, the founder of cell theory, worked in the laboratory of Müller, the founder of tumor cell theory. This, of course, is the tradition of pathological anatomy where observations of normal and pathological structures are pursued simultaneously. Simultaneity does not, however, imply identity or relevance. Despite constant attempts to relate pathological structures to normal structures, pathological anatomy could not be reduced to a phenomenological extension of normal anatomy. Observation of a normal structure did not necessarily hold in the realm of the pathological. Not only did the morbid structures require clinical correlations in order to "make sense," they also required their own vocabulary of description.[118] Moreover, when it came to the processes that generated the pathological structures, sharp differences separated the normal from the pathological. This was so at the tissular as well as the cellular level.[119] On a more pragmatic, and yet equally as vital level, Müller founded his original classification of tumors on the clinical distinction established by surgeons between those curable by extirpation and those that are not (similar to the benign and malignant division).[120]

Rudolf Virchow's cellular pathology offers a second possibility as an early form of biomedicine. The title of his major work, *Cellular Pathology as Based upon Physiology and Pathological Histology*, would certainly seem to indicate an intimate relation between biology and medicine. Indeed, as Virchow states in lecture 3: "I will nevertheless endeavour in the course of these lectures to furnish you with proofs that every pathological structure has a physiological prototype, and that no form of morbid growth arises which cannot in its elements be traced back to some model which had previously maintained an independent existence in the economy."[121] However, Virchow's notion of "based upon" in no way implied identity, for two reasons. In the first place, the physiology that Virchow foresaw as the basis of pathology furnished at best, prototypes, models, and "paradigms"[122] for the understanding of pathology. As a consequence, Virchow proposed the production of a special kind of physiology for the understanding of disease, a "pathological physiology." According to Rather, the clearest definition of cellular pathology and its relation to normal physiology can be found in an article published by Virchow[123] on the subject several years after the original work and which may be summarized as follows: all abnormalities of structure are degenerations, transformations, or repetitions of normal structure.[124] Now, these degenerations, transformations, and repetitions are those that are recognized by pathological histology and in this respect there is no new relation between the normal and the pathological. It is the same as that defined by the tradition of pathological anatomy except at the tissular and cellular level. Note that even the repetition of normal structures does not identify the normal with the pathological. According to Virchow

> Even new-formations [tumors] which very evidently follow the type of some definite normal tissue, still for the most part possess peculiarities, whereby they may be more or less distinguished from this tissue, so that in the majority of cases, at least, it is by no means necessary to see the whole of the new-formation in order to know that this is not the normal, regular development of the tissue, but that on the contrary there is something in it, although it does not lose the type, which deviates from the ordinary course of homologous development.[125]

The pathological form is first recognized as such and then analyzed in terms of repetition. Inexplicable in physiological terms, the generation of the morbid structure requires Virchow's "pathological physiology."

One of Virchow's followers, Gustav Speiss, realized this when he explained, "Insofar as cellular pathology deals only with changes of the form and the mixture of the living body it remains merely pathological anatomy i.e. not pathological physiology . . . the real pathology of the future." In other words, and this is the second reason, not only was Virchow's physiology dependent upon pathology, it remained of the future insofar as it was overshadowed by pathological morphology. Indeed, after Virchow's death, the editors of his celebrated *Archiv* dropped "physiology" from the title retaining only "pathological anatomy." Subsequently, "Cellular pathology itself became confused with pathological anatomy as both Bier and Aschoff were to complain in the nineteen thirties."[126] Cut off from wider notions of etiology and no doubt under "some pressure from their objects, the dead bodies,"[127] pathological anatomy came to rely on the autopsy to the extent that institutes of pathology such as that run by Jakob Erdheim performed thousands a year.[128]

As we saw in our discussion of Canguilhem, the *idea* that the pathological can be reduced to the normal is a common theme in nineteenth-century medicine. But, as we have just seen, despite these philosophical discussions, at the practical level the normal and the pathological remained the products of distinct experimental and institutional practices. Institutes of pathology were separate from institutes of physiology. Even so, historians have described numerous other programs that, in retrospect, might appear to be early forms of modern biomedicine. To see that this is not the case, consider the following description of a program of scientific medicine that proposed the replacement of pathology with physiology. According to Lenoir,

> Wunderlich's physiological medicine was based on the notion that illness and disease result from a disturbance in the normal functioning of an organ or system of organs. In his journal, the *Archiv für physiologische Heilkunde,* Wunderlich waged war against specific disease entities. He also opposed the view that pathological anatomy provided the sole source of scientific medicine. Rather he advocated the investigation through experimental physiology of the laws of normal organ function. . . . Wunderlich's central objective was to trace changes in organ function back to chemical and physical changes transpiring at their anatomical locus. In his program, therefore, pathology was only a tool to be employed in tracing the pathways of disturbed organ function.[129]

Note, as Lenoir does not seem to, that Wunderlich's pathology could not have been simply a tool of physiology since his "medical physiology" rests on the key notion of "disturbance." In this respect, Wunderlich's physiology could not have replaced pathology for there can be no physiology of disturbances. By definition, a disturbance is not a normal function of the body, human or otherwise. It is, rather, an infraction of the rules of physiology and therefore cannot be explained by physiology. The explanation lies in the realm of pathology. The reduction of medicine to physiology, in this case, we would argue, was purely syncretic and verbal.

Even today the central object of pathology remains the formation of a lesion, a process for which there is no corresponding process in biology. The products of the process, the cells of cancer and pathogenic bacteria, do, of course, have normal correspondents. In the nineteenth century, however, researchers identified these actors through their role in the pathological process. Pathogenic bacteria, for example, were isolated on the basis of their ability to produce clinical phenomena like tuberculosis and cholera. Virchow and the great German morphologists recognized distinctly pathological cells whose relationship to normal cells remained unknown or were postulated by the pathologists themselves.[130]

As noted repeatedly, since World War II there has been a concerted effort to marry experimental biology and medicine. These efforts have been expressed in a bewildering variety of institutions and projects explicitly devoted to the alignment and articulation of biology and medicine (as mentioned at the beginning of this chapter). To a considerable degree, these efforts have been successful. Indeed, biological and medical research are now integrated in the sense that it is no longer a question of construing clinical observations as a form of natural science, of inventing speculative programs to give medicine a scientific basis, or of funding research whose intent is the application of biology to medicine.[131] Whereas the scientific or rational medicine of the nineteenth century rejected the idea that disease was the expression of an underlying pathological entity, the twentieth century has separated the entities that accompany pathological processes from the pathological event itself. In other words, the existence of lesions as traces of distinct pathological events is no longer in question. The status of the products of these lesions (e.g., the presence of unusually high quantities of a given protein or the presence of a novel protein), however, often remains in play.

Exploration of these products within a biomedical experimental system can produce knowledge about biological or pathological entities. In addition, when pathologists do speak of pathological entities, they view them as discrete modifications of biological entities and not as quantitative extensions of normal physiological processes or as distinct members of a separate animal or vegetable kingdom. For example, bacteriologists describe discrete genes for virulence that render certain species of bacteria pathogenic. They do not think of those species of bacteria as individuating according to laws that lie above and beyond those of natural selection. Contrast this attitude with that prevalent before World War II. Here, bacteriologists tended toward two opposing and now obsolete points of view: either there were distinct species of pathogenic bacteria or there were no bacterial species whatsoever.[132] Simply put, before the advent of biomedicine two views of the relationship between the normal and the pathological dominated the field. The first, epitomized by Claude Bernard and sharply criticized by Canguilhem, held that the pathological could be reduced to (a quantitative extension of) the normal. Against this reduction, biomedicine has maintained a subtle distinction between these two categories. The second, championed by pathologists, held that the normal and the pathological corresponded to two discrete epistemic fields and consequently to separate domains of work. The study of either thus required both distinct institutional and conceptual-material frameworks of intervention. In overcoming this division, biomedicine has created new entities and events (of which several examples are discussed in chapters 4 and 5) that, without eliminating the distinction between the normal and the pathological, function within common experimental systems and a single space of representation.

Finally, the notion of biomedicine should not be confused with the belief, widespread before World War II, that medicine was a branch of biology. When, for example, Rufus Cole opened the Albert Merritt Billings Hospital at the University of Chicago in 1927, which was, to his mind, "the first hospital erected on the campus by a university with the analogy of the hospital and the laboratory clearly in mind," he counseled: "The student of disease, as the student in other branches of biological science, must bring to his aid the methods of the more fundamental sciences, physics and chemistry and physical chemistry, and even employ the methods of mathematics."[133] He nonetheless quickly added that pathology, or the study of disease, could in no way be reduced to the other sciences; physiology and pathology remained independent pursuits.[134]

Biomedicine as Practice and Policy

What Canguilhem described as a philosophical or epistemological problem in the 1940s has become a problem for public policy. Like scientific research in general, funding for medical research before World War II came mainly from private sources. We mentioned, at the beginning of this chapter, the contrasting exponential rise in public funds that has been made available to university and parapublic biomedical research since World War II. As with any large-scale change in public policy, there was opposition. Lewis Thomas recalls the initial resistance in the 1950s to his research-oriented pathology department at New York University:

> At the outset, there were some complaints about us from the national community of professional hospital pathologists, and a few hostile articles and editorials in the pathology journals. It was felt by some that we were skewing or trying to skew classical pathology away from its traditional objectives, training young people to do research instead of pathology, downgrading the field in general. [135]

Thomas's opponents became the losing side. Although the NIH's mandate was the conquest of disease, research administrators concluded that the latter presupposed the conquest of life. An NIH study committee of the Office of Science and Technology reported to President Lyndon Johnson in 1965:

NIH devotes its principal efforts to a broad program of investigation of life processes, rather than to search for a direct cure or prevention of disease. It employs this approach for a simple and valid reason: life science is so complex, and what is known about fundamental biological processes is so little, that the "head on" attack is frequently the slowest and most expensive path to the cure and prevention of disease.[136]

In France, needless to say, things were different, although the end result was more or less the same. Public funding of medical research is today assured mainly by INSERM (the French Medical Research Institute) which, in 1964, replaced the prewar National Institute of Hygiene, an organization mainly devoted to public health.[137] Jean-Paul Gaudillière described postwar French developments:

Between 1945 and 1970, the fortuitous encounter of major changes in medical and biological practices, alliances between (some) scientists and (some) physicians and, finally, the expansion of the role of the state in the reorganization of research had, as a result, the inversion of the equilibrium established between the clinic and the biological sciences leading numerous young clinicians toward a career in biology and establishing the cell and the molecule as the principal objects of medical research.[138]

As in the nonmedical sciences, a consistent problem for policymakers has been to hasten the movement of knowledge from the pure (biology) to the applied (medicine) domains. Arguing that following the discovery of microorganisms in the 1850s, it took thirty years for the first pathogenic human bacteria to be isolated, science administrators and biomedical researchers began wondering whether there was any way to speed up the process.[139]

Regardless of the plan or project, however, there is a problem common to any attempt to articulate biology and medicine: both are moving targets. Priorities in medicine respond to changing patterns of public health. The impact of AIDS on biomedical research is a case in point. Similarly, priorities in biology change and today's research frontier may be tomorrow's relatively mundane undertaking. The latter problem is particularly acute. While some diseases such as cancer can safely be assumed to remain priorities over the long run, it is often impossible to predict what fields and techniques in the fast-moving world of biology will ultimately prove significant for the study of a particular disease or class of diseases. Decisions about the future, nonetheless, have to be made and the interim attitude has generally been that something will turn up. The previously quoted study committee was quite aware of this lack of alignment between biological results and medical problems. Such a situation, they noted, favored a "reductionist type of research. . . . This follows naturally as the organs and their systems are dissected into even smaller components for study and as cellular biology receives greater emphasis today."[140] In other words, sooner or later, the medical explanation must be reduced to a biological explanation.

The hospital platforms discussed in chapter 2 are just one expression of this overall trend. These new relations between biology and medicine also trouble the division of labor within medicine. In France, for example, legislation passed in 1975 for purposes of medical insurance reimbursement created the domain of "medical biology," essentially a laboratory specialty that initially included pathology, although, in 1994, pathologists ultimately opted out of the system. Included in the payment schedules are a series of "biological acts," some of which can be considered pathology, while others fall under the heading of biochemistry or bacteriology. Consequently, pathologists have objected from the very beginning that the law does not clearly distinguish between what counts as a medical act and what counts as a biological act,[141] and while they admit that both pathologists and medical biologists share a common "technical platform" composed of techniques derived from fundamental biology, they distinguish themselves from medical biologists even when using the same technique in two ways.[142] First, their use of these techniques is generally "nonrepetitive" and "nonautomated." Second, even if the techniques overlap in terms of rate of repetition, pathologists bring special knowledge to the act and consequently draw different conclusions. In particular, before doing a test on a sample, pathologists must know the age and sex of the patient, their medical history, and the site of the biopsy and the technique used. In turn, their reading of the test is not simply an observation of a biological variable, but remarks concerning a pathological lesion. When pathologists do a test, they make a "lesional reading that is nonquantitative. The pathologists' report contains an explicit conclusion on which a therapeutic decision is based."[143]

Modified many times since it was first passed, the law has resulted in the possibility of the same test being carried out by at least four differently qualified practitioners in three different locales with varying interpretations. If the test is carried out by a pathologist who runs his or her own clinic, then the test may be either diagnostic or, if purely biological, complementary to diagnosis. If the test is conducted in a medical biology laboratory, then either a pharmacist or a physician with certified training in the discipline of medical biology carries it out. In this case, the test is generally nondiagnostic. Pharmacists simply do not have the right to diagnose and physicians trained to run a medical biology laboratory generally do not see patients. Finally, if run in a specialized university hospital center, then the practitioner may be even further specialized and run, for example, a hematology laboratory. The meaning of the test then, as in the first situation, depends upon whether the test is considered part of a screening biopsy or genuinely diagnostic of a particular disease.

The governmental attempt to synthesize biology and medicine within one system of prepaid "acts" has led, as one can imagine, to considerable friction. In addition to the opposition between pathologists and medical biologists, at the European level French pharmacists are opposed to allowing clinical chemists to conduct medical biology tests as they do in Britain and Germany. Pathologists that work in private laboratories resent those that work in specialized hospital laboratories, as acts performed in the hospital are covered by block grants and need not figure in the state nomenclature of reimbursable medical biology acts. They worry that medical biologists or, worse still, scientists with no medical training will ultimately monopolize technologies developed in university centers.[144]

The fears of the French pathologists have been partially realized in Germany where similar problems have arisen in the German medical specialty of laboratory medicine. Created in 1958[145] and roughly equivalent to the American specialties of clinical pathology and clinical chemistry, laboratory medicine has distinguished itself from pathology through the use of new techniques derived from biochemistry, immunology, and hematology. Morphology and cytopathology of solid tumors remain the exclusive domain of the pathologist. There is, however, overlap: cancers such as leukemia and some of the lymphomas, as well as cancerous growths such as cervical cancer and lung cancer, can be diagnosed prior to tumor formation on the basis of single cells. Training in laboratory medicine requires an MD and five years in clinical chemistry. Alternatively, if you have a PhD in chemistry, five years of training in a medical laboratory will get you a specialization in laboratory medicine. There are, consequently, two distinct professional societies for pathology in Germany: the larger, the Deutsche Gesellschaft für Klinische Chemie, includes both MDs and PhDs, whereas the smaller one, the Deutsche Gesellschaft für Laboratoriumsmedizin, has only MDs as members. As in France where pharmacists can run medical laboratories, the question arises: when a PhD runs the same diagnostic test as a medically trained pathologist, is he or she doing a diagnosis?[146]

France and Germany are not isolated cases. The situation in the United States is similar to that in Germany.[147] Prior to 1950, pathologists supervised most medical laboratories. That same year, the American Board of Clinical Chemistry was established to certify specialists which included both physicians and individuals with PhDs in the natural sciences. With the advent of Medicare in 1964 and federal regulation of clinical laboratories, a two-year battle ensued over the question: could nonphysicians run clinical laboratories? The answer was yes and coupled with a manpower crisis at the beginning of the 1970s, more and more nonphysicians found themselves heading clinical laboratories.[148]

The professional problems just mentioned are further expressions of the fact that medical research, including research in pathology, is no longer the exclusive domain of medically trained researchers. In 1995, for example, *The American Journal of Pathology* added the subtitle *Cellular and Molecular Biology of Disease.* An editorial announcing the addition explained, "During the last decade, studies of pathogenesis and diagnosis have relied, to an even greater extent, on the methods of molecular and cell biology. These new developments sharpened the focus of pathology and, at the same time, greatly expanded its horizons by removing artificial barriers among disciplines." A change in method, however, is hardly cause for modifying the title of a journal. Methods change all the time. The editors thus went on to point out that the name change followed upon a prior change in name that had taken place several years before. In 1992, the American Association of Pathologists,[149] the society that published the journal, had voted to change its name to the American Society of Investigative Pathology. The change had been made in recognition of the fact that cell and molecular biologists were making increasing contributions to pathology and that it was time to lower the "artificial barriers among disciplines" by discarding the exclusionary name.

Biology and medicine cannot, of course, be articulated by fiat. No amount of legislation or core courses in molecular biology can make biology clinically relevant. If the biological sciences are clinically relevant, it is in a large measure due to the fact that clinicians have sought out biology and biological techniques and adapted them to clinical problems just as biologists have chosen animal models of disease with which to pursue biological questions. If, moreover, governments and research administrators have continually looked for ways to bring the two together despite the obstacles inherent in such an undertaking,[150] it is because the failures have been overshadowed by the successes. For that is indeed the novelty of the postwar era: it has in fact been possible to create a biomedicine. Such is the context for the rest of this book insofar as we will henceforth concentrate on a particularly successful marriage of biology and medicine as embodied in the creation of the immunophenotyping platform.

4

Leukemia, Lymphoma, and Immunophenotyping: Building a Platform

We began this book with an example designed to introduce readers to the notion of biomedical platforms. Borrowing from a routine (albeit electronic) diagnostic discussion of an individual patient, we used the example to avoid tortuous explanations, and to simply point to the object in question and say: "Look here, this is what we mean by a platform." We then explored the use of the expression in the relevant fields (semantic and otherwise), such as hospital architecture and organization. In the ensuing discussion of the transformation of medical practices during the second half of the twentieth century, we described two main processes—the biologization of medicine and the trend toward automation—that, although highlighted by other commentators, acquire new significance when jointly investigated under the heading of biomedical platforms. We now return, in this and the next chapter, to the level of detail foreshadowed in the opening example by analyzing the development of a specific platform—the immunophenotyping, or "IPT," platform—as it emerged in the field of lymphoproliferative diseases and, in particular, leukemia.

We have divided this chapter into two sections. The first and shortest section focuses on the period—circa 1975—during which the IPT platform arose out of experimental procedures that had, until then, been confined to a few immunology laboratories. We begin this section by examining a project proposal submitted to the U.K. Medical Research Council (MRC) and aimed at the application of new immunological approaches to a series of major leukemia clinical trials.[1] The second section travels backward in time, exploring the constitution of the experimental system out of which the platform originally emerged.[2] The next chapter travels forward to the post-1975 era, exploring the implementation of the IPT platform both in its initial domain—lymphoproliferative diseases—and in other fields of application such as AIDS. Our analysis in this chapter thus revisits the biology-pathology division discussed in chapters 2 and 3 by providing a detailed case study of how this division operates in clinical and laboratory practice. While the degree of detail may occasionally seem tedious to the general reader, it is nonetheless crucial to our argument. It acts as an antidote to the abstract nature of many of the debates about recent and future trends of biomedicine and, more important, this is the level of detail necessary to provide an adequate description of the relations and translations between the material, instrumental, social, institutional, and epistemological components of biomedical activities.

A Proposal

In 1975, Melvyn Greaves, a researcher at the tumour immunology unit (TIU) of University College, London submitted a grant application entitled "Immunodiagnosis of Human Leukaemia" to the MRC.[3] In the application, he proposed using "cell surface marker tests"—a novel technique based on the use of antibodies and other immunological tools—to analyze blood samples of all new patients enrolled in the MRC UKALL IV chemotherapy trial (ALL stands for *a*cute *l*ymphoblastic *l*eukemia, a form of leukemia that mostly affects children). Initially termed "molecular morphology," Greaves later renamed his program of research "immunophenotyping." While short-lived,[4] the term "molecular morphology" nonetheless expressed Greaves's intention to create a metaphorical bridge between the traditional morphological techniques of clinical hematologists and the new molecular biological approaches championed by biomedical scientists.

Understanding how Greaves's proposal stood apart from traditional methods requires some understanding of the history of leukemia diagnosis and treatment. To begin with, morphology and gross anatomy had dominated early approaches to the study of the leukemias. In his classic description of the disease in the 1840s, Virchow had shown that the disease in a patient presenting with swelling of the spleen followed a fundamentally different course from that in a patient presenting with a swelling of the lymph nodes, thus giving rise to the distinction between splenic and lymphatic leukemia. With the introduction of differential blood staining, the organ distinction gave way to a cellular distinction so that by 1900 the term myeloid (marrow-derived cells) replaced the term splenic. In turn, the term lymphoid came to signify an increase in lymphocytes (a subset of white blood cells) in the course of the disease.[5]

This displacement instituted the long-standing division between lymphatic and myeloid leukemias.[6]

The clinical subdivision of the leukemias into acute and chronic also dates back to the nineteenth century. A temporary cellular basis for what is clearly a division of outcomes emerged around 1900 when Naegeli described the myeloblast (a precursor of myeloid cells) as the predominant cell type in acute leukemias. By the 1920s, however, that division had broken down. Textbooks of the time tell us that chronic and acute leukemia can be either lymphatic or myeloid.[7] Nonetheless, these four categories—acute, chronic, myeloid, and lymphatic—have remained the basic divisions of the leukemias to the extent that observers in the mid-1970s could claim that "by the 1930s nearly all recognized morphologic forms of leukemia had been described."[8]

Until the mid-1960s, leukemia was an inevitably fatal disease. Treatment options were explored through clinical trials which, in the United Kingdom, began in 1959.[9] By the mid-1970s, clinical researchers routinely divided leukemia trials into those for children, with most patients suffering from ALL, and those for adults, with most patients suffering from another form of the disease, AML or *a*cute *m*yeloid *l*eukemia.[10] Early trials, however, did not separate AML from ALL, nor did they, as a consequence, experiment with different treatments for the two forms of the disease.

More often than not, leukemia chemotherapy trials sought less to test new drugs than to experiment with different combinations and quantities of known therapeutic agents (including not only drugs but also irradiation). For instance, a 1984 review of the therapeutic trials conducted by the MRC's Working Party on Leukaemia in Childhood readily admitted that the principles of modern treatment had been established and generally accepted by 1972, and that subsequent trials focused on variations of the basic protocol. Trials conducted between 1972 and 1979 in the United Kingdom, however, produced disappointing results, showing little or no improvement in long-term remission rates. Given that U.S. and West German studies had managed to achieve unusually high and sustained remission rates, new protocols were established after 1980. These, however, did not radically alter the previous approach[11] and, in fact, as the trials continued throughout the 1970s and 1980s, it became increasingly obvious that the choice of optimal therapeutic combinations required that patients be subdivided into categories corresponding to subclasses of the disease. The tool of choice for distinguishing between AML and ALL, morphological diagnosis, was, in the words of a pioneer of leukemia trials, "less accurate than it is now." Indeed, "[o]f 100 sets of slides from consecutive cases of leukaemia circulated among the eight haematologists in the Medical Research Council's typing party, only 18 received the same diagnosis from all eight observers."[12] If one adds to the unreliability of morphological analysis the obvious limits to experimentation raised by the fact that one is dealing with human patients, it is easy to see why the whole endeavor often turned into a frustrating exercise in guesswork, tinkering, and ad hoc adjustments.[13]

From this point of view, the "immunodiagnosis" promoted by Greaves's 1975 proposal came to be seen as a godsend. As Dr. Kay of the UKALL trials enthusiastically argued in 1977, the new approach would classify the cases of ALL "in a way which must supersede the less reliable criteria of morphology."[14] Knowledge of the approach circulated in the popular press. In an article in *The Times* of London, the medical correspondent drew a sharp contrast between the new and the old, describing how pathologists had traditionally examined blood and bone marrow specimens looking for decisive clues as to the precise species of leukemia in the shape, size, numbers, and appearance of blood cells. Yet, as the correspondent pointed out, "on as many as one-third of occasions there [would] be some doubt." While not a genuine drawback with an invariably fatal disease, the correspondent continued, diagnostic uncertainty became a serious issue when the dramatic increase in the cure rate prompted clinicians to start looking for prognostic factors specific enough to warrant changes in treatment. The new immunological approach had demonstrated that ALL had at least four distinct subgroups, each with different prognoses. These results showed "very real practical importance since the use of new anti-leukaemic drugs of unknown potential (and hazards) [was] clearly much more justifiable in children with "high risk" leukemia than in those with the more favorable variant." Better diagnosis and classification thus meant a greater chance of finding the most effective therapeutic combination.[15]

Greaves had been a member of the TIU since its creation as one of two extramural units established in the early 1970s by Michael Stoker, the new scientific director of the Imperial Cancer Research Fund (ICRF). In the United Kingdom, the ICRF, the Cancer Research Campaign, and the MRC constituted the three major sources of funds for cancer research. Unlike the other two agencies, however, the ICRF mainly supported research in its own establishments[16] and could thus more directly control research priorities in its laboratories. Following his appointment, Stoker had let it be known that, while committed to the funding of short-term "tactical" investigations, he also intended to give increasing weight to long-term "strategic research." He defined the latter as research that "might have a bearing on cancer but which is just as likely to lead to benefits in other fields." In other words, Stoker was prepared to support research grounded in the booming biological sciences characterized by the use of new instrumentation and a "ruthless reductionist" (his term) approach. One of the means of achieving this end appeared to be the creation of extramural units.[17] In turn, Greaves's "molecular morphology" represented an early capitalization on ICRF's investment in strategic research.

Stoker's "strategic" approach participated in the turn to biomedicine we discussed in chapter 3 and was clearly consistent with initiatives taken by similar institutions in both Europe and North America. As an instantiation of Stoker's views, Greaves's proposal fell into an area—tumor immunology and studies of the surfaces of cancer cells—that appeared promising to funding agencies and thus worthy of selective support.[18] As such, it meshed easily with a wider series of investigations pursued on both sides of the Atlantic. We will have a closer look at the rise of "cell surface immunology" in the next section. For the moment, suffice it to say that the same year Greaves submitted his MRC proposal, the Leukaemia Research Fund (LRF) acknowledged the importance of his approach by inviting Maxime Seligmann, a French researcher from Saint-Louis Hospital in Paris (the most important leukemia research center in France) and a champion of clinical immunology, to London to deliver the fund's Eleventh Annual Guest Lecture. The title chosen by Seligmann was "Lymphocyte Membrane Markers in Human Leukaemias and Lymphomas."[19] Five years later, it would be Greaves's turn—in 1976 he had moved to the ICRF to head a newly created "membrane immunology laboratory"—to deliver the LRF annual guest lecture to a packed house under the revealing title of "*Biology* of Acute Lymphoblastic Leukaemia."[20]

The 1975 MRC application emerged at a turning point when an experimental system began mutating into a biomedical platform. The description of the proposed investigation, while quite short (two and a half pages), captures the essence of the transformation. Greaves's program sought not simply to apply new immunological procedures to an ongoing clinical trial but, also, to test them in the process. In other words, two things had to be determined that could not yet be taken for granted: the prognostic value of the new procedures and the possibility of standardizing them so that, if proved of value, they could be used routinely. Standardization, a constant theme of the proposal, stood as an urgent matter in this field. The year before, a workshop sponsored by the World Health Organization/International Agency for Research on Cancer and attended by an international roster from both sides of the Atlantic had been held in London "to standardise the various [cell-surface] tests available and to identify remaining problems and the direction of future research."[21] The resulting "special technical report" opened by highlighting the recent discovery of two major populations of human lymphocytes, B and T cells.[22] More than a matter of scientific interest, the report noted that the distinction had direct implications for several diseases. Those implications, however, had to be reduced to practice before the distinction could be routinely applied in the clinic. For this to happen, researchers had to agree on a set of reliable laboratory procedures able to distinguish between the two lymphocyte populations. Unfortunately, because of "uncertainty regarding technical procedures, interpretation of much of the published data [was] questionable."[23]

With the problem framed in this manner, "markers" emerged as a key notion. Researchers wanted to know which markers corresponded to the characteristic signature of each cell population and which laboratory procedures should be used to detect a given marker. The report contained a detailed assessment of all available marker tests. In the course of the assessment, it examined the shape of test tubes ("the reaction should be carried out in round, not conical, plastic or siliconized glass tubes"), the kind of equipment to be used ("the most efficient microscopes using epi-illumination are desirable"), and matters of interlaboratory control ("if possible, the specificity of antisera should be cross-checked in several laboratories"). Yet, the discussion went beyond the analysis of techniques to provide an overview of recent findings on the role of B and T cells in different diseases. Obviously, clinical value and standardization of the markers went hand in hand. There was no point in standardizing highly idiosyncratic procedures if they had no clinical value and yet the tests would have clinical value only if their performance could be sufficiently standardized to permit cross-clinical comparisons. Referring to the workshop report a year later, Seligmann pointed out that even if the marker techniques were "now relatively well standardized," their diagnostic use required "caution" and "critical evaluation."[24]

Although specifically targeting leukemia, Greaves's 1975 proposal raised similar issues with regard to the markers. Piggybacking on the large U.K. network for clinical trials, Greaves's proposal presupposed that large-scale patient screening would establish the prognostic value of the new cell-surface marker technology. Convinced of success, Greaves also projected the future "exploration of assay methods that might eventually be suitable for haematology laboratories with no special immunological expertise," as well as the "investigation of methods for large scale production" of the relevant immunological reagents "with a view to using [them] as standard reagents on a routine basis."

While, as previously noted, Greaves's laboratory was not alone in the development and testing of cell-surface marker reagents, part of its competitive edge derived from the use of a sophisticated and expensive electronic device, called the fluorescence-activated cell sorter (FACS), only two of which existed at that time in Europe (more on this later). The proposal described the FACS as a powerful tool for the "*automatic* evaluation of cell surface fluorescence— . . . for *standardising* tests and for bulk analysis" (our emphasis)—and hinted at the possible development of "a simple and less expensive instrument for this purpose." To appreciate the promise incorporated in an automating and standardizing device, recall that, in 1975, the production of immunological reagents (antisera) for cell-surface analysis was quite complex and time-consuming. A sense of the multifaceted nature of the operation can be gained from the following excerpt from the 1974–76 annual report of the French research group headed by Seligmann describing the production of their antisera:

> Heteroantisera were prepared using rabbits immunized with either fetal thymocytes, peripheral T cells from a patient with sex-linked agammaglobulinemia with no circulating B cells, or with human fetal brain. . . . After heat inactivation, a series of adsorptions were performed using human liver, human A and B erythrocytes, normal human serum, and immunoglobulin chains of different classes coupled with Sepharose 4B. Antisera were subsequently absorbed with cells from diagnosed B-chronic lymphocytic leukemia. The specificity of antisera was tested on normal human blood and tonsil lymphocytes, T lymphocytes obtained through nylon column filtration of blood and tonsil lymphocytes, and B lymphocytes from patients with chronic lymphocytic leukemia.[25]

In addition to access to the relevant clinical material, the production of antisera involved months of repetitious, dull, yet highly skilled laboratory work. As one of Greaves's coworkers recently recalled, the production of the antiserum against ALL took three months and "maybe 25 absorptions."[26] The fact that the immunized rabbits, the source of the prized reagents, do not live forever further constrained the entire process. Symptomatic of the idiosyncratic nature of the antisera reagents were the pragmatic, procedural definitions of the cell populations isolated through their use. For instance, the previously mentioned annual report describes a "rabbit anti-human fetal brain antiserum" with which researchers had isolated a group of cells "that are not to be equated with those that form active sheep red blood cell rosettes [another kind of immunological test; see below]" but, rather, are characterized by the fact that they "are retained on nylon filters . . . and cannot be stimulated by phytohemagglutinin or pokeweed [two substances known to induce cell division]."[27] As one can see, these are exceedingly narrow claims, characterized by a low degree of "externality."[28] Researchers at the time thus required complex interlaboratory arrangements to ensure consistency between the idiosyncratic reagents and the correspondingly idiosyncratic results produced in different laboratories. Compared to the reagents, a piece of sophisticated electronic equipment such as the FACS seemed far less problematic, both from the point of view of, and as a possible route to, standardization and automation. Yet, without standard reagents, even the FACS could not provide unchallenged, consistent results.

It just so happens, however, that 1975 was also the year that an MRC laboratory in Cambridge developed a technique for the production of a new kind of immunological reagent—monoclonal antibodies. In contrast to the old rabbit antisera, the new sera were secreted by cells that could be maintained indefinitely and through techniques that rendered the reagents tailor-made. The cells and the antibodies they secreted thus offered the "overwhelming advantage" of providing an "unlimited permanent supply of material" and, as a consequence, "worldwide standardization."[29] It would take only a few years for the new reagents to invade the cell-surface arena and, consequently, leukemia. Greaves began production of monoclonal antibodies to leukemic cells in 1978 and by 1979 he had already set up a panel of eight monoclonal antibodies obtained in part from British and American laboratories. As discussed below, he used this panel for routine leukemia immunodiagnosis and subclassification.[30]

With the convergence of monoclonal antibodies and the FACS, nowadays perceived as the prototypical components of the IPT platform, the latter took off. Indeed, it can reasonably be argued that the availability of monoclonal antibodies as off-the-shelf commercial reagents and the production of cheaper and simplified desktop versions of the FACS led to the widespread adoption of the platform. To use Fujimura's term, these two components combined to form a (relatively) standardized package that, as such, circulated easily.[31] As we discuss below, however, a platform is not reducible to a device or a package. Generally speaking, for equipment to function as a platform, one needs regulatory conventions that are incompletely embodied in the material components of the platform. Moreover, to work on the IPT platform does not require one to use a FACS or any version of that device: IPT is often carried out by typing the specimens under the microscope. Finally, if we take Greaves's 1975 MRC proposal as a starting point, then the IPT platform clearly took shape prior to the advent of monoclonal antibodies. We are thus faced with the somewhat paradoxical situation wherein some components of the platform can be described as typical yet dispensable. This apparent paradox holds the key to our understanding of the notion of a biomedical platform. To explore it, let us take a closer look at the experimental system that led to the 1975 MRC proposal.

Building a Platform

On the eve of his retirement in 1991, N.A. Mitchison summarized the work carried out under his direction at the ICRF's TIU since 1971:

> The twenty years of this Unit has seen an exciting time in immunology. At the start, one could picture the cells of the immune system as billiard balls, bouncing off one another with a minimum of interaction. At the end they seem softer and gentler to one another, touching and feeling and transmitting signals full of meaning, for purposes that we can begin to understand.[32]

Mitchison's metaphor resonates with a more recent one:

> The surface of a cell is not smooth and flat, like a ball bearing; it is more like a microscopic garden tended in darkness, bathed by warm salty fluid, a rounded and shaggy convex landscape with cellular vegetation waving like seaweed above the cell membrane. . . . It is constantly changing. New vegetation shoots up and old vegetation collapses as in a time-lapse film. . . . Certain receptors, like perennial flowers, grow on the surface, so permanent and unchanging a fixture that they can in essence serve as a reliable molecular landmark, or fingerprint, that reveals the identity of the cell itself. Indeed, they are known as clusters of differentiation (CD), or "markers," and were first reported in mice by Lloyd Old in the early 1960s.[33]

Whether described as a "garden tended in darkness" or as the means through which anthropomorphic cells touch and feel each other and exchange meanings, the cell surface has captured the imagination of scientists. As indicated in our discussion of the IPT platform, it has become a major focus of biomedical research. As an important node in the international network of cancer research establishments, and a locus of initial research on the cell surface, the ICRF offers a convenient starting point for exploring the emergence of the "new" cell surface.

Exploring the Cell Surface

As noted in the previous section, Michael Stoker's arrival at the ICRF in 1968 resulted in the adoption of a new cancer policy based on the distinction between strategic and tactical research. In his first introduction to the ICRF annual report, Stoker suggested that the uncertainty surrounding the real nature of cancer made a "general inquiry into living processes" a necessity. Such an inquiry had now become possible because of molecular biology's "intensive study of individual cancer cells and of their difference from normal cells." Key technological breakthroughs included cell culture, the separation of molecular components of the cell, the use of chemical and viral carcinogens, and the production of cell hybrids. Since patient treatment remained the primary rationale for ICRF's existence, the long-term strategy leading from the less complex (a "complete understanding of the cancer cell and the normal cell from which it arose") to the more complex (tissue, organs, and the patient) had to be complemented by a short-term strategy grounded in empirical research of the trial-and-error sort ("shortcuts"), yet profiting from breakthroughs provided by the long-term approach. In practical terms, the strategic turn entailed the expansion of research into the molecular biology and genetics of cancer cells, the establishment of cell culture facilities, and the creation of small, independent laboratories around experienced researchers rather than topics.[34]

Unsurprisingly, Stoker believed that "Medicine, as we all know, is one of the branches of biology," and that, in spite of the fact that the revolution in biology of the previous decades had so far had little impact on medicine, it was only a matter of time until its consequences would begin to be felt in the clinical wards: "[j]ust you wait!"[35] Yet, there were difficulties. The fact that scientists conducted long-term research mostly on nonhumans created the reciprocal danger of researchers losing contact with the hospital and of clinicians ignoring the new biology.[36] As noted in the Zuckerman report, commissioned by the British prime minister as a reaction to Nixon's 1971 "war against cancer," "clinicians who deal[t] with the patient [were] frequently as unconcerned with the basic research worker as the latter [was] remote from the hospital bed."[37]

To remedy the situation, in addition to such simple steps as the establishment of fellowships allowing clinicians to mix with scientists,

Stoker took the bold step of proposing the establishment of two extramural units: a medical oncology unit (MOU) to be housed in a hospital and focusing on clinical research, and a tumour immunology unit housed at University College, London and engaged in strategic research on "immunity in cancer and possibly on cancer vaccines." The plan projected interaction between the two units in order to establish "a chain of contact from the patient to at least some of the basic research laboratories."[38] In particular, while the MOU would conduct clinical trials of different forms of chemotherapeutic treatment as its principal mission, its work would also include the search for biochemical and morphological changes in patients in remission for early detection of relapse. Leukemia and lymphomas were to serve as a model case. This meant collaboration with other research facilities, like the TIU, for the supply of human tumor material for experimental research and, in return, for the testing of new assays and procedures on patients.

Why did the ICRF choose these two units? The choice of oncology appears, to a large extent, self-explanatory for a cancer research agency.[39] The choice of immunology, however, requires some explanation. As is evident from a variety of sources, ranging from scientific publications to popular accounts such as BBC correspondent David Wilson's *Body and Antibody. A Report on the New Immunology*, by the turn of the decade immunology had become established as a major biomedical discipline.[40] During the 1960s, the number of national immunological societies had risen from two to twelve, whereas the number of international immunological journals had more than doubled, rising from six to thirteen. The formation of an International Union of Immunological Societies in 1969 capped off a decade of remarkable growth.[41] To appreciate the spectacular rise of immunology in the 1960s, recall that before World War II, immunology had essentially been the science of antibodies: if one could not detect antibodies in the blood or tissues of the organism under investigation, then nothing immunological was going on. The presence of specific antibodies demonstrated an immune reaction to a particular disease, just as therapy for a number of infectious diseases consisted of the injection of antisera containing antibodies to the disease in question (serotherapy). Part of the increased importance of immunology in the postwar period resulted from a change in emphasis from antibodies and other soluble substances to cells.

The beginnings of "the rise of cellular immunology" have been located in the new theories and techniques of skin grafting developed in Britain by Peter Medawar and his associates. In a series of studies begun during World War II, they determined that lymphocyte cells and not antibodies caused the rejection of skin grafts in mice.[42] At the time, however, little was known about those cells.[43] James L. Gowans, another British scientist, filled that knowledge gap in the 1950s by setting up an experimental system that allowed him to follow the actors, i.e., the lymphocytes, as they moved between the blood vessels and the lymphatic system of vessels that run parallel to the blood system. According to the official story, by showing that the lymphatic cells (re)circulated between the two sets of vessels, he laid to rest the then dominant notion that the lymphocytes were merely transitory entities that eventually turned into blood cells. Combining this knowledge with Medawar's system of skin transplants, he subsequently demonstrated that the small lymphocytes in particular caused the rejection of skin grafts in mice.[44] This finding precipitated a whole new series of investigations in the 1960s that led to the dissection of what became increasingly described as the immune *system*[45] into "compartments" corresponding to distinct cell types and functions.

As evidenced by this brief description, British researchers made valuable contributions to the expanding field of immunology in the 1940s and 1950s.[46] They continued to do so in the 1960s. One such contributor, N. A. Mitchison, working at MRC's Mill Hill Institute on the outskirts of London, and under consideration for the chair of zoology and comparative anatomy at University College, was casting about for support for his research in the late 1960s. Word came to Stoker for whom it seemed too good an opportunity for the ICRF to miss. Stoker quickly drafted a proposal to create "a unit for tumour immunology (or some similar title)" and submitted it to the fund's council.[47] The status of TIU's research remained unclear. On the one hand, the very name of the unit—*tumor* immunology—and the fact that the initial proposal explicitly referred to "cancer vaccines" suggested the tactical dimension of the proposed endeavor. On the other hand, it quickly appeared that much of the unit's work would focus on the basic biology of the T and B lymphocytes—their interaction, development, and distribution—rather than on cancer per se, with most of the experiments performed on mice rather than on human material. As such, the operation looked like strategic research.

Further signs of this ambiguity can be read in the program statement formulated by the head of the TIU, Mitchison.[48] Having just been entrusted with the direction of the unit, he openly wondered why, "since nothing revolutionary [had] come up by way of ideas and technology, and there has been little clinical success," research agencies had provided such lavish support for the field of tumor immunology. Mitchison's own answer suggested that the field had outgrown a disreputable history of outrageous claims[49] and profited from rapid progress in cellular immunology. Funding agencies assumed that these successes would be followed by applications in clinical medicine. Immunology's success, moreover, coincided with the failure of radio- and chemotherapy to provide long-term cures for cancer. Despite this optimistic introduction, in his subsequent discussion of the three principal domains of tumor immunology (cancer prevention through vaccines, cancer detection by immunological tests, and immunotherapy), Mitchison remained cautious: "Let me not conclude on a note of pessimism. What matters is that these problems have been identified: much better to have a clear-cut difference, and the tools available for further work, than vague uncertainty." With the benefit of hindsight, one can easily surmise that "further work" meant the elucidation of basic immunological mechanisms, or, were we to adopt the then current ICRF terminology, strategic research.

We would not, however, say that Mitchison willingly or unwittingly entertained confusion between distinct kinds of research. The experimental system adopted by the TIU had a tendency to generate precisely this kind of ambivalence. As Mitchison noted, the very idea of tumor immunology presupposed that tumor cells produced tumor-specific antigens or, in other words, *markers* (the term, as we will see, is decisive) able to distinguish cancer cells from normal cells. The markers simultaneously signified pathological processes—i.e., they pointed to an oncological lesion setting cancer cells apart from normal cells—and biological processes—i.e., "markers for cellular differentiation . . . shared in common by normal and tumour cells of the same differentiated type."[50] We have here the crux of the matter: markers were expressions of pathology and thus qualitative tools, and yet they were biological, and thus opened the door for quantitation and, further on down the road, automation, as maintained, for instance, in Greaves's 1975 MRC proposal. Because of this polarity set up between pathology and biology, cell-surface markers qualified as a prime example of strategic research:

> Of course there are a number of changes in the cell surface which are considered to be characteristic of cancer cells, or at least of transformed cells; on closer examination, however, many, even of these, have been found to be manifestations of rapid growth and are almost certainly secondary rather than

causal phenomena. This has led to an increasing concentration on the role of the surface in normal cell functions, in relation to both growth and differentiation. It does not diminish the possibility that a change in the cell surface is a primary event in a cancer cell nor should one forget the particular importance of the tumour-specific surface antigens, but the main thrust of cell membrane research seems now to be much more concerned with normal cell biology.[51]

As the above excerpt suggests, by the mid-1970s the cell surface had become a focus of biomedical inquiry, one believed to contain the secrets of cancer. The ICRF had been at the forefront of this research since the late 1960s. As Stoker noted in his introduction to the 1969–70 ICRF annual report, "research has been turning increasingly to the surface membrane of cells." In the following year's report, Stoker commented on the recent hiring of Renato Dulbecco (a future Nobel Prize winner) by noting that Dulbecco's interest in surface changes in cancer cells might ultimately lead to techniques producing modifications in the surface so that cells could regain their normal properties. In sum, Stoker had become convinced early on that "studies of cancer cell membranes [would] become a major research theme of the Fund's laboratories."[52] By the mid-1970s, he was not alone. In the United States, the official recommendations for Nixon's National Cancer Program plan devoted a special section to the following objective: "Study cell surface and cell surface membranes."[53] Indeed, as noted in the following mix of biological and social topographies, the cell surface had become "a meeting ground of interest for various disciplines in biology."[54] More than biology, however, the surface had become a going concern in medicine. A 1975 article on the cell surface in the prestigious *New England Journal of Medicine*, for example, opened with the following lines: "There is little doubt that there are important differences in the biologic behavior of tumor cells and normal cells that can be correlated with altered surface properties."[55] Similarly, a review article significantly entitled "A New Look at the Cell Surface" noted that "It is hoped that the nature of the cell alteration responsible for malignant behavior may be elucidated by focusing on the outer part of the cell surface."[56] Finally, a review of "the contributions of cell biology to clinical medicine" listed the improved understanding of cell membranes as the first of five such contributions.[57]

Proof of this improved understanding lay in a technical achievement, namely the isolation of membrane proteins, and in the acceptance, at the beginning of the 1970s, of the so-called fluid mosaic model "as a paradigm" of membrane structure.[58] The new model constituted a significant departure from previous models. Indeed, until the middle of the 1960s the standard model of cell membranes, the "lipid bilayer model" initially formulated by chemists in the 1920s,[59] had portrayed the cell surface as a relatively static and ultimately monotonous sheet of fatty acids. In contrast, the "fluid mosaic model"[60] transformed the cell membrane from an uninteresting *place*, a mere inside-outside boundary, to "a highly dynamic fluid *organelle* which may have unique subunits at specialized sites related to discrete biologic functions."[61] Not only did proteins perform different biological functions (receptors, markers, determinants) while sitting on the membrane, but they were (relatively) free to move around.

But where did the cell-surface markers come from? The "microscopic garden" excerpt opening this section mentioned that Lloyd Old first reported markers in the early 1960s. Yet, we have looked in vain in modern histories of immunology for Old's contribution.[62] Given that Old (and coauthor Boyse) apparently uncovered the foundations of cell-surface immunology (the first markers), this seems rather odd. Nonetheless, it does make sense. How, for example, could Old have discovered markers of a particular kind of immune cell before it had been established in the late 1960s that those cells existed? How could he have known, as is now widely accepted, that those markers allowed one to distinguish between the two interacting arms (as they became metaphorically known) of the immune system, each arm featuring its own functional subclasses of cells? How, in other words, is it possible to say that Old discovered markers when he could not possibly have deciphered the meaning of those markers? Yet, we can treat Old as the "discoverer" of markers if the standard view of the history of immunology, according to which the detection of the components of the immune system followed an orderly biological logic, is supplemented with a view that shows that the proliferation of types of immunologically competent cells grew out of cancer research.

A View from Pathology

Once again, there are British roots to this work or, rather, Anglo-American roots, if we bear in mind not only the humans but also the experimental mice that crisscrossed the Atlantic both before and after World War II.[63] Old and Boyse's program of work had originated in Britain under the auspices of Peter Gorer, Boyse's research supervisor from 1957 to 1960. Boyse had left Britain in 1960 bringing with him mice from Gorer's laboratory and a problem initiated by Gorer, that of cancer antigens. Gorer, in turn, had been a student of the British geneticist J.B.S. Haldane and had begun working with inbred mice—the first available in Britain—imported by Haldane from the Vackson Laboratory in Bar Harbor, Maine, in the 1930s.[64] The investigation of the rejection of transplanted tumors with a genetically purified line of mice led Gorer to isolate what became the first transplant tumor antigens. In particular, he showed that the transplantation of a cancer[65] consistently produced the same kind of antibodies in the recipient mouse. He concluded that there must be an antigen on the surface of the cell that produced the antibodies that then provoked the graft rejection.[66]

But Gorer had worked in the 1930s. Transplanting cancer differed from transplanting normal tissues and, in retrospect, we can see Gorer's work as part of a longer line of therapeutic research directed toward the production of anticancer sera. In the 1950s and coincident with the rise of cellular immunology, skin transplanters such as Medawar overshadowed Gorer who entered into a long-standing dispute with Medawar over the role of antibodies in the rejection of transplants.[67] At the time, mouse skin grafts served as the major model of the transplantation process and Medawar had shown that experimental transplants did not require antibody for rejection. Moreover, since transplanters would not be transplanting cancer, Gorer's antigens remained of interest mainly to cancer specialists with the result that antibodies resurfaced as an important factor in graft rejection only with the advent of kidney transplants in the mid-1960s.[68]

Despite this partial eclipse of the significance of Gorer's work in the biology of the 1950s, Gorer's work had garnered interest in the cancer field. Notably, Gorer's student Boyse had taken up the technique and the C57 strain of mice and recast the transplantation problem as one of tumor antigens. The shift here was vital. Rather than representing the antigens formed upon the injection of cancer cells as transplantation antigens, Boyse and his American collaborator Old presented them as cancer antigens. Note here that in a transplanted cancer there are two forms of the "other" against which antibodies may be formed. The transplanted cancer may be perceived by the host as a normal yet foreign tissue in which case it is no different from a skin transplant. On the other hand, the cancer may be perceived as pathological, like a virus or bacteria. In the second case, it really should not matter whether the cancer is transplanted or homegrown: pathology is presumably foreign whether from home or away. The potential clinical significance of this fact is that one should be able to find antibodies to cancer in cancer patients; ineffective antibodies to be sure (i.e., they did not stop the cancer), but antibodies nonetheless. Conceivably, one could use these substances for diagnosis or, by somehow boosting their efficiency, therapy.

Boyse and Old, however, managed to extract cancer antigens from the transplantation problem without sliding into the world of cancer therapy. Using Gorer's line of mice and leukemia as an antigen, they produced experimental leukemias. Then, using the leukemia cells as the antigen, they produced antibodies. Because they used inbred mice—defined procedurally as mice that accepted intrastrain skin grafts—they excluded in advance the possibility that the antibodies recognized transplantation antigens.[69] But ambiguity haunted the enterprise from the beginning. The antibodies had a dual specificity: they recognized both leukemic cells and cells of the thymus. In other words, they recognized the pathological cells as well as the normal cells within which the pathology originated. Boyse and Old had found a cancer antigen that was also normal, which they designated accordingly TL, for *t*hymus *l*eukemia antigen.[70] Out of this initial identification, there emerged a new object of study: the cell surface as the site of biological *and* pathological differentiation.[71]

In 1967, the American Cancer Society sponsored a conference on "Tumor-Specific Antigens."[72] Just six years before, in 1961, a conference sponsored by the same society bore the title "The Possible Role of Immunology in Cancer."[73] As the change in titles suggests, tumor antigens and their antibodies had gained a certain degree of legitimacy. Certainly Boyse and Old felt so, for as they pointed out at the 1967 conference, "Not long ago the question '*Are* there specific tumor antigens?' was still topical and debatable. It would hardly arouse much discussion today because the existence of tumor antigens is no longer a subject of controversy."[74] Less the result of the discovery of tumor-specific antigens, the disappearance of the controversy followed the redefinition of what could possibly appear on the surface of the cell. The production of the TL antigen now meant that there were tumor-specific antigens that were not necessarily specific to tumors. The question of specificity, in other words, had become irrelevant. As Boyse and Old argued, the question "'Are these antigens, demonstrable in tumors of laboratory animals, specific for the tumor cells in which they are found?' [was] also somewhat archaic if it [was] meant to imply that the lack of such specificity mean[t] lack of relevance to cancer."[75]

To understand this change in perspective, note that prior to the TL antigen, two things had been found on the surface of the cell: transplantation antigens and cancer antigens. Now, there was more, much more in fact. In October of 1967 Boyse and Old announced the discovery of an entire series of completely normal antigens on the cells of the thymus (the thymocytes or thymic lymphocytes).[76] This was the celebrated Ly series, originally named Ly-A and Ly-B and later called Ly-1, Ly-2 and Ly-3.[77] At first, Boyse and Old thought they had isolated transplantation antigens, "although final proof awaits tests with the congenic [inbred] strains now being prepared."[78] But it turned out that the new antigens were merely "associated" with them. Reviewing the whole situation a year later in the *Annual Review of Genetics*, Boyse and Old concluded that one could characterize thymus cells with "six known systems of surface antigens demonstrable by the cytotoxic test with specific antisera."[79] By using the neutral term *surface*, Boyse and Old signified that they no longer studied transplantation antigens or cancer antigens. They now studied "normal and abnormal cell surface genetics."[80] In other words, what had begun as a problem of grafting—the formation of normal antibodies in the course of rejection—and had been seen as clue to the study of cancer—the cancer (pathological) antigen—had been refashioned as an object of study in its own right: the genetics of the proteins on the surface of the normal or pathological cell.

Three classes of things now sat on the surfaces of cells: transplantation (histocompatibility) antigens, tumor antigens, and an entirely new entity, "differentiation" antigens, the only instance of which had, so far, turned up in Boyse and Old's experimental system.[81] Mixed function distinguished the differentiation antigens from the first two: unlike the biological status of transplantation antigens and the pathological status of cancer antigens, differentiation was at once a cancerous and a biological process. Differentiation antigens "associated" themselves with cancer and yet appeared on normal cells. Since they could not be transplant antigens because they arose in identical individuals, researchers wondered what their function could possibly be. That question raised greater interest than the question posed by transplantation antigens, for, as Boyse and Old pointed out, "the antigenic differences which offer most in the way of biological implications, in all probability, are not those that distinguish between two individuals but those that distinguish between the tissues of one individual."[82]

The switch was now complete. Having begun the investigation of cancer as a form of foreign invasion, using transplantation as a model,

Boyse and Old had by 1970 accumulated a series of biological questions concerning the surface of the normal cell. Cancer could now be described in terms of the failure of normal cell-surface structures to perform properly. In particular, the three major manifestations of malignant growth—disordered histoarchitecture, invasion, and metastasis—could all be termed "defects of identification."[83] The problem of pathology thus became a problem of biology: to know what constitutes a defect in identification, one must first know the normal, biological mechanisms of identification. The reduction of the pathological to the normal was not, however, complete. For cancer to be described in entirely biological terms, the failure in communication had to be described not in terms of different receptors, but in terms of quantitative variations of the same kind of receptor.

For the discoverers of differentiation antigens, the idea that cells recognized each other through the presence of distinctive surface molecules seemed, somewhat paradoxically, inadequate.[84] There were, to put it bluntly, too many functions and not enough genes to account for all the molecules needed to carry out those functions. Rather, it seemed reasonable to argue that the "individuality" of cells depended not upon the "presence of one or another of a very large range of unique [molecules]" but "upon surface displays whose individuality is conferred by unique arrangements of relatively few [molecules]."[85] Boyse and Old thus set about devising a system that, by using labeled antibodies and an electron microscope, would allow them to visualize and investigate topographic differences in the organization of antigens on the cell surface.[86] In so doing, Boyse and Old had, one could say, discovered and then discarded differentiation antigens.

The View from Biology

Meanwhile, according to standard histories of the discipline, immunologists had been quite busy setting up new cells, new functions, and new organs, all drawn together under a new term: the immune system.[87] In other words, despite the fact that anomalies or problems in pathology (skin burns in RAF personnel led to Medawar's initial interest in skin transplants; leukemia and cancer of the thymus led to the development of the two-compartment view of the immune system) often suggested immunological experiments, immunologists had been producing biological facts. Pathology, in other words, was less the context for this production than the excuse. Histories of immunology have consequently detected the following trend: begin with an anomaly—an experiment of nature—and set up an experimental animal system to find out what is really happening at the level of biology.[88]

From the biological point of view, the American pediatrician Robert Good is a perfect example of this kind of research. He and his collaborators began work in the 1950s in Minneapolis on the relationship between different diseases affecting tissues known to be related to the immunological response.[89] Prompted by a chance encounter with a patient suffering from both a tumor of the thymus and a disease (agammaglobulinemia) where the subject is unable to produce antibodies, by the early 1960s Good and his collaborators were claiming that patients affected by different types of cancers of the blood cells showed different impairments of immune functions. Those afflicted, for instance, with myeloma easily succumbed to bacterial infections and yet remained relatively resistant to viral infections, whereas patients with Hodgkin's disease were more sensitive to viral infection.[90] Good's decisive step, at least the one most often mentioned by historians, was, however, to show that these differences held in a biological way by experimenting with mice, rats, rabbits, chickens, and hamsters, and not humans.

In 1959 Good read a 1956 report from a relatively obscure journal, *Poultry Science*, according to which antibody production in chickens stopped if one removed a small sac arising from their intestines and known as the bursa of Fabricius.[91] Triangulating clinical observations with this kind of biological evidence, Good came to the conclusion that there must be an organ, and hence cells, for the production of antibody, and that a related, "appropriate experiment" would be "to take the thymus out of rabbits and mice, and later out of rats and hamsters, in the immediate neonatal period" and see what happened.[92] The role of the thymus was being investigated independently with similar methods by other researchers, namely the Australian Jacques Miller, then working in London. He had noticed that mice whose thymus had been removed failed to reject skin transplants and had concluded that the thymus controlled the cells that controlled the ability of the organism to accept or reject transplants.[93] A whole new series of animal experiments by Good and coworkers led to the proposition that the immune system had two cellular components. One consisted of B cells (so named after the *b*ursa) that produced antibodies and protected against bacteria, and another consisted of T cells (so named after the *t*hymus) that protected against viruses (and, one may add, transplant surgeons).[94] Both types of cells were lymphocytes.

The data did not convince everybody: James Gowans (as we saw, a major player in the field of lymphocytes) for years doubted the existence of T and B cells.[95] Others, such as Ivan Roitt of the Middlesex Hospital Medical School in London, jumped quickly on the bandwagon. According to Greaves, one of his former students, Roitt stood out in the conservative milieu of British academic medicine as a card-carrying biochemist who had somehow managed to become head of a medical department.[96] Roitt and Greaves coauthored a 1969 survey of the new "cellular basis of immunology." Published in *The Lancet*, then as now one of the two most important clinical journals (along with the *New England Journal of Medicine*), the article contained no new information. It nonetheless attracted considerable attention because it presented a coherent synthesis of scattered findings and systematically reviewed interpretations of clinical manifestations in terms of the two lymphocyte populations.[97] Less than three years later, Good published an editorial in the *New England Journal of Medicine* that ended with the following words:

> In summary, these studies promise that a new pathology is developing that will include precise immunochemical analysis of surface receptors and markers that will be useful in defining malignant neoplasias, including different forms of all lymphomas. With the development of such new and potentially precise markers, the search for the site of action and location of the oncogenic agent (or agents) and the nature of the oncogenic event can be further focused. It is hoped that such studies will lead to new information that can lead toward better diagnosis and better treatment, and ultimately even to prevention of these diseases.[98]

Good's editorial made liberal use, in the title and text, of the notion of *marker*, a term presupposing the acceptance of the T-B distinction: only if one took that distinction for granted did it make sense to speak of and to look for markers separating the two cell populations. By the early 1970s, many clinicians willingly accepted not only the reality of that distinction but also its clinical usefulness.[99] As we will see below, one could argue that the notion of "marker" took on a life of its own, not so much because markers gained independence from the kinds of cells (T, B, and subsequently an increasing array of subkinds) they supposedly marked—a marker obviously remained a marker of something—but because that very notion, as embodied in an increasing array of diagnostic and prognostic tests, acquired its own technological momentum.

We can easily visualize this momentum. Figure 4.1 shows the number of papers listed in MEDLINE as using the terms "cell-surface marker(s)," "surface marker(s)," or "cell marker(s)" in their title or abstract.[100] The

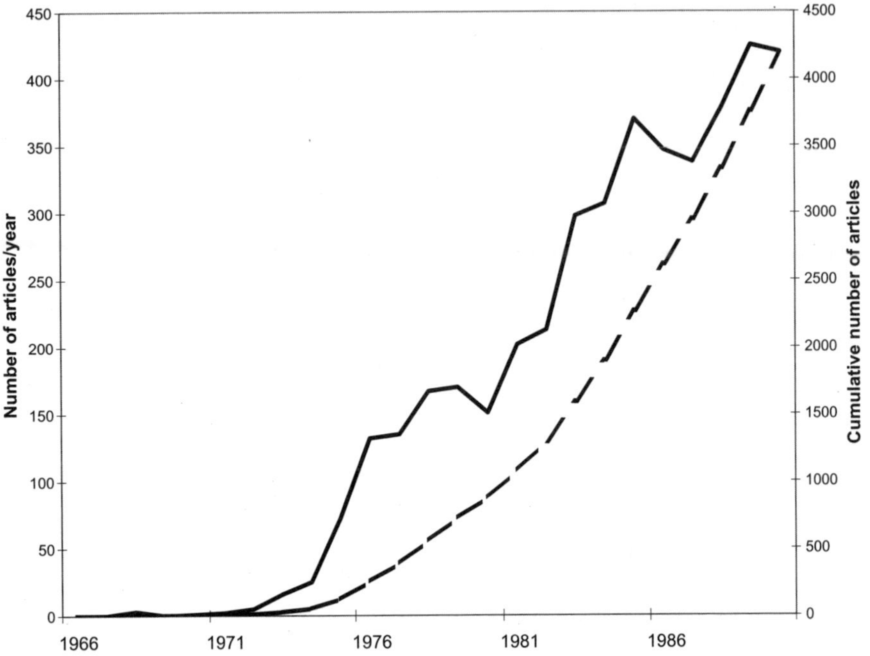

Figure 4.1
Yearly (*solid line*) and cumulative (*broken line*) number of articles using the terms "cell-surface marker(s)," "surface marker(s)," or "cell marker(s)" in their title or abstract. (Data source: MEDLINE.)

trend is clear. The figure shows exponential growth, starting with the early 1970s, in the number of papers per year coded by the notion of "cell-surface marker," a trend that becomes even more apparent when, instead of the number of papers per year, we use the cumulative number of papers.[101] To be sure, the number of publications discussing or using markers is only a pale indication of the even more dramatic increase in the number of routine clinical analyses performed in thousands of laboratories. In a paper polemically entitled "Lymphocyte Markers: Diagnostic Help or Costly Vogue?,"[102] one of the pioneers of lymphocyte marker research, Louis Preud'homme (a collaborator of Maxime Seligmann), denounced this very trend several years later, by the same token documenting the growing importance of markers in diagnostic practice.

Markers Steal the Show

Another British immunologist quick to hop on the T-B bandwagon was Mitchison. He had been joined by Martin Raff, a Canadian postdoc at

Mill Hill in 1968. Funded by the (U.S.) National Multiple Sclerosis Society, Raff had no previous training in immunology. To get the ball rolling, Mitchison showed Raff a 1963 paper by Reif and Allen describing an antigen they had named theta (in 1970, it was renamed Thy-1).[103] The Reif and Allen paper had been published just a few months after Old and Boyse had reported their work on the TL antigen. Like Boyse and Old, Reif's findings had resulted from work on cancer, more specifically from the search for a leukemia-specific antigen. Reif had linked theta to thymus-derived leukemia lymphocytes, as opposed to normal lymphocytes.[104] Now armed with the new T-B distinction, Mitchison asked Raff to verify whether theta could be used as a marker for normal T cells.[105] Raff responded to the request with two seminal papers. Here is how a scientist turned historian describes the results: "It was M. C. Raff who in 1969 identified a cell surface marker (theta) on T lymphocytes and thereafter it became possible to distinguish between T and B cells on morphologic as well as functional grounds. . . . A year later Raff provided evidence for the existence of two distinct populations of peripheral lymphocytes—T cells with the theta marker and B cells carrying naturally occurring immunoglobulin determinants on their membranes."[106]

One might easily surmise that Raff's work had been conceived in biology and eventually moved into the clinic. Yet, as we have seen, both of the substances available for the identification of T cells—Reif's theta antisera and Boyse and Old's TL antisera—had come from pathology. Once again, then, it was not simply a question of applying biology to medicine. The nature and existence of the markers had been established simultaneously in experimental systems in both biology and medicine. True, pathological phenomena frequently became a means of modeling biological problems[107] just as researchers sought solutions for the problems of pathology in biology. However, with the rise of cell-surface markers, it just so happened that by 1970, a new space of representation offered itself to researchers in *both* biology and medicine.

But the story has a further twist. Independently of Raff, an Israeli researcher, Michael Schlesinger, had performed essentially the same experiment and published his results several months earlier. Both publications appeared in prestigious journals (Raff's in *Nature*, Schlesinger's in *Science*) and yet Raff has generally been credited for these findings. In fact, by 1984 his paper had been cited 415 times, Schlesinger's only 80 times.[108] Figure 4.2 shows the number of citations of the 1969 papers by Raff and Schlesinger. One can easily see, in Raff's case, a sharp rise

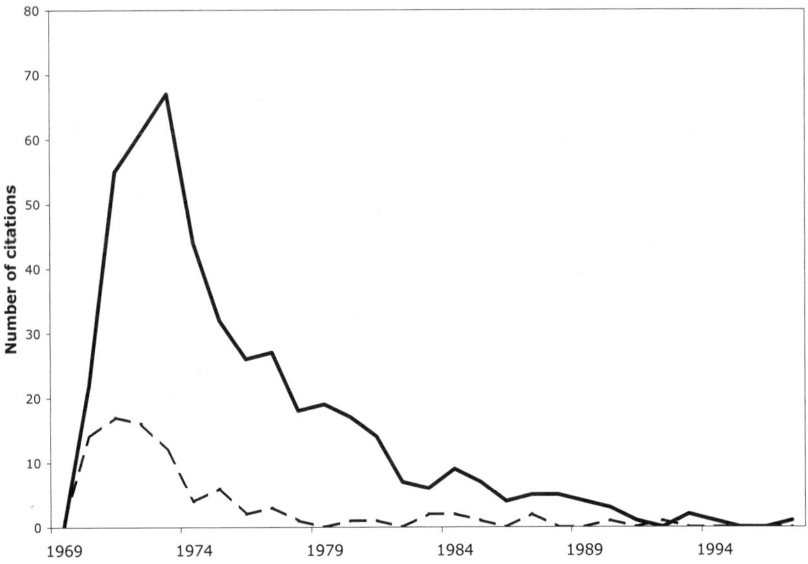

Figure 4.2
Number of citations to the 1969 articles by Raff ("Theta Isoantigen as a Marker of Thymus-Derived Lymphocytes in Mice," solid line) and by Schlesinger and Yron ["Antigenic Changes in Lymph-Node Cells after Administration of Antiserum to Thymus Cells," broken line]. (Data source: *Science Citation Index.*)

in the number of citations, as well as the persistence of a high citation rate, as compared to the less successful citational performance of Schlesinger's paper. A similar fate lay in store for two reviews of the field published by Raff in 1971 and by Schlesinger in 1972.[109]

Both Raff and Reif, who later played Schlesinger's advocate, have provided the same explanation for this puzzling turn of events: "What distinguished Raff's paper was its title and interpretation," and, as for the reviews, "As in the earlier reports from their laboratories, Schlesinger's title . . . was far more conservative than Raff's fetching title."[110] Raff used the term *marker* in his titles ("Theta Isoantigen as a Marker of Thymus-Derived Lymphocytes in Mice" and "Surface Antigenic Markers for Distinguishing T and B Lymphocytes in Mice"); Schlesinger did not ("Antigenic Changes in Lymph-Node Cells after Administration of Antiserum to Thymus Cells," "Antigens of the Thymus"). Terminology, it would appear, made a difference. Figure 4.2 reminds us of that. But, one could ask, how so? What's in a word? Simply put: different perspectives, different kinds of interventions can be prefigured in a word.

For instance, when working with "surface antigens" one might wonder whether one has more or less of a given antigen, or what the distribution or configuration of the antigen is on the surface of the cell. A "marker," on the other hand, singles out a cell, marks its unique identity; it is a matter of quality, not quantity. A marker sits somewhere between pathology (tumor antigens) and biology (differentiation antigens). As such, it functions as an operator, marking (both on cells and in the social space) a specific place, in this case the place of biomedicine.

At the end of the previous section, we raised the apparent paradox whereby the two prototypical components of the IPT platform (monoclonal antibodies and the FACS) could, in fact, be described as dispensable, since they did not figure in the initial platform. We argued, in other words, that the platform could not be described as a specific device or set of reagents coming together in a standardized package.[111] What, then, defines the platform? Our narrative points in one direction: markers. In other words, that set of practices, reagents, tools, and so on organized around a new *biomedical* entity that links the normal and the pathological and thus connects in complex, new ways clinical and laboratory interventions. Individual elements of a platform, some of which can be and often are absent in any given instantiation, are, per se, irrelevant. What matters is the flexible, yet clearly identifiable combination of elements.

In 1969, shortly after Raff's arrival, another researcher joined Mitchison's group at Mill Hill: Melvyn Greaves. As we have seen, Greaves had done his doctoral work under Ivan Roitt and had published an important review of the clinical implications of the T-B distinction with him. According to Greaves, working under Roitt had "a big impact on me because it illustrated that it was possible to do really careful, interesting science in a clinical environment or with clinical material." Many of Greaves's colleagues "thought I was crazy not to work on *Drosophila* flies or worms or something more amenable."[112] "[S]cience in a clinical environment or with clinical material" accurately characterizes Greaves's subsequent career.

Following his doctorate with Roitt, Greaves spent a year doing postdoctoral research in another temple of biomedical research, the Karolinska Institute in Stockholm. There, he worked with Göran Möller, another pioneer of cell-surface antigens.[113] Back in London, he set out to apply his knowledge of markers to human leukemia. He knew he could perform "really careful, interesting science" at Mitchison's laboratory where players followed relatively strict rules of the game. Mitchison, for instance, had stated that the best way to reach the unit's goal of unraveling the nature of the immune response to tumors in experimental animals was to restrict oneself to a simple experimental system meeting a few selected criteria. Some of these criteria were heuristic (the immune response must be strong and repeatable and it must take place in *animals* whose immunological mechanisms are already well understood), while others were decidedly more practical (the unit should be able to profit from in-house expertise).[114] But what about research with the more refractory and undomesticated *human* material? Here, they conducted studies using well-defined antigens and substances known as mitogens (i.e., substances causing cells to undergo mitosis or cell division) with the aim of characterizing variation in reactivity between different lymphocyte populations. Greaves started with mice and ended up with humans.[115]

At the time, two antisera—the theta/Thy-1 antiserum initially developed by Reif and transformed by Raff into a T-cell marker, as well as the Old and Boyse TL antiserum—could be used to single out T cells. Contrary to today's easily accessible commercial reagents, the 1970s antisera could not be purchased off-the-shelf as standardized reagents from a commercial supplier. In some cases, limited quantities of homemade antisera could be obtained from colleagues and in other cases they had to be painstakingly produced in one's own laboratory. As already mentioned, production involved a series of complex and delicate operations (immunization, absorptions, etc.) and required access to particular kinds of patients, for instance, individuals suffering from agammaglobulinemia (lacking B cells, their lymphocytes consisted entirely of T cells) or chronic lymphocytic leukemia (CLL) of B-cell origin.[116] This of course raised issues of equivalence between the reagents and thus of the comparability of results from different laboratories.

As for B cells, the presence of immunoglobulins (Ig or antibody molecules) on the cell surface had been proposed as an appropriate marker. As in the theta/Thy-1 case, the initial observation that some lymphocytes carried Ig on their surface, went back to the early 1960s. The idea that one could use Ig as a B-cell *marker* emerged, as previously noted, only several years later in Raff's and Greaves's work.[117] In the meantime, another technique—known as E-rosette formation—had quickly become a significant and somewhat controversial player in the marker field.

The *E* in E rosette refers to erythrocytes or red blood cells. The rosettes themselves are the striking visual pattern produced when a lym-

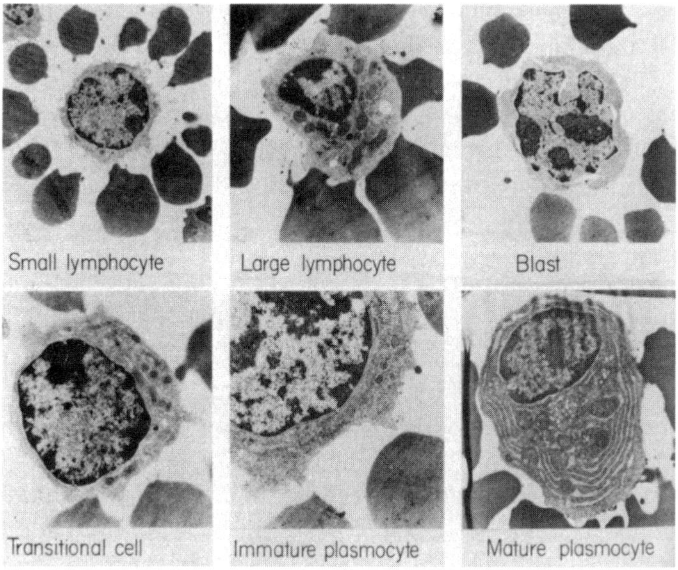

Figure 4.3
Ultrastructural (electron microscope) images of E rosettes. (From Biozzi et al., "Morphology and Differentiation of Rosette-Forming Cells during the Immune Response," 340. © 1972, reprinted with permission from Elsevier Science.)

phocyte exposed to sheep red blood cells (SRBCs, a very common reagent in immunology) combines with five to ten erythrocytes and appears under a microscope as a flower or rosette (see figure 4.3).[118] In 1970, a number of laboratories reported that the reaction, previously observed in the mouse, could also be produced with human lymphocytes.[119] Since only a proportion of the lymphocytes reacted in this way, researchers surmised that the reactive lymphocytes corresponded to "a separate sub-population of cells." Which one? Several inconclusive reports followed. In 1972, Fröland in Oslo suggested T cells as the most likely subpopulation, thus making the binding of sheep erythrocytes to human lymphocytes a "probable marker of T lymphocytes."[120] At about the same time, Borella and Sen, two researchers at St. Jude's Children's Research Hospital in Memphis, Tennessee, the major center for the study and treatment of childhood leukemia in the United States, published the results of a study of a small cohort of patients (four) arguing that although none of the patients had B-cell markers (surface Ig), one of them formed rosettes and was thus presumably afflicted with a leukemia composed mainly of T cells.[121] Considerable uncertainty surrounded the significance and performance of the technique and an international roundtable convened to settle "the technical aspects of the rosette test." The proceedings of the conference appeared in a 1972 issue of *Transplantation Proceedings*. After stating, somewhat vaguely, that "it is likely that rosette formation is not the most reliable measure for T-cell receptors," the report concluded that "From the discussion it was clear that a general outline for the technique on rosette formation cannot be given, as the procedure depends upon the use of the rosette test in connection with the problem to be solved."[122] Yet, E-rosetting soon joined the list of marker tests.

The various markers did not lead an isolated existence. Rather, they reinforced each other's significance and reliability. So, for instance, Greaves's contribution to the 1972 special section on E-rosettes in *Transplantation Proceedings* consisted in analyzing "the cell surface antigenic characteristics of rosette-forming cells."[123] In other words, he investigated rosetting by using other marker techniques. A 1974 article by Brown and Greaves confronted the relations between markers and their individual status in a more explicit manner.[124] After prophesying, in no uncertain terms, that "the enumeration of T and B cells in blood [would] become a routine clinical assay" and listing the different "marker systems that [had] already been used to selectively label human T and B cells," the authors were forced to admit that "several difficulties [had] already emerged with these marker systems which might limit their wide clinical application." The difficulties included the annoying fact that "evidence that most of them [were] unequivocally specific for T and B cells [had] been lacking" and that it remained an open question as to whether the markers labeled all or only part of T and B cells. Test reports from a number of laboratories showed considerable variation and nobody knew if the variations were the result of faulty techniques or biological processes.

To work around these problems, the authors developed "a series of presumptive markers for T and B lymphocytes *which could be tested in parallel*" (our emphasis). In other words, while any individual marker was an uncertain parameter, a set of markers all pointing in the same direction added robustness to the enterprise. Moreover, the authors quickly preempted possible objections by stressing that "these markers are only operationally specific and it would be rash to conclude that a particular antigen or receptor is completely absent from either T or B lymphocytes." To use a pragmatic definition such as "operationally specific" restricted, implicitly, the markers to those domains in which they could work as markers for a specific purpose. As we have seen, by 1974 the clinic constituted a horizon of possible purposes.[125]

The Markers of Leukemia

The year 1973 had been a very busy year for Greaves. His name appeared on eleven of the twenty-four projects featured in the scientific report of the TIU. Nine of those projects had, as their main title, "Cell-Surface Markers on Human Lymphoid Cell Populations."[126] These projects included the development of a *panel of markers* for T and B lymphocytes, the analysis of the expression of cell-surface T and B markers in leukemia (in collaboration with St. Bartholomew's MOU), and attempts to identify leukemia-specific markers in collaboration with the Institute for Child Health, this last project described as being of "possible diagnostic and prognostic value." In addition, another joint project with the MOU and involving approximately sixty patients with non-Hodgkin's lymphoma focused on the prognostic significance of surface markers and the testing of a simplified lymphoma classification based on the new technology.

Greaves was not alone in this pursuit. As we have seen, between 1964 and 1973 other researchers, many of whom would attend the 1974 London meeting devoted to the standardization of marker technology, pursued antibodies to cellular antigens. Their research, too, had oscillated between the normal and the pathological. First thought to be cancer-specific, the antigens or receptors on the surfaces of cells had by then become biological markers of functional subsets of cells implicated in the immune response, but also prospective clinical (diagnostic and prognostic) markers. The initial clinical implications of markers had been slightly disappointing partly because of the variable and often highly local results obtained through the new techniques (a problem researchers attempted to address through standardization). Part of the poor performance resulted from the fact that some of the initial attempts to use markers in clinical medicine (and not simply in pathology) sought correlations rather than articulations. In 1973, for example, Aiuti and collaborators at the University of Rome selected a cross section of patients with lymphoproliferative disorders and measured the percentage of T and B cells in the peripheral blood of the patients.[127] Using the various techniques for the differentiation of T and B cells,[128] they produced a spectrum of differences. They observed decreased numbers of T cells in CLL, Hodgkin's disease, and ALL. B-cell counts went up in CLL and lymphosarcoma. Further differences emerged when correlating percentages and stage and treatment of disease: B cells, for example, were significantly reduced in patients with CLL following treatment. In studies such as these, immunology functioned as a handmaiden to pathology insofar as researchers mapped the T-B distinction onto standard diagnoses and standard treatments in a search for confirmation and precision.

Maxime Seligmann (his team included Jean-Louis Preud'homme and Jean-Claude Brouet) and Mel Greaves (collaborating with, among others, George Janossy) carried out work with greater potential for innovation. Both teams worked along very similar lines in keeping with the fact that formal links and exchanges between France and the United Kingdom went back to at least 1963, when the newly established Leukaemia Research Fund inaugurated its series of annual guest lectures with Jean Bernard, the distinguished French hematologist. In 1971, the LRF took advantage of a joint meeting of the British and French societies for hematology to organize an informal "think-in" on leukemia.[129] The think-in led to increased cooperation between French and British researchers, including the establishment of a series of symposia and a fellowship scheme.[130] A 1973 meeting on "The Immunology of Leukaemia"[131] led, in 1975, to another meeting on the "Characterisation of Cells in Leukaemias and Lymphomas,"[132] attended by both Seligmann ("B and T Cell Membrane Markers in Human Leukaemias and Lymphomas") and Greaves ("Surface Antigens of Leukaemic Cells").[133] In other words, both teams closely followed each other's work and people and ideas moved freely between London and Paris.

Several important differences, however, separated the Paris and London teams. To begin with, while Greaves focused almost exclusively on leukemia, Seligmann studied, in addition to leukemia and the lymphomas, several other diseases and, in particular, a rare pathology he initially described in 1967, affecting patients of eastern Mediterranean origin and characterized by the presence of abnormal antibody proteins in the blood.[134] In other words, Seligmann's initiatives rested on the implicit hypothesis that the new immunohematological approach would provide greater dividends when applied to the whole spectrum of "blood diseases." In this respect, both researchers faced a well-known dilemma. By changing techniques—in this case, by replacing morphology with immunology—they both hoped to subvert traditional nosological distinctions by showing, for example, that a single disease concealed the existence of two or more distinct disease entities or that different diseases were in fact the same.[135] In practice, however, one had to use existing clinical distinctions in order to apply the new tools. In any event, and herein lies the dilemma, one had to decide between casting the net widely (as Seligmann did)[136] or narrowly (as Greaves did). In this case, Greaves's choice resulted in a better payoff.

Second, a distinct political aura surrounded Seligmann's career. His early work at Saint-Louis Hospital took place within Jean-Bernard's Research Center on Leukemias and Blood Diseases, established in 1955–56 and initially sponsored by the Claude Bernard Association, an organization spearheaded by French "neoclinicians" who sought the transformation of medical practices through the introduction of laboratories into hospitals.[137] In keeping with this reform tradition, Seligmann drew unfavorable contrasts between the scientific opportunities offered by immunological diagnosis and the time-honored, impressionistic morphological methods used by pathologists. Accordingly, clinical colleagues at Saint-Louis endured recurrent accusations of maintaining an outdated confidence in "the science of (clinical and morphological) observation."[138] Other researchers mocked the morphologists' internal battles as marked by "glancing blows with microscopic artifacts," and announced the dawn of a new era: "hematology without a microscope."[139] For sure, Greaves also criticized pathologists, but without the political overtones heard in France. In the 1970s, for example, Seligmann proposed that an immunology unit be established in every medical department, not merely as a technical resource for performing complementary diagnostic tests, but as a source of inspiration for other medical disciplines.[140] In the early 1980s, Seligmann temporarily entered politics, ending up at the Ministry of Education—overseeing, among other things, the introduction of immunology as an autonomous discipline in university science faculties—before returning to research and devoting himself, in more recent years, to the human immunodeficiency virus.

Finally, and of most interest for us, Seligmann maintained close connections with clinical activities in immunohematology. From the outset, his training had been both clinical and scientific: clinical at Saint-Louis under the hematologist Jean Bernard, and scientific at the Pasteur Institute under the immunologist Pierre Grabar. His research thus focused simultaneously on the antigenic structure and products of both normal and pathological cells,[141] and his approach to research consisted in shifting between fundamental and clinical immunology, looking at theoretical questions with their possible clinical applications in mind, and profiting from clinical activities to ask questions about fundamental immunological mechanisms.[142] Janossy noted, in this respect, that "Seligmann . . . was always interested in the clinical, the total picture, he never had the ambition of running an immunodiagnostic service. . . . Seligmann is a much more wider brain, . . . he instilled the ideas into Mel Greaves' head and they communicated rather than being worried [about who was] going ahead or not."[143]

Greaves, as mentioned earlier, had a narrower focus. Nonetheless, he pursued the translation of his results into a routine, clinical-diagnostic IPT platform. Seligmann resisted the appropriation of his results for routine hematological diagnosis even within his own hospital, Saint-Louis. As he recalled recently, he did not believe that one could transfer such preliminary research results to a diagnostic laboratory.[144] Seligmann's resistance ultimately forced the head of the Saint-Louis hematology laboratory to send one of his collaborators across the Channel to Mason's laboratory in Oxford to learn IPT.[145] Partly due to Seligmann's reliance on his prized antisera, the product of esoteric skills and thus not something one could hand over to less specialized workers, this attitude was also consistent with the group's initial resistance to monoclonal antibodies, construed as an instrument for the "proletarianization of immunology" and as necessarily inferior to antisera harvested from one's own rabbits.[146] It also jibed with the group's delay in using flow cytometry to automate cell analysis.[147] As such, Seligmann's stance stood in contrast to Greaves's quick embrace of automation and monoclonals, a strategy that, by providing extensive clinical data, was designed to test the bold hypotheses concerning leukemia devised by the British team.

In spite of these differences, Seligmann and Greaves covered much of the same ground. They shared, for instance, the notion that *normal* human lymphoid cells could be identified and characterized by membrane markers selectively expressed by T and B cells (and their subsets). Seligmann also maintained, however, that while a classification based on markers was "relatively safe" for normal lymphocytes, it "may not be valid when extrapolated to cancer cells."[148] In other words, he had, up to a certain point, the same reservations as pathologists and hematologists concerning the extent to which the normal could be mapped onto the pathological. As he noted in 1976, "if the validity of the markers used to distinguish B cells and T cells has been demonstrated for normal human lymphocytes, it is necessary to be prudent when applying the same interpretation to poorly differentiated malignant cells."[149] To be prudent, however, did not mean to reject the whole project as misguided. It simply meant that one had to use a *panel* of membrane markers, a "methodological" solution that, once again, and as previously discussed, Seligmann shared with Greaves.

The panel would have been unneeded had researchers found specific markers of malignancy, i.e., markers present only on leukemic cells. As we have seen, Boyse and Old had initiated this work in the 1960s.[150] Between 1971 and 1974, at least four alleged cancer antigens had been found.[151] Whether or even to what extent the antigens appeared specifically on leukemic cells remained questionable and much of the work done had been intended to eliminate the possibility that the antigens occurred normally.[152] Greaves dismissed the "plethora of claims for tumour specific antigens," saying that "much of this evidence [for tumor-specific antigens] is misinterpretation based upon ignorance of the cell *biology* of the tissue and cells involved in the cancers studied."[153] By the early 1980s, Old himself had to admit that "despite vast effort aimed at demonstrating such [cancer] antigens, their existence in the generality of cancer remains unproved."[154]

Although both Seligmann and Greaves rejected the search for tumor-specific antigens as misguided, they did so not simply because of the abysmal record of unproven claims, but because it contradicted their understanding, grounded in marker technology, of the etiology of blood diseases. Pathologists' traditional perspective represented cancer cells as normal, mature cells that had somehow degenerated or dedifferentiated (i.e., lost their mature cell status). From within this perspective, one might hope to find "degenerated" antigens singling out those cells. An alternative view had begun to emerge according to which leukemic cells were in fact primitive cells, whose development had been arrested at some early stage. Their surface markers represented normal antigens of primitive cells. According to this view, one should look for tumor-*associated*, as opposed to tumor-*specific*, markers. Those markers would prove in fact to be "preserved" or "frozen" differentiation antigens of early maturation stages of the kind promoted, for instance, by Seligmann.[155] While Greaves would later refine this theory by claiming that rather than a "blunt-ended maturation arrest or freezing," cancer resulted from the "uncoupling of proliferation and differentiation,"[156] at the moment the new perspective combined the methodological need for a panel of markers with an etiologic rationale.

Both Seligmann and Greaves spoke of maturation arrest and both set out to establish, on that basis, new classifications of blood diseases. In both cases, one finds harsh words for their morphology-minded colleagues. Greaves blasted the traditional perspective of pathologists saying that it "reflected a naïve overinterpretation of morphology in ignorance of cell lineage and maturation stage relationship."[157] Seligmann noted that when confronted with a set of increasingly contradictory and confusing clinical and morphological findings, pathologists reacted by proposing new, "fashionable" designations that "do not really solve the problem since they are mainly based upon morphological similarities which have been misleading in the past."[158] Clearly, clinicians and researchers needed "new classifications of leukemias and lymphomas which will not be based merely upon morphological criteria and will thus become more accurate and reproducible."[159] This meant an immunology-based classification.

The new maturation arrest perspective did not come together all at once. It grew slowly out of a dense series of technical engagements with human pathological material. Initial work in Greaves's laboratory resorted to plant mitogens, i.e., substances known since the beginning of the 1960s to stimulate cell growth in culture. With the establishment of the T-B distinction in the late 1960s, it became possible that the mitogen effect could be selective, i.e., that a given mitogen might act only on either B or T cells. Combined with markers that provided "a logical direct approach to establish the precise selectivity of [mitogens] for different populations of human lymphocytes,"[160] mitogens became a tool to analyze differentiation pathways, i.e., the normal development of cells from an early to a mature stage. Greaves and Janossy felt that they could develop them into "a clinical tool for monitoring the immunological competence of lymphocytes from both patients with various immunological disorders and those undergoing immunosuppressive therapy."[161] Between 1971 and 1975, they published approximately fifteen papers on the separation of B cells and T cells using the experimental system they had set up to this effect. Initially, then, the cell-surface markers participated in the plant mitogen system. Markers, however, soon became independent of the mitogen system and entered directly into the study of leukemia, a step already taken by Seligmann, without the detour through the mitogens. Yet, it is possible to claim, retrospectively, that Greaves's detour, rather than being useless, did settle him on the course of an etiologic account of leukemia (the maturation arrest perspective he would soon develop in considerable detail).

As we have seen, both Greaves and Seligmann fashioned the immunology of cell-surface receptors into a tool for the study of leukemic cells mobilizing individual markers as members of a panel to discriminate between B-cell and T-cell populations. In a lengthy review article explaining his approach to hematologists, Greaves, after recalling that "methods for identifying individual cell surface components on intact cells" had been developed by immunologists, went on to explain that "the principle involved [in his approach was] straightforward enough: with a panel of markers or probes, we can hope to define a cell surface phenotype that will at least suggest, or at best determine, the identity and/or origin of the cell of interest."[162] Unlike previous work, this program combined biology and medicine within the same experimental system. Although he treated methods in immunology as technology, he did so in order to generate facts about both biology and medicine. The purpose of the project was thus twofold: "I can see two applications of this new technology. First, it provides an approach to investigating basic questions of biological organization, particularly within the immune system, but in principle in other heterogeneous cellular systems also. Second, it provides a highly discriminating tool for identifying interrelationships of cells in disease and for separating subpopulations or rare cells for analysis."[163]

Associated or Specific? Making Sense of cALLA

Like Seligmann's, Greaves's first panel of "markers" contained seven different antibody tests that, together, separated lymphocytes into T cells and B cells. The panel, as we have already noted, overcame possible objections concerning whether individual markers for T and B cells identified these cells alone. Further, openly acknowledged potential pitfalls of the panel approach included the necessary assumption that the marker sites existed on B and T lymphocytes throughout the course of their development and that the sites found on normal cells could be found on cancerous cells.[164] Undeterred by these complications Greaves and coworkers, combining technical with semantic innovation, concluded the aforementioned review by naming the new approach and predicting a bright clinical future for it: "We are encouraged by these investigations to suggest that further cell-surface 'phenotyping' of leukemias and lymphomas will aid diagnosis and eventually therapy and prognosis."[165] And indeed, with their system they confirmed Seligmann's results, namely that the chronic form of leukemia (CLL) is essentially a B-cell disease.[166] As for the acute form (ALL), they once again confirmed Seligmann's results and, in so doing, were confronted with the following puzzle: a tiny minority of ALL cells originated in the B-cell line, a more sizable minority were of T origin, but a majority (around 70%) lacked both B and T markers.[167] The obvious question, prompted by their approach, was: what was the cellular origin of the non-T, non-B cases of ALL? The related clinical question boiled down to: did the new categories of ALL (especially the T vs. non-T, non-B) correspond to some clinically relevant difference, one that could separate different *kinds* of acute leukemias on the basis of, for instance, prognosis?

In the absence of significant correlations between markers and clinical outcomes, supporters of the new approach could do little more than maintain optimism: "There is some hope that [the immunological subclassification of ALL] will not remain purely academic and that it will help not only to improve the accuracy and reproducibility of acute leukaemias, but also to identify the target cell for the leukaemic process and to provide new tools for treating and monitoring patients with acute leukaemias."[168] With regard to the phenotypic identity of the majority of ALL cells, the findings were not purely negative. As previously discussed, "phenotyping" panels used not only reagents that detected antibody molecules on the surface of B cells or E-rosette tests, but also laboriously produced rabbit antisera that had been raised in each laboratory by complex immunization and absorption schedules. The antisera produced a distinct pattern of reactivity for non-T, non-B ALL cells showing that those cells also had cell-surface antigens that could be used to characterize them. There were, however, further problems. First of all, given the idiosyncratic nature of antisera raised in different laboratories, comparisons between the resulting patterns of reactivity were fraught with complications. Second, nobody knew what to do with the non-T, non-B markers. Were they leukemia-specific, the peculiar product of pathological processes? Or were they simply leukemia-associated, i.e., markers corresponding to the phenotype of a normal counterpart, a rare kind of cell from an early stage of lymphocyte differentiation?

Seligmann, while prudently leaving both possibilities open, clearly indicated that he thought the latter the more likely, and consistently spoke of leukemia-associated antigens.[169] Greaves, around 1973, decided to run an experiment that, according to the director of his unit, Mitchison, should not have worked, but, surprisingly, did. He took ALL cells, coated them with rabbit antibodies directed against normal T and B lymphocytes so as to block the normal T and B markers, and immunized rabbits in the hope that they would develop antibodies against the non-B, non-T receptors that had been left uncoated.[170] Because of his strategic position at the ICRF/TIU, Greaves was able to test the resulting antiserum against different types of leukemic blood.[171] A pattern of positive reactions to the anti-ALL antiserum emerged indicating that the antibody detected either a leukemia-specific or a leukemia-associated antigen. The hesitation between these two interpretations is reflected in the titles of two papers published almost simultaneously by Greaves's group in December 1975: "Leukemia-Associated Antigens in Man" and "Candidate Leukemia-Specific Antigen in Man."[172] One paper announced the existence of "an antigen found thus far only on non–T-cell ALL and in some acute undifferentiated leukemias, which we therefore regard as a strong candidate for a leukemia-specific antigen."[173] The other paper, however, reported that "After initial absorptions with red cells, liver and tonsil lymphocytes, the antisera seemed to be ALL specific; however, careful analysis using the FACS-I revealed that reactivity remained against a small population of mononuclear cells in non-leukemic bone marrow samples."[174] In other words, the marker could also be found on a normal population of rare cells. It received a name, cALLA (for *c*ommon *ALL* antigen) and sharply increased the visibility of Greaves's work.

In the following years, the focus of Greaves's group shifted to cALLA and, as shown by the last quotation, another key player, the fluorescence-activated cell sorter (FACS), entered the field (see figure 4.4). The initial role played by the FACS can be understood as follows. Antisera developed by Greaves and Seligmann could be used in connection with functional (cytotoxicity) tests or by using immunofluorescence. For several reasons, including the possibility of simultaneously examining different markers and standardizing the procedure, Greaves, Seligmann, and others chose immunofluorescence.[175] This meant, initially, using a fluorescence microscope, under which the stained cells could be analyzed. Developed around the mid-1970s, the FACS, on the other hand, gave, in principle, the same results as looking under the microscope. Yet, the apparatus did more than substitute for the microscope. It allowed researchers to count the number of cells that reacted to the antibody. Widely considered a gain in "objectivity" insofar as it provided a quantitative alternative for the troubled classification of the leukemias, the inscriptions produced by the FACS, either in the form of numbers or of graphic representations (histograms, dot plots) of cell populations, allowed, moreover, for interlaboratory inspection of the results, as opposed to the expert (and ultimately idiosyncratic) appraisal of slides under a microscope by a skilled hematologist.[176]

In 1974 the TIU acquired one of the first two FACS machines to be sold to Europe, as well as David Capellaro, a member of the California team that had developed the device. Given Capellaro's expertise, the

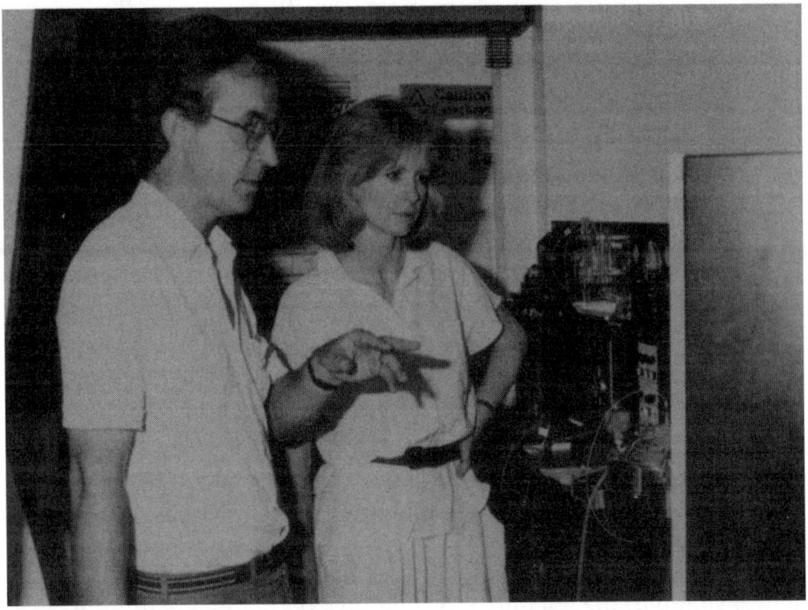

Figure 4.4
Dr. Greaves, c. 1986, showing the then current model of his FACS machine to a supporter of the Leukaemia Research Fund, with actress Jane Asher. (From: *Leukaemia Research Fund Yearbook 1986*, 17. Reprinted with kind permission from the Leukaemia Research Fund.)

FACS became immediately operational. Greaves quickly monopolized the machine and put it to work in tandem with cALLA[177] (see figure 4.5). Analysis of the ALL antigen enabled him to claim that "ALL is in fact two separate diseases, one a neoplasia of the T-lymphocyte axis and another (constituting the majority) a malignancy of either stem cells or very early erythroid cells." He also expanded his collaboration with the MOU at St. Bartholomew's and with the Institute of Child Health not only to the diagnosis of patients at presentation, but also to the search for rare leukemic cells in bone marrow: "the FACS has proved invaluable for these analyses and has enabled us to detect a variable number of leukaemic cells in a proportion (5/14) of patients considered to be in complete 'haematological' remission."[178]

In describing the role of FACS, we are not advancing a technological determinism. We are not saying, for example, that without the FACS, Greaves's group would have been led to believe that they had a

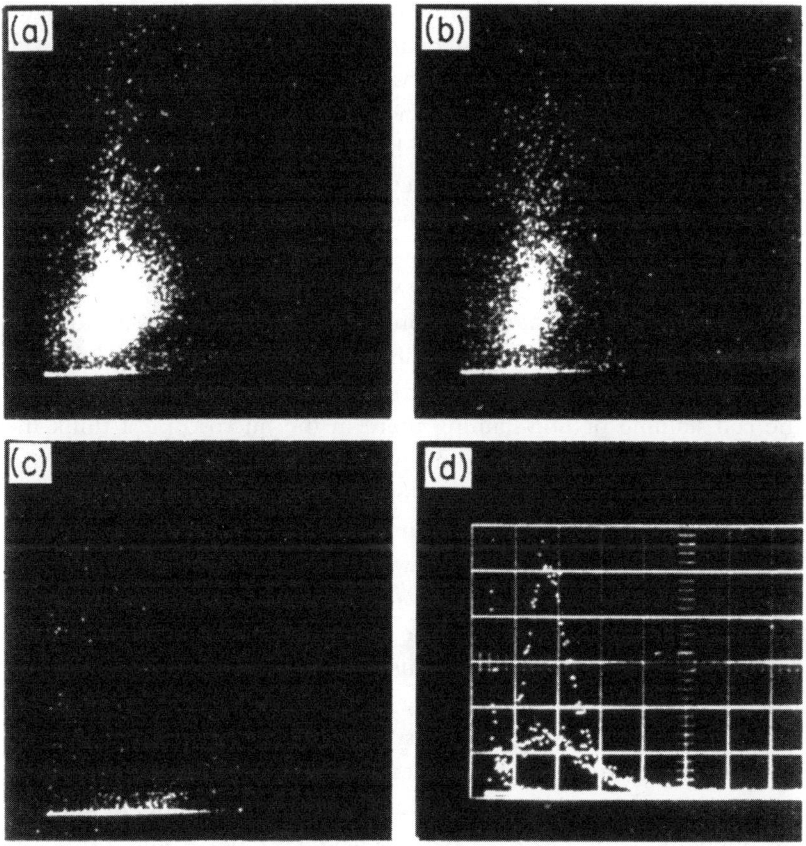

Figure 4.5
Examples of early FACS analysis of leukemia by Greaves: FACS analysis of ALL with rabbit antisera specific for the common ALL-associated antigen. (From Greaves, "An Immunological Window on Leukemia," 57. Reprinted by permission of Blackwell Science Ltd.)

leukemia-specific antigen. Not only did they go to further lengths to show the opposite, but several years later in 1980, when Stuart Schlossman claimed to have found a leukemia-specific antigen using a similar automated cell sorter, Greaves's group reverted to fluorescence microscopy to show that he had not. As Greaves recalled back then, "If the cell population of interest was less than 5%, you ran into problems."[179] Greaves claims that Schlossman failed to detect a minor population of normal bone marrow cells (1% to 2%) that were reacting positively to his monoclonal antibody, thus indicating that the antigen populated cells other than leukemic cells. Under the microscope, the population was visible. The lesson was clear: "Ever since then I've told people in the lab, they still do it now, whatever you do in flow cytometry, you look down the microscope because you miss rare events unless you've got everything beautifully set up with controls."[180] Retrospectively, Greaves maintains that the instrument did not play a crucial role: "we would have drawn much the same conclusions in terms of clinical relevance and biological understanding without flow cytometry." Yet, he also admits that the FACS added a convincing quantitative edge to their work: "we found flow cytometry really quite helpful and I think it helped us persuade people that things can be quantified. It wasn't just seeing the cell staining or non-staining there in the microscope. I think the hematologists were fairly convinced by that."[181] And, as shown by the insistence on the role of FACS in both his papers of the time and his 1975 MRC application, FACS figured prominently in the rhetorical structure of Greaves's argument. It would figure even more prominently in the routinization and standardization of the platform.

By 1975, Greaves could describe the diagnostic value of cALLA as "well-established." Over 300 patients had been tested (immunophenotyped) including patients entering the national MRC chemotherapy trial.[182] Then, according to Janossy's recollection, something "totally unexpected" happened. Having heard about the new diagnostic tool, hematologists around the United Kingdom started sending in samples: "we suddenly started to have 10–15 leukemias a day from all over the UK and we couldn't understand what the hell was going on."[183] In 1976, Greaves could report that cALLA had been applied to the diagnosis of 700 untreated patients from all over the United Kingdom.[184] And then, in 1976, Greaves, Janossy, and Capellaro, as well as the FACS machine, left the TIU to become the head of a newly established membrane immunology laboratory set up by the ICRF. The IPT platform was up and running.

5

Running the Immunophenotyping Platform

Between 1974 and 1984 Melvyn Greaves and coworkers set up and operated an immunophenotyping platform. According to a quasi-official history of the Imperial Cancer Research Fund, the platform had produced an "acceptable 'biological' subclassification" of acute leukemia into four major categories each of which displayed distinctive hematological and prognostic features.[1] Widely adopted in other countries, the IPT platform entered diagnostic routines in hematological laboratories in hospitals around the world, creating the basis for further biomedical research in hematology, immunology, and epidemiology. Most important, the platform freed itself from its initial dependence on leukemia and spread to other diseases, assuming different technical configurations.

The spread of the IPT platform had, nonetheless, its limits. First of all, the platform has been added to and not replaced other platforms. Moreover, its adoption was confined to specific diseases. The 1997 edition of the *Primer on Allergic and Immunologic Diseases,* a special issue published every five years (for the last twenty) by the *Journal of the American Medical Association,* tells us that while "quantitation of lymphocyte populations has proven to be invaluable in certain clinical situations and a useful research tool in many others," those clinical situations remain essentially the diagnosis and treatment of the leukemias and the lymphomas (or what are collectively known as the "lymphoid malignancies" or lymphoproliferative diseases) and HIV prognosis. As for other applications, although IPT has been used in research, the reader is warned that "these data have provided useful insights into many of these disorders but have generally not provided diagnostic or prognostic information."[2] Rather than unqualified success or utter failure, we are confronted with several nuances.

Consequently, in this chapter we take a closer look at the early years of the platform, concentrating on its initial stabilization as a diagnostic tool and the work taken to position it with regard to more traditional diagnostic practice, namely morphology. In addition, we compare two different career trajectories of the key players in the establishment of the platform—Melvyn Greaves and George Janossy—and their evolution with regard to the platform. In particular, we follow Greaves's career as he moves from the IPT of leukemia to the molecular biology of the same disease and Janossy's career as he adapts the IPT platform to clinical contexts outside of leukemia. Let us begin with a brief comparison of Greaves's and Janossy's publishing record so as to provide a formal context for their career decisions.

Figure 5.1 shows the number of articles published each year by Mel Greaves and George Janossy, as well as the number of articles they coauthored. A close analysis of the figure reveals several instructive facts. First, joint publications are concentrated in the 1971–82 period. The initial date corresponds to Greaves's and Janossy's arrival at Mill Hill,

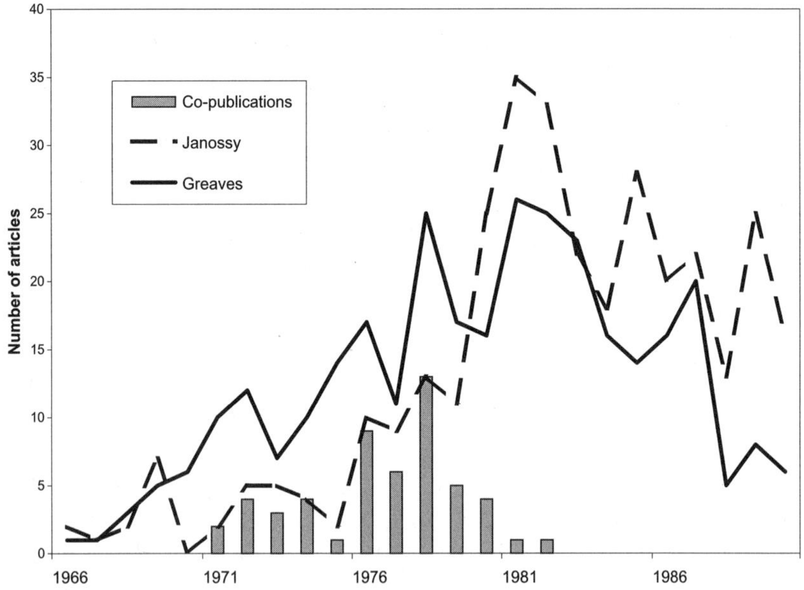

Figure 5.1
Number of articles published between 1966 and 1990 by Greaves and Janossy, and number of coauthored articles. (Data sources: MEDLINE for the 1966–73 period, *Science Citation Index* for the post-1973 period.)

the former from his postdoctoral work in Sweden and the latter from his native Hungary. Although he had a medical degree and had already published several scientific articles,[3] upon his arrival in the United Kingdom Janossy, with support from the Royal Society and the Wellcome Trust, enrolled in a PhD program under the joint supervision of G.L. Asherson (Division of Immunology of the Clinical Research Center at University College) and Greaves (tumor immunology unit).[4] Janossy's doctoral work, completed in 1974, focused on the mitogen experimental system discussed in chapter 4 and resulted in several papers cosigned with Greaves, which account for most of Janossy's publications for that period. In 1975, the TIU officially hired Janossy and when Greaves established the Membrane Immunology Laboratory (MIL) in 1976, Janossy (and the fluorescence-activated cell sorter) followed him. The productivity of both researchers increased over the next few years with, once again, Janossy's total output restricted mainly to the articles coauthored with Greaves. Their joint publications coincided with the further refinement of the IPT platform in the field of leukemia. Greaves's non-Janossy publications included the seminal articles on (common acute lymphoblustic leukemia antigen) that "proved to be a springboard for what then developed as a cottage industry of immunophenotyping in leukaemia."[5]

Then, in 1978, at the peak of their joint publications, Janossy left the MIL for the Royal Free Hospital to head the department of clinical immunology. As can be easily seen, in addition to marking the decline of the collaboration between Greaves and Janossy, the end of the 1970s coincided with a period of high productivity for both researchers. A close analysis of their publications shows that this burst of activity reflects two different strategies. Greaves, on the one hand, continued work on leukemia and, moving away from IPT, adopted molecular biology in his search for the etiology of the disease. Janossy, on the other hand, continued working on the IPT platform and, extending its reach, applied IPT not only to leukemia—successive three-year Medical Research council grants, from 1984 to 1994, allowed Janossy to conduct routine service work for leukemia diagnosis for 127 hospitals, with reporting to UKALL (U.K. acute lymphocytic leukemia) and UKAML (U.K. acute myeloid leukemia) trials[6]—but also to a raft of other diseases (including arthritis, graft-versus-host disease, hepatitis, Hodgkin's disease and, later, AIDS) and sites (bone marrow, gastrointestinal tract, kidney, and lung).

Returning now to the collaboration between Greaves and Janossy, we learn from the 1977 report of the MIL that six of the laboratory's sixteen projects for that year involved both researchers. Among these figured the application of markers to the clinical diagnosis of leukemia, using a collaborative network initiated three years earlier.[7] According to the report, the practical value of the testing (by then involving more than a thousand patients) resided in the differential diagnosis of ALL and AML (requiring different treatment) and in the subclassification of ALL into different subgroups. In addition, always on the lookout for support for cALLA and the other members of his panel of markers, Greaves applied the IPT platform to the study of *cultured* cell lines of human leukemia and lymphoma. Cell culture is a difficult art, fully mastered by only a few research centers. Accordingly, Greaves enrolled researchers from Buffalo, Paris, and Uppsala who were leaders in this field.[8]

The grafting of cell line technology onto the IPT platform offers an interesting example of the entrenchment of a platform through its articulation with preexisting techniques whose robustness it enhances. The process began when Pulvertaft established the first hematopoietic cell line in 1963 at the University of Ibadan (Nigeria) with cells derived from African Burkitt's lymphoma patients. In the early 1970s, the list of available cell lines quickly expanded with the development of cell cultures derived, inter alia, from ALL patients.[9] In spite of optimistic initial reports, the hope of finding a "magic" (i.e., tumor-specific) marker using the homogeneous cell lines that had recently been made available soon gave way to a more practical goal. Cell lines, because of their homogeneity, could be used to test and characterize the specificity of poorly defined antisera. In turn, once characterized using better-defined antisera, homogeneous cell lines could be used to raise improved antisera. The markers characterized the cell lines and the cell lines stabilized the markers.[10] Researchers on the IPT platform were thus able to put cell lines to work as a new kind of experimental material, acting as a model system of normal and malignant hematopoiesis.

With the availability of permanent cell lines, including those isolated and found to be cALLA positive by a leading researcher in this field, Jun Minowada (then based at Roswell Park Cancer Institute in Buffalo), the IPT platform became fully operational. The individual parts of the platform began to function as an integrated, organized whole. Immunological markers were tested as a panel, the measurements conducted in a quantitative manner using flow cytometry, and the analysis extended by sorting the cells of interest for further morphological and biochemical studies and for culture. The platform also included a range of biochemical markers.[11] Moreover, researchers performed these measurements on permanent cell lines, comparing the results with the features of rare, immature normal cells in fetal tissues and bone marrow taken from individuals of different ages. As we describe below, the rapid solution of a long-standing biomedical dilemma, namely the cellular origin (referred to as the "target cell") of chronic myeloid leukemia (CML) and its relationship to the different forms of acute leukemias, provided eloquent testimony to the power of the platform.

The biomedical problem first arose when clinicians noticed that lymphoblasts (i.e., cells classified as of lymphoid, as opposed to myeloid, lineage) could occasionally be seen in large numbers during the acute phase—referred to as "blast crisis"—of CML. The phenotypic features of these cells were unknown and it was difficult to see how mature lymphocytes—if this was indeed what lymphoblasts were—could be part of the pathology of a myeloid disease. Researchers ignored this problem, regarding it as an anomaly, until Mike Beard, a hematologist at the ICRF MOU Unit, informed Greaves of his suspicion that at least three cases of the frozen samples deposited in the unit's cell bank had lymphoid morphology. He wondered whether these cells expressed cALLA, suspecting that their phenotypic features might not be those of mature lymphocytes but, rather, those of cells in their early stages of differentiation, as in the case of ALL. Greaves agreed and both subsequently argued that if there were phenotypic features shared by *immature* cells during the development of two different diseases,[12] these features could not be regarded as specific for either *pathology* but, rather, as features of *normal*, immature cells (target cells) involved in both types of leukemias.

Soon after the formulation of this hypothesis, interested hematologists quickly provided cell samples from all over the country.[13] Further help came from across the Atlantic when Minowada sent his permanent cell lines from Buffalo. Surface and biochemical markers showed that blast crises in CML were indeed heterogeneous: 60% to 70% were myeloid but a substantial minority, 25% to 30%, were lymphoid reflecting the phenotypic features of blasts seen in common ALL and not those of mature lymphocytes. Patients suffering from a "lymphoid" blast crisis even responded, albeit transiently, to ALL-like therapy. Using his cell line collection, Minowada redefined CML as a stem cell disease involving cells from the early hematopoietic lineages. Finally, cALLA expression was also detected on lymphoid-like precursor cells present, in moderate numbers, in fetal as well as infant bone marrow, and in lower numbers in adult bone marrow.

Now, all these observations could be used to support the view that the ALL antigens were "normal progenitor stem cell gene products rather than leukemia specific markers," or, in other words, that they could be found both in human leukemia cells and normal bone marrow stem cells. This claim had both theoretical consequences—it offered a new etiology for leukemia—and practical consequences for the analysis of the early relapse of patients following antileukemia treatment. Moreover, the two conflicted. As acknowledged in the 1978 MIL report, the "unexpected" presence of normal cells bearing the leukemia marker in the regenerating bone marrow thwarted the hope that accurate enumeration of leukemic cells would lead to better management and insight into disease evolution. That observation, however, lent further support to the etiological view suggesting that cALLA was a normal differentiation antigen of lymphocyte precursors. Janossy's later work, discussed at the end of this chapter, would in part be devoted to the development of technical modifications allowing the platform to circumvent these difficulties and enabling it to be used in the early detection of relapse, by documenting, quantitatively, the asynchronous expression of normal differentiation antigens.

Looking for Clinical Significance

The stabilization of the new platform depended heavily on the establishment of its clinical significance. Despite repeated claims that the latter had been unquestionably demonstrated, clinical significance had to be continuously reaffirmed and reassessed. It should be noted that postwar biomedicine has a particular view of clinical significance that leans heavily toward prognosis.[14] Now, to determine the prognostic value of a given test is no simple matter. As noted by one of Seligmann's collaborators in the specific case of leukemia markers, it requires the comparison of so-called survival curves of significant numbers of patients who have been classified according to traditional prognostic factors (age, blood count, etc.) and according to immunophenotype.[15] The technology for the production of survival curves engenders its own series of unique problems, whose difficulty cannot be underestimated.[16]

The prognostic significance of the immunological analysis of ALL had purportedly been shown in a test conducted by Seligmann's group shortly after Greaves isolated cALLA.[17] Greaves and his collaborators also maintained that they had something prognostic, even though, in 1977, only the initial results of a prognostic study carried out with the

Institute for Child Health (ICH) were available, and no results had yet been obtained from an MRC-UKALL follow-up study and from a separate analysis of adult ALL cases carried out in collaboration with the MOU. Nonetheless, the 1977 MIL report claimed that marker analysis had "prognostic correlates." An article published by Greaves's group that same year concluded that from the therapeutic point of view, common ALL cases fared better than T-cell ALL (T-ALL) cases.[18] Prognostic success did not, however, lead the authors to call for the substitution of immunological diagnostics for morphological techniques. Asking whether the immunological divisions provided "better guidelines for prognosis and management than the traditional prognostic features," they prudently concluded that "it seem[ed] clear that both need[ed] to be taken into consideration to improve the results of treatment."[19] They restated their belief that the IPT platform would produce valuable prognostic information in 1978 when they reported that further results on the prognostic value of the immunodiagnosis of leukemia showed, for instance, that common ALL had superior remission duration to "null" ALL. As a result, "it [was] now considered imperative at diagnosis to subdivide ALL into its subclasses in order to rationalize therapy and the design of new trials."[20]

When, only a few years later, the statisticians had tabulated the complete results from the phenotyping of the 1974–78 ALL clinical trials, the prognostic value of immunological classification turned out to be less significant than expected. Clinicians already knew that the higher the white blood cell count (WBC), the worse the prognosis. Did the phenotypic subclass add further information in this regard? Greaves had to concede that the phenotypic subtype did "not provide an unequivocally independent prognostic factor."[21] Knowing the WBC sufficed. More precisely: "Overall in this series and also within the major cALL (common ALL) there is a strong correlation between high WBC count and poor clinical response (remission induction and duration). When the three major immunological subclasses are adjusted for WBC count, the prognostic correlation of antigenic phenotype is reduced and statistically insignificant."[22] Subsequent papers reached a similar conclusion: in 1984, for instance, Greaves admitted that "in many, probably most, cases, immunological subtyping makes little if any contribution to patient management besides confirming the hematological diagnosis."[23]

This admission, however, did not reduce IPT to clinical insignificance. One could still argue that knowledge of the normal cell of origin conditioned knowledge of the subsequent development of the cancer. One could say, for example, that because T-cell and B-cell leukemias originated outside the bone marrow, they would be less likely to interfere with bone marrow function.[24] In this case, they would be less "symptomatic" or, in other words, they would be diagnosed later in their evolution than the cALL leukemias. The late diagnosis would, in turn, make them more resistant to therapy.[25] Markers, then, insofar as they brought the clinician closer to the biological nature of the disease (in this case, the relevant cellular entities and, thus, the disease's etiology) presumably had some clinical significance. A mutually reinforcing mechanism came into play in instances such as these: since the prognosis for a given disease category was, for all practical purposes, modified by the medication given to patients diagnosed with that disease, and since clinicians adjusted treatment to the disease category as diagnosed and classified according to IPT, diagnosis became attached to prognosis. This mutual interaction has allowed Greaves to claim a measure of prognostic success for the classification he introduced.[26]

Note here the dynamics of self-vindication and, in particular, how researchers and clinicians raised and answered questions concerning the platform's prognostic value or its role in developing etiologic accounts.[27] By combining the normal and the pathological, the platform established a new space of representation and intervention. This space, in turn, allowed prognostic questions to be asked and answered outside of the traditional categories of valuation. In other words, arguments about prognostic value were not raised against some absolute, external standard. Rather, they implied explicit or implicit comparisons with alternative approaches and standards.

Morphology and Immunophenotyping

Morphology remained the "gold standard" against which the IPT platform had to prove itself. While morphological inspection of neoplastic cells goes back to the nineteenth century, when leukemia researchers and clinicians think of morphological analysis today, they usually have in mind a set of practices specified in a relatively recent classification of these diseases and referred to as the FAB (Franco-American-British) classification. Crafted in the mid-1970s, the FAB did not attempt to incorporate the newer immunological approaches, although it can be seen, in part, as a reaction to the latter.[28] At the time, hematologists justified the search for a uniform morphological nomenclature by noting the absence of common methods for distinguishing lymphoid from myeloid leukemias. The rapid development of improved therapies, moreover, lent a sense of urgency to the project. Finally, the establishment of the clinical significance of the B and T division in the late 1960s had already begun to affect the field.

So, when French, British, and American researchers met in 1974 and 1975 to create a new classification on the basis of classic morphological and cytochemical characteristics by comparing slides and diagnostic criteria, they were quite aware of the immunological developments.[29] Although their system eschewed the new cell-surface markers that distinguished B and T cells, the FAB group claimed that the common nomenclature based on common diagnostic practices would serve as a reference standard that would subsequently facilitate the entry of the surface markers into leukemia diagnosis. They thus presented the FAB classification as an interim measure leading to the "final" etiologic classification to be provided by immunology.[30] The FAB classification however, outlived the immunological turn and is still used today in combination with the IPT and other, more recent platforms. This survival is not simply the result of the entrenchment of morphological practices in hematological circles. The FAB classification has undergone several revisions that have incorporated comparisons between morphological data and IPT and cytogenetic results.[31] According to Janossy, once clinicians learned to associate the morphological categories with the diagnostic categories provided by IPT and cytogenetics, they relearned morphology on a new basis.[32]

Thus, in the field of leukemia, morphology was being reinvented as an integrated platform at approximately the same time as the development of the IPT platform and in interaction with the latter. We therefore suggest that the development of the IPT platform transformed perceptions of previous practices and precipitated their consolidation into a morphology platform that was both dependent upon and in competition with the IPT platform. Greaves and Janossy emphasized the competitive aspects of the relationship in a series of papers published in hematology journals between 1977 and 1984. As advocates of the IPT platform, they criticized traditional (read pathological-morphological) views and explained how the new "molecular morphology" or membrane immunology emanating from their and other laboratories would be useful to clinicians.[33] The phenotyping platform would, for example, dispel a few "myths" concerning the characterization of leukemic cells. In a presentation of his program in *Blood Cells,* Greaves explained:

Some acute leukaemias are considered to be "poorly differentiated," "undifferentiated," "de-differentiated" or "stem cell." The actual proportion of total acute leukemias benefiting from these labels appears to vary according to "local" combinations of folk-lore, technical wizardry (or the lack of it) and "intuitive" hematological knowledge (whatever that is—perhaps "experience"): however, it is usually around 5%–15%.[34]

This belief, based on the visual inspection of leukemic cells, camouflaged the fact that the true cell types had been determined by other means that bore the marks of high technology as opposed to folklore and intuition:

The advent of monoclonal antibodies, cell sorter (e.g., FACS) and stem cell culture techniques should enable us to determine the phenotypes of those numerically rare haematopoietic precursor or stem cells from which acute leukaemias originate: this will then provide the proper framework for a molecular analysis of acute leukaemic cells versus their normal counterparts.[35]

High technology (and its correlates such as standardization, quantitation, objectivity, and collegial inspection) opened the way to the redefinition of the pathological on the basis of the normal or, rather, to the definition of a new domain where the normal and the pathological no longer stood in opposition.

The previous quotation listed three factors: monoclonal antibodies, FACS, and cell culture techniques. We have already discussed the role of the FACS in the initial development of the platform. Recall that, in 1974, Greaves had noted how the FACS had proved "invaluable" in detecting leukemic cells in patients thought to be in complete remission.[36] Soon after he arrived at the MIL in 1976, he modified his FACS to allow, for instance, for the simultaneous detection of two markers (double-stained cells). In 1978 he again reported that the FACS had "greatly facilitated the dissection of the complexity of cell types observed in rapidly evolving [chronic myeloid leukemia]."[37] In 1980, an external assessor of the MIL vindicated Greaves's initial investment in the technology, praising him for his "early recognition of the power of the FACS for detecting membrane antigens."[38] We have also briefly alluded to the role of cell culture techniques in the production of the first IPT platform. We are now in a position to say more about monoclonal antibodies and their role in the stabilization of the platform.

In the second half of the 1970s the development of a way of producing in vitro tailor-made reagents (monoclonal antibodies) made it possible to standardize the reagents used in the cell sorter.[39] Once standardized, the instrument and the reagents could be used to standardize the surface of leukemic cells. As we have seen, before the advent of monoclonal antibodies, the reagents used to separate leukemic cells consisted of antisera (polyclonal antibodies) obtained through complex artisanal, and ultimately idiosyncratic means. Monoclonal antibodies, on the other hand, resulted from a technology developed in 1975 that, as we have already observed, produced bulk reagents of identical makeup, at least in principle. These mutually reinforcing advantages suggested that immunological reagents could be transformed into something like chemical reagents. Industrial production by commercial enterprises such as Becton-Dickinson and Ortho Diagnostic Systems (to cite two companies active in the field of lymphocyte markers), as well as the establishment of public or semipublic centralized repositories such as the American Type Culture Collection (ATCC), soon put the principle into practice.

Greaves and coworkers quickly jumped on the monoclonal antibodies bandwagon. They first mentioned the use of monoclonal antibodies against leukemic cells and purified leukemic antigens (cALLA) in the 1978 annual report of the MIL. In 1979, the MIL reported a panel of eight monoclonals to be used in studies on human leukemia. As previously noted, some members of the panel had been obtained from other ICRF laboratories, Oxford, and from the United States (Stanford and the University of Pittsburgh). Results obtained with the panel against normal and leukemic cell lines using the FACS found "selective patterns of reactivity that correspond[ed] to previously defined phenotypic subclasses of leukemia." The monoclonals could thus safely replace the heterologous antisera, and the report proceeded to affirm that MIL already used the antibodies "routinely for leukemia immunodiagnosis and subclassification and also . . . to investigate phenotype or progenitor cells." This initial use expanded in the early 1980s when a series of international workshops reorganized the leukemia markers and their dual status—pathological and biological—into a system known as the CDs (clusters of differentiation). Commercial enterprises produced reagents for their detection making the CDs available off-the-shelf to any researcher, biological or clinical, so inclined to detect them.

We discuss the CD nomenclature in greater detail in the next chapter. For the moment, we note that it originated as a reaction to the proliferation of locally produced monoclonals that had resulted in problems of interchangeability and nomenclature. Researchers spoke of "considerable confusion"[40] and this confusion clearly threatened the standardizing properties ascribed to the monoclonals.[41] The combination of these two events—the development of monoclonal antibodies and the establishment of the CD nomenclature—created a third one: once linked to a panel of markers, the flow cytometer became more than a cell counter. It classified as it counted. More than measuring the property of a cell, the IPT platform registered classificatory events. At this point, the standards for its performance could no longer be measured by reference to what could be seen under the microscope. They now depended upon the conventions incorporated into the platform.

A Normal Account of Pathology

In 1980, the ICRF undertook a quinquennial review of its immunology research units, including the TIU and Greaves's MIL. In addition to British referees, the review process called upon leaders in the field from the United States (MIT, Stanford, National Institutes of Health) and France (Seligmann) as outside assessors. Greaves's group received very high marks. Referees and assessors emphasized its pioneering role in the redefinition of human leukemia, noting that its approach had "differed from other groups', particularly in their effort not only to characterize the phenotypic heterogeneity of leukemic cells, but also to relate this heterogeneity to clinical prognosis on the one hand and to normal hematopoietic differentiation on the other." Thus, "in addition to its pioneering contribution to the diagnosis and prognosis of some human leukemias, a considerable achievement in itself, the work of the laboratory [had been] of fundamental significance in revealing new facts about the normal early hemopoietic differentiation in humans."[42] One assessor, while faulting Greaves for "lacking in a mechanistic approach to leukemias" [sic], nonetheless praised him for having been "among the first to actively pursue the leukemia-lymphoma problems in terms of membrane markers in a highly organized matter," and also praised, as already mentioned, the group's pioneering use of the FACS. The recent adoption of monoclonal antibodies for those same purposes had "markedly increased the reliability of this work." The outcome had been a "greater precision of diagnosis in the leukemias and the extension of the concept that leukemias can be thought of as fixation through malignant transformation of a given differentiated state of a normal cell."[43] Both comments are noteworthy insofar as they describe the markers, as developed by Greaves, as both an indicator of a pathological event and of new biological entities.

As a *biomedical* novelty, then, markers had become independent of pathology and biology. A further indication of the biomedical nature of Greaves's research appears in a short presentation of the MIL published in the 1979 *ICRF Scientific Report*. Greaves noted here that the laboratory focused on the investigation of the relationship between normal differentiation and malignancy using human leukemia as the main model. This analysis had led to "new and precise criteria" for leukemia diagnosis and subclassification as well as to insight into the etiology of the disease, now understood in terms of "target cells, intraclonal evolution and level of maturation arrest." In addition, the platform now gave access, in both a figurative and literal sense, to a rare and important biomedical entity—numerically infrequent stem cells with two or more developmental/cell lineage options and their leukemic counterparts—that provided a system to explore biological and pathological mechanisms of differentiation, proliferation, and malignancy.[44] The mutually reinforcing references to both normal and pathological processes concurred in establishing a *biomedical* space of representation and intervention. And indeed, as previously mentioned, Greaves generalized his findings into a doctrine that has since been associated with IPT, namely, that the different leukemias did in fact correspond to different stages of the development of the lymphocytic and myelocytic cells of the blood.[45] The doctrine essentially stipulated that the understanding of the pathological passed necessarily through the normal: leukemic cell phenotypes could only be "meaningfully interpreted" if one had access "to the normal equivalent cell type."

Greaves and Janossy often expressed the continuity of the relationship of the normal to the pathological in terms of "lineage fidelity." They maintained that malignant cells retained the capacity to further differentiate (defined as lineage commitment) and mature (defined as residual development within a given cell lineage). In other words, there could be no "dedifferentiation" or reversion to a "fetal phenotype," as pathologists had claimed. Rather, the leukemic cells remained "'frozen' in a particular cell lineage compartment but ha[d] an essentially normal cell surface phenotype."[46] Lineage fidelity or the consistent correspondence between normal phenotypes and leukemic phenotypes thus supported the view that "no qualitatively unique and consistent leukaemia 'markers' may exist or be required."[47] And, for the sake of consistency, since the cell surface remained essentially unchanged during the leukemic process, one need not look for mutant genes that grossly changed the molecular architecture and gave rise to "foreignness":

"Rather, it [was] suggested that subtle alterations uncoupling the controls that integrate[d] proliferation and differentiation [were] all that [was] required."[48]

Of course, relating a leukemic cell to its normal equivalent only made sense if one could show that the leukemic cell retained some of the key characteristics of the normal cell. If the leukemia changed its phenotype from B to T, for example, or if it expressed a combination of B and T phenotypes or some other unexpected markers, then there would be little point in knowing the normal *past*, as the pathological *present* would have been entirely different. That leukemic cells retained the immunophenotypic properties of normal cells was not universally accepted. One of the foremost American experts in leukemia therapy, Donald Pinkel at St. Jude's Children's Research Hospital in Memphis, Tennessee, for instance, did not agree with Greaves: "Leukemia cell phenotypes are disorderly and asynchronous, not just arrested in maturation. For example, B-cell leukemia lymphoblasts combine a highly primitive appearance with the differentiated function of immunoglobulin synthesis. At no stage of normal B-lymphocytic differentiation can one find cells that look like those of B-cell leukemia." It followed, for Pinkel, that "we cannot extrapolate from leukemia to normal hematopoietic differentiation. Attempts to draw conclusions about normal lymphocyte differentiation by study of leukemia cell populations can yield erroneous results. On the other hand, leukemia cells can be good sources of antigens and genes involved in growth and differentiation. Leukemias are useful tools for study of hematopoietic differentiation but not models." In short, "[t]he expression of T- or B-cell features in lymphoid cancer cells could not be equated with corresponding normal lymphocytic lineage."[49]

Undeterred, Greaves and coworkers insisted that they had "not seen a single T plus B phenotype cell in something like 2000 cases of lymphoid leukemia examined over 7 years," noting that it was "remarkable that such a high proportion of leukemias [had] a phenotype consistent with normal gene expression and that 'mixed' or 'illegitimate' phenotypes occur[red] so infrequently."[50] In fact, they did not have to look in order to see: the FACS had done the counting, and its quantitative output made for a convincing claim. Reports of empirical results pointing to lineage "infidelity" or lineage "promiscuity" nonetheless demanded a reply. Greaves's team did so in two ways. First, they raised doubts about the competence of the researchers reporting those results. For instance, when asking whether these results corresponded to an "identity crisis for cells, monoclonal antibodies, or investigators," Greaves noted that the last-named often made erroneous presumptions about the specificity of the markers and reagents that they used.[51] As he put it in a slightly different context, "many antibody-defined structures turn out to be not quite what one at first presumes or what their arbitrary name implies to innocent observers. Specificity is very much in the eye of the beholder and an awful lot depends upon what sort of an experimental window you look through."[52] Second, for those data that could not be clearly ascribed to methodological errors, Greaves's team offered an alternative explanation that "saved the phenomenon." Essentially, the explanation was this: since all cells in a chain of development can potentially develop into subsequent cell stages down the chain, then a single leukemic cell could express antigens from two different lines of development if it became cancerous at the branching point of these lines.[53]

Regardless of the outcome of this debate, we note that the implementation of the IPT platform related in many substantive ways to the development of an etiologic approach that could be literally termed biomedical in the sense that it associated normal and pathological events in a new way. This association was more than representational since the IPT platform operated by isolating (counting and sorting) hybrid (biological-pathological) entities, namely cells on which further laboratory manipulations could be performed. The platform and the entities it generated provided the basis for new diagnostic and prognostic interventions on patients that in turn translated into therapeutic decisions.

The transformation from a pathological to a biomedical phenomenon is probably best illustrated by a comparison between two visual representations of normal and pathological hematopoietic differentiation pathways. Figure 5.2 shows diagrams corresponding to the traditional pathological approach denounced by Greaves (*a* and *b*) and a diagram generated by the IPT platform (*c*). Two striking differences appear. First, in the hematopathological scheme, in spite of the fact that cells, arranged in a circular pattern, are schematically drawn, there is an obvious attempt to represent their morphological characteristics. In contrast, in the biomedical scheme, the cells are all represented as identical circles: one does in fact wonder why the illustrator bothered to draw them, since the only difference between them lies in the list of surface (CD) molecules appended to each circle. Second, in the hematopathological scheme we see two kinds of differentiation pathways, normal and

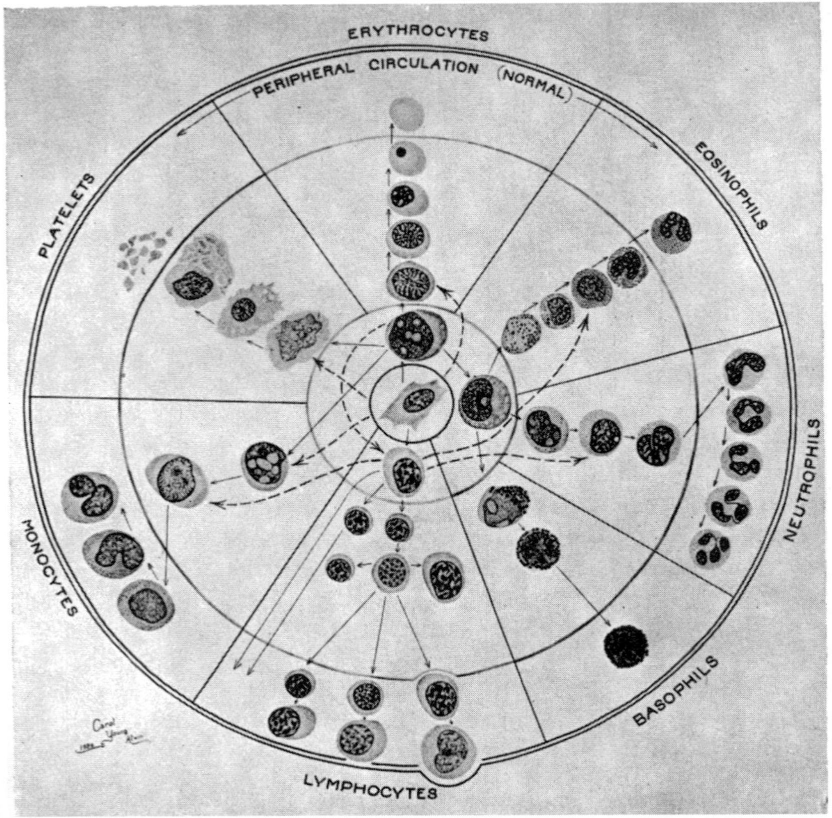
ERYTHROCYTES
PERIPHERAL CIRCULATION (NORMAL)
EOSINOPHILS
NEUTROPHILS
BASOPHILS
LYMPHOCYTES
MONOCYTES
PLATELETS

(*a*)

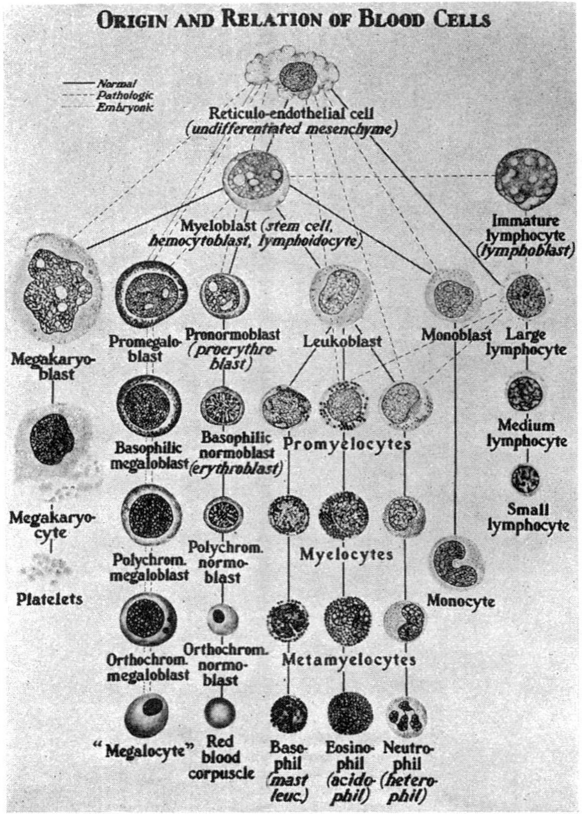
ORIGIN AND RELATION OF BLOOD CELLS
Normal
Pathologic
Embryonic
Reticulo-endothelial cell
(undifferentiated mesenchyme)
Myeloblast (stem cell, hemocytoblast, lymphoidocyte)
Immature lymphocyte (lymphoblast)
Megakaryo-blast
Promegalo-blast
Pronormoblast (proerythro-blast)
Leukoblast
Monoblast
Large lymphocyte
Basophilic megaloblast
Basophilic normoblast (erythroblast)
Promyelocytes
Medium lymphocyte
Small lymphocyte
Megakaryo-cyte
Platelets
Polychrom. megaloblast
Polychrom. normo-blast
Myelocytes
Monocyte
Orthochrom. megaloblast
Orthochrom. normo-blast
Metamyelocytes
"Megalocyte"
Red blood corpuscle
Baso-phil (mast leuc.)
Eosino-phil (acido-phil)
Neutro-phil (hetero-phil)

(*b*)

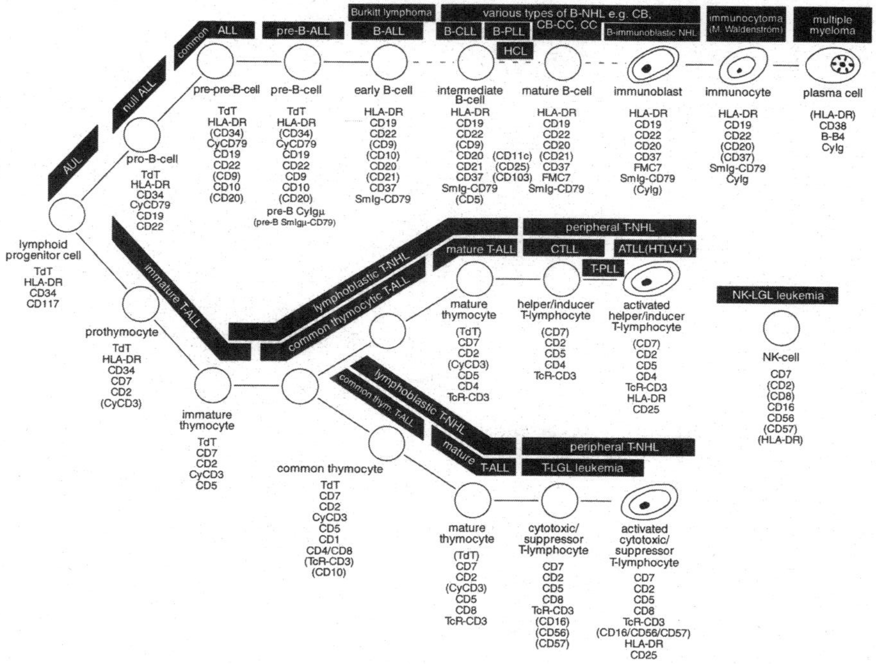

(*c*)

Figure 5.2

Morphological representations of normal and pathological blood cells: Solid lines indicate normal relations (*a* and *b*); broken lines indicate pathological relations. (From Downey *Handbook of Hematology*, 2026 and 2021. Reprinted by permission of Lippincott Williams & Wilkins. (*c*) Immunophenotypic representation of normal and pathological lymphoid differentiation. (From Van Dongen and Adriaansen, "Immunobiology of Leukemia," 91. Reprinted by permission of W. B. Saunders Company.)

pathological, represented, respectively, by a solid and a dashed line. The biomedical illustration consists of a single line of descent; the pathological event lies only in the correspondence between a given disease entity and a given stage of maturation along a single differentiation pathway.

Stepping off the Platform

As our previous analysis should have made clear, for Greaves the IPT platform was not an end in itself. It is true that Greaves devoted a major part of his early work to the establishment of immunodiagnostic tests for U.K. hospitals and that he had therefore devoted a significant proportion of laboratory space and time to the running of the platform for the analysis of human blood specimens. In fact, Greaves's former head at the TIU, N. A. Mitchison, had misgivings about this line of work. He suspected that it was too clinically oriented or, in other words, too far removed from strategic research on the immune system.[54] Yet, it is also true that, especially after the successful establishment of the platform, Greaves came to see the latter as subservient to the higher goal of pursuing a biological-etiologic understanding of leukemia (on which it was, qua platform, in fact based). He thus moved from an exclusive focus on immunological markers to a multiparameter approach, one that associated immunological markers with enzyme and cytogenetic markers. In 1979, for instance, while promoting the value of immunological methods he also added that the latter were "limited in their applicability and [that] the optimal cell identification program incorporate[d] multiparameter analysis."[55] He further noted that same year that "the selective use of a battery of investigative techniques result[ed] in a better definition and classification of all forms of leukemia," singling out chromosome analysis as especially important.[56]

In the short presentation of the MIL published in the 1979 *ICRF Scientific Report* that we just mentioned, Greaves spoke of interfacing immunological features with enzymatic and karyotypic markers to compile "a composite phenotype" characteristic of each subclass of leukemia. The phenotype would then ideally be related to patterns and sequences of phenotypes seen in normal hematopoiesis. This project required analysis of the biochemistry of cell-surface, leukemia-associated antigens in order to develop better immunodiagnostic assays. The long-term objective projected the discovery of the regulatory role of some cell-surface structures in early hematopoietic differentiation. In other words, rather than simply a means to an end (cell identification), markers became an object of (biochemical) inquiry. Simultaneously, markers (the molecules on the cell surface), rather than the antibodies used to detect them, became the focus of attention.

Greaves's next step took him to molecular biology. As he noted in a 1983 paper, "the next few years will see an increasing emphasis on the molecular biology of leukemia."[57] And indeed, most of Greaves's post-1985 work falls within that category. Retrospectively, he faulted the IPT approach for "lack[ing] the directness of molecular biology,"[58] a corollary of this statement being that "it [was] doubtful that any such essential descriptive cataloguing, whether biochemical, biophysical or immunological, [was] capable in itself of revealing anything of causal significance."[59] This did not mean, however, that Greaves discarded the IPT platform. While less significant, surface markers still played a key role in defining "real" disease entities on which molecular biological and related epidemiological studies could then be performed. Greaves made this very clear in a 1985 paper. Noting that "epidemiological studies [had] in the past been considerably compromised by lack of diagnostic precision and uniformity," and that the situation had been transformed by the development of immunological, enzymatic, and molecular markers, Greaves went on to "emphasize the importance of identifying distinct disease entities in the search for etiological clues, a point long ago acknowledged by epidemiologists who [had] been at the mercy of hematologists and pathologists in this respect!"[60]

It is not the purpose of this chapter to follow Greaves's work into the field of the molecular biology of leukemia. We note, nonetheless, that molecular biology led to modifications of the classification established through IPT. More important, it led to a revision of the claim that no basic differences existed between a leukemic cell and the corresponding stage of maturation of a normal lymphocyte. Beneath the similarities generated by the immunophenotypic profiles lay significant molecular genetic differences. According to Greaves

> [IPT] changed the way we thought about leukemia, completely, because it led us to the view that we published in '78 that all these leukemias could be mapped onto the developmental pathway of the normal blood cell production and that childhood leukemia was not a disease of the lymphocytes of the blood, but was coming from these rare progenitors, stem cells in the bone marrow. . . . The principle that [leukemias] could all be mapped onto the normal developmental structure of the system . . . didn't change until molecular genetics came in. There was a new classification, then things started to change . . . ten years ago, in the 80s.[61]

These changes did not challenge the distinctly *biomedical* nature of the new research and diagnostic practices. Even if one could now speak of a molecular genetic lesion by analogy to a tissular lesion and thus contrast the normal with the pathological, the molecular analyses were played out on a field where it was no longer possible to say whether a particular research project would result in biological or medical facts.

It is noteworthy, in this respect, that when putting together his new molecular genetic platform, Greaves adopted the successful strategy he had previously used with IPT, namely by turning his LRF center into a national referral laboratory for childhood leukemia, where all the diagnosed cases were sent for genetic marker analysis. As with IPT, where standardization led to decentralization ("once it was monoclonal we could farm it out"), Greaves similarly expects that regional centers will subsequently—that is, when the basic biomedical elements of the platform are sufficiently stabilized—take over the genetic marker work.[62]

At the end of the 1970s and the early 1980s, then, Greaves's work underwent significant changes which, in turn, were related to similar transformations at the ICRF and the Leukaemia Research Fund (LRF). To begin with, strategic research had found further reinforcement. In his introduction to the 1977 *ICRF Scientific Report*, Stoker had reaffirmed his belief that "whereas miraculous discoveries may turn up at any time, the final solution to the [cancer] problem will probably depend on new knowledge and understanding of order and disorder in living cells, which form the constituent of healthy tissues and of any cancer." More specifically, he had claimed that "the importance of the outward surface of cells constantly recurs in relation to differentiation and growth control, in the stimulation of immunity, and, not least, in the abnormalities of cancer cells." When writing those lines, however, Stoker knew that Walter Bodmer would replace him in July 1979. As every new director brings new orientations, Bodmer's 1979 program statement focused on genetics and the cell surface. At first sight, these new directions seemed pretty much in line with those of his predecessor. Bodmer, however, was able to stipulate in advance the tools that would be deployed in the program, i.e., new techniques such as recombinant DNA, cloning, and monoclonal antibodies. In turn, this meant a shift not so much in terms of disciplinary emphasis—say, from immunology to molecular biology—but, rather, in experimental systems and associated technologies. In other words, there was a general move toward molecular biological approaches within different fields, including immunology.[63]

Of special interest to us is Bodmer's remark that "the search for specific tumour-associated cell surface changes, or tumour antigens, has proved frustrating, whereas the use of the surface properties of cells to characterise their origins has proved to be of great value."[64] An obvious reference to both the false hopes that had surrounded the establishment of the TIU and to the unexpected spinoff represented by Greaves's work, Bodmer added that the recently developed technique for producing monoclonal antibodies would play an invaluable role in a variety of studies, including the general characterization of cell-surface determinants, and advanced the following speculation:

> I do believe that it should be possible to mount a unique attack on the cancer cell by using a combination of some of its properties. These might for example include cell type, as determined by surface properties; and growth properties or drug sensitivity. Each of these attributes may vary independently in different normal tissues, but the unique combination may not occur together except in one particular type of cancer cell.[65]

Markers would play a secondary role in the broader picture defined largely by molecular biology. The IPT platform, however, could be expanded to include the new molecular biological entities. The FACS–monoclonal antibodies tandem could, for instance, be used to detect both immunologically relevant surface markers and protein products of disease-related genes.

While at the ICRF, Greaves had played an active role in the LRF.[66] The fund's founders had initially felt that a cure for leukemia would quickly be found.[67] In the 1970s, however, fund managers realized that such optimism was somewhat premature and that the LRF should create "a climate for more worthwhile research and a genuine attack . . . on the problems of leukaemia with strong encouragements for new ideas and initiatives." This meant that "large research projects could be entertained as suitable opportunity arose."[68] The idea of funneling more LRF funds into biological research also resulted from lobbying by scientists involved with the organization.[69] In 1979, in a decidedly biomedical turn, the fund's Medical Advisory Panel (MAP) changed its name to Medical and Scientific Advisory Panel (MSAP).[70]

In a 1982 report to the executive council of the fund, Gordon Piller, the LRF director, explained the need to create a "centre for molecular and cellular biology of human leukaemia" by arguing that the future lay in molecular biology. He pointed out that all the meetings co-organized by the LRF, including a world summit meeting held in 1981 in Leeds,

UK, had reached this conclusion, as had articles published in journals ranging from the *New Scientist* to *Lancet*.[71] The proposal to create an LRF center constituted a major change from the policy initially established in 1962. Back then, the MAP had advised against the creation of LRF centers, arguing that the most fruitful way of furthering knowledge on leukemia was to encourage collaboration between existing research centers.[72] Once the LRF decided to go ahead with the new approach, things moved quickly. In June 1982 the LRF director notified the MSAP that the LRF would set up a major new research unit in London to study the molecular and cellular basis of human leukemia. In November of that year, LRF told the panel that the new center would probably be funded solely by the LRF. In early 1983 the panel learned that Greaves would direct the new center at the Institute for Cancer Research at the Royal Marsden Hospital (RMH).

The center opened in 1984 with a total investment of £4 million for the first six years, making it one of the largest leukemia research units in Europe.[73] The new institutional scheme was reinforced by the adoption, in 1985, of an official research development policy hailed as "the beginning of a new and important cycle of expansion." While LRF involvement in clinical work would continue, LRF now wanted to tighten the connection between basic science and the clinic.[74] In 1985, the LRF established an "applied leukaemia and lymphoma diagnostic laboratory" at Oxford.[75] Subsequent years saw the establishment of an LRF Centre for the Study of Viruses in Human Leukaemia in Glasgow and an LRF Centre for Clinical Epidemiology of Human Leukaemia and Related Diseases in Leeds, both inaugurated in early 1987.[76]

When Greaves moved from the ICRF to the new LRF center "for molecular and cellular biology," the question immediately arose of how to dispose of the immunodiagnostic activities. The problem was not new. In 1980 the ICRF committee reviewing the MIL had noticed the dual function of Greaves's laboratory, namely its "fundamental research on the differentiation of the haematopoietic cells" and its status as the national immunodiagnostic laboratory for ALL. The committee had taken note of the decentralization of the diagnostic service—six other centers had been added—but had also mentioned the importance of not severing all links since "invaluable material" for the fundamental research came from involvement in diagnostic work.[77] At the new LRF center, Greaves hoped to jettison the routine IPT work to concentrate on his other research activities. He nonetheless wished to maintain access to reliably characterized clinical material for his research, which meant that a "friendly face" had to "run the show" (i.e., routine IPT).[78] The two goals conflicted.

In 1985, noting that his center had "an expanding interest in the use of monoclonal antibodies, flow cytometry, molecular probes and computer programming in leukaemic diagnosis and monitoring" as part of a number of collaborative studies with colleagues in hospitals in the U.K. and abroad, Greaves was forced to admit that he "face[d] the dilemma that this activity, though undoubtedly interesting and worthwhile, [was] beginning to compete seriously for space and resources with the basic cell biology activities of the lab."[79] He thus proposed that the LRF establish a new molecular diagnostic laboratory in a hospital setting to be run by one of his collaborators. The LRF scientific director replied that the proposed new laboratory would be in competition with the new applied diagnostic laboratory that the LRF had just established at Oxford. Since the LRF needed to use resources effectively, they could only support programs "free of duplication or 'stamp collecting.' "[80] Greaves insisted that he needed to maintain a clinical research/diagnostic activity to ensure an efficient input of leukemic samples and that it was precisely because of its success that the activity now compromised the more biological research.[81]

As a biomedical platform, IPT had become essential to Greaves's clinical work and an input and condition of possibility for Greaves's new molecular biological experimental system. The latter needed blood: reliably characterized blood, i.e., blood that had passed through the IPT platform. We can illustrate the importance of the latter in the following episode. In the past, and as previously mentioned, Greaves's long-standing collaboration with researchers from the ICH at the Hospital for Sick Children in London constituted a major source of experimental material. With the establishment of the new LRF center in 1984, one of Greaves's senior technicians at ICRF had moved to the hospital's hematology department to provide the IPT services previously carried out in Greaves's laboratory. At the time, Greaves had understood that collaborative work and thus the flow of samples would continue. Yet, relatively few samples arrived, a state of affairs that would have stopped his work on ALL were it not for help from Manchester Children's Hospital and old samples in a freezer. Counting on the fact that the LRF supported both the ICH and his center, Greaves requested that LRF's scientific director intervene to mediate what had now developed into a dispute and he listed possible institutional arrangements designed to secure a regular supply of blood.[82]

The ICH clinician rejected the proposed institutional arrangements, noting that the institute took as much blood and bone marrow as possible from patients, but obviously gave priority to local diagnostic demands. The remaining material ended up either in a local research project, the Royal Free Hospital (in charge of IPT for the UKALL clinical trials) or, what little remained, with Greaves.[83] Two years later, the situation remained unchanged. Talking to outside experts during a site visit to his center, Greaves pointed out that he still experienced problems obtaining pediatric material since most of the cases from the Hospital for Sick Children were shipped to the Royal Free Hospital and he thus had to use samples from other parts of the U.K. and from as far away as St. Jude's in Memphis.[84] Correspondence in 1989 indicates that the discussion about the availability of samples for research had become "somewhat acrimonious," thus further underlying the critical role of access to properly characterized blood supplies.[85]

Staying on the Platform

As we have just learned from the debate over the distribution of pediatric blood samples, the Royal Free Hospital received a significant share of that material as part of the MRC UKALL clinical trials. George Janossy, as readers will recall, had left the MIL in 1978 to establish a department of clinical immunology at the Royal Free Hospital. Once there, he pursued a strategy quite different from that of Greaves: instead of focusing on the disease (leukemia), he focused on the platform, using it to analyze a host of other conditions. The difference between these two strategies lay not only in the number and variety of diseases targeted but also in how the platform was used. For instance, several of Janossy's articles after 1980 had titles including terms such as "immunohistologic diagnosis [or analysis, study, characterization, monitoring] of . . . ," indicating the systematic application of the IPT platform to different kinds of biomedical analysis. In addition to studies of the development of normal and leukemic white blood cells, Janossy investigated the therapeutic use of monoclonal antibodies (e.g., in bone marrow transplantation, to purge the bone marrow of leukemia patients of the few remaining cancerous cells, or to prevent graft-versus-host disease, as well as in the prevention of kidney or liver rejection after transplantation), the immunohistology and tissue distribution of subpopulations of T cells and macrophages (as part of the investigation of diseases such as rheumatoid arthritis, myasthenia gravis, biliary cirrhosis, inflammatory bowel disease, leprosy, hepatitis, etc.), and HIV infection and AIDS, a field that in the 1990s would become the almost exclusive focus of Janossy's publications.

After his move to the Royal Free Hospital in 1978, Janossy had been forced to abandon his previous work on leukemia, since Greaves's laboratory continued to perform the IPT work for MRC leukemia clinical trials. Looking for other subjects to which he could apply his experience with the IPT platform and monoclonal antibodies, Janossy took advantage of the Royal Free Hospital's Hemophilia Center (later to prove of strategic value for HIV-related work) and its hepatitis unit. The situation changed in 1984 when Greaves moved to the newly established LRF center and began looking for ways of delegating the basic IPT work to a trustworthy laboratory. His former collaborator was an obvious choice for this task, and so Janossy was able to devote a large part of his time to the MRC UKALL and UKAML trials, an activity that resulted in sixty publications. In 1984, Janossy's laboratory analyzed a total of 350 leukemic samples for 23 hospitals; in 1985 the number rose to 550 samples (including 25 for the UKALL trial) from 43 hospitals, and, in 1986, to 720 samples (including 53 for the UKALL trial) from 49 hospitals.[86] The work used the monoclonal antibody–flow cytometry instantiation of the IPT platform, and, rather than a routine application of standard methods, involved the methodological development of the platform (five-parameter flow cytometry, quantitative flow cytometry), in collaboration with American and European colleagues.

Before transferring the IPT responsibility to Janossy, however, Greaves had initially attempted to partially decentralize the process. As a member of the Working Party on Leukaemia which supervised the trials, Greaves was quickly confronted by those who feared that decentralization would lead to interlaboratory confusion.[87] He countered by maintaining that the withdrawal of his centralized services would not have serious repercussions since "the reagents for a comprehensive and complete diagnosis were now generally available and the tests were relatively simple," and could thus be performed at any participating center. Despite these assurances, other members of the Working Party on Leukaemia raised the specter of a minority (5%) of difficult cases that would create problems.[88] To assuage these fears, Greaves, in collaboration with the U.K. agent of Becton-Dickinson, drafted a document setting up criteria for minimal screening and providing guidelines for difficult cases.[89]

Problems, nonetheless, arose. In 1986, for example, an ad hoc meeting had to be convened to discuss concerns about the validity of the immunological classification of ALL "in view of the discrepancy sometimes observed between the interpretation of cell marker analysis and the clinical features present, and also the occasional different interpretation of results by the trial participants and the CTSU [central trial service unit]."[90] Participants at that meeting learned that, in 1984, 106 (57%) of the 186 patients enrolled in the UKALL VIII had not been immunophenotyped because the assays had not been performed or the results could not be interpreted. The CTSU representative pointed out that the reporting of results varied considerably between participating centers and did not appear to be consistent.

Thus, the MRC moved swiftly to transfer the responsibility for Greaves's former IPT activities to Janossy who was awarded an initial, six-month special grant, beginning in October 1984, and who subsequently applied for, and was granted, three-year extensions of this initial support.[91] "Swiftly," however, does not mean without reservation. In particular, the MRC cell board expressed a number of concerns over the hybrid nature of Janossy's funding applications. According to a reviewer of Janossy's 1990 MRC application, the latter contained "a rather unusual mixture of service work, clinical research and basic research," which made it difficult to judge by "conventional criteria." The issue was not the quality of Janossy's work, which was unanimously praised, but its socioepistemic status: the service work was a vital component of the clinical trial machinery, but other parts of the proposal qualified as, and were indeed explicitly presented as, research. While research activities had to be properly emphasized in order to obtain funding from the MRC cell board, the applicant was also urged by a senior colleague with whom he discussed the most effective way of presenting his application not to be "coy" about the project's service component. The ultimately successful applications were thus the object of a series of careful revisions designed to provide an optimal balance of their different components. The award recommendations, in turn, displayed a keen awareness of these issues, thus bearing witness to the distinct *biomedical* nature of postwar clinical research in general, and the IPT platform in particular.[92]

In addition to transferring responsibilities for MRC IPT to Janossy, the leukemia committee members sought a partial solution to the problem of quality control by sponsoring a series of workshops. The first took place in September 1986 (33 participants), and was followed by other workshops in November 1987 (120 participants), October 1988 (71 participants), and January 1990 (54 participants).[93] The 1990 workshop, for instance, discussed a variety of issues, ranging from discussion of the most important markers, to discussion of their commercial sources, their standardization, and related quality assurance issues. Starting in 1988, the workshops also included "practicals" at the bench and a quiz, targeting those centers that, on the basis of their returns, seemed most in need of training. The workshops thus tried to enforce "reliability" by combining standardization with the necessary flexibility, given that local circumstances such as available equipment, the number of samples, and personal preferences influenced technical choices.[94] While the workshops remained a major strategy for enforcing uniform standards, they occasionally had to be complemented by ad hoc measures. When, for instance, central trial organizers discovered in 1988 that only a small number of centers had performed a newly required IPT assay, they sent a memo to the delinquent centers explaining the value of the assay and urged them to either perform it or to send the samples to Janossy's laboratory where the assay could be performed.[95]

The MRC acute leukemia trials restricted official IPT work to Janossy's laboratory. Routine hospital IPT was another matter. As a result of the flow cytometry companies' strategy of offering free equipment to institutions purchasing their reagents, many hospitals began doing their own IPT work. Janossy thus embarked on the training of hospital personnel. Between 1982 and 1987, Janossy's laboratory trained 90 visitors from 24 countries to perform the immunodiagnosis of leukemia, and between 1984 and 1987 it supplied the necessary reagents to 19 hospitals in London and 47 in the rest of the United Kingdom, while continuing to perform diagnostic work for 24 London hospitals and 39 hospitals in the rest of the country.[96] In contrast, Greaves resisted the introduction of flow cytometry into smaller hospitals since he believed that expert performance required the concentration of IPT in a few centers to ensure, first, that IPT was competently performed at the technical level, and, second, that clinicians could make (clinical) sense of the reports submitted by the IPT service.[97]

For Greaves, the issue of competent technical performance was particularly acute in the case of his international studies. In the 1980s, for instance, in an attempt to identify leukemia-associated environmental or genetic factors, he launched an international collaborative study of changing patterns of incidence of subtypes of childhood ALL. The study, it goes without saying, required use of the IPT platform with the diagnostic markers developed by the LRF team. By 1986, more than six hundred cases of ALL from around the world had been entered into the London database, to be used as a basis for etiologic hypotheses.[98]

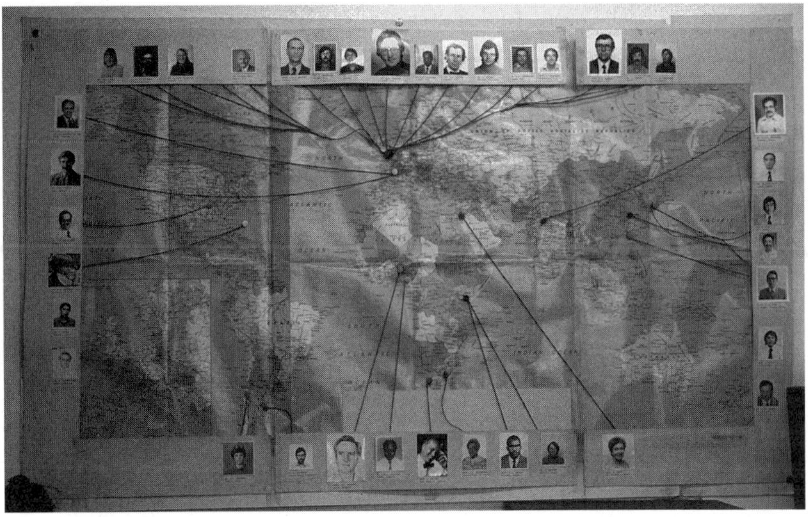

Figure 5.3
World map on the wall of Greaves's office, featuring the location and photograph of his collaborators. (Photograph: A.C.)

Regulations required researchers wanting to join the study to file a detailed report on the laboratory facilities at their disposal and the structure and selection of their patient population.[99] More important, and certainly more effective, was, however, the fact that most of the members of the international team, from South America, Africa, and Asia, had been trained at the London LRF center, as pictured on a map hanging in Greaves' office (see figure 5.3).

The other key regulatory issue, as just mentioned, consisted in providing clinicians with the "correct" diagnostic or prognostic interpretation of the results of IPT. As noted by Greaves, "particularly in the [United] States, with pathology labs doing these things, you send your blood sample to a pathology lab, back comes a report saying it's CD7 positive, CD3 negative and nobody interprets it."[100] To obviate this problem, he engaged in the development of a computerized system designed to provide clinicians with an "expert" interpretation, in terms of relevant diagnostic categories, of laboratory reports.[101] Janossy was similarly aware of the importance of finding proper ways of guiding clinicians through the maze of IPT results. Instead of resorting to computer analysis, however, he sought to establish bridges between IPT and more traditional nosological categories already familiar to clinicians.

For his MRC work, for instance, rather than reporting "complicated 'phenotyping' details" (such as lists or percentages of positive and negative markers), he provided visual information, including color-coding and morphological correlations. We analyze visual representations of IPT results (and their regulation) more closely in chapter 9. We note here that cells analyzed by flow cytometry are often represented as dots on a two-dimensional display. These displays can be organized so as to take into account not only surface markers, but also the "morphological" characteristics of the cells, such as their size and granularity as determined electronically by the cytometer.[102] By color-coding each dot according to cell lineage as determined by phenotype (green for myeloid cells, blue for B cells, red for T cells), by including the morphological information as elicited by the flow cytometer, and by adding the diagnostic category as defined by the FAB classification, it is possible to create a composite picture that provides clinicians with the relevant IPT information *and* links it to familiar nosological categories (see figure 5.4). This is yet another instance of the previously mentioned process by which clinicians relearned morphology on the basis of IPT. As shown again here, morphology and IPT do not necessarily compete. Although sometimes presented as competing methods, they also entertain complex relations of coexistence, cooperation, and mutual dependence.

"Making IPT simpler" presupposed the joint development of flow cytometric equipment and reagents capable of simultaneously measuring several parameters. Clinicians, scientists, and technicians from hospitals, research institutions, and commercial companies participated in this collective, international endeavor.[103] A manager of a flow cytometry company noted that in the course of this process, "we have always seen the situation where the biology will always move to fill in whatever the hardware is capable of doing, we have never been to the point where the hardware is so far ahead of the biology that there is no use for a parameter that we put on the instrument."[104] As an expression of a technologically deterministic understanding of the process, the speaker suggests that hardware comes first and that "biology" will subsequently and inevitably "move in to fill" the new hardware capabilities. Yet, as we have tried to show in this chapter, this linear evolution exists only insofar as the hardware in question is already a component of a biomedical platform.

Extending the hardware capabilities of the platform has as a consequence, but is also a consequence or an extension of, for instance,

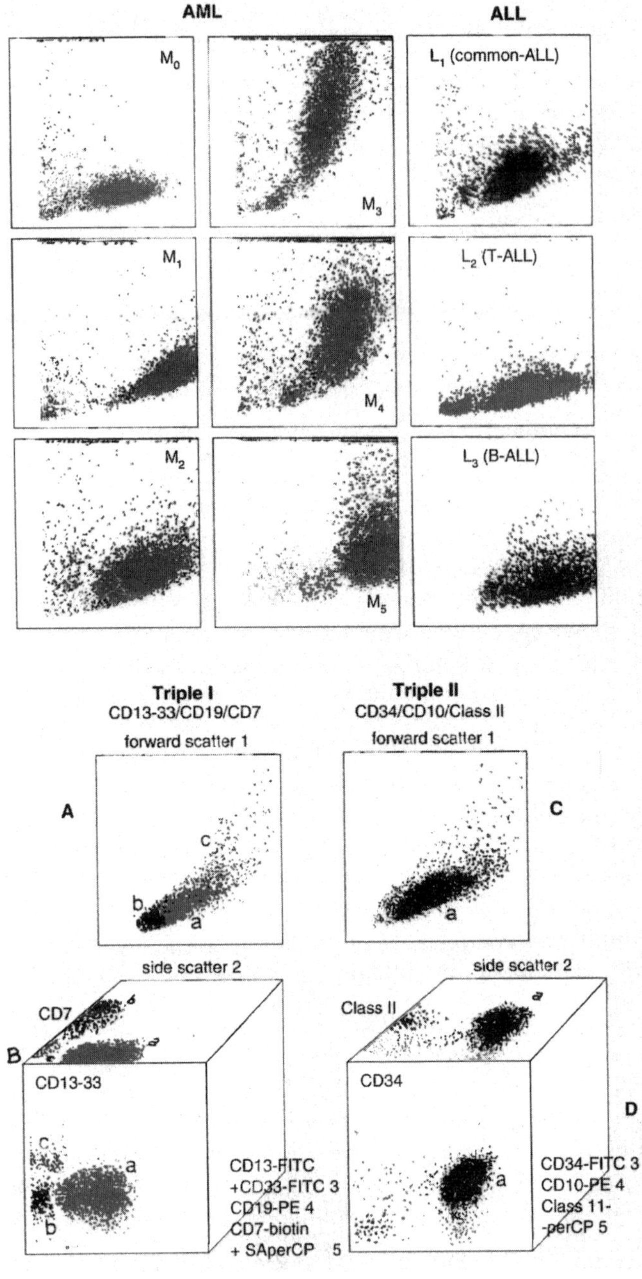

Figure 5.4
Visual representation of patient assessment results for the Medical Research Council clinical trials, displaying both immunophenotypic and morphological information (original in color). (From Janossy, unpublished MRC grant report [c. 1994]. Reprinted with kind permission from Dr. G. Janossy.)

clinical correlations. Among the examples of clinical projects generated by Janossy's revamped IPT platform, two bear mention: the detection of minimal residual disease, namely detection of leukemic cells after intensive chemotherapy (an early indication of relapse), and the detection of minimal leukemic contamination of bone marrow transplants used in the treatment of leukemia. Both of these projects participated in a larger European concerted action project linking six laboratories from five different countries.[105]

Projects such as these constitute typical uses of the IPT platform. The new multiparameter hardware, for example, developed into a system capable of simultaneously detecting several markers. On this basis, and for the express purpose of detecting residual disease, one could thus elicit unique antigenic profiles showing "aberrant antigenic expression" that distinguished leukemic cells from their normal counterparts.[106] In keeping with the elision of the normal/pathological distinction that, as we have seen, accompanied the development of IPT as a *biomedical* platform, "aberrant antigenic expression" now meant "aberrant" expression of "normal" antigens. One of the consequences of accepting the notion of an aberrant expression of normal antigens has been to identify minimal residual disease by investigating the combination of immunological markers in a *quantitative* manner.[107]

Starting in the mid-1980s, staying on the platform took on a renewed sense of urgency as several key figures who had participated in the events we have just analyzed turned their attention to AIDS. IPT's immediate utility drew on the fact that the platform was constitutive of CD4 cells whose depletion, as previously noted, marks the progress of the disease. By then, the IPT platform had left the restricted circle of researchers we have been following in this chapter. Indeed, one of the key issues for AIDS-related IPT and its circulation beyond Western laboratories has been the development of "affordable" CD4+ cell counting for developing countries, a challenge taken up by, among others, Janossy.[108] In keeping with this change of scene, the next two chapters will replace the diachronic approach adopted in this and the preceding chapter with a more structural view of the extended operation of the platform.

6

The Core of the Platform: Markers

In the preceding chapters we described the emergence and initial success of the immunophenotyping (IPT) platform. We now break the platform down into its component parts and discuss some of the processes that allow these parts to function together in clinical situations. Before going any further, note that dividing the platform into separable, functioning parts shows that most of the components can be described as *activities* that consist of "organizing markers," "sourcing material," "preparing specimens," "detecting markers," "counting markers," "displaying data," "interpreting data," "diagnosing diseases," or "isolating syndromes." Since a number of instruments or devices can perform these functions or tasks, the platform itself can be instantiated in several ways. There are thus two limits to this functional description. First of all, it leads to an endless description of the many possible instances of the platform. We therefore need some order other than function. Second, given a purely functional definition of platform components, readers may rightly object that if all the parts of the platform can be described in terms of function, then they all have substitutes. But if each and every part can be alternatively described, then one might legitimately ask: wherein lies the innovation? Is it not merely organizational and thus disconnected from the material components of the platform? What, in other words, is new and special about the IPT platform?

As we have already pointed out, there is a component of the platform for which there can be no substitute: the cell-surface marker. In particular, while one cannot perform IPT with markers alone, they are nonetheless common to all instances of IPT. So, although the platform cannot be reduced to markers, the latter are essential to its existence. Note that markers are more than a notion or concept. They exist in a material sense as standardized reagents (the so-called CD reagents, already mentioned in chapter 5, to which we return below) and as

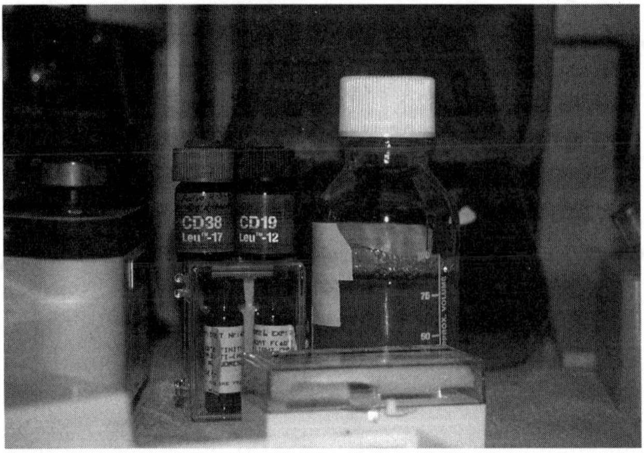

Figure 6.1
Markers in a bottle: CD38 and CD19 on a laboratory bench. (Photograph: A.C.)

procedures and guidelines surrounding their proper use. To be blunt: markers are bottled concepts (see figure 6.1). We can thus impose a minimum of order on our description of platform components and divide them into the essential or core components—the markers—and the peripherals—all those items necessary for the conduct of IPT but which lack the specificity of the markers in the sense that, for any particular peripheral item, one can find, in principle, a substitute. In chapter 7 we will look at two major types of the IPT platform based on differing peripherals: microscope/slide-based peripherals and flow cytometry–based peripherals.

In this chapter, we focus on markers. They are more than the novel component of the platform, as they also provide the basis for comparisons within and between laboratories and thus function as a source of platform stability. In this respect, they do not exist in isolation, but in relation to each other or, in other words, as part of a system of markers. More precisely, before clinicians and researchers could use the markers on a routine basis, they had to standardize the two constituents of the markers: the antibodies and the sites on the cell surface that they recognize. To do so, researchers involved in the biological and clinical study of cell-surface markers set up an international regulatory system at the beginning of the 1980s to collate, manage, and name the markers. This system, referred to these days as the CD (for "clusters of differentiation") system, has since grown to the extent that the cell-surface markers used in IPT are now a subset of a larger system of markers. In particular, the CD system now includes not only the original cell-surface structures that identified different stages of normal and pathological cell development, but also a number of additional structures unrelated to the process of cellular differentiation and development. The new structures include, for example, those that participate in the adhesion of one cell to another or in communication between cells.

In addition to requiring standardized reagents, routine IPT also demands that such reagents be readily available. And, indeed, markers circulate as commercial products—namely, as industrially manufactured, ready-to-use antibodies—that mark cell surfaces. The easy availability and standardized nature of these reagents allow for the previously mentioned interlaboratory comparisons and retrospective studies that would otherwise be impossible. Figure 6.2 shows laboratory posters listing commercial preparations for each component of the CD family. The proliferation of commercial sources of CD markers resulted in problems of comparison between the various studies using them. The establishment of equivalences—a process to which we return in detail below—eliminated these problems by creating identities between different products. These arrangements were not ex ante standards imposed on already existing products. Rather, as we will see, they were constitutive of these reagents qua reagents. In turn, the amount of "reified theory," to use a Bachelardian term, and the number of universally recognized conventions borne by these reagents are such that their use in some form easily qualifies as an instantiation of the IPT platform.

The first commercially produced markers—the first members of the CD system—differentiated between subsets of T cells. Before turning to the development and structure of the system, however, we describe the process that led from the production of these T-cell subsets in the laboratory to the market. We do so for a number of reasons. First of all, such a description necessarily details the amount of work condensed into these biomedical reagents. Second, given that we have already analyzed the constitution of B-cell markers and their clinical and research applications, a discussion of the production and use of markers for T cells and their subsets will complete our immunological tableau. In addition, however, to reinforcing the themes raised in the previous chapters, studying the development of T-cell subsets and their markers allows us to discuss actors and arrangements absent in Greaves's case. In particular, the production of markers for T-cell subsets brought together

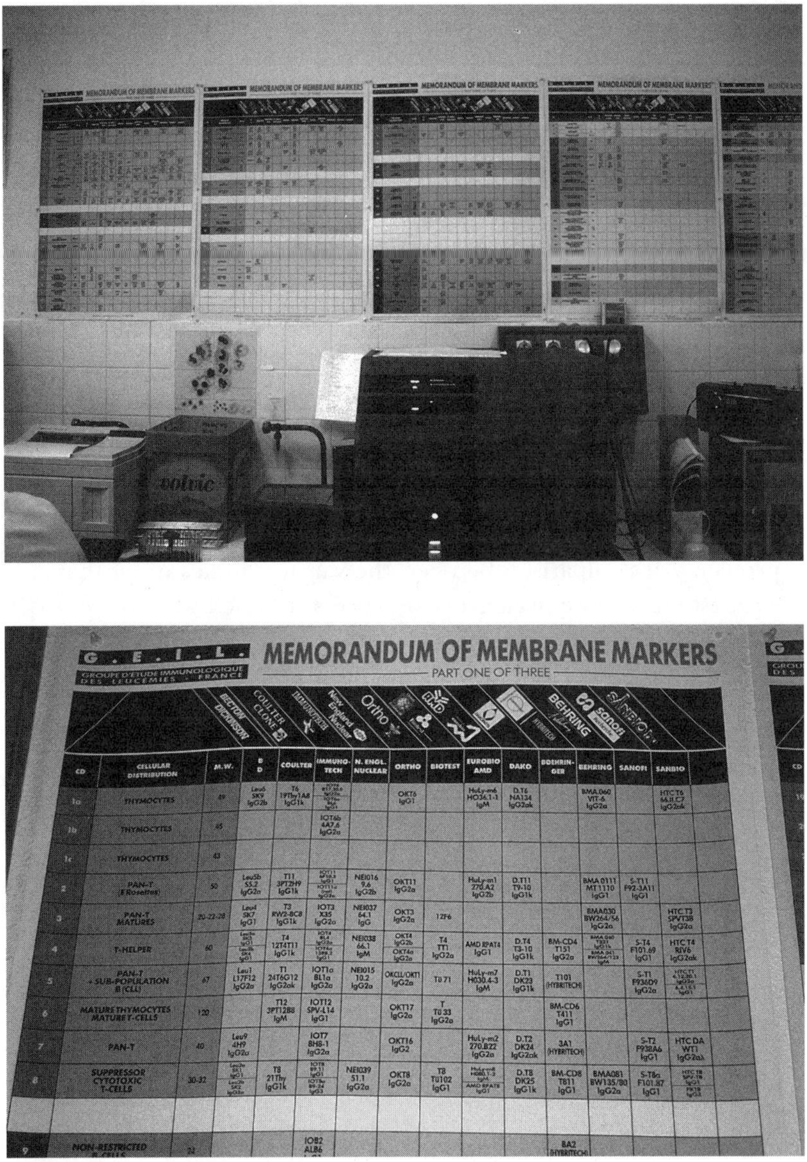

(*a*)

(*b*)

Figure 6.2

(*a* and *b*) Posters showing equivalences between commercially produced marker reagents. The machine beneath the posters on the wall (*a*) is a Coulter flow cytometer. (Photographs: A.C.)

previously unrelated networks of commercial biotechnologists, mouse researchers, and human researchers in a new field of biomedical research. In other words, we will see some of the many ways in which modern biomedicine in its multiple, mutually constitutive forms—in the laboratory, in the biotech factory, and at the bedside—can be defined as the crossing of boundaries between the normal and the pathological.

Constituting T-Cell Markers in Mice

Before describing the laboratory work carried out on T-cell markers, let us recall that by the beginning of the 1970s, immunologists generally believed that, unlike B cells, which were devoted to antibody production, T cells could perform a variety of functions. For instance, they could destroy other cells such as those introduced by surgeons' grafts and by biologists experimenting with transplanted cancer cells, or they could cause allergic ("delayed hypersensitivity") reactions when challenged with the appropriate substances. Moreover, and in keeping with the emerging notion of an immune *system* consisting of interacting cellular and humoral components,[1] researchers knew by the mid-1960s that T cells cooperated with B cells in the production of antibodies,[2] and, by 1970, that T cells controlled the immune system to the extent that they could, ultimately, suppress the immune response.[3] Resorting to a rich metaphorical language, immunologists referred to the T cells that performed these operations as killer, cooperator, helper, and suppressor cells according to the function carried out. Alternatively, they spoke of T cells as having helper, killer, and suppressor functions.[4] Immunologists generally believed, in this respect, that the same T cells performed different functions when called upon to do so.

The function performed depended upon the context (experimental or, by extrapolation, natural) within which the cell was found or found itself. If a B cell looking for help came across a T cell, for instance, then the T cell activated its helper function. If, on the other hand, a cancer cell bearing a cancer antigen came looking for trouble, then the T cell activated its killer function. It is true that "Nobody ever said it that way, nobody ever said T cells [could] do everything"[5] but, then again, nobody said they could not. This is why when, in 1975, Harvey Cantor and Ted Boyse explicitly rejected the hypothesis that a given T cell could perform all sort of functions, they subtitled their paper with the following affirmation: "The Generation of Functionally Distinct T-Cell Subclasses Is a Differentiative Process Independent of Antigen."[6] In other words, the

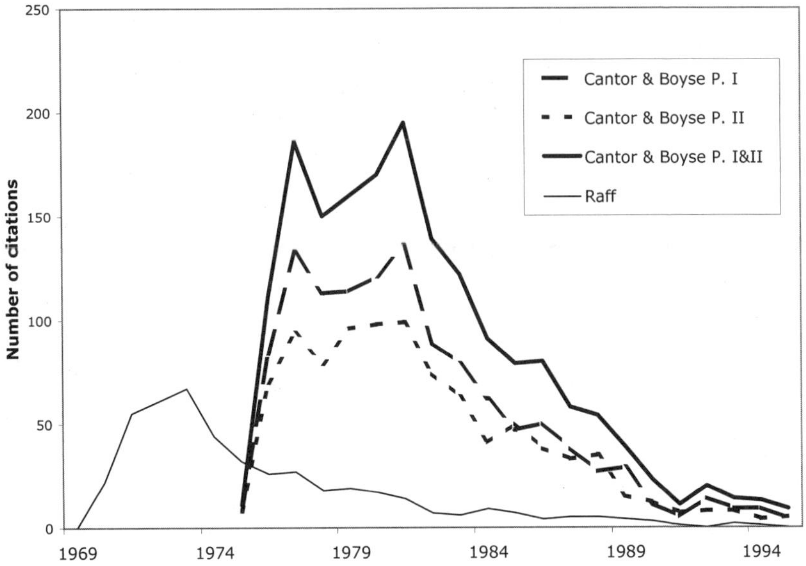

Figure 6.3
Number of citations to Cantor and Boyse's 1975 article "Functional Subclasses of T Lymphocytes Bearing Different Ly Antigens." The article was published in two parts: the diagram shows the number of papers citing either part I, part II, or both. As a comparison, the diagram reproduces the number of citations received by the Raff article as shown in figure 4.2. (Data source: *Science Citation Index.*)

existence of various kinds of T cells each carrying out a different, specialized task predated the actual performance of that task and the antecedent encounter with an antigen. The paper became a citation classic (see figure 6.3).

Readers may by now suspect that where one finds a differentiative process involving human cells, there is no doubt some "marker" signaling that process. And they would be right. Cantor and Boyse did indeed separate the functionally distinct subclasses on the basis of T-cell surface antigens. In addition, they correlated different markers with the different biological functions that emerged along the developmental pathway. Both of these claims were considerable novelties. Originally termed Ly antigens in the mouse, the corresponding markers were later defined as CDs in humans. Helper cells became CD4 cells, whereas suppressor cells became CD8 cells. Now, we saw in chapter 4 that Boyse and Old had produced the original differentiation antigens back in 1968. We can therefore ask, why did Boyse and Cantor not correlate the different T-cell functions with the different antigens until 1975?

Part of the answer lies in the fact that the antigens belonged to pathology, whereas the functions belonged to biology. In particular, coming from pathology and tumor antigens, Boyse and Old's explanation of differentiation, transplantation, and tumor antigens had had to overcome a pathobiological paradox. Differentiation antigens signaled stages in cellular differentiation and also appeared on fully developed cells. The antigens appearing on tumor and transplanted cells, on the other hand, triggered an immune response leading to the destruction of the cells bearing the antigens. Since transplanted cells are just normal cells in an unusual situation, it had to be assumed that the antigens on the transplanted cells were of the same nature or kind as the normal, differentiation antigens. How, then, was it possible for the immune system to distinguish between colonies of normal cells and colonies of transplanted or cancer cells since they both had the same kind of markers?[7]

One possible solution to the paradox was to isolate additional variables such as number and location when characterizing the antigens. The same antigen could then generate two different patterns (signals or marks) based on the number and location of the antigen on the cell surface and thus be seen as foreign and destroyed, or domestic and ignored. Boyse called this form of identification "configurational specificity"[8] as opposed to antigenic specificity. At bottom, the receptors were the same; only their quantity and arrangement made the difference. The idea of configurational specificity, quickly endorsed by other researchers in the field, created a short-lived need for a topographic visualization of the cell surface. Martin Raff had taken the initial step in this direction by developing a technique that coupled an iron-containing protein with antibody, thus allowing one to view the antibody bound to the cell surface under an electron microscope.[9] Seligmann and Preud'homme used fluorescent antibodies and a fluorescence microscope to visualize the "patterns" of antibodies on the surface of lymphocytes.[10] Boyse and his associates developed yet another electron microscopy technique to visualize antigens on the surface of mouse sperm.[11] Pernis and coworkers' call for "a complete mapping of the lymphocyte surface, with regard to the relative location of the immunoglobulin receptor" was symptomatic of the kind of work that would be required to carry out this visualization of the cell surface.[12] Cantor and Boyse's argument that cell surfaces in general and T-cell surfaces in particular differed qualitatively rather than quantitatively and spatially, however, rendered the program obsolete. Separating functional subsets could now be carried out on the basis of sets of specific antibodies rather than on the basis of a visual pattern.

The research that led to the correlation of structure and function in T cells did not flow directly from the claim that T cells had different functions and that T cells had distinctive markers on their surfaces. Nor did it follow directly from the availability of the equipment that would ultimately be used routinely to sort functionally distinct subclasses of T cells on the basis of cell-surface markers. In fact, despite the availability of both the biological information and the scientific equipment, putting biological structure and function together required yet another detour through pathology and the use of the "sick" as a variable within several experimental systems that spanned two continents and four different institutions in the period 1970–75.

Harvey Cantor carried out the initial steps in this line of work in one of the core institutions of the U.S. biomedical system, the National Institutes of Health (NIH) or, more precisely, at the National Institute for Allergy and Infectious Diseases (NIAID). Cantor's work originated in pathology both in the sense that he used pathological material—a line of mice that after the age of 4 months spontaneously developed anemia and, subsequently, lymphoid neoplasms—and in the sense that the experimental system he used required distinguishing between the healthy and the sick.[13] The experiments themselves consisted in harvesting lymphocytes from the spleens of sick and healthy mice and comparing the capacity of those cells to generate an immune response. Somewhat unsurprisingly, the healthy lymphocytes provoked a fivefold greater response than the sick lymphocytes. But the system also produced an unexpected result. Mixing the sick and the healthy cells together prior to injection gave a greater response than injecting the two types of lymphocytes separately.[14] In a second series of experiments, while retaining an assay system firmly grounded in pathology, Cantor and his colleague Richard Asofsky switched to healthy mice, transferring to biology the conclusion that they had drawn from pathology: there must be "two [distinct biological] cell types."[15] But, as Harvey Cantor recalled, "it took us about two more years before we could say with certainty that they were both T cells."[16]

In 1970, after the mouse experiments, Cantor left the NIH and traveled to England as an NIH fellow to work in Avery Mitchison's laboratory at Mill Hill (by now a familiar place to our readers; see chapter 3). There he met another familiar figure, Martin Raff, who enrolled him in his emerging "cell-surface" immunology. The two of them set about looking for antibodies that would separate mature from immature T lymphocytes. Note that they were thus not looking for a way to separate mature T cells into functional subsets. Rather, by adopting an anatomical and developmental division, they sought to separate T cells in the peripheral blood from the cells in the thymus (known as thymocytes) that gave rise to them. To reach that goal, they initially used the two better-known antisera produced so far: Old and Boyse's thymus leukemia (TL) antisera and Reif's theta antisera (see chapter 3). These tools, however, enabled them to only partially correlate their anatomical and developmental division with cell-surface characteristics: TL-positive cells appeared only in the thymus, whereas theta-positive cells appeared in both the thymus and peripheral tissue. How, then, could one distinguish T cells from thymocytes? In other words, as Cantor and Raff explicitly recognized, "Clearly it would be helpful to have a surface antigenic marker which is present on the T-like cells and absent from immature thymocytes." As luck would have it, "Recently, we have accidentally stumbled upon such a marker."[17]

The new antiserum allowed Raff and Cantor to complete the anatomical breakdown and to map the synergistic effects discovered by Cantor and Asofsky onto a speculative developmental scheme that went like this: there are two populations of lymphocytes. The first, T2, is young and immature and lives in the thymus. On contact with an antigen, T1 becomes T2 or thymus-independent and acquires the properties of being long-lived and capable of recirculation. Most important: "T_2 cells alone are responsible for the T-lymphocytes component of the immune response seen after overt primary or secondary immunization."[18] Note that this scheme did not by itself call into question the belief that, prior to immunization, all T cells were capable of performing a variety of functions. It did, however, meet with some puzzlement, as illustrated by a contemporary exchange between Martin Raff and James L. Gowans at a conference on immunologic intervention.[19] Gowans, the chairman of the session and originator of the notion of T-cell circulation, found it difficult to distinguish the new model from the old. After having repeatedly questioned Raff, he finally confessed that "I must admit to still being confused about these T1, T2 and T3 lymphocytes. I assume they bear no relation to the old scheme of an immature lymphocyte entering the thymus, a mature one leaving it, and the progeny of the latter being generated by antigen stimulation in peripheral lymphoid tissue."[20] In response Raff admitted that a good deal of work remained: "We have not attempted to place the different immunological functions of T cells . . . into the scheme. However, if the hypothesis has any validity, it should not be difficult to fill in the gaps."[21]

The difficulty in "filling in the gaps" resided mainly in the fact that the populations were "more or less separable."[22] As it stood, the only populations that had been separated were the mature and the immature, whose existence had not been doubted. Immunologists still had to learn how to separate, for example, helper populations from killer populations, and they thus complained that "recognition of the diverse functions and interactions of T cells has not been matched by the development of techniques for identifying and separating the different T-cell subpopulations involved."[23] The availability of technical means for separating these various functional subsets appeared to be a necessary, although not sufficient, condition for ensuring their existence qua stable, reproducible biomedical entities. And, once again, researchers had a choice between a quantitative or a qualitative strategy, often hesitating between these two possibilities, as when stating that "subsets of T cells with different immunological functions may exhibit qualitative or quantitative differences in surface antigens."[24] They could also, in each case, opt for a more or less technology-intensive approach.

Stanford immunologist Len Herzenberg embarked on what was decidedly the high-tech route and he did so by initially endorsing a quantitative approach. He had a "cell-separator" or, more precisely, a "fluorescence-activated cell sorter" (FACS), that he openly contrasted with the then-current separation techniques such as antigen-coated columns, by claiming that "ours is an engineering approach."[25] When, still looking for a solution to the separation problem, Cantor left Mill Hill in 1972 and moved to Stanford Medical School as a resident, he initiated a collaboration with Herzenberg's group. The latter had begun analyzing T cells with the FACS in 1971, with a view toward standardizing and quantifying these entities.[26] As noted in a 1975 review article, "The FACS analyzes a cell preparation with respect to two parameters in a quantitative rather than a qualitative manner."[27] In line with the quantitative techniques developed by Raff, Boyse, and Seligmann, the Stanford team had based its T-cell studies with the FACS on the amount of fluorescent antibody absorbed (the "quantitation of cell antigens") and not the kind of antibody to which the fluorescent molecules were attached (the detection of novel cell antigens). What the FACS offered in this instance was not the means of producing new entities but the means of quantifying a known phenomenon.[28]

As far as the sorting aspect of this line of work was concerned, the Herzenberg team, using the FACS and antibodies to the theta antigen, had managed to separate the T cells from the other lymphocytes such as B cells, but at no time prior to Cantor's arrival had they produced any new T-cell subsets nor had they construed the cell-surface markers as signs of immunological function.[29] Herzenberg's collaboration with Cantor did little to change this situation despite the fact that, as previously noted, one could retrospectively argue that all the equipment necessary for change was present. Rather than look for an antibody to subdivide the T cells marked by theta antigen, Herzenberg and Cantor used the FACS in a quantitative manner, once again sorting the T cells based on the amount of fluorescent antibody absorbed: the "dull" (less) and the "bright" (more).[30] At this point, Herzenberg and Cantor parted ways in two senses. Cantor moved to Boston where he encountered an antibody that would qualitatively discriminate between T-cell subclasses. Herzenberg remained in California and pursued his quantitative strategy of using the FACS to measure physical parameters such as amount of antibody absorbed.[31]

Once in Boston where he had moved to take up a position at Harvard Medical School, Cantor learned that Ted Boyse had produced yet another line of T-cell antibodies, the Ly series. Entering into collaboration, within a year Cantor and Boyse isolated the first T-cell functional subsets in mice using Boyse's Ly antisera. On the surface, the papers simply described a technique for separating different classes of T cells defined according to their function (helping, killing) using antigens that appeared on the cell surface as markers of these functions. Cantor and Boyse did more, however, than show that the Ly antigens were "markers." They used the markers to choose between two alternative schemes for the generation of the diversity of T-cell function. Figure 6.4, taken from their landmark 1975 article, neatly summarizes these competing accounts. The article presented a strong case favoring the second alternative, namely, that "subclasses of T cells are programmed for different T-cell functions during differentiation *before* contact with antigen."[32] Thus, and this is the crux of the matter, by showing that the marks existed before the T cells established contact with antigen, they demonstrated, in effect, that the T-cell functions were preprogrammed and not a function of context. This, in turn, established the markers not simply as means for identifying cells, but also as significant signs of function. In mice. Whether an equivalent phenomenon could be found in humans remained an open question, but not for long.

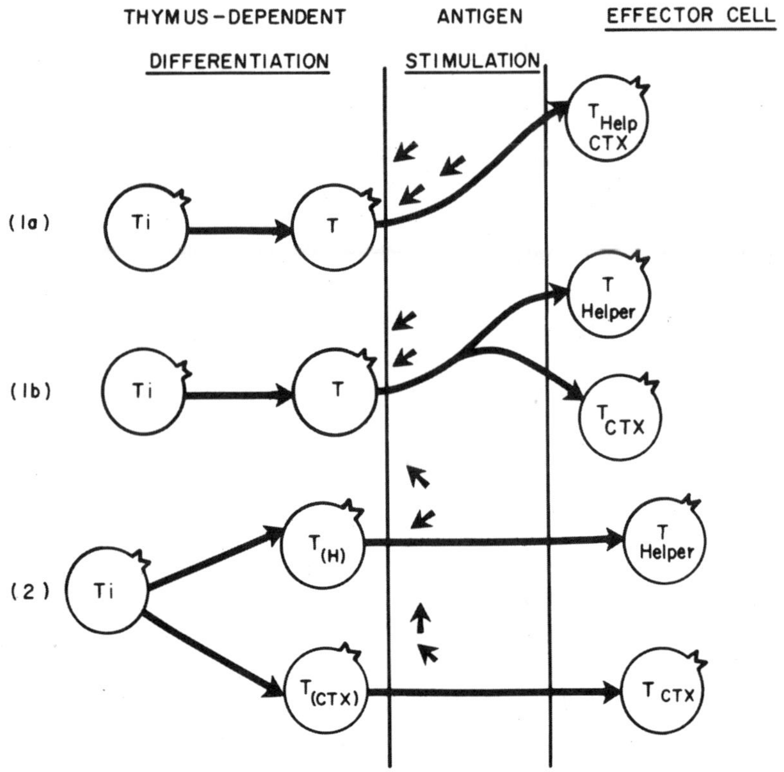

Figure 6.4
Alternative schemes of the generation of the diversity of T-cell function. (From Cantor and Boyse, "Functional Subclasses of T Lymphocytes Bearing Different Ly Antigens I," 1378. Reprinted by copyright permission of The Rockefeller University Press.)

Constituting T-Cell Markers in Humans

In biomedical research, the mouse/human distinction has come to epitomize the ambiguous relations between the laboratory and the clinic insofar as it symbolizes the presence of different sociotechnical networks that only partially, yet necessarily—insofar as humans remain the biomedical horizon—overlap.[33] The distinction can be expressed in terms of rivalry and competition, as when an interviewee claimed that, before the mid-1970s, "mouse immunologists" had "always thought that the human immunologists were a bunch of losers taking care of patients."[34] It can also be expressed in terms of experimental opportunities or the lack thereof. For instance, research performed on humans obeys different temporalities and regulations than research on mice: reproduction times are not the same, humans cannot be too openly experimented upon; in short, ethical, technical, and practical considerations result in different experimental configurations. In this book, however, we are interested less in the boundaries that separate than in the interfaces that connect, for biomedical work commonly travels back and forth between humans and mice, often within a single laboratory, and the establishment of new platforms depends upon the successful development of these articulations.

In 1972, Stuart F. Schlossman, an expert in hematologic malignancies working at the Beth Israel Hospital, an institution affiliated with Harvard Medical School, moved to Harvard's Dana Farber Cancer Center, after spending the previous year in England on sabbatical in (yet again!) Av Mitchison's laboratory. There he had met Harvey Cantor, whom he subsequently invited, in 1973, to join the Dana Farber. As suggested by his choice of location for a sabbatical, Schlossman shared the growing interest in the clinical role of B and T cells. He had already worked, both with mouse and human material, on the separation of these two kinds of lymphocytes, even giving his name to a device—the Schlossman column—specially designed for this purpose. Back in Boston, he began searching for ways to overcome a key problem of research on human B and T cells: contrary to Cantor and Boyse, he could not use standardized, genetically identical organisms such as inbred mice as experimental material.[35] How, then, could he obtain purified sources of experimental material? The solution Schlossman devised consisted in setting up a large human cell bank containing, inter alia, samples of cells from patients with forms of leukemia known to express relatively homogeneous lines of T cells. Schlossman alerted pathologists "from all over the city" and they began sending "wonderful samples . . . , exciting different kinds of leukemias, lymphomas," so that, in the end he could say:

> I have twenty thousand leukemic samples frozen away or something like that. We used to be on call, from the early 70's on, for every accident that happened in the city of Boston to get a spleen if there was rupture, to get an extra lymph node of someone. I paid technicians to cover for seven days and seven nights a week, we had people available that would be on call. Because I never believed that we should ever miss a sample in the city. And we had people standing outside of the operating room, when they were doing cardiac operations so we could get a piece of thymus, that was prior to the monoclonal antibodies, so we would do those sort of things.[36]

This systematic collection of "experiments of nature" acted as a substitute for inbred laboratory animals.

In 1973, Schlossman coauthored a grant proposal whose principal investigator was Emil T. Frei, the newly elected director of the Dana Farber and a pioneer of leukemia combination chemotherapy.[37] In his section of the proposal, using a trope by then widespread in cancer research circles on both sides of the Atlantic (see chapter 3), Schlossman proposed "to translate developments in basic immunology, generated here [Harvard] and elsewhere, to clinical problems in cancer emphasizing both immunodiagnosis and immunotherapy."[38] The clinical part of the translation process sought the improvement of therapy through the refinement of diagnosis. As a member of the Acute Leukemia Group B, one of the original cooperative oncology groups that controlled clinical cancer trials in the United States, Schlossman worked with a definition of "complete hematologic remission" of acute lymphocytic leukemia (ALL) that required "bone marrow containing 5% or less leukemia blasts." Biologists use the term "blast" (from the Greek *blastos,* meaning germ or offspring) in a generic sense to designate immature or precursor cells. In the context of leukemia, it refers to the cancerous cells that, according to the now superseded pathological view, had regressed to an immature stage, or, according to the new immunological understanding, had stopped maturing at an early stage and had entered a phase of uncontrolled proliferation. The problem with this diagnosis of remission lay in the determination of what cells fell into the "blast" category and in the morphological techniques used to distinguish normal immature cells from leukemic blasts. Given the morphological approach then in use, questionable cases arose "not infrequently."[39] Thus, Schlossman found himself in a similar, although not identical, diagnostic situation as Greaves and developed a similar aspiration: cell-surface immunology would replace an outmoded cellular morphology and its attendant ambiguities.

Unsurprisingly, given the biomedical nature of the grant application, the "translation process" proposed by Schlossman worked in both directions: basic immunology mirrored the clinic. On the one hand, the grant proposal drew upon work done on animals, in particular the guinea pig, to support the contention that similar work could be done in humans.[40] On the other hand, Schlossman planned to use the T-cell antiserum described in the cited animal work[41] to separate functional (biological) subclasses of T cells by measuring the "density" of the antigens on the cell surface.[42] Moreover, while Schlossman obviously had no doubt about the functional plurality of T-cell subpopulations, he nonetheless believed that their cell-surface differences resulted from variations in the number or quantity of "determinants," i.e., their density, not their quality. Thanks to his connection with Cantor, Schlossman had become aware of the potential usefulness of Herzenberg's FACS, a commercial version of which had recently been produced by Becton-Dickinson under a license from Stanford University. In order to pursue his density measurement project, he requested a FACS, a momentous decision, since, as he would later recall, "the big difference between progress of what was done in the mouse and humans was that everything we did was related to the bloody flow cytometer."[43] In the meantime, Schlossman received the grant and the sixth FACS ever produced.[44]

Back on the clinical side of the proposed translation, Schlossman hoped to be able to quantify the determination of "complete hematologic remission" from ALL and thus reduce clinical ambiguity. As we saw, Greaves, the biologist, had found cALLA (common acute lymphoblastic leukemia antigen), an antigen that allowed for the clinical quantification of ALL cells, without removing, however, all uncertainty surrounding the complete remission diagnosis. Schlossman, the clinician, found in the course of the investigation something that may have had greater biological significance than Greaves's cALLA: antibodies that distinguished between functional subclasses of T cells, namely human helper and cytotoxic/killer T-cell populations. Doing so required joining forces with a commercial biotechnology company in a productive effort that combined Schossman's collection of human pathology samples with the recently developed technology of monoclonal antibodies. The result was of obvious clinical significance, but it also provided human immunologists with an edge over mouse immunologists: "We [the human and the mouse immunologists] started out at a similar time and I would argue strongly that ultimately they [the mouse immunologists] haven't caught up with us because once the [monoclonal antibody] technology became an available tool, then we ran away with the thing."[45]

In his initial attempt to separate functional subclasses of T cells, Schlossman had pursued the following strategy. Take a cell sample from patients suffering from immunological disorders known to be a T-cell disorder: the sample will presumably consist largely (though not exclusively) of T cells. Inject the human cells into rabbits. Take the antiserum raised in the rabbit, mix it in with a normal lymphocyte sample, and test the resulting mixture to see if it performs one of the known functions of T cells. In principle, the antibodies should have selectively depleted the mixture, leaving only specific lymphocyte subpopulations. By 1975, Schlossman had separated T and B cells and little else.[46] Then, one day in late 1975, Schlossman walked into an unusually purified source of human T cells. In his own words:

I was still practicing medicine. I walked down the ward and there was a patient of mine by the name of H.S. and he had what was known as mycosis fungoides [a variety of lymphoma] and he had these big red lumps on his skin and he had a hundred thousand white count lymphocytes. I said, that's going to be a T-cell leukemia, because the only cell that gets into the skin, puts red bumps on the skin is a T cell that has migrated. It looks like a hypersensitivity reaction. So I said to Robby Evans [a collaborator], let's get a pot of H.S.'s cells. . . . And we did that and what we got was what was then the TH2 antiserum. And the TH2 antiserum proved to be CD8, and the TH2 negative, which still reacted, was CD4.[47]

But that was in retrospect and at this juncture the commercial alliance proved crucial. The problem lay not in the experimental system or in the claims generated by the system. Indeed, using a purified rabbit polyclonal antiserum against H.S.'s cells and the FACS, Schlossman's group was able to claim to have isolated the first human T-cell subclasses early in 1976, barely a year after they had been isolated in the mouse.[48] The problem lay in sustaining the claim. A year after the publication of their initial findings, Schlossman's group produced a second rabbit serum that added confusion rather than clarity to the nature and status of the original antibodies.[49] Although subsequently referred to as the "cleanest antibody that we had ever made,"[50] the new rabbit antihuman T-cell serum pointed to "two distinct drawbacks to the method."[51] Identically prepared antisera did not produce identical results in terms of the functional subclasses isolated.[52] Moreover, the group suspected further variation within a single antiserum. In sum, whatever the Schlossman team had isolated in 1976, it was not easily reproducible. At this point, Schlossman crossed paths with Patrick Kung, a researcher hired by Ortho Diagnostic Systems. (a subsidiary of Johnson & Johnson) to work on T cells.

After obtaining a PhD in cell biology at the University of California, Berkeley and a three-year postdoc in David Baltimore's laboratory at MIT from 1974 to 1976, Kung had switched to industry, joining Ortho in 1977 after a brief, ten-month intermezzo at Du Pont de Nemours. While Baltimore's laboratory was then known for its work on tumor viruses, Kung, during his postdoctoral stay at MIT, had worked on T-cell differentiation in leukemia, lymphoma, and myeloma, investigating the role of an enzyme known as TdT (terminal deoxynucleotidyl transferase) as a T-cell marker.[53] Moreover, using Baltimore's dense scientific network (he was a recent cowinner of the 1975 Nobel Prize), Kung had insider knowledge of the newly established technique for producing monoclonal antibodies.

Kung's background turned out to be quite useful at Ortho where he had begun working with Gideon Goldstein on a project dealing with immunoregulation and the thymic hormone. At the time of Kung's arrival, Schlossman was already a consultant with Ortho and he had suggested that Ortho develop antisera against human T cells. By allowing one to dissect lymphocytes into subsets, the antisera would have been useful tools both for Goldstein's work and as potential products for an emerging clinical market. In other words, following Boyse's work in the mouse and Schlossman's work in humans, it had become clear that sera distinguishing different functional classes of T cells could be produced and that they had a potential clinical interest.

Instead of following Schlossman's more traditional approach of purifying antisera, Kung had taken a chance and decided to produce the anti–T cell antibodies using the new monoclonal antibody technique. We say "chance" because, at the time, even though initial reports on the production of monoclonal antibodies against various antigens had been published, many researchers still doubted that the procedure would work for all kinds of antigens and that satisfactory monoclonal antibodies could thus be made against T cells. Moreover, even if the technique did work, there was uncertainty or even skepticism concerning whether the hybrid cells (known as hybridomas) used to produce the new kind of antibodies would prove to be stable (an important question for industry).[54] Kung's approach was doubly innovative: not only did he opt for hybridoma technology but, in order to perform the fastidious yet crucial task of screening thousands of hybrid cells, he used a flow cytometer developed and marketed by Ortho under the trade name Cytofluorograph. His bet paid off when, in 1978, he obtained stable hybridomas producing the right kind of antibodies. Ortho quickly informed Schlossman of the results, and a "natural collaboration" evolved.

The natural part of the collaboration flowed from the fact that without Schlossman, Kung and Ortho had the monoclonals and little else. Schlossman, on the other hand, had the human cell bank and the cellular immunoassays needed to characterize the antibodies and show that they were indeed what Ortho claimed them to be.[55] The acceptance of the "emerging monoclonal reagents" as bona fide reagents depended on the demonstration that they "detected determinants recognized by the conventional antisera with which cells responsible for various aspects of immune function had been identified"; their target antigens, in other words, had first to be "mapped . . . onto the set of determinants identified with conventional reagents."[56] And this is why the Ortho and Dana Farber teams joined forces. A number of landmark papers describing the first series of monoclonal antibodies against human T cells, nicknamed OKT (for *O*rtho-*K*ung-*T* cell), ensued.[57] Products containing the OKT antibodies began to be sold in 1980. Ortho marketed most of the antibodies, including OKT3, OKT4, OKT8, and OKT11 in kits known under the trade name of Ortho-mune. Ortho subsequently developed OKT3, renamed Muromonab-CD3 (Orthoclone OKT3) for therapeutic purposes for the prevention of transplant rejection.[58]

The Commercial Production of Markers

It is tempting to analyze the commercial development of markers such as the OKT series as part of a broader context, namely the development of a new biotechnology industry. By the late 1970s to early 1980s, public and private reports heralded the latter as the harbinger of a new industrial revolution.[59] The two most often cited pillars of the new industry were the gene splicing, recombinant DNA (rDNA) techniques, first developed in 1973, and hybridoma technology, developed in 1975.[60] While perceived as less wide-ranging than rDNA techniques, reports singled out hybridoma technology as the one most likely to lead to commercial products in the short run. By the mid-1980s, industry observers could point to the numerous commercial enterprises that had emerged to exploit hybridoma technology (150 in the United States, 20 in the United Kingdom).[61] NIH funding for R&D involving monoclonal antibodies had grown from $78 million in 1981 for a total of 768 funded projects to $206 million in 1983 for a total of 1940 projects.[62] In 1984, the U.S. Office of Technology Assessment predicted that the U.S. market for monoclonals—estimated to sit in the $5 to $6 million range—would lie between $300 to $500 million by 1990.[63]

According to a 1985 report, by that date over seventy monoclonal diagnostic kits had been approved by the U.S. Food and Drug Administration (FDA) and these kits alone accounted for sales of $30 to $50 million a year.[64] Both critics and supporters of the emerging biotech industry saw this growth as the beginning of a new chapter in university-industry relationships. As noted by Löwy and others, although close relationships between university, clinical, and industrial actors in the biomedical field can be traced back to the second half of the nineteenth century, it was only after World War II that these ties became an integral part of academic research and clinical practice. Two periods in particular mark this transition: the one immediately following the war, and the 1980s.[65] Thus, the OKT story and the Kung-Schlossman collaboration could be seen as products of the new climate linking university and clinical researchers to commercial-industrial interests.

As tempting as such an interpretation may be, we cannot endorse the "broader context" trope. While there are theoretical reasons for this,[66] in the present case a simple empirical remark will suffice: Kung did not walk into a context: he had to create it. When Kung developed the OKT antibodies, Ortho administrators asked whether the antibodies were mere tools for another project, namely Goldstein's work on the thymic hormone, or whether they should be pursued as ends in themselves. Kung chose the second solution which entailed the exploration of commercial options. When Ortho's marketing department produced a survey showing that there was no prospective market for the OKTs,[67] Kung replied that while the company's marketing people were very good at assessing the market for "me-too" products, i.e., for products with an existing market, they were notoriously bad at discerning new markets. In the ensuing confrontation, and with the recently garnered support of Ortho's chairman, Kung's view prevailed. As we now know, the development of the IPT platform as a clinical tool (not only for leukemia but also, and more importantly in terms of commercial outcomes, for AIDS after 1980) proved him correct.[68]

To keep the OKT story in its proper perspective, it is thus important to understand that these reagents are not simply another example of a commercial product based on monoclonal antibodies. True, one might represent the situation as such retrospectively. Early observers of the biotech industry have indeed tended to treat monoclonal antibodies as a discrete, albeit heterogeneous field of production. They have even subcategorized commercial enterprises in this sector according to a range of strategies, some companies specializing in the mass production of monoclonals, other companies improving already established diagnostic test kits for soluble antigens (pregnancy tests, antihepatitis tests, and so on) by substituting monoclonals for polyclonals, and a third group of companies, the one of interest to us, targeting cell-surface antigens of lymphocyte subclasses.[69] Although this a posteriori classification makes sense for venture capitalists, from a sociological-historical point of view it is an ex ante categorization. OKTs signal the emergence of a new field, one predicated upon the development of monoclonal antibodies to be sure, but also, and, we would argue, at least as decisively, predicated on the emergence of the IPT platform as defined by the markers. OKTs, in other words, killed two birds with one stone: they opened the way to the widespread, routine performance of IPT, the domain to which they owed their genesis, *and* they simultaneously served as grounds for testing the commercial and legal (see below) possibilities of hybridoma technology.[70]

The circulation of the Kung-Schlossman antibody as a commercial marker both for routine IPT and for research generated significant advantages. Schlossman's painstakingly collected cell bank had functioned as one of the few sources of well-defined human T cells and thus as a basic resource—an obligatory passage point—for the characterization of conventional antisera. As we have seen, a few laboratories such as Schlossman's produced the latter, which were always in short supply. Rabbits, mice, and guinea pigs did not create enough serum on a single occasion nor did they live long enough to supply even a restricted research market. "Once it was gone," a good antiserum was "essentially impossible to duplicate."[71] The supply problem created a significant obstacle for researchers considering the switch from fluorescence microscopy to flow cytometry. While the cytometer promised decisive gains in terms of automation and "objectivity," its "collegial" functioning depended upon the shared availability of high-titer, high-specificity antisera, a limiting condition.[72] Monoclonal antibodies changed all this: once produced and properly characterized, unlimited supply of a given reagent was, at least in principle, available.

In addition to short-circuiting the need for repeated and tedious characterizations, the commercial production of OKTs entailed widespread availability. As already noted, the production of antisera by traditional methods used procedures often equated with "art" (as opposed to "science") and was thus restricted to those laboratories skilled in the art.[73] Moreover, as we also saw, even the most artful hands could not prevent antisera from showing unpredictable variations. Having mapped the antigens detected by monoclonals onto those previously detected by antisera, researchers agreed that monoclonal antibodies could indeed be used to isolate cell-surface markers.[74] Then, "other people could get their hands on them and they then became a very powerful tool for dissecting the heterogeneity of the human T cell response."[75] Increased circulation, in turn, boosted the value of the new antibody reagents for potential users. Indeed, following a pattern well described by economists of innovation, once convinced of the superiority of the new reagents users turned it into a de facto market standard by both massively adopting it (a "bandwagon" effect) and by increasing the costs (economic and otherwise) of using alternative approaches.[76]

Examination of the use of the markers in the transplantation field shows how OKTs and similar products circulated. In 1981, following contact with Kung at Ortho,[77] a research team at Massachusetts General Hospital began testing OKT antibodies for monitoring kidney transplant patients by measuring the "relative and constantly shifting populations" of T4 cells vs. T8 cells. Dr. Robert C. Burton, a member of the team, commented on the research in the following terms:

> Until these subtle cell measurements became possible, . . . the only way the surgeons knew whether they were giving too little immunosuppression was when the donor organ was rejected. Infection was the only signal that they were giving too much. With the monoclonal monitoring . . . it's possible to fine-tune the delicate balance between the two extremes. It's astounding to us. . . . We now expect the day-to-day management of these transplant patients to depend on these measurements.[78]

Burton and coworkers presented similar claims in different words in the scientific literature of the early 1980s.[79] Some clinicians agreed and called for determinations of T-subset levels to be made "on a frequent basis (3 times a week)."[80] Other researchers remained unconvinced, saying that the promotion of routine determinations was "premature" and "unjustified."[81] Still others called for further studies, improved methods of data analysis, and increased attention to various interpretative pitfalls.[82] By 1984 Burton had to admit that "there is controversy as to whether the OKT4 OKT8 ratio can predict either the onset of acute cellular rejection or the reversibility of [renal failure episodes] in the early posttransplant period," but, qualifying his early statements, he maintained that "nonetheless, T cell subset monitoring is clearly a useful *addition* to the diagnostic tests."[83] The flow of papers supporting and questioning the clinical usefulness of lymphocyte subset monitoring continued unabated throughout the 1980s. The debate evolved along with the increasing sophistication of the flow techniques used, and, correlatively, with the number and combination of subset markers. Toward the end of the 1980s some researchers suggested that the improved techniques provided "valuable information for the monitoring, and possibly the treatment, of allograft recipients," and promoted "closely spaced immune monitoring (at least twice a week)" as offering "a very reliable early indicator of impending transplant rejection."[84] Other researchers continued to speak of the "lack of sensitivity" of IPT when used to correlate rejection with antigenic expression.[85]

Controversy did not prevent the widespread adoption of the IPT platform in this field. A 1992 survey of the international membership of the Transplantation Society concerning the availability, use, value, and critical assessment of lymphocyte subset monitoring showed that this technology was available in most clinical settings surveyed and regularly used by about half of the respondents associated with a clinical transplant program (another 25% used it "rarely").[86] Although they described the measurement as useful, respondents attributed low diagnostic value to the technique and about two thirds believed that its absence would not affect their clinical judgment. Even more surprisingly, 25% of the respondents sent blood for subset measurements although they did not think the technique was useful.[87] Unlike the diagnostically significant biopsy (the "gold standard"), subset measurements belonged to a complex of different indicators that provided a "fuller picture" and were thus performed to this end. Moreover, unlike biopsies, markers were noninvasive. Thus, despite a lack of consensus concerning their usefulness, once commercially available, markers generated clinical interest and entered into clinical-diagnostic routines.

Other companies soon joined Ortho in the commercial production of IPT markers. Among them were flow cytometer manufacturers. Here, competition was so fierce that the original Orthoclone markers were almost immediately countered, unsurprisingly, by Becton Dickinson which marketed its own line of B and T cell antibodies under the trade name of Leu (for leukocyte). Leu-3, for example, competed directly with OKT-4 in the recognition of the helper subset of T cells (later renamed CD4). Becton Dickinson's product line derived mostly from work carried out in Leonard Herzenberg's laboratory at Stanford.[88] Following Boyse and Cantor's publication, the Herzenberg laboratory had also searched for antibodies to human T cell subsets and had quickly found them:

> We got thymocytes from normal people, I mean: not normal, but people who had been operated on to correct a heart problem. They often take out the thymus to get it out of the way. So you can get thymuses if you're in a major medical center and that's what we did. We had the pathologists help us.[89]

In the case of the Leu antibodies, the initiative came from Herzenberg rather than Becton Dickinson. Understanding that the future of FACS and thus of his own research depended on the development of reagents, at the end of the 1970s Herzenberg and his team had put their energy into developing such reagents. They also urged Becton Dickinson to develop a production center to supply fluorochrome-coupled monoclonals to laboratories that did not have access to the technology; the center began operating in 1981.[90] Herzenberg explained his involvement in the commercial field as follows:

> I think that [the fact of] the companies being involved and making these antibodies was actually very important to the development of the whole field because it was very difficult for one laboratory to develop a whole library or battery of reagents that it needs for its work. . . . The idea of hybridomas was that everybody should have the same specificity, reactivity, same amount of color, and reagents. So if everybody made their own there was great difficulty logistically in everybody making their own. It also defeated the purpose, the great advantage of monoclonals. So I felt it should come from central sources. [Becton Dickinson] agreed that I could train their people so they would be very good at making standard reagents and keep the quality up.[91]

In other words, by putting a large number of marker antibodies on the market, commercial enterprises would not only increase the availability of these reagents but also create a de facto standard.[92]

Compared to Becton Dickinson, the other major producer of flow cytometers in the United States, Coulter Electronics, focused more closely on the clinic than on research and was thus less sensitive to the needs of and inputs from university scientists. In spite of this, Coulter quickly realized not only the economic potential of the reagents, but also their strategic role with respect to the hardware, and followed Becton Dickinson with a series of reagents entitled simply T1, T2, and so on. Like Becton Dickinson, Coulter obtained its first monoclonals through collaboration with university and clinical researchers, including Schlossman's group which had in the meantime severed its ties with Ortho.[93] Still, compared with Becton Dickinson, Coulter initially banked more on the hardware and on a limited set of major markers than on the joint development of an extensive set of reagents. Surmising that such a strategy put the company at a disadvantage—insofar as consumers increasingly treated the hardware as a black box, concentrating instead on the reagents and the molecules they recognized—in 1996 Coulter acquired Immunotech, a company in Marseille with a large catalog of IPT reagents.[94]

As noted above, in the early 1980s a number of companies were created to exploit the new monoclonal antibody technology. The startups included Immunotech, created in 1982 as a spinoff of the Centre d'Immunologie de Marseille-Luminy (CIML).[95] A joint initiative of INSERM (the French Medical Research Council) and CNRS (the French National Council for Scientific Research), the CIML had been established in 1975 as part of the French government's development plan for immunology and soon became an immunological powerhouse.[96] In addition to breaking with the traditional centralization of immunological research institutes in Paris, research at the CIML was expected to lead to medical applications and the establishment of an industrial interface. The creation of Immunotech—a somewhat belated response to the interface requirement—had been championed by the founder and director of the CIML, who had introduced hybridoma technology to the center after a sabbatical at Oxford, and a CIML researcher specializing in immunoassays. INSERM supported Immunotech by providing the new company with privileged access to CIML equipment, laboratories, and researchers, and by signing a ten-year contract giving first right of refusal for all hybridomas produced by INSERM laboratories.

While the company had initially targeted the large market of diagnostic kits, replacing conventional, polyclonal-based assays with monoclonals, their lack of experience with industrial production modified this plan. Looking for a quick profit, in 1983 Immunotech began selling more specialized monoclonals for cell analysis that had been obtained from various public laboratories. By the end of 1984, Immunotech's catalog featured seventy reagents, including a large selection of leukocyte markers, thus placing the firm in competition with Ortho, Becton Dickinson, and Coulter for a share of the French market estimated at 5 to 10 million francs.[97] The AIDS crisis and the ensuing development of the cell-markers field reinforced this shift in production so that by 1997, contrary to initial expectations, about 60% of the catalog consisted of IPT reagents. The acquisition of Immunotech by Coulter in 1996 amounted to open recognition of the key role of reagents in the IPT platform.

The growth of the CD markers market precipitated intellectual property conflicts given that Ortho had already patented the OKT series. Further problems of privileged access to materials and reagents emerged[98] when, for example, Kung's team at Ortho and Schlossman's team at Dana Farber squared off concerning the distribution of the OKT series. Although Ortho's team had sought patent protection, they also wanted to make antibodies available to a large number of investigators in order to multiply their uses. Schlossman's team preferred to restrict the initial use of the antibodies to maintain their lead over competitors.[99] Such an attitude was hardly idiosyncratic since, as Herzenberg recalled: "For the most part everybody was playing very close to the bat [sic]. They gave their friends some antibodies but they were not going to give the antibodies out. They were generally not going to make them publicly available."[100] The "private ethos," so to speak, motivated the academic researchers more than the commercial research team. When the connection with Schlossman's team faded, Kung and his colleagues at Ortho signed several papers with other researchers—including, between 1980 and 1982, articles with Janossy and Greaves in the United Kingdom—providing many institutions with the new monoclonals prior to sale.[101]

Meanwhile, Ortho aggressively pursued its proprietary rights, having filed for patents for the antibodies and the related hybridomas concurrently with the publication of articles in 1979 reporting production of the OKTs. The patent office issued the patents in 1981[102] and in September 1984 Ortho filed a patent infringement suit against Becton Dickinson who, as we have seen, had been selling its own version of the marker antibodies.[103] In so doing, Ortho once again broke new ground, for, at the time, considerable uncertainty surrounded the possibility of patenting new life forms in general, and antibodies in particular.[104] In addition to issues of novelty and obviousness, the suit raised the problem of the breadth of antibody patent protection. Since one could, in principle, generate, against the same antigenic marker, a large number of monoclonal antibodies that differed, chemically speaking, from each other, would Ortho's patents cover only the antibodies Ortho had produced (in which case the patent had no real value) or all possible antibodies against the markers targeted by their reagents? Ortho claimed that their patents covered all *functionally equivalent* (albeit chemically distinct) antibodies.[105]

Ortho and Becton Dickinson settled out-of-court in Ortho's favor: Becton Dickinson agreed to pay $5 million for damages and royalties in return for nonexclusive licenses for the patents. So armed, Ortho turned and sued Coulter, reaching another favorable out-of-court settlement. Although no court issued a judgment, the settlements constituted a de facto enforcement of Ortho's patents. Other companies, such as Immunotech, took note and requested licenses.[106] Commentators have noted that the decisive factor in these cases appears to have been that the OKTs detected previously unknown antigens and therefore contributed to the development of a new field of practice.[107] Their innovative character, in other words, lay not in their intrinsic properties (from the fact, for instance, that they were monoclonal antibodies) but derived from their participation in the constitution of the IPT platform.

The increasing sophistication of the components of the IPT platform—the development of flow cytometric equipment for the simultaneous measurement of a growing number of fluorescent labels and the related development of markers tagged with different colors—opened new avenues of commercial diversification. As noted by a flow cytometry marketing manager:

> I've been on both sides of the hardware and the reagents. Usually it's driven by one or the other. For example, if you know that a new [fluorescent tag] is going to be available, then the knowledge of that [tag] drives the design. Or in some cases we didn't know that a [new fluorescent tag] was going to be available but we assumed that it would at some point and then we made the hardware; in most cases we've made hardware capability before the reagents were available for it. . . . As soon as that hardware is available then people automatically gravitate towards designing reagents that will take advantage of those hardware capabilities. . . . So, you know, there, the market is continually getting more and more complex and adding more capabilities to the system . . . we haven't seen an end yet to the number of colors, the number of parameters, all we're seeing is that you're putting more and more capability in a smaller and smaller box and trying to keep costs down, and making all more user-friendly, more automated.[108]

Thus, for instance, companies began selling prepackaged reagents, i.e., antibodies conjugated with specific labeling molecules, and competing on that basis. Here is an example. When the American-based multicenter AIDS cohort study (MACS) set out in 1984 to define the natural history of AIDS through IPT, in order to improve comparability of results across the centers and over time, MACS organizers decided to use identical flow instrumentation, reagents, and analytical procedures in each center. For instrumentation MACS chose a two-color instrument. Although Coulter won the contest with its Epics C cytometer, MACS decided to purchase monoclonal antibodies from Becton Dickinson as it was the only company selling the relevant antibody reagents labeled with phycoerythrin.[109] The luminescent compound belonged to a whole new family of fluorescent tags that enabled flow cytometry manufacturers to exploit the multicolor possibilities of their instruments. Stanford University had quickly filed for a patent for the new fluorochromes after they had been developed in 1981 by a joint team from Stanford and the University of California, Berkeley.[110] One of the three coinventors named on the patent, issued in 1985, had been working in Herzenberg's laboratory and he subsequently moved to Becton Dickinson. Realizing the advantage of the new reagents, Coulter, rather than acquire a license from Stanford, quickly developed its own conjugates, so that when another multisite study launched toward the end of 1985 decided to improve comparability by using identical hardware and reagents, it was able, this time, to purchase both the hardware and the phycoerythrin-labeled reagents from Coulter.[111] In 1986, Stanford sued Coulter for patent infringement. Coulter settled out-of-court in 1987 and acquired a license.[112]

By now, readers might be wondering about the present size of the market for CD reagents. Data concerning the flow cytometry subfield of the market (thus not including reagents used for slide-based immunocytochemistry, the other major instantiation of the IPT platform) show that the worldwide market for these reagents amounted, in 1999, to $500 million per year, as compared to a mere $2 million between 1978 and 1981.[113] The 1999 estimate is consistent with figures provided by another source, according to which the 1998 sales of in vitro diagnostic products (IVDs) for flow cytometry amounted to $405 million.[114] As a comparison, worldwide IVD sales during the 1996–99 period were in the range of $18 to $19 billion annually, with an average growth rate during the 1990s of approximately 6%. In 1998, North America constituted the largest segment (43%) of the market, followed by Europe (33%) and Japan (12%). The largest share of the market (approximately $4 billion) went to immunoassays, followed by clinical chemistry (approximately $3.2 billion) and glucose monitoring (just below $3 billion). Flow cytometry reagents thus represented a relatively minor market share (2.2% of the total). Nonetheless, with an expected annual increase of 13% in the 1999–2004 period, this category also represents the area with the second greatest growth potential in the IVD field after nucleic acid testing (23%), as compared to a meager 3% for immunoassays. The relatively slow growth of the IVD sector in the 1990s, as well as small profits, have resulted in numerous mergers so that in 1999, seven companies controlled 70% of the market. Two of the seven companies (Becton Dickinson and Beckman Coulter) are the major players in the field of flow cytometry instrumentation and reagents.

Data concerning the routine use of CD reagents in hospitals are difficult to obtain because statistics are not collected according to this category.[115] In Quebec, the Ministry of Health has collected data concerning cell surface marker tests performed by hospital laboratories since 1996. Data concerning the number of medical diagnostic acts related to the broader diagnostic category within which these tests fall (thus, an indirect and imperfect measure of the number of tests performed) are available for a longer period. They show that while from 1980 to 1986–87 the number of diagnostic acts remained relatively stable, marked growth began after 1987, attaining in 1995 an almost sevenfold increase over the early 1980s.[116] Most of the growth is due to AIDS testing. Data from a major Montreal hospital show that in 1995 87% of the IPT tests performed by flow cytometry were for AIDS, 7% for the diagnosis of leukemia and related lymphoproliferative disorders (mainly for confirmatory diagnosis after morphological and cytochemical investigations), and 6% for the monitoring of stem cell transplant cases.[117] In the case of leukemia, while the morphological analysis of bone marrow biopsy remains the gold standard in diagnosing acute leukemia, as noted at the beginning of this book, IPT and cytogenetic tests have become significant components of the routine "diagnostic algorithm." As the epidemiology of leukemia has remained relatively stable in recent years, differences in the incidence and prevalence of the disease reflect mainly demographic changes and are thus likely to be relatively minor factors in the spread of the IPT platform.[118] In other words, changes in the number of IPT tests performed in leukemia reflect developments in the IPT technology itself, such as the development of multicolor equipment, the availability of new markers or marker-panels, and so on.

American hospital data concerning the use of IPT for AIDS are consistent with Quebec data: a 1990 CDC survey of 100 hospitals chosen randomly from among 550 hospitals treating HIV patients showed that 16% had begun performing IPT during 1980–83, 31% between 1984 and 1987, and 53% between 1988 and 1990.[119] A majority (61%) performed IPT testing through outside laboratories, but the number of hospitals using their own laboratories increased steadily, clearly correlating with the number of HIV patients admitted to these hospitals. Hospitals performing in-house IPT (35%), for example, had treated 64% of the HIV patients. The large variation in costs and charges among hospitals reflected the fact that some institutions used abbreviated antibody panels while others used full panels that, in addition to identifying all the lymphocytes and distinguishing between CD4 and CD8, provided internal quality checks. The frequent use of IPT in AIDS stems from the fact that CD4 counts have been used as a basis for therapeutic decisions (both for antiretroviral therapy and for the treatment of opportunistic infections), as a part of the criteria (in the United States) for determining disability in HIV-positive persons and, after 1993 (as noted in chapter 1), as the cornerstone of the CDC classification and staging of AIDS.

The CD System

The production of a growing number of markers by public laboratories and private, competing commercial companies generated considerable confusion at the beginning of the 1980s. The proliferation of proprietary names and idiosyncratic names of "homemade" antibodies that began circulating at about the same time served as the initial impetus for the standardized marker nomenclature produced and regularly updated by an ongoing series of workshops. To understand the sense of confusion that led to the nomenclature, one need merely ask: was Leu-3 really the same as OKT4? Initial attempts to answer this question led to dubious solutions such as using the term L3T4 as a mnemonic conflation of the two commercial designations.[120]

The above "solution" attempted to paper over two related but distinct issues. Did different antibodies indeed target the same antigen, and how could one characterize the physicochemical features of those antibodies? Only by first establishing that a given set of different antibodies did indeed target the same antigen—by establishing, to use the terminology of the patent dispute mentioned earlier, the presence of "functional equivalence"—could cumulative knowledge about that antigen (and the processes in which it was involved) be produced. The second issue has special relevance for those who wished to select the most promising antibody for a given project from a variety of antibodies targeting the same antigen. Such a selection was ultimately an empirical problem and did not flow ineluctably from any standard criteria. Consider the following example. In the early 1980s several groups reported the production of antibodies that, when tested against several normal and leukemic blood samples, showed a similar, though not identical, pattern of reactivity. The research groups consequently questioned whether or not those antibodies were directed against the same surface molecule. The answer in this case drew upon a mix of procedural, biological, and sociocognitive reasons. In particular, the laboratories decided that the different antibodies did indeed react with the same antigen (later called CD9), and that variations in reactivity patterns were due to differences in technique, the antibodies' strength of reaction, and "possibly interpretation."[121]

Given the tentative, open-ended character of this line of work, how did researchers manage to reach agreement? As always in these cases, the solution came from a technical and institutional procedural innovation. As noted above, monoclonal antibodies presented several advantages over traditional antisera. Their use, however, generated new coordination issues and called forth the establishment of interlaboratory conventions and agreements. Generally speaking, and as noted by Fortanier and associates in their analysis of the therapeutic use of CD34, the definition and regulation of the objects at the center of a given set of practices provides a way of working around the uncertainties surrounding the coordination of these practices.[122] The burden of agreement, in other words, is shifted from human actors to the objects themselves. In the present case, the design of a mechanism for the establishment of equivalences between the antibodies produced by different laboratories provided a solution to several concerns: the circulation and exchange of materials, as well as the validation of results produced by different researchers. Here is how.

Confronted with a profusion of antibodies emanating from both private and public sources that recognized cell-surface antigens of both known and unknown function, in 1982 French, American, and British researchers launched a series of workshops, whose results are published as an ever-expanding CD system of cell-surface markers. The main organizers of the first workshop, Laurence Boumsell and Alain Bernard from the Saint-Louis Hospital in Paris (a major center for leukemia research and treatment in France) brought together a highly symbolic organizing committee that included, in addition to themselves, Jean Dausset, Stuart Schlossman, and César Milstein. Milstein, an immunogeneticist at the U.K. Medical Research Council, was soon to share the 1984 Nobel Prize for his role in the development of monoclonal antibodies. Schlossman, as we have seen, played a key role in the development of human T-cell subsets and his team was engaged in collaborative research with the Saint-Louis team.[123] Dausset, a Saint-Louis hematologist and immunogeneticist, as well as a 1980 Nobel Prize winner for his research on the HLA (human leukocyte antigens) system, had been instrumental in the establishment of a previous series of workshops. Begun in the 1960s in the United States, these workshops had been devoted to the systematization of human transplantation antigens used in tissue matching for transplantation. The HLA workshops acted as a model for the CD workshops since they, too, had sought to domesticate recalcitrant work materials by using the collation, confrontation, and correlation of results from different and often competing laboratories to generate collective results more robust than the original findings.[124]

Before describing the mechanics of the workshops, several preliminary remarks are in order concerning the CD terminology. To begin with, some confusion surrounds not only the actual meaning of the abbreviation CD (most often translated as "clusters of differentiation" but also as "cluster determinants" or "cluster designation") but, more decisively, the issue of whether the CDs refer to the object marked (the antigens allegedly sitting on the cell surface) or to the object doing the marking (the antibodies recognizing those antigens, in which case one would speak of anti-CDs as one speaks of, say, hepatitis antigens and anti-hepatitis antibodies). Indeed, this terminology issue has become a minor irritant, for, in spite of the fact that common usage accepts both senses of CD—the context supplying the correct referent of the term—some journal editors insist that prospective authors use the term "anti-CD" to describe a given antibody.[125] Far from being a question of sloppy terminology or overzealous editors, the issue has interesting sociological implications.

First, the origin of the confusion alerts us to the fact that scientists continuously switch between procedural and ontological interpretations of the products of their activities. Recall that cell-surface markers are, by definition, physical sites on the surfaces of cells that are recognized by antibodies raised against these sites or, in immunological parlance, antigens. Note that because of the way antibodies are produced, the antigen is the source of the antibody or, in other words, the mark is the source of the marker. Immunization procedures imply a contact between a particular antigen and the cells of the immune system responsible for the production of antibodies; this "contact-by-design" (a lot of work goes into the establishment of proper immunization schedules and procedures) leads to the production of antibodies that, in return, can be used to locate and isolate that same antigen. Are the antibodies or the antigens that generate them the markers? Clearly, the object marked is the antigen, and, in that case, the antibody acts as the marker, but one could just as easily say that if that particular antigen was picked out by scientists and clinicians as a target for antibody production, then it is because it marked some cell of interest to them, in which case the marker is the antigen residing on the cell surface waiting for some other substance to connect with it.

The situation becomes even murkier if one takes into account the historical fact that, in the late 1960s, the presence of antibody on the surface of certain white blood cells served as a marker that distinguished these lymphocytes from other, morphologically identical, lymphocytes that did not produce antibodies. In other words, antibodies acted both as the object to be marked and as marking tools. The ambiguity also expresses the dual nature and origin of the markers as signs of normal differentiation and as signs of pathology. For diagnostic and therapeutic reasons, clinicians initially sought the antibodies and not the antigens. From the biological point of view, however, researchers used antibodies as a tool to isolate a "deeper" reality, the antigens or sites on the cell surfaces.

Textbook definitions, far from clarifying the issue, simply restate it. Abbas, Lichtman, and Pober, for example, tell us that "a surface marker that identifies a particular [white blood cell] lineage or differentiation stage, that has a defined structure, and that is recognized by a group ("cluster") of monoclonal antibodies, is called a member of a cluster of differentiation."[126] Here "CD" clearly refers to the antigen that marks particular cells. However, more historical and procedural definitions can also be found that turn antibodies into the initial referent of the term: "The term CD (cluster designation) was derived by computer analysis of monoclonal antibodies raised in different laboratories worldwide against human leukocyte antigens. . . . Monoclonal antibodies with similar specificity characteristics were grouped together and given a CD number. This number is now also used to indicate the specific molecule recognized by a group of monoclonal antibodies."[127] In other words, both the mark and the marker have been assigned the same number and the same name, "CD." We are thus provided with a quasi-historical account, according to which the CD number initially referred to the antibodies insofar as they (or, more precisely, their worldwide proliferation) provided the original rationale for the endeavor as well as the focus of the statistical and laboratory interventions. But, once the proper equivalences had been established, antibodies (or rather the antibodies tamed by the various workshops) could be turned into "mere instruments" for the isolation of the antigens. As noted by the chair of the most recent (2000) workshop:

> The primary focus . . . should be on the functional molecules (the "antigens"); the antibodies are merely tools used in their study. Whereas in the late 70s and early 80s the question behind many studies was "What does my antibody react with?," we are now able to focus on much more fundamental questions about intercellular interactions and cell : molecule interactions.[128]

Second, the use of antibodies as markers of unknown cell-surface components signaled an "important departure" from the traditional approach according to which one proceeded from function to molecule, i.e., having defined a phenomenon of interest, one would proceed to isolate the molecules participating in the function.[129] Although the initial CD meetings presupposed functions before classifying the antibodies (after all, this work began as an investigation of the involvement of B, T, and myeloid cells in normal and pathological events), subsequent workshops inverted the epistemological order, so that "the definition of a new CD [became] the starting point of the definition of its function, and not the other way around."[130] Consequently, "dozens of CD antigens . . . waiting for a function to be defined," suddenly confronted researchers, a somewhat troubling prospect since "[f]ashionable journals are not interested in new molecules of unknown function."[131] The previous, rather tart remark was perhaps prompted by the fact that the *Journal of Experimental Medicine* had refused to even referee a paper describing a monoclonal antibody to detect a human differentiation antigen.[132]

Nonetheless, organizers of succeeding workshops expanded the CD nomenclature to include any surface marker that could be detected by monoclonal antibodies, thus severing the link between the definition of a new CD and the existence of a functionally defined subset of cells. Some workshop participants brazenly suggested that the traditional division of lymphocytes into B, T, and myeloid cells no longer reflected a "biological outlook." And indeed, while maintaining "for organizational reasons" the classic subdivision of the workshop into T, B, and myeloid cell sections, the organizers of the 1989 Vienna workshop quickly added that "the borders between these cell types are no longer as rigid as originally thought."[133] In addition to the cell-surface structures that marked out different immunological functions,[134] researchers found that some cell-surface structures participated in the "normal," nondevelopmental functioning of nonimmune cells such as cell adhesion. These structures could not be construed as markers as they did not signal differentiation along a pathway to immunological function or an emergent pathology. Cell-based divisions could thus be deemed, from a "radical" phenotypic point of view, as "completely arbitrary, without biological basis," insofar as similar or identical structures appeared on different cells.[135] The upshot of the transformation of the cell-surface markers has been a reorientation from molecules directly related to immunology and pathology to a more physiological focus on the multifarious surface structures of the cells of the hematopoietic system.[136]

The international workshops freight CDs with a number of conventions that transform antibodies produced in different laboratories into mutually equivalent substances. Indeed, journal referees will question the use of an antibody that "has not been officially 'blessed' by one of the Workshops."[137] Workshops, in other words, provide both truth and trust: they define the true target of the antibody and produce confidence in the latter. To understand how this is so, it is necessary to understand the conduct of the workshops. Although the term "workshop" normally refers to a group of individuals sitting in the same room, in the present case the meaning has been stretched. Borrowing a metaphor from computing, we can describe the CD workshops as more "virtual" than real and consisting of a network of laboratories. How was the network put together? The organizers of the first workshop selected participating laboratories on the basis of two criteria. First, the laboratories had produced antibodies that the organizers would distribute to the other laboratories as part of a panel of anonymous antibodies.[138] Second, the laboratories agreed to test the antibody panel. The organizers then centralized the results of these blind tests for statistical analysis.

Centralized in Paris, the first workshop comprised 54 research groups from 14 countries and resulted in the establishment of 11 CDs. Since then, the endeavor has grown considerably. Figure 6.5 shows that by the

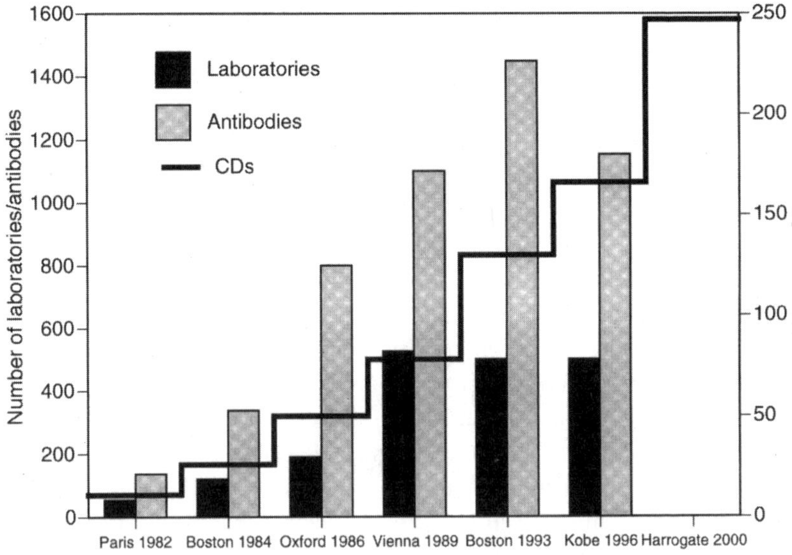

Figure 6.5
Cumulative number of CDs defined as number of laboratories taking part in and number of antibodies tested at each HLDA workshop.

time of the seventh workshop held in Harrogate (UK), the cumulative number of CDs had increased from the original 11 defined in 1982 to over 247. By 1989, the number of participating laboratories had risen from the initial 54 to over 500, although it has since stabilized at that level, having no doubt saturated the field. Similarly, the number of antibodies tested increased from the original 137 in 1982 to 800 in 1986 (with more than 150,000 assays being used to characterize them).[139] That number plateaued at 1450 in 1993 and dropped to about 1100 in 1996, a decrease that is largely due to the fact that the workshops have increasingly adopted molecular-biological techniques, as opposed to antibodies, for determining new CDs. Figures 6.6 and 6.7 show the geographic distribution of the participants who attended the final meetings of the first and the fifth workshops. They illustrate the growing entrenchment of the Human Leukocyte Differentiation Antigens (HLDA) workshops in the 11 years between 1982 and 1993.

An even more dramatic representation of the growth of the HLDA workshops is provided by figures 6.8 and 6.9, which display the institutions that submitted antibodies to the various sections of the first and the fifth workshops (the producers, as opposed to the mere participants). The figures have been generated using software for the analysis of heterogeneous relational data.[140] Each institution appears only once in each map. The square nodes correspond to the workshop sections (B, T, etc.) and their size is proportional to the number of antibodies submitted to each section. Similarly, the round nodes correspond to the submitting institutions and their size is proportional to the number of antibodies submitted by each institution. Figure 6.8 indicates that only six institutions submitted antibodies to all three sections of the first workshop, and that Schlossman's Dana (then Sidney) Farber Institute in Boston was by far the most important producer. In fact, there seems to have been a deliberate (and, we would add, rewarding) strategy on the part of the Bostonians to cover the entire B, T, and myeloid field.[141] The fine detail of figure 6.9 is, admittedly, difficult to decipher but the point in reproducing it is to show, in addition to the marked growth in the number of producers, the overall pattern, with a few central institutions contributing to all or, at least, a majority of sections, and a larger number of more specialized institutions. Among the core institutions we find several commercial companies (such as Becton Dickinson, Coulter, Immunotech) that were not permitted to officially submit antibodies during the first workshop.

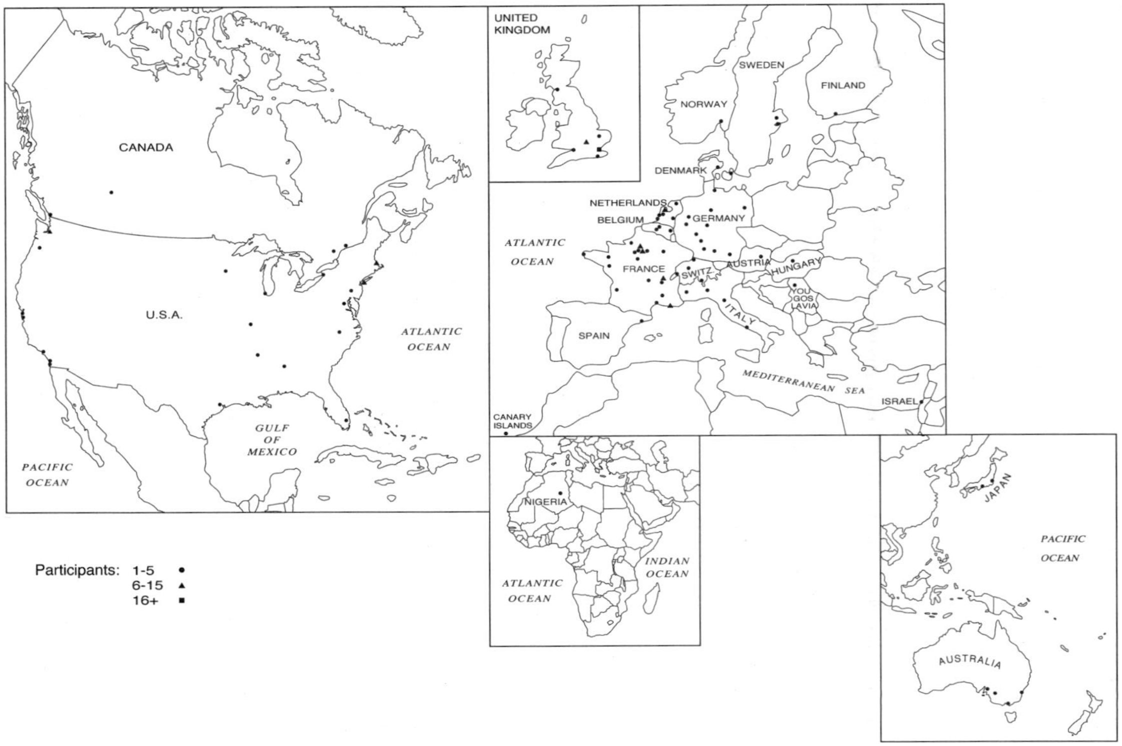

Figure 6.6
Geographic distribution of the participants at the first HLDA meeting, Paris, 1982. (Computer graphics by Richard Bachand.)

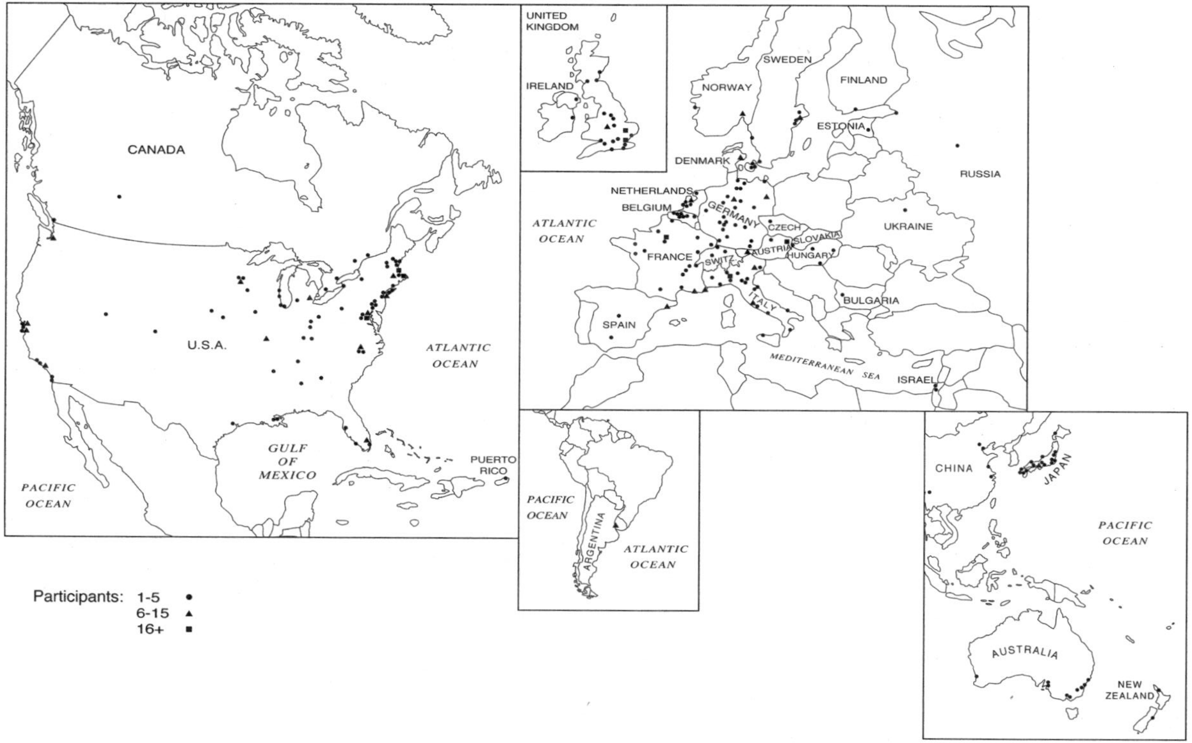

Figure 6.7
Geographic distribution of the participants at the fifth HLDA meeting, Boston, 1993. (Computer graphics by Richard Bachand.)

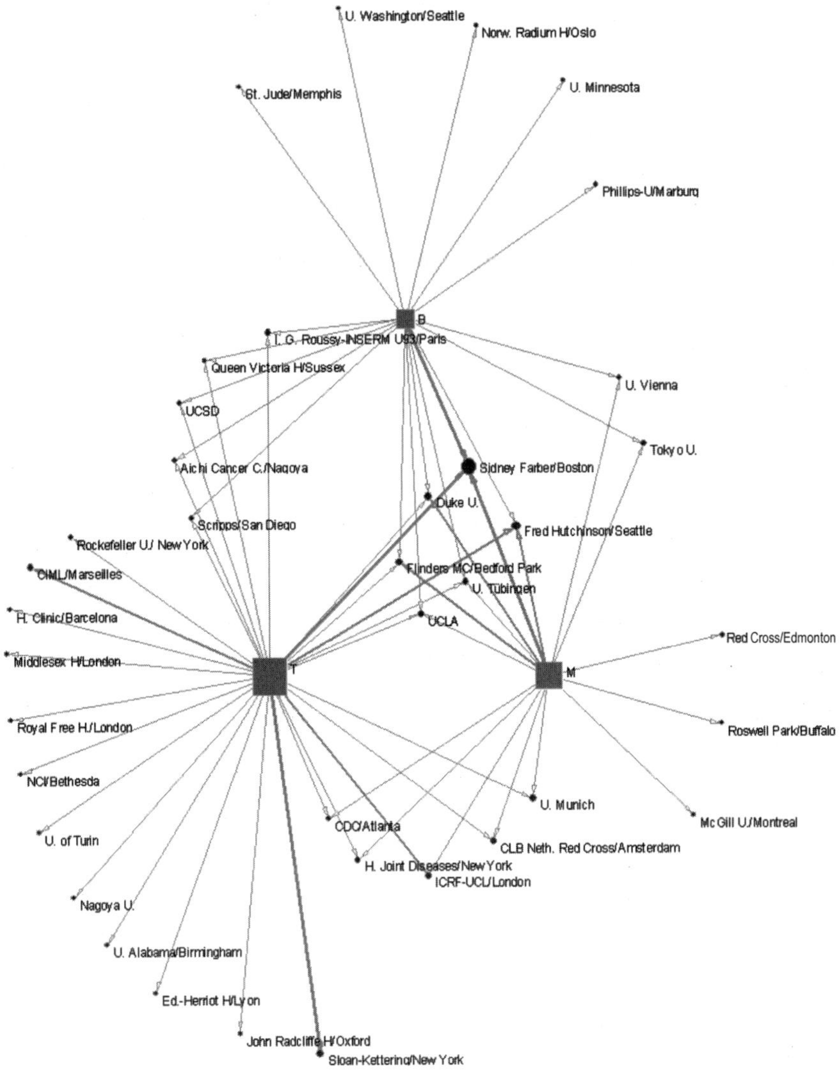

Figure 6.8
A map of the network of institutions that submitted antibodies to the first HLDA meeting, Paris, 1982. See text for explanation.

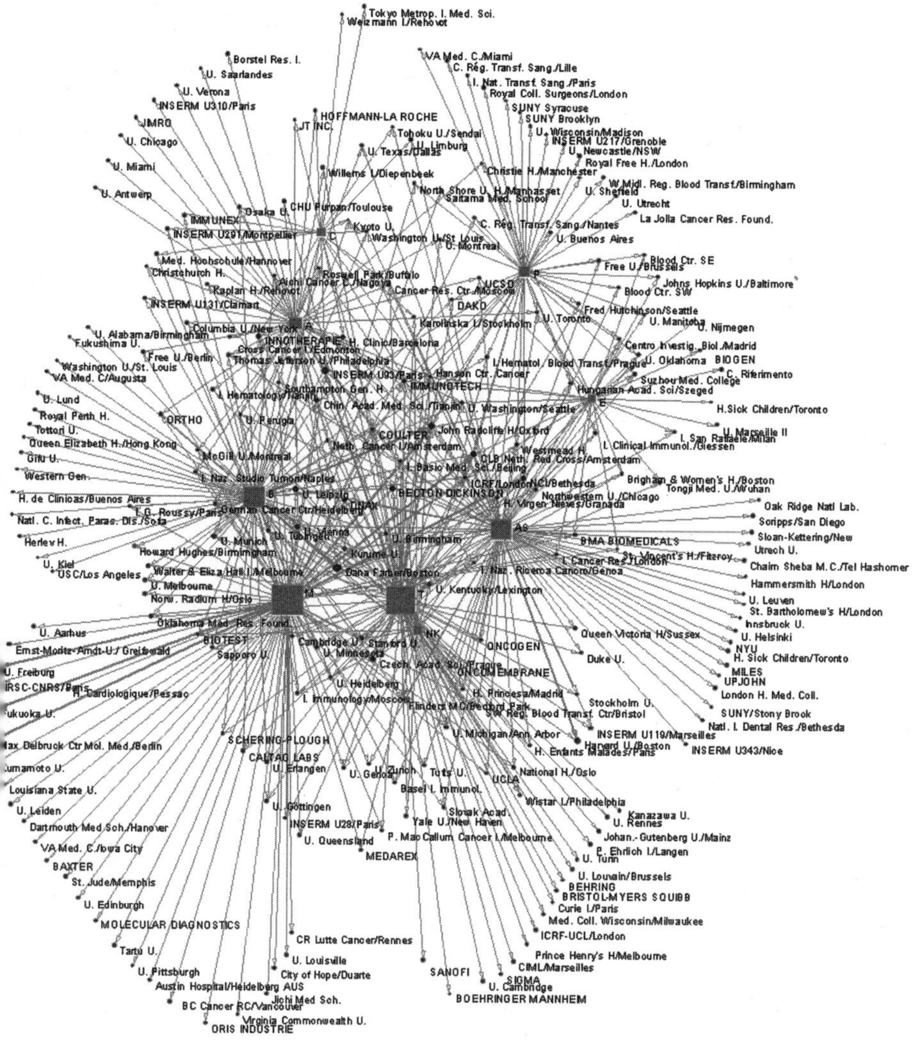

Figure 6.9
A map of the network of institutions that submitted antibodies to the fifth HLDA meeting, Boston, 1993. See text for explanation.

To see how the final products of these workshops, the CDs, took form, note that the latter are statistical constructs based on the clustering of the reactivity data supplied by the various laboratories. The clustering, in other words, reveals similarities in reaction patterns when the antibodies are tested on multiple tissues. Initially, statistical analysis was the only criterion for classifying an antibody within a particular cluster, even though the availability of "some molecular data" was expected. In more recent workshops, molecular data, i.e., data obtained from gene cloning and experiments with recombinant proteins, have begun to play an increasingly important role, to the point that "solid molecular data" have now gained the upper hand. For instance, based on the assumption that molecules coded by similar genes may have different cellular expressions, it is now deemed appropriate to assign molecularly related molecules to the same cluster even when their expression pattern is dissimilar.[142] In this sense, one could argue that the system has freed itself from its original status as a central component of the IPT platform.

Let us have a quick look at the original statistical criteria that formed the basis of the CD nomenclature. A 1984 matter-of-fact description of the statistical procedure reads as follows:

> The statistical analysis relied on the distance between antibodies. The distance between 2 antibodies for a given target cell type is the average of the absolute difference between the reactivities of the 2 antibodies for all target cells of the type considered. Then, cluster analysis of the matrix of distances between all pairs of antibodies and algorithmic computation permitted the definition of groups of antibodies that were similar, and those that were clearly different, on each type of target cell. The clusters of differentiation were then readily delineated from summing-up tables of groups of antibodies obtained for each target cell type; these clusters included the antibodies that always had very similar reactivities. Moreover, the confrontation between blind studies on the relative molecular mass ("molecular weight"), performed with the antibodies, and cluster analysis showed an almost perfect correspondence. These final clusters were termed clusters of differentiation (CD).[143]

While this description implies the unproblematic implementation of an algorithmically defined procedure, a considerably more complex process ensued. Once participating laboratories had sent the results of the first workshop back to Paris, decisions had to be made regarding statistical treatment. These choices, in turn, required six months of collaboration between a biomedical statistician and two biomedical scientists experienced in the distribution of the reagents and the collection of laboratory results.[144] In the course of the collaboration, the team decided, for example, to conduct an initial analysis using medians instead of means, because, according to the statistician, "the median is a more robust estimate than the mean when there are erroneous values."[145] The choice took into account both social and technical variables insofar as the choice of median over mean implied that "human" and "technical" errors produced as much statistical variation as biological factors.

Subsequently, workshop participants examined the resulting patterns to see if "they made sense biologically." This maneuver was made possible by the fact that lymphocytes had already been classified on the basis of morphological and functional criteria. Moreover, a limited amount of phenotypic information had been gathered in the premonoclonal antibody era using polyclonal antisera. "Making sense biologically" thus entailed correlating the existing knowledge of function, morphology, and phenotype, and the extensive phenotypic information now being gathered with monoclonal antibodies. The strength of the correlations varied according to the different classes of cells. While relatively extensive knowledge concerning T cells and B cells, for example, existed, other types of leukocytes were less well characterized. Nonetheless, if the new data could be shown to "make sense biologically" for the best-known cells, then participants felt that statistically generated information concerning the less-known cells could not be dismissed as a mere artifact of statistical algorithms.

In addition to the biological questions, a number of sociotechnical questions plagued the early workshops. At the time of the first workshop, monoclonal antibodies were relatively new and uncertain reagents. Moreover, flow cytometry had not been universally adopted by workshop participants as slide-based methods continued (and continue) to be used by workers in the field of the lymphomas. It could thus be asked: how did the results obtained with these two different techniques compare? Furthermore, the reliability of the research groups participating in the workshop could not be taken for granted. Did they master the new techniques and instruments? Did they properly prepare and handle the cells against which the antibodies had to be tested? And what about the secondary reagents, i.e., reagents other than monoclonal antibodies, including, for instance, traditional serological reagents (i.e., reagents obtained by immunizing animals against a given substance and collecting the serum from the immunized animals) used to detect the presence of the monoclonal antibodies? Were they correctly produced and used and did laboratory differences in secondary reagents influence the outcome of the tests? If this were so, could laboratories and the results they generated be compared?[146]

Largely because of these uncertainties, the workshop organizers had to assess two kinds of reliability: the reliability of the laboratories performing the tests and the reliability of the tests. As one depended on the other, organizers of the first workshop asked each laboratory to test the panel of 137 reagents not only against a set of cells of its own choice but also against specific types of cells. Consequently, in addition to analyzing a set of frozen cells sent from Paris, participants had to analyze a set of cells prepared locally. Organizers also asked participating laboratories to indicate "the procedures used to separate the cell populations as well as the results of local controls made to check the purity of a preparation."[147] As a result of this design, the organizers of the first workshop categorized laboratories that were unable to implement techniques successfully used by the other research groups as unreliable. The first workshop allowed organizers to conclude that, despite the novelty of the biological materials and techniques, the results did not show unpredictable local variations and could thus be properly compared.

The workshop organizers also built into the system ways of dealing with uncertainty, such as provisional designations (so-called CDw) that have to be confirmed at the following workshop. The system is admittedly not foolproof, as "dead CDs" and, more frequently, the splitting of CDs into sub-CDs show. But the overall scheme has turned out to be remarkably robust, and has been able to survive even the major change in focus from reactivity patterns to molecular analysis that, as already mentioned, has characterized the more recent workshops.

The success of the CD system cannot be accounted for solely in terms of the structure and organization of the workshops; without proper enforcement, the proposed nomenclature would have remained just a proposal. While companies continued to market markers under proprietary names, by the end of the 1980s the major scientific journals had imposed the CD nomenclature as standard, and the nomenclature had become a standard feature in major immunology and hematology textbooks. The *Bulletin of the World Health Organization* published the report of the first CD workshop, thus giving the CD designations the endorsement of a major international institution that is well-known for its work in the field of medical classifications.[148]

However, no conquest is entire and no single nomenclature can capture the complexities of scientific usage. Journal policies reflect this reality. In February 1987, *Nature* published a "Note on Nomenclature"[149] stating that "in the interest of consistency, *Nature* [would] in future use the CD nomenclature for all T-cell differentiation antigens between CD1 and CD8." In order to facilitate the task, the journal included a list of the alternative, commercial designations for humans (e.g., CD4 = T4/Leu-3) and mouse (e.g., CD4 = L3T4). By restricting this initial enforcement of the CD nomenclature to the CD1–CD8 range, *Nature* adopted a pragmatic approach. Alternative designations for higher CD numbers often conveyed information about the function of the molecule. CD25, for example, was also known more tellingly as the interleukin-2 receptor. Recent policy statements emanating from the CD workshops express the same pragmatism.[150]

Nature's pragmatic policy set the tone for other journals. In 1988, for instance, the *Journal of Immunology* added the following passage to its "Information for Contributors" notice: "For the purpose of consistency in the literature, *The Journal* will follow the style proposed in *Nature* 325: 660, 1987, which uses CD designations for all T-cell differentiation antigens between CD1 and CD8." As was the case with *Nature*, the *Journal of Immunology* included a table that correlated CDs and previous human and mouse designations. The initial statement was revised several times in the following years. Some of these revisions simply took into account the periodical revisions of the CD nomenclature itself as applied to human molecules. The relevant passage in 1994 reads: "For the purpose of consistency, *The Journal* will utilize the CD nomenclature. . . . [F]or human molecules, standard CD nomenclature will be used as updated." Others reflected attempts to work around classificatory inconsistencies such as those resulting from the development of different approaches for human and mouse nomenclature. In 1993, for example, the *Journal* began enforcing a recently proposed style that joined the CD system (from CD1–CD74) and the so-called Ly system used for the mouse.[151] The two systems differed insofar as the latter was genetically based, whereas the human nomenclature was based on the nature of the antigen recognized by the monoclonal antibodies. The joint system used uniform CD designations for both mouse and man when genetic counterparts existed for both species, retaining the Ly designation for those mouse genetic loci with no human counterpart.[152] The fact that the mouse nomenclature adopted the designations initially used for the human nomenclature signals the changing fortune of human immunologists with respect to mouse immunologists and, in turn, represents a significant example of the new *biomedical* configuration that now defines this domain.

To sum up: the formation of consensus, the collation of results, and the industrial production of the antibody reagents led to a major transformation. A biomedical purity replaced the purity of pathology manifested by the populations of patients and animals with the "same" immunological disease that had launched the initial investigations into cell-surface markers in the 1950s and 1960s. The development of a way of producing monoclonal antibodies that, contrary to traditional antisera, could be produced and supplied in large, unchanging quantities had made it possible to standardize the biological reagents used on the slides or in the flow cytometer. The standardization of these reagents through the CD workshops made it possible, in turn, to approach the epistemological object of study, the cell surface, with a standard technique. Researchers then completed the purification process by separating biomedical variation from technical variation through the normalization of biomedical practices. And, as we saw, commercial enterprises subsequently mass-produced these reagents and made them available to any researcher, biological or clinical, inclined to use them.

7

At the Periphery: Flow and Slides

Framed by an internationally accepted nomenclature, buttressed by workshops that coordinated the results of hundreds of laboratories and commercial concerns, and mass-produced by biotechnology companies, by the late 1980s cell-surface markers, redefined and reorganized as CDs (clusters of differentiation), could be used as standard clinical-diagnostic reagents. This could be done in a number of ways. We have chosen to distinguish two major variants of the platform in terms of the peripherals used to read the signals generated by the markers. This division corresponds both to divisions within the market of peripheral suppliers and to divisions within the field of clinical research and practice. Simply put, the division boils down to the difference between flow cytometry–based immunophenotyping and slide-based IPT. The difference between the two approaches is quite significant as each has its advantages.

Slide-based IPT initially allowed immunology researchers to maintain continuity with the older, morphology-based tradition of slide and microscope and the work routines entrenched in surgical pathology. At the same time, it allowed pathologists to gain access to the phenotypic knowledge, practices, and tools generated by immunology: old networks could be connected to new. This articulation was impossible using flow cytometry. In particular, cellular arrangement and the numerous subtleties of tissue and cellular morphology that appeared in biopsy samples on the microscope slide disappeared in the flow cytometer, for the operator saw only a dot on a computer screen and no longer the cells themselves. Flow cytometry, however, had its own advantages, especially in the case of diseases where cells in suspension, such as peripheral blood cells, rather than tissues, were the diagnostic target. In part because of its automation potential and high-tech cachet, flow cytometry greatly contributed to the circulation and public image of the IPT platform to the point that it was often identified with the latter. But the reverse is also true: the advent of the CD system of markers radically transformed the flow cytometer. By combining a panel of markers and the flow cytometer, the apparatus became more than an automated cell-counting device. As previously pointed out, it classified cells into types based on their cell-surface characteristics as it counted them. More than measuring some physical property of a cell then, the flow cytometer, as part of the IPT platform, registered classificatory events.

Given these diverging advantages, it is easy to see that the choice of peripheral is related to divisions within the field of clinical research. Because of the wide variety of configurations of peripheral and the ever-expanding categories of use, however, it is not easy to show exactly how these two forms of peripherals map onto use. In order to gain a more nuanced understanding of how they do, we compared the publication patterns of two highly productive British researchers, D. Y. Mason and G. Janossy.[1] Although they both experimented with the entire spectrum of techniques related to IPT, Janossy worked mainly with flow cytometry and Mason with tissue slides. In particular, Mason developed a slide-based technique known as APAAP (*a*lkaline *p*hosphatase–*a*nti-*a*lkaline *p*hosphatase) that allowed researchers and clinicians to conduct IPT with common hematologic preparations such as blood and marrow smears without recourse to flow cytometric equipment.[2] Since the technique interfaced so easily with existing hematologic routines, Mason and his collaborators initially suggested "that APAAP labeling should become the method of choice for immunophenotyping neoplastic samples in many haematology laboratories not equipped with specialized immunological diagnostic facilities."[3] As for Janossy, we have already examined his role in developing new flow cytometric techniques in relation to the IPT platform (see chapter 3). In comparing the two, we asked: Given the choice of peripheral, is it possible to spot different patterns in the reception of their work by the scientific and clinical community?

Using the *Science Citation Index* we first selected two years in the mid-1980s and the early 1990s during which Janossy and Mason received numerous citations.[4] Thanks to a comprehensive list of publications obtained from both researchers, we then created a database containing all the articles citing their publications during the two peak years.[5] For each of the four files, we compiled a list of the titles of the journals containing the cited articles. Finally, using this list and data on "journal-to-journal" citations, we constructed a co-citation matrix and analyzed it with standard statistical methods.[6] Tables 7.1 and 7.2 contain a summary of the relevant results, showing for each author for a given year a list of journal clusters (or "factors") which, taken together, make up the "citational environment" characterizing that author at that time. By looking at the journal titles making up each cluster, the latter can be further assigned to a given discipline or specialty, thus providing a hierarchical list of the various fields according to the response to the techniques promoted by the two authors.

An initial comparison of Janossy 1984 and Mason 1986 shows that several factors overlap, confirming that the same technology (IPT) finds application in roughly similar biomedical domains. In both cases, and unsurprisingly (since we are dealing with the use of antibodies), immunology heads the list of factors (factor 1 for Janossy, factor 2 for Mason). There are, however, interesting differences in the contribution of the various factors to the overall variance. For instance, in Mason's case, pathology is factor 1 (contributing 21.7% of the total variance), whereas in Janossy's case it is factor 4 (8.8%). Hematology, on the other hand, is factor 2 for Janossy (17.7%), but only factor 4 for Mason (10.1%). This suggests that Mason's work found wider reception within pathology and Janossy's within hematology.[7] Comparing Janossy 1991 and Mason 1993 confirms this initial analysis, showing that while some similarities remain, the original differences are accentuated in 1991–93. Although factors such as immunology, pathology, and hematology feature in both Mason 1993 and Janossy 1991, Mason's two top clusters are pathology, thus showcasing the importance of this discipline to his citational environment.[8] Immunology (31.8%) and Hematology (22.6%) top Janossy's list.[9]

We must be cautious, when interpreting these findings, concerning the different audiences for the two different instantiations of IPT. On the one hand, as we saw in the previous chapter, IPT created new lines of work: rather than simply "diffusing" into preexisting contexts, it established new contexts. On the other hand, IPT had to contend with the resilience of preexisting practices. The new contexts were in part constituted by elements of the older ones: networks merged rather than emerging de novo, and they continued to evolve. For instance, and as previously noted, Mason and his coworkers had initially promoted APAAP as an ideal technique for the hematology laboratory (at least for those lacking sophisticated immunological equipment), yet the citational evidence suggests the technique did not manage to cross the hematology/pathology divide. For sure, our results do not concern the

Table 7.1
Citational environment of Janossy's 1984 and 1991 publications.

	Janossy 1984			Janossy 1991		
	Topic	% var	Cum %	Topic	% var	cum %
Factor 1	***Immunology***			***Immunology***		
	Clin. Immunol. Immunopathol.	29.3		Scand. J. Immunol.	31.8	
	Scand. J. Immunol.			Immunology		
	J. Immunol.			Cell. Immunol.		
	Cell. Immunol.			J. Immunol.		
	J. Clin. Immunol.			Clin. Immunol. Immunopathol.		
	Clin. Exp. Immunol.			Eur. J. Immunol.		
	J. Immunol. Methods			Clin. Exp. Immunol.		
	J. Clin. Invest.			Neth. J. Med.		
				Am. J. Pathol.		
Factor 2	***Hematology***			***Hematology***		
	Br. J. Haematol.	17.7	47.0	Leukemia	22.6	54.4
	Scand. J. Haematol.			Blood		
	Blood			Br. J. Haemat.		
	Blut			Leuk. Res.		
	Leuk. Res.			Bone Marrow Transpl.		
	Semin. Haemat.			Crit. Rev. Oncol. Hematol.		

Factor 3	***Cancer***			***Gastroenterology***		
	J. NCI	13.9	50.9	Gastroenterology	14.1	68.5
	Cancer Res.			Gastroenterol. Clinics N.A.		
	Intl. J. Cancer			Gut		
	Br. J. Cancer			Hepatology		
	Br. Med. Bull.					
Factor 4	***Pathology***			***Pathology***		
	Human Pathol.	8.8	69.7	Histopathology	10.5	79.0
	Am. J. Clin. Pathol.			Am. J. Clin. Pathol.		
	Cancer			Cancer		
	Am. J. Pathol.			J. Clin. Pathol.		
	J. Clin. Pathol.					
Factor 5	***Transplantation***			***Transplantation***		
	Transpl. Proc.	6.9	76.5	Transpl. Proc.	7.2	86.2
	Transplantation			Transplantation		
Factor 6	***Gastroenterology***					
	Gut	5.2	81.7			
	Sem. Liver Disease					

Table 7.2
Citational environment of Mason's 1986 and 1993 publications.

	Mason 1986			Mason 1993		
	Topic	% var	Cum %	Topic	% var	cum %
Factor 1	***Pathology***			***Pathology***		
	Histopathology	27.1		Modern Pathol.	29.8	
	Am. J. Surg. Pathol.			Am. J. Clin. Pathol.		
	Cancer			Am. J. Surg. Pathol.		
	J. Pathol.			Human Pathol.		
	Human Pathol.					
	Virchows Archiv A					
	Onkologie					
Factor 2	***Immunology***			***Pathology***		
	Immunology	24.3	51.4	Path. Res. Practice	13.3	43.1
	J. Immunol.			J. Pathol.		
	Eur. J. Immunol.			Virchows Archiv A		
	Immunol. Invest.			Histopathology		
	Clin. Exp. Immunol.			J. Clin. Pathol.		
	J. Immunol. Methods			Acta Pathol. Jap.		
	Pathology					

Factor 3	***Cancer***			***Hematology***		
	J. NCI	11.5	62.9	Br. J. Haemat.	10.6	53.7
	Cancer Res.			Blood		
	Br. J. Cancer			Leukemia		
	Cancer Surveys					
Factor 4	***Hematology***			***Oncology***		
	Blood	10.1	72.9	Seminars Oncol.	8.9	62.6
	Scand. J. Haematol.			Cancer		
	Leuk. Res.			Med. Pediatr. Oncol.		
				N. Engl. J. Med.		
Factor 5	***Pathology***			***Immunology***		
	Lab. Invest.	8.8	81.7	J. Immunol.	7.1	69.7
	Am. J. Pathol.			Eur. J. Immunol.		
	Virchows Archiv B					
Factor 6	***Dermatology***			***Pathology***		
	Br. J. Dermatol.	6.8	88.5	Am. J. Pathol.	5.4	75.1
	J. Am. Acad. Dermatol.			Int. Rev. Exp. Pathol.		
	J. Invest. Dermatol.			Cancer Res.		
				J. Histol. Cytochem.		

actual performance of diagnostic routines in clinical laboratories, but Mason himself has recently conceded that "we [had] suggested that the APAAP technique should lend itself to use on leukemia samples, but in practice it has never really overtaken other methods. I think it needs rather more care than flow cytometry."[10] If APAAP, once presented as a simpler alternative to flow cytometry, turned out to require "rather more care," this was due not simply to a flawed assessment of the skills actually required to perform it, but, at least in part, to the fact that highly automated, benchtop flow cytometers appeared in the mid-1980s at about the same time that Mason developed his technique. Whereas in the early 1980s Schlossman could still, half-jokingly, report that he needed forty engineers to run his flow machine,[11] the development of user-friendly, compact equipment geared toward specific clinical applications changed the range of the instrument. The new equipment brought flow-based IPT "to the masses," so to speak. We therefore turn to the development of flow cytometry–based IPT, before moving to the slide-based instantiation of the platform.

Flow Cytometry Immunophenotyping

When, in the early 1970s, Becton Dickinson began manufacturing flow cytometers, the company initially forecast sales of 50 machines worldwide.[12] And indeed, companies sold fewer than 40 flow cytometers between 1973 and 1975. By 1993 there were approximately 7000 flow cytometers worldwide. The total number of machines sold between 1973 and 1999 totaled 15,000 and, in 1999, estimated sales were 1500 instruments per year.[13] Given that France did not play a pioneering role in this field, the following figures are particularly relevant. French researchers bought their first flow cytometer in 1978.[14] By 1983 there were approximately 30 cytometers in the country, a number that rose to about 60 in 1986 and to over 400 by 1995.[15]

Obviously, and in spite of their esoteric-sounding name, flow cytometers have become common instruments in both basic and clinical biomedical laboratories. As already noted, early models—large, expensive pieces of equipment—needed a dedicated room with special electricity, water, and air supplies. In addition to counting cells, these instruments were able to physically sort them. New generations of flow cytometers now include benchtop models that can simply be plugged into standard electrical power outlets, and thus usable in the routine clinical laboratory. These instruments do not sort; they only count. Flow cytometers of the first kind are often likened to a Rube Goldberg device, and cytometers of the second to a black box, an equation that, as least as far as the black box analogy goes, has been actively promoted by producers of the instrument (see figures 7.1 and 7.2).[16]

As noted by the author of a flow cytometry textbook, "[t]he field really exploded because 'black box' flow cytometry became available."[17] It is estimated that only one out of ten flow cytometers in use by the mid-1990s was of the larger, more elaborate kind, and these were mainly used in research laboratories rather than in clinical settings.[18] French data confirm this trend. Two thirds of the approximately thirty instruments available in 1983 were high-end, cell-sorting models located mostly in the public sector (which, in France, includes hospitals and the research laboratories of the two major scientific agencies, INSERM and CNRS). By 1995, slightly less than 80% of the 400 instruments then available were of the low-end, counting-only kind (66% of these having been acquired by laboratories located outside Paris). About 80% of the high-end, sorting instruments were in the public sector, private pharmaceutical companies having acquired most of the remainder.[19]

The mere availability of affordable, user-friendly versions of the instrument does not, of course, explain its clinical and commercial success. One must take into account its relation to the developing platform and to the entities generated by the platform, in particular the CD4 cells, whose measurement quickly became a central concern in the effort to understand and monitor the evolving AIDS pandemic. AIDS, in other words, thrust flow cytometry into the spotlight. The author of a major flow cytometry textbook pointed out in 1988 that the sales of flow cytometers peaked just prior to the discovery of the HIV in 1985 (and thus of the development of antibody tests), when T-cell subset ratios were believed to be an appropriate screening test for AIDS.[20] This claim is supported by the results of a survey of 174 practitioners from another field—transplantation—who used flow cytometry to perform lymphocyte subset measurements to monitor their patients for signs of graft rejection.[21] We asked respondents to tell us when flow cytometers had become available in their institution. Their answers, summarized in figure 7.3, show that cytometer acquisition peaked in 1985, indicating that cytometers that had initially entered hospital laboratories to diagnose AIDS were subsequently being used by researchers in other fields.

The converse is also true: laboratories working on AIDS recruited clinical researchers who had developed prior expertise with the IPT

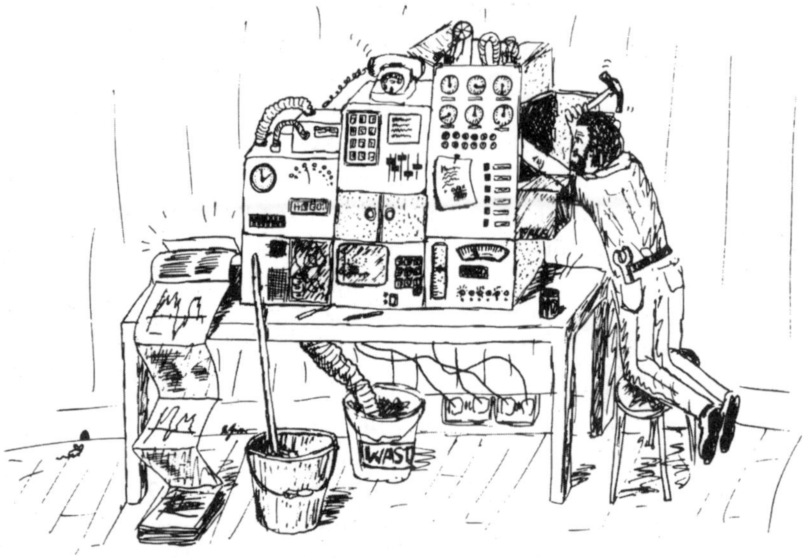

(*a*)

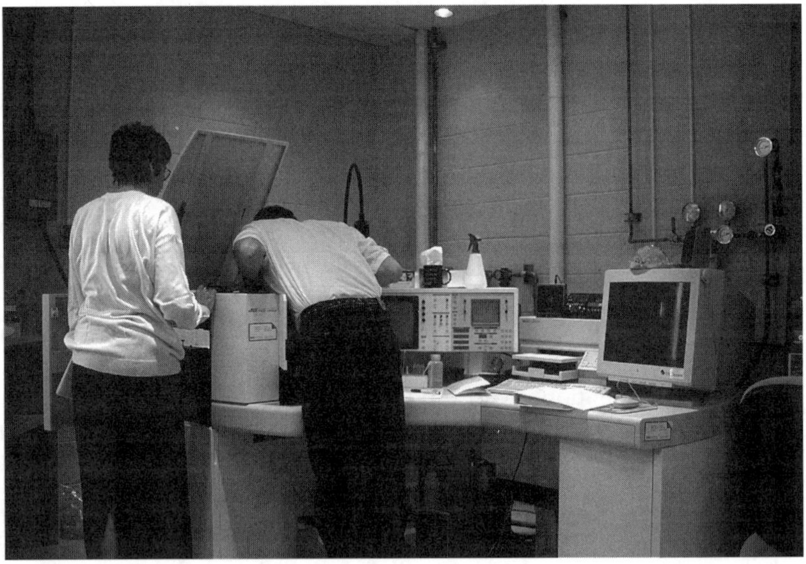

(*b*)

Figure 7.1
High-end flow cytometers as a Rube Goldberg device. (*a*) Cartoon from a flow cytometry textbook. (From Givan, *Flow Cytometry: First Principles*, 136. Copyright 1992 by John Wiley & Sons, Inc. Reprinted by permission of John Wiley & Sons, Inc.) (*b*) Scene from a training session in a flow cytometry laboratory. (Photograph: A.C.)

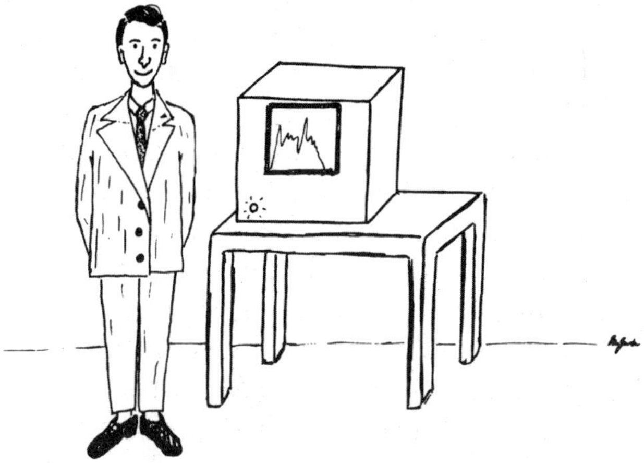

(*a*)

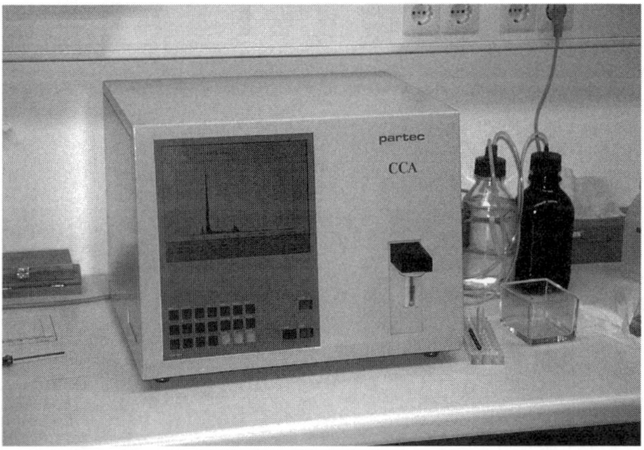

(*b*)

Figure 7.2

Desktop flow cytometers as black boxes. (*a*) Cartoon from a flow cytometry textbook. (From Givan, *Flow Cytometry: First Principles*, 136. Copyright 1992 by John Wiley & Sons, Inc. Reprinted by permission of John Wiley & Sons, Inc.) (*b*) A Partec desktop cytometer. (Photograph: A.C.)

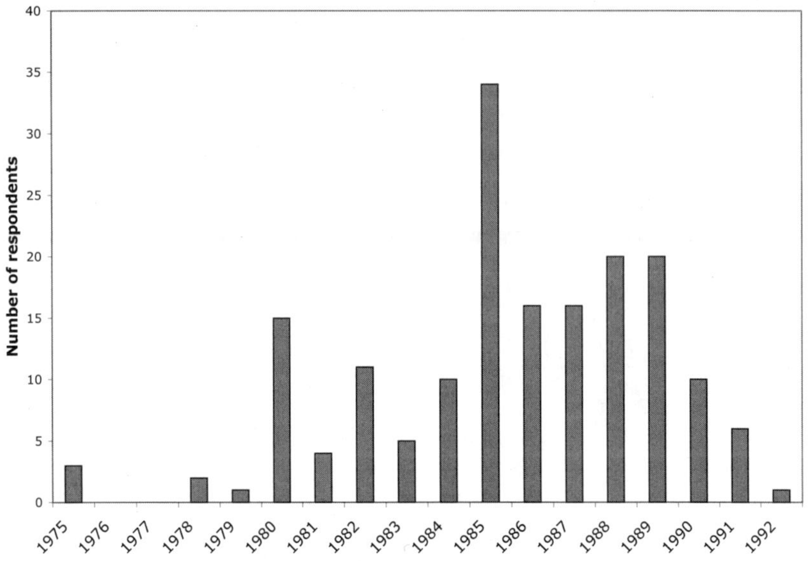

Figure 7.3
Date of acquisition of a flow cytometer by respondents to a survey of the members of the Transplantation Society. (From: Cambrosio, Keating, and Guttmann, "New Medical Technologies and Clinical Practice," 535. Reprinted by permission of Blackwell Science Ltd.)

platform in other diseases. Take the case of Dr. Janis Giorgi. Before 1985, she had published on a variety of immunology-related conditions, including leukemia and transplantation. These publications used data generated by flow cytometry, a technique she had learned in the late 1970s as a postdoctoral fellow in Noel Warner's laboratory in Albuquerque, New Mexico.[22] Her expertise in immunology and flow cytometry earned her, first, a position in 1981 at the Massachusetts General Hospital to work on transplantation monitoring with the OKTs, and, subsequently, in 1984, a position at the UCLA School of Medicine, where she was recruited by a team of prominent AIDS researchers.[23] As shown by her post-1985 publications, from then on she worked on the development of the IPT platform in AIDS, both in substantive and methodological terms (see figure 7.4).

A qualitative sense of the overall development of flow cytometry is given in the following excerpt from a 1992 introductory textbook:

> . . . flow cytometry has itself become a "field" . . . that has captured the imaginations of many people . . . [and where] there exists a spirit of camaraderie; flow

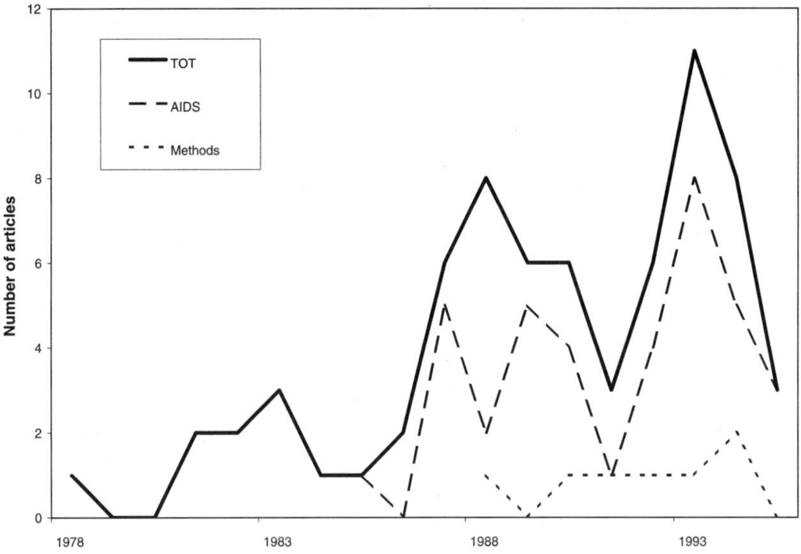

Figure 7.4
Articles published by Giorgi by category: total number of articles (*TOT*), articles devoted to AIDS, and articles concerning methodological issues related to flow cytometry. (Data source: MEDLINE.)

cytometry societies, clubs, meetings, journals, courses, and books abound. . . . What began as a clever technique for looking at a very limited range of problems is now being used in universities, in hospitals, within industry, at marine stations, and on board ships; plans exist for future use on board space ships as well. The applications of flow cytometry are proliferating rapidly, both in the direction of theoretical science, with botany, molecular biology, embryology, marine ecology, genetics, microbiology, and immunology, for example, all represented; and in the direction of clinical diagnosis and medical practice, with hematology, dermatology, bacteriology, pathology, oncology, obstetrics, surgery, genetics, and immunology becoming involved.[24]

These remarks are consistent with quantitative data. For instance, a MEDLINE search for publications related to flow cytometry revealed a dramatic growth from about 120 articles per year in 1980 to almost 4000 articles per year in 1999 (see figure 7.5). The results of the MEDLINE search actually underestimate the number of articles involving the use of flow cytometric techniques, as shown by the growth in the percentage of articles containing flow cytometric imagery. According to a manual search of two leading immunology journals, *Immunology* and the *Journal of Immunology*, by 1992 approximately 20% to 25% of the articles

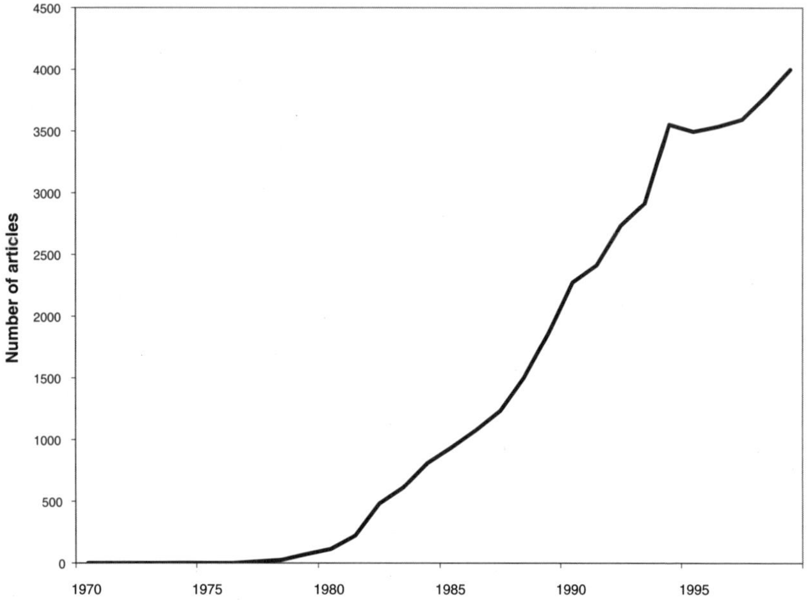

Figure 7.5
Number of articles indexed by the keywords "flow cytometry." (Data source: MEDLINE.)

displayed such imagery (see figure 7.6).[25] While the initial percentage of articles indexed with the keywords "flow cytometry" was equivalent to the percentage of articles found to contain flow cytometric images, a gap between these two percentages subsequently developed. Flow cytometry, in other words, became a background technique, no longer worthy of explicit indexing: it is now common to find illustrations recognizable as using flow cytometry without explicit reference to flow cytometry. Largely represented in immunology journals, cytometric data, reaching beyond that field, were by 1997 present in close to 1% of all biological papers.[26]

Clearly, then, the applications of flow cytometry cut across disciplines and specialties. In other words, the cytometer, as a piece of equipment, is not platform-specific. In addition to applications outside the field of medicine, early medical applications of flow cytometry include cell cycle and DNA (ploidy) analyses in oncology that measure the DNA content of solid tumor cells to detect chromosomal aberrations and tumor proliferation. It would indeed be possible to follow the instrument around and compare different applications of flow cytometry in a number of

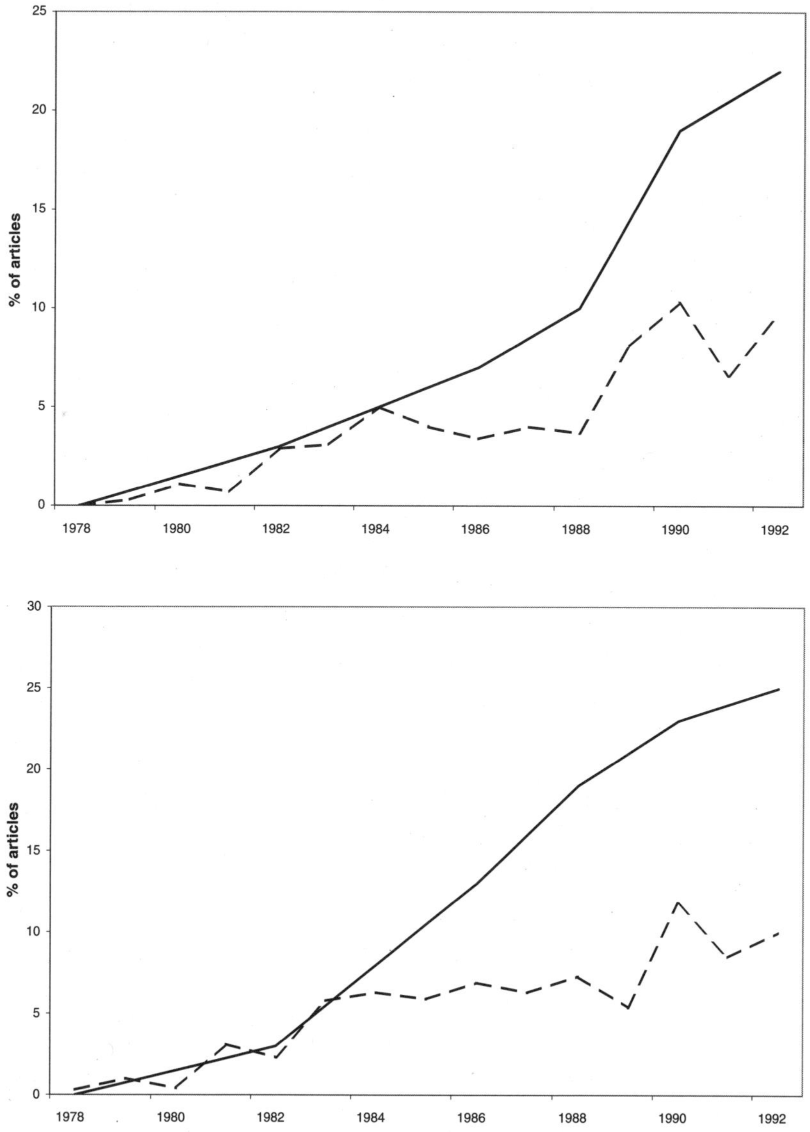

(*a*) (*b*)

Figure 7.6
Percentage of articles in *Immunology* (*a*) and the *Journal of Immunology* (*b*) containing flow cytometric imagery (*solid line*) as compared to the percentage of articles indexed by MEDLINE with the keywords "flow cytometry" (*broken line*).

fields, including fields outside biomedicine. This is not, however, the purpose of this book, and in the following paragraphs we focus mainly on how the instrument came to be part of the IPT platform.

Flow Cytometry: From Device to Platform Peripheral

Before proceeding further, we must describe the workings of a flow cytometer. Review articles define the instrument as a device that individually identifies (counts) and (optionally, depending on the model) separates thousands of cells per second "according to how much fluorescent dye is bound to each cell."[27] A more detailed definition reads as follows: "A flow cytometer measures physical and chemical characteristics of single cells and organelles passing through the apparatus in a fluid stream. On the basis of measurements of light scattering and of the fluorescence of labeled antibodies and other dyes, subpopulations of cells in mixed populations can be identified, counted, subjected to quantitative analysis, and physically separated (sorted) for further study."[28] Thousands of cells labeled with fluorescent antibodies flow each second through a laser beam and the light-scattering and fluorescence measurements are electronically stored and available for real-time or subsequent offline analysis. Each cell flowing through the apparatus is thus characterized by (or represented as) a set of computer-stored parameters. As a result of this complex series of translations, flow cytometry allows one to quantitatively manipulate individual cells in statistically significant quantities according to multiple parameters.[29] In less technical terms, this means that scientists now work with machine-defined, digitally represented cell populations.

What does this mean, in practice, for an operator handling a flow cytometer? Consider the following contrast. By looking through a microscope at, say, a blood smear slide, clinicians "see"[30] and recognize cellular shapes (stained or fluorescent, depending on the technique used); the investigator's experience, albeit mediated by the instrument, takes place in the visual domain. A flow cytometer does not "see": it takes measurements that are subsequently translated into optical events on a computer screen. As noted by an interviewee, this has caused some trouble:

> I remember the resistance of a highly regarded technician, who was an expert in phenotyping lymphocytes by two-wavelength fluorescence microscopy to the use of the FACS for this purpose because one could not see what one was doing. The latter comment I have heard rather frequently and seems to indicate a basic problem that morphologically trained medical investigators may have in thinking of cells in terms of fluorescence signals and frequency distributions.[31]

"Fluorescence signals and frequency distributions": how are these abstract notions translated into operational parameters? Results of a flow cytometry run are represented on a computer screen using different representational techniques that increasingly resort to sophisticated software. They include single-parameter displays or histograms (where the relative number of cells is plotted on the vertical axis and the fluorescence intensity or light scatter on the horizontal axis); two-parameter displays (a combination of two measurement values, e.g., red and green fluorescence, rendered as either dot plots or contour plots); and, more rarely, three-dimensional renderings (perspective plots, resembling three-dimensional peak-and-valley maps) (see figure 7.7). We will return to the regulatory problems raised by these different representational techniques. For the moment, suffice it to say that the development of flow cytometry implied the establishment of a complex set of continuities and discontinuities with previous visual and instrumental practices.[32]

Present-day flow cytometers have many roots. Different "origin" narratives are thus possible, depending on how one defines the instrument in terms of its present uses and components. For instance, one might want to trace the flow cytometer back to the blood cell counting instruments developed in the 1950s on the basis of the "Coulter principle," according to which blood cells flowing through an orifice generate an electrical signal as they displace a saline solution.[33] Instruments based on this principle soon colonized hospital hematology laboratories and formed the basis of the spectacular growth of Coulter. Alternatively, one could focus on developments in fluorescence microscopy, especially after researchers began fitting cameras and photodetectors onto these microscopes. Such an account would make more room for European (as opposed to North American) contributions. Coming to more recent times, one might emphasize the radical novelty of the FACS, the instrument that came out of Herzenberg's laboratory at Stanford in the early 1970s or, to the contrary, depict the FACS as one of many similar instruments developed in various U.S. and European locations during the 1960s.[34] In short, an instrument has no unique genealogy, in part because notions such as novelty and innovation do not mean the same thing in scientific, technical, clinical, and industrial regimes and yet each contributed to the development of flow cytometry.

All is not confusion, however. More than a platform peripheral, and before becoming one, the flow cytometer clearly participated in a class of instruments devoted to the quantitative analysis of cell properties that

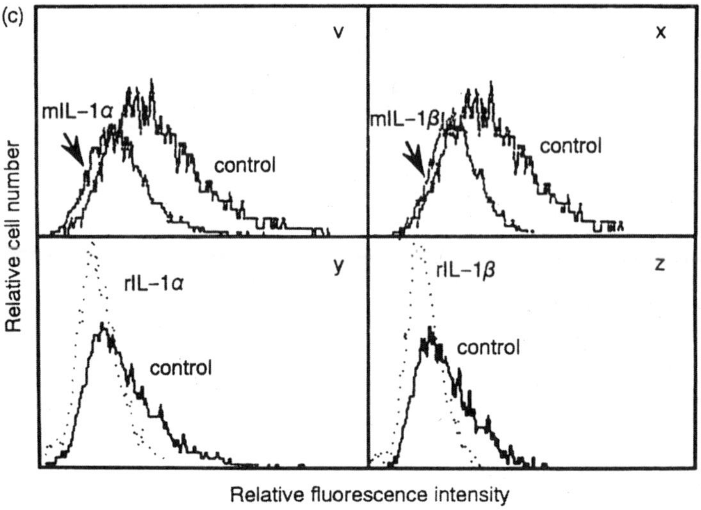
(c)
v
x
mIL-1α
control
mIL-1β
control
y
z
rIL-1α
control
rIL-1β
control
Relative cell number
Relative fluorescence intensity

(*a*)

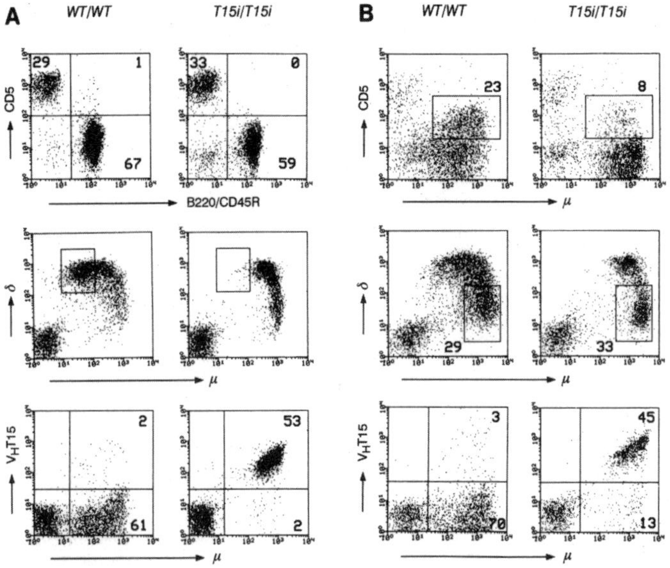
A
WT/WT
T15i/T15i
B
WT/WT
T15i/T15i
CD5
B220/CD45R
δ
μ
V_HT15
29
1
67
33
0
59
23
8
29
33
2
61
53
2
3
70
45
13

(*b*)

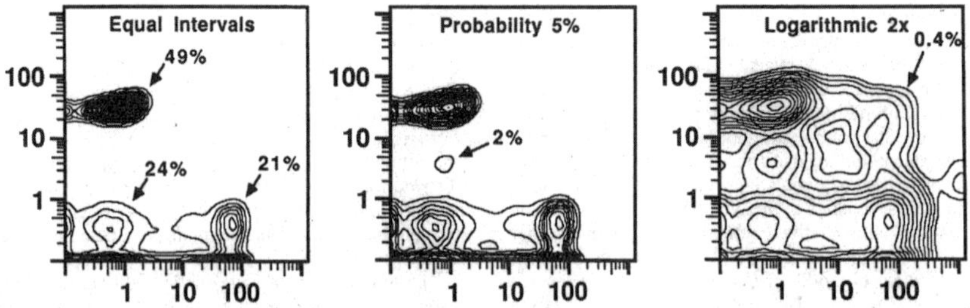
Equal Intervals
49%
24%
21%
Probability 5%
2%
Logarithmic 2x
0.4%
100
10
1
1
10
100

(*c*)

were developed in a variety of contexts in the 1950s and 1960s and that had a common purpose: automation. Now, as a device devoted to the automation of a laboratory task, the flow cytometer does not, in the immediate context, merit particular interest. In the course of its development in the 1970s, however, the flow cytometer radically changed its vocation. As previously mentioned, when combined with cell-surface markers the flow cytometer began to classify cells rather than merely count them. It consequently began to produce unexpected results and generate highly valued data. In this respect, then, the history of the device and its transformation into a platform peripheral is instructive on several counts.

To illustrate this transition, we present a series of vignettes of the early, preplatform days of the instrument. These vignettes exemplify the manifold yet intertwined trajectories that resulted in the present-day instrument. They also allow us to underline a common theme in this process of instrument development. Even though undetermined "biomedical" applications remained the ultimate intention of the instruments produced, we will see that all the early devices initially targeted a continuous, biological variable as opposed to a discontinuous, pathological variable. We contend that the flow cytometer became an integral part of the IPT platform once it ceased to count and separate cells on the basis of the measurement of physical quantities and began to classify and separate cells based on the presence or absence of discontinuous biomedical entities, namely specific cell-surface markers. In other words, we will show that, in the course of the 1970s, the instrument ceased to be either a medical device devoted to the automation of diagnostic tests or a biological instrument devoted to the quantification of physical parameters.

Figure 7.7

Examples of flow cytometric displays. (*a*) Single-parameter histogram. (From Ye et al., "Interleukin-1 Down-regulates Gene and Surface Expression of Interleukin-1 Receptor Type I," 429. Reprinted by permission of Blackwell Science Ltd. (*b*) Two-parameter dot plot. (Unpublished illustration courtesy of Dr. Karl Rajewsky, Center for Blood Research, Harvard Medical School. (*c*) Two-parameter contour plot. The illustration also shows the effect of different algorithms (equal intervals, probability, and logarithmic) on contour displays of the same data. (From Parks, Herzenberg, and Herzenberg, "Flow Cytometry and Fluorescence-Activated Cell Sorting," 791. Reprinted by permission of Lippincott Williams & Wilkins.)

IBM, Sloan-Kettering, and the Pap Test An early prototype of the flow cytometer followed attempts to automate the Pap test in the 1950s.[35] In the wake of the failure of the cytoanalyzer described in chapter 2, a large market had, nonetheless, been created for a device capable of automating all or part of the Pap test. Among others, IBM had become convinced that automating the Pap test would be a profitable venture and, in the early 1960s, had set one of its researchers, Louis Kamentsky, the task of developing a machine to do so.[36] Following studies in physics at Cornell (PhD 1956), Kamentsky had begun his professional career in the late 1950s working for Bell Telephone Laboratories on the development of optical scanners to read accounting documents in order to computerize Bell's revenue department.[37] In 1960, Kamentsky had joined IBM where, through continued work on optical scanners and pattern recognition, he developed a machine capable of reading Internal Revenue Service forms.

To learn about the Pap test, Kamentsky entered into collaboration with Myron Melamed, a pathologist at the Sloan-Kettering Institute. According to Melamed, things moved very quickly in the beginning:

> So Kamentsky came down, we met and talked and we got along very well right away. He came in the lab and I tried to explain to him what we were looking at and what the differences were and he looked at slides with me for a few days and then he kind of disappeared into the lab, into the library and I didn't see him again for about 3 weeks. . . . When he came back he said . . . this is not going to work this way.[38]

Kamentsky had seen the cytoanalyzer and had an entirely different solution to the problem:

> So he said, I have an idea of another way to do this . . . instead of measuring the cells on slides why can't we not measure them in flow as they go through a light source and measure the absorption that way. . . .I remember the analogy he made was to weighing the people in an audience in an auditorium. He said, if you have a scale and you go around and weigh each person one at a time, it takes forever. If you put the scale at the door and have people walk over it when they come through, you get it easily and right away.[39]

By the summer of 1963, Kamentsky's group had developed the method outlined above. Rather than have a microscope move over a slide and scan the cells, they had inverted the process by forcing the cells to flow, in single file, through a microscopically small orifice where they were examined by a beam of light. In the orifice, once analyzed by a computer, the light readings discriminated between the different kinds of cells, and an electrostatic field deflected droplets containing "suspicious cells."[40] Tests carried out at the end of 1963 using normal and cancerous cells were "very encouraging." It was clear at the time that the possible application of such a device went far beyond cervical cancer screening and included the study of the properties of cells in general.[41] Indeed, Kamentsky described the principle purpose of the device as one that would "selectively separate the components or constituents of a biological sample according to type or condition."[42] The project to automate the Pap test had therefore inadvertently resulted in the production of a biomedical apparatus—a "rapid cell spectrophotometer"—that screened normal cells for both biological and pathological purposes.

After leaving IBM, Kamentsky became one of the recognized "technical gurus" of flow cytometry. Following the development of the rapid cell spectrophotometer in the mid-1960s, he went on to develop, in the early 1970s, a series of instruments (the Cytograf and Cytofluorograf series), commercialized by a new company—Biophysics Systems—that he had established in 1968 and that Ortho (Johnson & Johnson) acquired in 1976. Kamentsky's team at Ortho developed the instrument used in the original OKT work and in the early 1980s they built a new instrument—the Spectrum III—specifically designed for *clinical* use with the OKTs.[43]

Los Alamos: From Low-Level Radiation to Red Blood Cells Other biomedical projects afoot in the mid-1960s also needed an apparatus for "screening" and "separating." Nuclear weapons testing and its fallout had created a global population subject to the effects of radiation. Shortly after Kamentsky developed his device, researchers at the Biological and Medical Research Group (H-4) of the Los Alamos Scientific Laboratory (also mentioned in chapter 2) developed a similar device in the context of a project to monitor the environmental and human effects of low-level radiation.

Following the ban on atmospheric nuclear weapons testing, the group decided at the beginning of the 1960s to reorient itself toward "more fundamental and long-term investigations,"[44] and its low-level counting section began to look for "research uses of low level [radiation] counters."[45] Medicine offered several opportunities. Marvin Van Dilla, a physicist and member of the group, set up a whole-body counter to measure isotope uptake as a means of studying various conditions and functions in humans and rodents. Studies of thyroid function (iodine retention) and anemia (iron uptake and retention) were performed in the early

1960s in collaboration with Clarence Lushbaugh, the Los Alamos pathologist.[46] Part of the experimental protocol for the anemia study required the establishment of normal values for the number of red blood cells as a background for the analysis of anemic blood. To count the blood cells, Lushbaugh used the commercially available Coulter counter. Unsurprisingly, normal individuals had more or less the same number of red blood cells. But there was lots of other equipment around, so "one day our group leader [Wright Langham d. 1972] asked me [Marvin Van Dilla] if I could hook up one of the 100-channel pulse height analyzers I was using for gamma ray spectroscopy so that the pulse height distribution from the Coulter instrument could be measured."[47]

Van Dilla obliged and found himself involved in a "tricky" controversy.[48] Lushbaugh, using blood cells from a number of different species, had observed that the larger the red blood cell, the larger the number registered on the pulse height analyzer. Assuming that the readout from the pulse height analyzer measured cell volume, he became convinced that the new instrumentation had produced an unexpected finding. The red blood cells in normal humans appeared to be of two different sizes indicating two different kinds of red blood cell which, lacking any known function, he labeled "A" and "B."[49] He published his findings in a series of articles in *Blood,* the leading hematology journal.[50] Neither Langham nor Van Dilla believed that the readings should be interpreted in that way. Consequently, Van Dilla started running "very uniform"[51] polystyrene spheres through the counter–pulse height analyzer system.[52] He obtained the same bimodal distribution produced by the blood cells, suggesting that Lushbaugh's results were "spurious."[53] Simultaneously, Mack Fulwyler, a physicist who had joined the group in 1962, came up with the idea of attaching a cell separator to the Coulter counter. By separating the two groups of cells, each subset could be run again through the counter; if the same bimodal distribution occurred, Lushbaugh's claim could be branded as an artifact. But Fulwyler did not have a cell separator, so he had to invent one.

At that point, Fulwyler came across a potentially useful device developed by the Stanford engineer Richard Sweet in 1964 and subsequently reported in the *Review of Scientific Instruments.*[54] The device consisted of a vibrating nozzle that sprayed ink onto paper for high-speed computer printers, the vibrations of the nozzle causing the ink to exit the nozzle in droplet form. Sailing through the air, an electrostatic field directed the drops to their proper place on the paper. Thinking of blood as just another liquid, Fulwyler applied the nozzle to the cell-sorting problem.

A solution of blood cells flowing through a vibrating nozzle could be broken up into a series of droplets. Adjusting the rate of vibration to the appropriate level would make it possible to obtain droplets the size of single blood cells and electrostatic deflectors could then separate individual cells into groups based on some characteristic detected in the counter, such as size or volume.[55] The trick worked, and the immediate result was to relegate the two blood cell populations to the category of machine artifacts. In doing so, however, Los Alamos had produced the world's second "cell separator." A patent, granted in 1968, was filed in June of 1965.[56] By 1969, the apparatus was in routine use and could, in fact, be operated by a technician. The problem, at that point, became application. In his 1964–65 report, Fulwyler had spoken of an electronic *particle* separator with *potential* biological applications.[57] The following year, the instrument had become a *cell* separator suitable for routine application to a variety of biological and nonbiological problems. Preliminary applications included the separation of human leukocytes and mouse bone marrow cells.[58] But the device was obviously looking for a problem.

Meanwhile, on the European Side On the other side of the Atlantic, in institutional circumstances similar to those prevailing in Los Alamos, Wolfgang Göhde put together the first European flow cytometer in 1969 as part of his doctoral thesis in radiobiology. From 1962 to 1965 Göhde had performed single-cell DNA measurements as part of cell cycle studies at Uli, one of the largest nuclear research centers in Germany.[59] Unlike Los Alamos and Livermore, the biological program did not monitor the environment for the effects of nuclear fallout. Instead, it emphasized the positive contribution of ionizing radiation to cancer therapeutics and plant breeding. In 1965, Göhde joined the Radiobiology Institute at the University of Münster, where he completed his thesis, later becoming a professor at that university.[60]

During his initial experiments, Göhde had used a scanning cytophotometer produced by Zeiss. Originally developed in 1955 and presented, with unwarranted hype, as a "cancer cell detection machine,"[61] Zeiss's UMSP (Universal Microspectrophotometer) apparatus had grown out of the work performed in Sweden by a team headed by Torbjörn Caspersson at the Karolinska Institute or, more precisely, at the Nobel Institute for Cell Research, where many instruments for quantitative cytochemical work had been produced in the aftermath of World War II.[62] A whole new technoscientific domain developed in the 1950s and

1960s from these initial contributions. The groups that followed Caspersson's lead in the expanding field of absorption cytophotometry[63] included a number of German commercial companies and academic groups such as Sandritter's team in Freiburg (Germany) working on tumor material.[64] The cytophotometric approach led to a number of new instruments and methods and generated some genuine enthusiasm—in Göhde's words, it was a "most fantastic technique"—insofar as it allowed for single-cell measurements of minute quantities of DNA. Unfortunately, it took an hour and a half, sitting in a dark, air-conditioned room, to do so. After a month and a half, one had generated enough data for a "small histogram of some 100 cells, or maybe 200."[65] Flying back from Stockholm, where he had acted as a consultant for a German firm interested in the Celloscope—a Swedish competitor of the Coulter machine—Göhde realized that he did not want to spend years doing cell analysis,[66] and that one way out of this situation was to apply flow principles to cell measurements.

After initially refusing, Göhde's superior, Dittrich, agreed to join him in the project. With immediate support from the Volkswagen Foundation, who saw the project as leading to new ways of detecting cancer, by October 1969 Göhde and Dittrich had their first flow cytometer up and running, using parts from the cytophotometer and a flow chamber designed by Göhde. According to Göhde, he was then unaware of similar American developments, a claim supported by the fact that the instrument embodied several original features—such as a flow chamber design that led cells to flow through the focal plane[67]—and a mercury arc lamp rather than a laser, as was the case with the Los Alamos models.[68] The German microscope manufacturers, Leica and Zeiss, both came looking for licenses. Göhde refused both offers, suspecting that they would have promoted his device as a microscope accessory, a view consistent with their primary manufacturing interest. He turned instead to Phywe AG of Göttingen who, in 1970, put the first Impulscytophotometer (ICP11, later followed by the ICP22) on the market (see figure 7.8).

Looking for ways to promote the instrument, Phywe offered to lend the cytochemistry laboratory of the Leiden Pathology Institute an instrument for testing. Leiden accepted and the instrument became the first flow cytometer installed in a European laboratory (outside Göhde's prototypes). Phywe had chosen Leiden as it had become an important center for quantitative and fluorescence microscopy, due, in large part, to the contributions of Johan S. Ploem, who worked in close collabora-

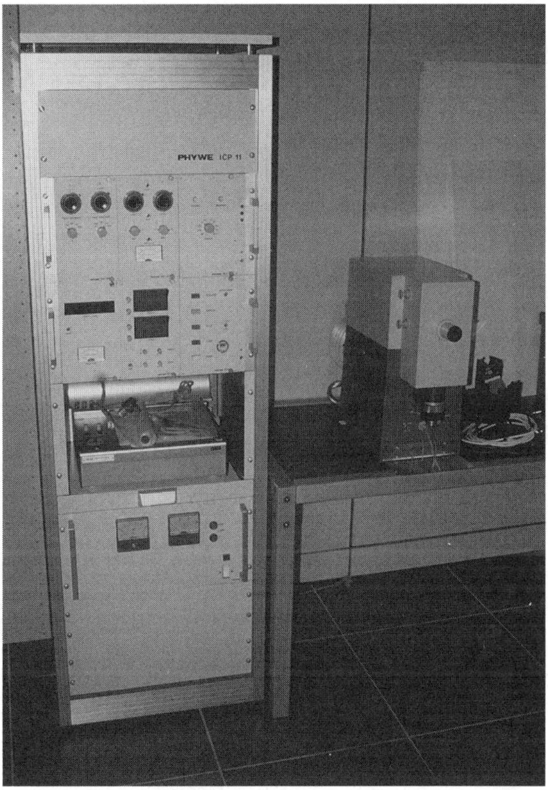

Figure 7.8
An early model of Göhde's Impulscytophotometer (ICP) commercialized by Phywe. (Photograph A.C.)

tion with the German microscope industry (in particular, with Leitz), and had developed in the late 1960s a technique known as "epi-illumination" which is employed by all modern fluorescence microscopes.[69] A Leiden pathology professor who was skeptical of the instrument asked a small committee, including the future founder of Eurotransplant, to assess its prospects: the committee concluded unanimously that flow cytometry had no future in immunology and hematology, and the instrument was returned to Phywe. A few years later, realizing that they had missed an early possibility to work in the field of flow cytometry, the pathology institute bought a Phywe instrument, and the transplantation laboratory followed suit, albeit buying Becton Dickinson's.[70]

In spite of this initial setback, over the next five years Göhde's instrument captured Europe's somewhat limited research market. The first international conference on flow cytometry held in 1975 actually took its name from Göhde's apparatus. Held in the Netherlands, the First International Symposium on Pulse-Cytophotometry brought together instrument builders and clinicians from both sides of the Atlantic.[71] Leukemia was singled out as a major field of application.[72] Over the next few years, the pulse cytophotometry symposia became one of two annual meetings for the presentation of research findings concerning instrument development and clinical applications. The latter consisted mainly of the characterization of normal and abnormal cells through the measurement of physical parameters such as light scatter, fluorescence, and DNA, and further exploration of the cell cycle and related themes. Then, following the 1976 meeting held in Münster and the 1978 meeting in Vienna, the 1980 meeting, held in Norway, changed its name to "Flow Cytometry," thus yielding to North American pressures.[73]

In 1978, Ortho acquired rights for the IPC from Phywe and quickly took it off the market, favoring its own instruments. While pursuing his academic career at the University of Münster, Göhde got involved in another company, Partec, that produced the orifice jewels for Coulter counters, but he was prevented from developing a flow business in North America and most of Europe, since his patents had been sold to Ortho. The company could nonetheless continue to develop flow cytometers in Switzerland where the patents were not valid. Following expiration of the old patents, Partec moved to Münster in 1989 where it now produces an array of high-precision but low-cost flow instrumentation for niche markets.[74]

Stanford: From Exobiology to Immunology Back on the other side of the Atlantic, yet another impetus for the development of an automatic cell-sorting machine grew out of the U.S. space program, in particular the initial Mars landers: in an unmanned spacecraft, somebody or, rather, something had to do the work. To this end, the Stanford University Instrumentation Research Laboratory (IRL), in concert with the department of genetics of the medical school, received a substantial NASA grant to develop an "automated computer-controlled biological laboratory for planetary exploration."[75] Thus, in the mid-1960s, the head of the department of genetics and director of the exobiology laboratory at Stanford University—the Nobel laureate Joshua Lederberg—entered into collaboration with Elliott C. Levinthal of the IRL. Since the conventional cell separators, such as centrifuges, used by the IRL were considered too heavy for use in outer space, the Stanford team began looking for alternative approaches and became interested in the separation equipment developed by the Van Dilla team at Los Alamos and by Kamentsky and his colleagues at IBM.[76]

The Stanford group and IBM thus entered into a "working relationship" for the development of "laboratory automation and instrument concepts for space missions."[77] IBM loaned the Kamentsky device to Stanford for 1967–68 on the condition that if Stanford obtained a patent on any improvements made on the machine, IBM would be granted a "world wide royalty-free license."[78] When Kamentsky left IBM to create his own company in 1968, however, he also ended his collaboration with Stanford. Consequently, the two prototypes that were eventually developed by the Stanford team were based on the Fulwyler–Los Alamos apparatus. The first prototype ran into difficulties in replicating Fulwyler's nozzle and was finally abandoned. William Bonner, a self-taught engineer hired for the project by Levinthal, developed the second, successful prototype in parallel with the first. Bonner redesigned the apparatus incorporating the notion of taking readings of the cells as they came out of the nozzle and not while they were in it.[79]

Unfortunately, the initial success was followed by failure for, by the end of 1968, the "high speed fluorescent cell separator" showed a "manifest lack of reproducibility of results."[80] So, the following year, the team built a third prototype incorporating two improvements developed by Van Dilla at the Los Alamos laboratory: laminar flow (allowing for the alignment of cells at the core of a wider stream before they were counted) and a blue (argon) laser to increase light intensity.[81] By all accounts, these two technical "adjustments" made the apparatus "workable."[82] In the meantime, however, about 1969 support for cell separation research shifted from NASA to the NIH, and simultaneously, the focus shifted from the search for life on other planets to medical applications. The latter had, in fact, always been present. For instance, when H. R. Hulett of the Stanford team reported back to IBM in the fall of 1968, undefined clinical applications loomed behind the work described in the report.[83] But biomedical concerns now shifted to center stage and this shift was made official by transferring leadership of the cell-sorting team from Levinthal and Lederberg to Herzenberg.

With the instrument up and running in his laboratory (see figure 7.9),[84] Herzenberg quickly began looking for ways of making it available to other laboratories so that the scientific results he had obtained could

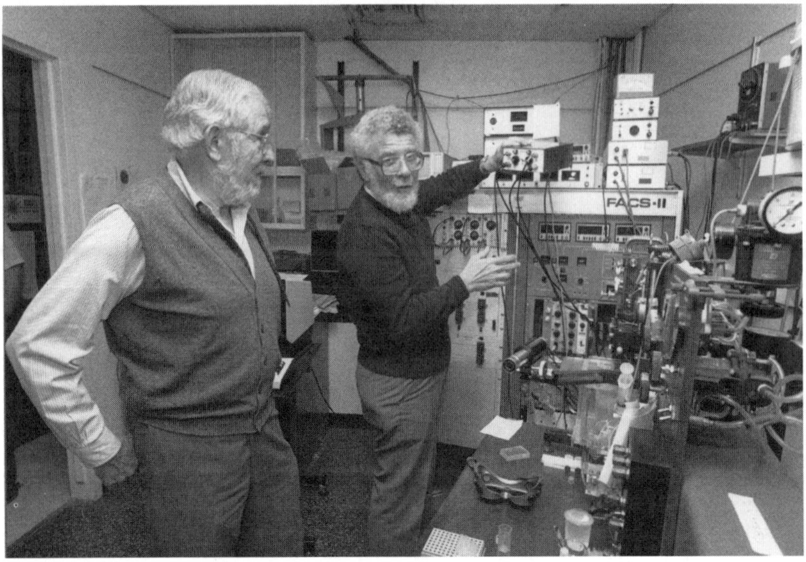

Figure 7.9
Bernard Shoor (*left*) and Leonard A. Herzenberg (*right*) with one of the early commercial FACS models. (Photograph Courtesy of Edward W. Souza, Stanford University News Service. Reprinted by permission.)

be generalized. After unsuccessfully approaching several companies, he finally found a sponsor in Bernie Shoor, a Becton Dickinson employee who also had problems convincing his company to commit itself to the commercial development of what eventually became known as the FACS.[85] Becton Dickinson reluctantly conceded, planning initially to produce instruments only on order. News of the impending production was accordingly circulated among a selected number of immunologists and geneticists deemed capable of using the instrument. The focus on biologists, as opposed to clinicians, was not fortuitous. Participants in the development of the flow cytometer at Stanford repeatedly pointed out in interviews that their work had been "biology driven." The latter meant that the project had aimed to *sort* rather than to type, characterize, or otherwise diagnose cells. Unlike clinicians, they, as immunologists, needed living cells upon which further biological analyses could be undertaken. Commercial development began in 1973 and production in 1976.

Los Alamos and Stanford: Flow Cytometry before IPT The developments we have just described all took place before the establishment of the IPT platform. What did the various teams do with their prototypes? Rather than use antibodies that marked cell functions or signs of differentiation, the early studies explored a number of physical measurements running from the amount or density of the antibody absorbed on the cell surface to the way that cells scattered the light shone upon them.

At Los Alamos, for example, the "biophysics" of light scatter became the major concern. In an extensive research program, researchers attempted to develop a whole new cell morphology and classification (both normal and pathological) through the study of the light-scattering properties of cells. In the beginning, the technique relied mainly on computer algorithms extracting meaning from the masses of data generated. Here is a typical procedure: "After the light-scatter signatures [statistical patterns] are collected for several thousand cells, pattern recognition and feature extraction algorithms are applied to the data to determine the number of distinct classes into which the light-scatter signatures may be divided and to determine the minimum number of scattering angles needed to achieve these classifications."[86] While these classifications did not necessarily generate new species of cells, they did generate new subpopulations, potentially harboring distinct biological characteristics. Applied to algae, for example, the light-scatter "signatures" managed to distinguish between two populations of *Clamydomonas* that, on examination, demonstrated differences in their growth cycle.[87]

The investigation of light scatter as a novel physical measurement of some unknown biological parameter remained a priority throughout most of the 1970s, both in Los Alamos and in the field of flow cytometry in general. Researchers took the first measurements of light scattered by cells at two angles (0° and 90°). From that point on, the number of angles steadily increased. In 1972, Herzenberg's team at Stanford measured light scattered at ten different angles,[88] although, as John Steinkamp pointed out in a lengthy review of flow cytometry a decade later, even though such measurements allowed them to distinguish between live cells and dead cells, "it was unclear as to what differences were being detected."[89] By the mid-1970s, the Los Alamos group had developed an instrument for measuring scatter from 0° to 32°.[90] While, theoretically, an infinite number of angles can be measured, researchers at Los Alamos initially measured about twenty-five different angles between 0° and 30°. Even as Greaves's group perfected their IPT platform and as Herzenberg turned to work on T-cell subclasses, at Los Alamos the light-scatter research strategy continued unabated. In 1977, Los Alamos announced plans to develop an instrument that would measure light scatter between 2.5° and 177.5°,[91] and the following year the circle was completed when trial runs on a 360° flow system prompted the following declaration: "This instrument will be utilized ultimately for identification and discrimination of biological cell types based on the sensitivity of light scatter to external and internal morphological properties."[92] As we know, this did not happen.

Given that the National Cancer Institute (NCI) funded much of the flow instrument development in the United States, the Los Alamos researchers had simultaneously pursued light scatter as a way of distinguishing the abnormal from the normal. In this case, the results had introduced several quandaries. Things had begun well. Abnormal cell samples generated several additional classes of light scatter other than those generated by normal cell populations. The problem, however, was one of overlap. Groups of normal cells sometimes contained classes of light scatter that usually appeared only in the abnormal groups. Since the flow cytometer could not sort cells based on this multiangle light scattering, the source of the overlap remained unknown.[93] To solve the problem, the Los Alamos group instituted two lines of research: the first consisted in improving the mathematics that produced the classes of cells through the light-scatter patterns; the second led to a sort of mathematical morphology of the single cell.[94] Neither of these possibilities worked out and at this point NCI support for research based on light scatter ceased.[95]

As for the Stanford group, they had attempted to use yet another general biological characteristic of cells: their ability to generate a fluorescent substance within the cell when grown on a particular substrate (fluorescein diacetate).[96] Indeed, from the beginning of the project, as had been the case at Los Alamos,[97] fluorescence was seen as one of the possible light sources to be used for discriminating between cells.[98] Ben Papermaster, one of Herzenberg's postdoctoral fellows, had imported the technique into the Stanford laboratory from the NIH.[99] Based on the possibility that the test could be automated and used to type tissues for the diagnosis of graft rejection, Herzenberg obtained NIH funding in 1968.[100] These possibilities were never realized.[101] Why some cells generate more fluorescein than others was not known; nor was the clinical relevance. Initial studies done with Kamentsky's apparatus revealed differences: Chinese hamster cells generated more fluorescein than ascites tumor cells which generated more than spleen cells.[102] The team surmised that the differential generation could be given a medical spin. On the assumption that living cells would generate more fluorescein than dying or dead cells, the difference could be used for what was termed a "viability test." While not of any specific interest, distinguishing life from death would presumably have had some clinical application. In any event, the difference itself turned out to be too variable to achieve the status of test.[103]

What happened next has been discussed in detail in chapter 3 and in the first half of this chapter: the researchers and clinicians who had developed IPT adopted flow cytometry and turned it into a platform peripheral. There were, of course, other more "medical" applications of the instrument. The authors of a 1981 review claimed that the main *clinical* application of flow cytometry in the previous decade had been measurements of cellular DNA content.[104] This is not surprising in view of the fact that many of the European researchers involved in quantitative microscopy had used this approach to perform precisely that task, in particular with tumor cells.[105] The early work by Caspersson had focused on differences in DNA content between normal and malignant cells[106] and this work had been pursued in various directions by several teams, using both microscope-based photocytometric techniques and, as soon as they became available, the newly developed flow cytometric techniques.

These studies included the analysis of "tumor ploidy"—the presence of abnormal DNA content in malignant subclones—leading, for instance, to attempts to develop a "DNA index" that could be used in the diagnosis and prognosis of cancers. They also included cell cycle analysis, allowing, for instance, for the determination of yet another index (called SPF) estimating the *f*raction of cells in the *S* *p*hase (i.e., the DNA synthesis phase). SPF values were also used as a prognostic factor. Moreover, cells in their division phase (or M phase, for *m*itotic) were particularly sensitive to chemotherapeutic drugs, and further studies were initiated in this domain.[107] This is not the place to analyze these complex fields of inquiry, except to note that, unlike IPT, and in spite of repeated attempts to establish quality-control procedures and several consensus conferences, they continue to be marred by controversy about the value, clinical usefulness, and methodology of the various measurements.[108]

As shown by obvious trends in the literature, DNA research was performed before the advent of flow cytometry, and, although a good proportion of investigators in that field soon adopted flow cytomety, investigations using a variety of other devices—all including a combination of microscopy with computer-based automation—continued in parallel until recent years, when the field as a whole underwent a crisis and a transformation.[109] In other words, flow cytometry, as far as tumor DNA was concerned, functioned as one among several other *devices* for the automation of the field. In contrast, flow cytometry became deeply entrenched in the IPT platform, functioning as a part of the latter in the production of *qualitatively* new results, rather than as a more or less autonomous tool for the automation of tedious tasks. Regulation of the apparatus was implicated in the regulation of the other platform components leading the platform to function as a whole.

As the preceding vignettes should have made clear, instrument manufacturers and commercial considerations influenced the field of flow cytometry from the very outset, and, upon reflection, it is indeed difficult to imagine how it could have been otherwise. While the first edition of Howard Shapiro's influential flow cytometry textbook published in 1985 contains a somewhat curious section on how to build a homemade flow cytometer, subsequent editions (1988, 1995) feature only commercial versions of the instrument,[110] for by the time the first edition appeared, sales of the instrument had increased rapidly and its main application had become that of a peripheral on the IPT platform, for which commercial manufacturers had already come to play a crucial role.

Manufacturing Flow Cytometers

We provided some quantitative data on the commercial development of flow cytometry at the beginning of this chapter. In what follows, we present an overview of the strategies followed by manufacturers in this domain, focusing on the aspects relevant to our platform analysis.

Two companies have dominated the market during the 1990s, and they are both American: Coulter (acquired by Beckman Instruments in 1997 to give birth to Beckman Coulter)[111] and Becton Dickinson (BD). A third player, Ortho Diagnostic Systems, has been in and out of the market since the late 1960s. Coulter, Becton Dickinson, and Ortho, as we have seen, have also commercialized a variety of CD reagents, as well as other products, such as beads and calibrators, to regulate the instruments. A minor American producer is Cytomation, a company established in 1988 to develop powerful flow cytometers for niche markets. Cytomation's initial strategy came to fruition in 1993, when, after signing an agreement with the Lawrence Livermore National Laboratory (operated by the University of California for the U.S. Department of Energy) it began commercializing a high-speed cytometer targeting specific users and tasks.[112]

European companies (e.g., Bio-Rad and Göhde's Partec) have managed to secure only a minor share of the market, also confined to particular market niches. Some have secured even less than a niche. The French government, for example, worried by the American quasi-monopoly, attempted to promote a French alternative to the American instruments in the early 1980s. With the support of the immediate ancestor of the Ministry for Scientific Research and the Ministry of Industry, researchers from the Atomic Energy Commission developed a prototype of a machine—called ATC—that was initially tested in the cancer research laboratories of the Institut Gustave Roussy (just outside Paris) and subsequently commercialized by ODAM, the Alsatian subsidiary of Brücker, a private firm involved in medical instrumentation.[113] The endeavor ended in a commercial failure.[114]

If we now look at instruments evolution, we can distinguish several generations:[115]

1. The *precommercial period* of the 1960s saw the development of Kamentsky's rapid cell spectrophotometer (RCS), Fulwyler's Los Alamos cell sorter, and the prototypes of Göhde's impulscytophotometer (ICP) and Herzenberg's fluorescence-activated cell sorter (FACS).

2. In the *early commercial period* of the early 1970s, instruments (including the Phywe ICP, the Biophysics Cytograf and Cytofluorograf, BD FACS-I, and Coulter TPS-1) varied considerably in their characteristics, available measurements, and applications. Data analysis was typically with a pulse height analyzer. Of these instruments, only the FACS had the sensitivity to measure immunofluorescence and do sorting. It was, in a sense, the prototype for the instruments that followed.

3. The *first generation of research instruments* (late 1970s, early 1980s) has been characterized by Shapiro as manifesting "laser machismo." The instruments (BD FACS-IV and FACS 440, Coulter EPICS and EPICS 541, Ortho Cytofluorograf System 30/50) had dual-laser systems, which was the only practical way to do two-parameter fluorescence studies at the time. The lasers were typically large water-cooled models. Endowed with computer-based data management systems, the high-end units had the ability to sort, although manufacturers also offered nonsorting configurations.

4. For the *first generation of clinical instruments* of the early 1980s, manufacturers offered smaller, nonsorting models aimed at the clinical research market (BD FACS Analyzer, Coulter EPICS C, Ortho Spectrum

III). Instruments typically used a single light source of lower power (arc lamp or air-cooled laser). They all measured four parameters, and integrated extensive computer control of instrument function. The EPICS C was closer to a research machine, offering sorting capability and using a higher-power water-cooled laser.

5. The *second generation of research instruments* of the mid-1980s was a group of sorting instruments (BD FACStar, Coulter EPICS 750 series, Ortho Cytofluorograf II) that retained a dual-laser configuration while employing smaller lasers and more efficient optics. They typically had four- to five-parameter capability, and incorporated microcomputer systems and software for instrument control as well as data analysis.

6. The nonsorting models of the *second generation of clinical benchtop instruments* of the mid- to late 1980s, (BD FACScan/FACSTrak, Coulter EPICS PROFILE), designed for the clinical research and routine laboratory work market, were the first to incorporate a true "plug-in benchtop" design. They used single small air-cooled lasers and measured five parameters. There was increased use of software applications and autopreparations for routine work and "user-friendliness."

7. The *third generation of research instruments* of the late 1980s included sorting instruments (BD FACStar Plus, Coulter EPICS ELITE) that continued the trends of the previous generation. They had six-parameter capability and a choice of lasers. They also marked the start of an ergonomic, "stylish" design for research cytometers.

8. The *third generation of clinical benchtop instruments* of the 1990s followed the trends laid down by the previous clinical generation, especially with respect to increasing automation. This group of nonsorting instruments (BD FACSCalibur, Coulter EPICS XL, Ortho Cytoron Absolute, Cytomation MoFlo Desktop Analyzer) had five- to six-parameter capability and incorporated PC-based computers. The EPICS XL was the first benchtop with four-color capability, and used full digital electronics.

9. Again continuing the trend of adding lasers and parameters, the *fourth generation of research instruments* of the 1990s (BD FACS Vantage, with up to three lasers and seven parameters; Coulter EPICS ELITE ESP with up to four lasers; Cytomation MoFlo High-Speed Sorter with up to three lasers and eight parameters) incorporated increased automation and were built with a sleek ergonomic design. The FACS Vantage uses a Macintosh computer system; all the others use IBM PC systems.

This generational instrument chronology highlights three topics, all related to the design of the equipment, on which we would like to comment further, namely, the research-clinic dichotomy, the race for additional parameters, and the increasingly sleek appearance of the instruments.

Since the first devices entered the market in the 1970s, the central design question confronting manufacturers of flow cytometers has been the dichotomy between the clinic and research. An additional twist has been that one of the particularities of IPT concerns its role in developing clinical research, i.e., a "third category" that overrides the division between clinical practice and basic research. So, while there has indeed been a trend to produce, at one end of the spectrum, simplified, black-boxed cytometers for the routine clinical market and, at the other end, sophisticated, highly flexible equipment for the research market, manufacturers have tended to blur this distinction by focusing their activities on what they conceive of as "cytometry products." They have thereby maintained a studied ambiguity between the "research platform" (as they call it) and its possible uses, including its transposition into an IPT platform.[116] This trend became even more visible toward the end of the 1990s, after manufacturers began selling "hybrid" models such as the FACSCalibur, which, because of its modular design—additional elements, including a sorting module, can be added to the basic model—somehow sat between the clinic and research, targeting "clinical research."

As shown by our chronology, in the early 1980s, just before the full impact of the AIDS epidemic, the "big three" put a series of new machines on the market.[117] All three companies offered relatively low-cost, desktop instruments small enough for the crowded clinical laboratory. Most did not have sorting capacity; at the time, potential buyers considered this a sign that a cytometry instrument was destined for routine clinical use. Finally, all three incorporated considerable automation. As already noted, AIDS put a lot of flow cytometers into a lot of hospital laboratories, first as research instruments, then as routine diagnostic instruments for AIDS diagnosis and the monitoring of therapy. While any one of these features—automation, size, lack of sorting, price—might have characterized the instruments as clinical, their status at the time was somewhat more problematic. First of all, Ortho, Becton Dickinson, and Coulter comarketed their instruments with their new lines of monoclonal antibodies, which, in 1980, were more experimental than clinical, and were thus often labeled as "for research use only."[118] Second, since there were no "proven" clinical applications, the intended market for such devices was less the clinic and clinicians than clinical research and clinicians with research ambitions.[119] In other words, the new instruments sought to develop a new market either by bringing university research to the clinical laboratory through automation or by taking the clinical researcher to a higher level of research.

Commercial advertisements such as those circulated by Coulter in the early 1980s reflected these strategies. Promising to turn routine clinical work into research through a device described by its designers as "a flow cytometer without knobs,"[120] Coulter claimed to have packaged high technology for use in the clinical laboratory, thus making research possible at the clinical level. The pitch in a 1983 EPICS C advertisement was: "Today's lab is a very busy place, usually too busy for you to spend hours analyzing a single specimen. So the emerging technologies of flow cytometry and monoclonal antibodies were confined to university campuses and research foundations. At Coulter, we're changing all that." Now clinicians would be able "in minutes instead of hours . . . to analyze and separate cells based on differences in cell surface receptors (such as B and T lymphocyte subpopulations)." In 1987 Coulter announced that its new machine was "the world's first clinical flow cytometry analyzer . . . created specifically for clinical flow cytometry." The other manufacturers made similar claims.

Now, it was not simply a question of the instrument following "needs" as determined by an independently defined clinical or research market. The "co-construction" of market and devices was achieved by "interiorizing" the market. According to a Coulter senior product manager:

> We had a meeting that was held here in [name of place] last October where we invited 14 customers from around the world and we picked them strategically to represent the whole world . . . and we picked people that did clinical as well as research work . . . and we asked them to tell us what do they see in the future, what needs are going to be needed to be addressed by a company, and where would they like us to go. And those are very valuable types of conferences because we can have all of the people, the engineers, the software people, the scientists, and everyone can be there in the same group and be asking them questions and then get a real live type of feel as to why they need certain things and how it fits into their work.[121]

Thus, manufacturers and their clients constantly extended and redefined the market while simultaneously renegotiating the relation between the electronic and biological components and thus the potential uses of the device. As noted by the same interviewee, when asked to comment on the increasing number of lasers and color parameters added to the instruments:

> We've always seen the situation [as one] where the biology will always move to fill in whatever the hardware is capable of doing. We've never been to the point where the hardware is so far ahead of the biology that there's no use for a parameter that we put on the instrument.[122]

And indeed, as shown again by our chronology of instruments, both the high-end and the low-end machines have continuously added new parameters, in a strategy apparently shared by all major manufacturers. Following the initial commercial period, each company quickly adopted the innovations introduced by its competitors. In fact, as noted by Shapiro, one could argue that, by the end of the 1980s, all the major technical breakthroughs had taken place. When one of the commercial manufacturers introduced a minor technical improvement, its competitors would quickly add it to their own models, a clear manifestation of a largely shared technical basis. Manufacturers, of course, insisted on the "unique features" of their own instruments, either in terms of specific core hardware features—such as analog vs. fully digital signal processing, or different optical configurations—or in terms of bundled software and minor added components. But if one looks at debates on a major online flow cytometry discussion forum concerning choice of model,[123] it appears that customer support[124] and the availability of a wide range of integrated products—including CD reagents, quality control, and calibration tools—were just as important as the actual hardware and software in decisions to switch from one instrument to another.

Still, if one compares the instruments produced by Coulter and Becton Dickinson in recent years, one cannot help but notice a distinct evolution, from complex-looking apparatus, full of knobs and switches (as in the cartoon of figure 7.1a), to sleek, almost sporty-looking equipment, even at the high-end side of the spectrum. We illustrate this trend in figure 7.10 by comparing a 1984 Becton Dickinson model (the FACStar) with a 1992 model (FACS Vantage). Similar comments could be made concerning the recent Coulter benchtop and research models, with their all-black, curved surfaces. The choice has been a conscious one: as noted by a Coulter engineer, the company decided "to have an instrument that looked aesthetically correct" and hired industrial

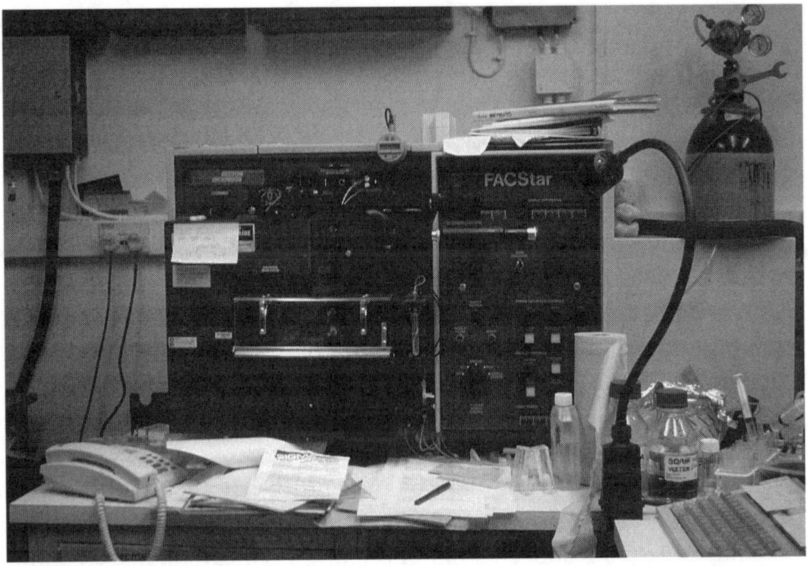

(*a*)

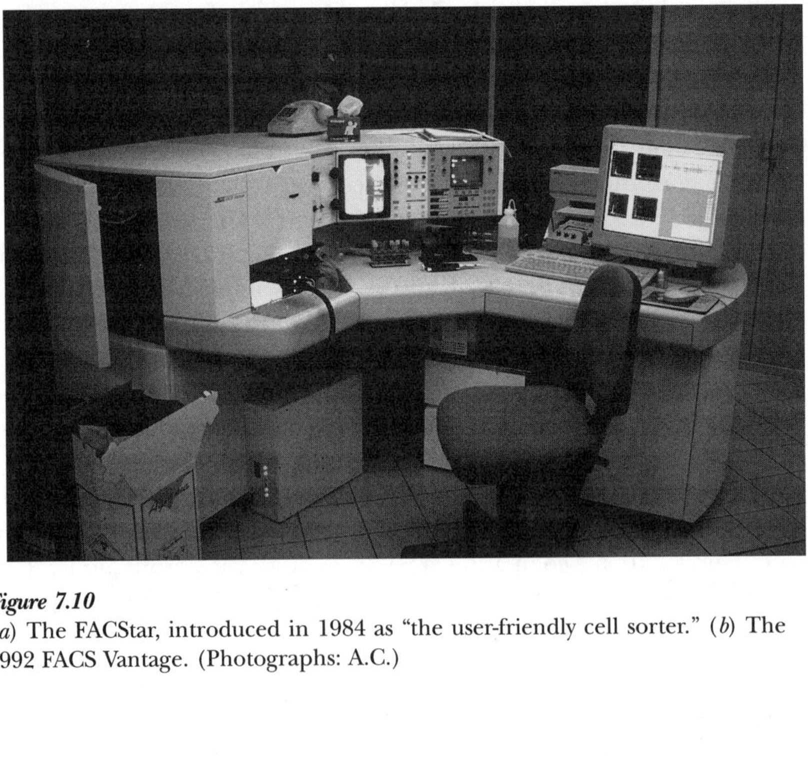

(*b*)

Figure 7.10
(*a*) The FACStar, introduced in 1984 as "the user-friendly cell sorter." (*b*) The 1992 FACS Vantage. (Photographs: A.C.)

designers to reach that goal.[125] But why pursue the "aesthetically correct?" We would reply that, in part, the design of (biomedical) instrumentation plays a major role in facilitating the practical and symbolic interpretation of the function and importance of a given piece of equipment, for instance, by establishing links with other pieces of equipment that share a similar design.[126] Clearly, the design of recent flow cytometers has moved away from the engineering look that scared clinicians toward the look of the other pieces of equipment that have come to characterize the modern biomedical laboratory.

The role of design, however, is far from limited to esthetic features; rather, it can be more broadly characterized as an attempt to articulate users and objects. In other words, the designers' task is to anticipate future uses and markets and this requires a conflation of esthetic, technical, functional, and commercial considerations, with no guarantee of success in spite of the previously mentioned attempts to "interiorize" the market.[127] Particularly telling in this respect has been the market failure of highly dedicated, fully automated instruments able to perform only a specific task, namely CD4 and CD8 determinations for AIDS. Given both the number of existing blood banks and the number of HIV-positive patients that had to be followed at three- to six-month intervals, such a stripped-down instrument would have seemed to make eminent marketing sense, but the downside was a lack of flexibility and, apparently, this was a fatal flaw.[128] A different example concerns decisions to embed some functions in the hardware (less flexible but controlled by the manufacturer) as opposed to the software (more flexible but open to modifications by customers). In other words, design decisions often imply a redistribution of activities between human operators and machines, between the operators themselves, and between the manufacturer and its customers.

This said, manufacturers do not completely control the game since it obviously takes more than advertisements and clever design choices to translate a device into a component of a biomedical platform. The translation involves, among other things, establishing a set of regulatory links between the device and biomedical practices in clinical fields. In this respect, some academic and clinical institutions are more important than others. Take, for instance, the University of Leiden. Site of the world's first medical clinic (Hermann Boerhaave, 1668–1738) and the world's first commercial microscopes (Johan van Musschenbroek, 1687–1748), the university boasts a long tradition of combining medicine and biology through the development of instrumentation. In more recent times, Leiden's Laboratory of Cytochemistry and Cytometry, initially formed in the 1960s as a cytochemistry subgroup of the department of pathology, has developed clinical uses for a variety of biomedical systems, including one intended to automate the Pap smear. We already met the laboratory when Phywe offered them the initial model of Göhde's IPC machine. A few years later, in 1978, Becton Dickinson sent a prototype of their FACS IV model to the same laboratory. The collaboration between Becton Dickinson and J.S. Ploem of the Leiden group resulted in the addition of a special illumination system to the apparatus, although it did not end there. Rather, it was extended, perhaps more importantly, to the testing of the instrument and the design of improvements for specific clinical purposes, thus contributing to the transformation of cytometers into components of the IPT platform.[129]

Aside from technical expertise in the field of instrumentation, Leiden offered several institutional advantages from a clinical point of view, some generic, others more specific. On the generic side, Leiden, like most hospitals in the Netherlands and unlike the United States where pathology specimens are usually centralized in general reference laboratories, had its own pathology laboratory. Access to pathological tissues was consequently easier and clinical laboratories often collaborated on quality-control studies. On the specific side, Leiden was the birthplace and head office of Eurotransplant, established in 1967 by one of its professors.[130] Hans Tanke, a PhD student at the time and now a professor in the same laboratory, recalls the relationship with Becton Dickinson:

> We had a nice contract with Becton Dickinson in those days. We used their cell sorters in combination with suitable monoclonals to look at all sorts of clinical applications. There are three or four theses from the department of transplantation where we monitored renal transplantations and also bone marrow transplantations using [lymphocyte] subsets to predict graft rejection. We also developed a clinical method to measure reticulocytes by flow cytometry, and that is now a rather important test that is routinely done on a flow cytometry.[131]

Although the objective was neither instrument development nor clinical research, both figured largely in this kind of research:

> There is a minimum amount of instrument development, but not zero. Sometimes it starts with buying some equipment, putting the equipment together, changing somewhat in the hardware and developing software, then investigating certain applications, doing cytochemistry, developing tests, making probes, investigating certain things in cells, and then applying it to patients. That would be the entire line, from developing the cytometry instrumentation, developing

cytochemistry, the probes, and the immunocytochemical stain, doing a pilot study and then going through a clinical study.[132]

Of course, the Leiden Cytochemistry and Cytometry Laboratory was just one of several institutions implicated in the fine-tuning of components of the IPT platform. What made Leiden particularly attractive to the cytometry division of Becton Dickinson was its combination of strong clinical departments and an instrumentation laboratory.

Meetings and Institutions

As we have seen, the tension between clinical and research applications, with all its ambiguities, was a key element of the flow cytometry manufacturers' strategies. A similar tension, albeit with a different twist, informed the development of professional organizations that went hand in hand with the development of the domain.

In discussing early European contributions to flow cytometry, we mentioned a series of meetings held in the late 1970s under the general title of impulscytophotometry. A previous forum for interaction between members of the emerging flow cytometry community grew out of a series of American Engineering Foundation research conferences that had begun in 1962 with the objective of isolating "gaps in engineering knowledge."[133] Entitled Engineering in Medicine, the third and fourth conferences held in 1967 and 1968 focused on screening instrumentation.[134] No longer restricted to the Pap test, the idea of screening had been extended to medicine as a whole in the form of a series of pilot projects known as "community automated multiphasic health testing (AMHT) centers."[135] From our present viewpoint, it is possible to see multiphasic screening as somewhat of a fad for which enthusiasm died out at the beginning of the 1970s.[136] However, a smaller, more focused group devoted to automatic cytology emerged from the shambles of the multiphasic screening project when, in 1970, the Engineering Foundation organized the last of its conferences devoted to AMHT in Davos, Switzerland. Participants in a workshop devoted to automatic cytology saw themselves as fundamentally different from the "screeners." This is how one of the participants, Mortimer Mendelsohn, described the atmosphere:

In our little group we were, I don't know, fifteen people maybe. We met in a separate room; we had nothing to do with the rest of the conference and we didn't think like them at all and we never thought we were into multiphasic testing. We thought we were in this gung-ho biophysically oriented new field that had all kinds of things to discover by itself and it brightened the future. . . . It certainly wasn't ready to plug into a machine and read five things and tell you whether you were healthy or not."[137]

The following year, the sixteen original workshop participants applied to the Engineering Foundation to hold their own conference. In 1971, the first conference on "Automatic Cytology," held in Henniker New Hampshire, drew participants from seven countries, giving a growing sense that there was indeed an international research effort under way. The field had grown from "less than a dozen in 1966 into a body of well over 100 workers."[138] With the exception of the Germans, the 1972 conference brought together representatives of the heterogeneous screening and automation community. Some had met before, some hadn't. George Wied and Louis Kamentsky from the Pap smear automation days were present, along with Len Herzenberg from Stanford, van der Ploeg from Leiden, Marvin Van Dilla from Los Alamos (then in the process of moving to the Lawrence Livermore National Laboratory where, in collaboration with Mendelsohn, he would develop yet another prototype of a flow cytometer),[139] and the Lawrence Livermore people—in addition to Mendelsohn, Brian Mayall—then attempting to develop applications in the field of chromosome sorting, a domain that would not truly find its niche until the advent of the Human Genome Project in the late 1980s. These meetings are indicative of the development of a sort of "technological underground" connecting the various protagonists of the cytometry projects we summarized in a series of vignettes.

The annual Engineering Foundation conferences became the basis for the Society for Analytical Cytology (SAC), formed in 1976 during the fifth conference. Although it began mainly as an American society, by the beginning of the 1980s SAC's annual meetings, sometimes held in Europe, had absorbed the participants of the pulse cytophotometry symposia. In 1979, the same year that it decided to discontinue its association with the Engineering Foundation, SAC commenced publication of the journal *Cytometry* and went on to become the premier professional organization devoted to flow cytometry and its clinical applications, adding "International" (ISAC) to its name in 1990. A 1994 survey conducted by ISAC showed that the society spanned the spectrum from basic biology to clinical medicine, passing through, unsurprisingly, instrument development. A breakdown of the 1365 respondents gave their disciplinary affiliations as natural science (439), research medicine (469), and clinical medicine (370). In keeping with the technical nature of the association, almost half of the respondents identified their research area as "flow cytometry" as opposed to the two slightly more popular categories of "immunology" and "DNA."[140] Wondering, a few years before, why members of the latter categories, as opposed to the technology-oriented members, would participate in ISAC's activities, the editor of *Cytometry* claimed that they often used the society as a source of technical information since "[t]he primary scientific and engineering literature is too technical and obscure to introduce the topic" and, as those who turned to the "private sector" for help found out, "[m]anufacturers manuals are focused specifically on considerations of their own products."[141]

The 1994 survey results glossed over an essential tension within the society. As early as 1984, noting that "cytometry was growing as a diagnostic and monitoring technology in the clinical laboratory," a group of biomedically oriented members had decided to establish an ongoing series of meetings on the clinical applications of cytometry.[142] The purpose of these meetings was to explore new clinical applications while "fostering close collaboration with industry." The first meeting took place in 1986 and by 1995 over five hundred participants attended the annual meeting. While clinical cytometrists took special care not to antagonize ISAC, presenting their endeavor as complementary because directed at a special audience, by 1992 they had reached a stage where they could claim that "a constituency, clearly different from that of ISAC, had been formed," and, as a result, established the Clinical Cytometry Society. A journal, *Communications in Clinical Cytometry*, followed in 1994.

The summer 1999 "State of the Society" report by ISAC's president contained another sign of growing dissonance within the society. The report called attention to the "recognition that our Society has a technological basis," adding that "over the past decade or so [ISAC's] efforts have been becoming increasingly diffused in the cell biology and clinical arenas," and that "as a Society we cannot compete with the best in these areas and we should not try to do so; we cannot be all things to all people all the time."[143] The proposed solution was to strengthen and enlarge the society's technological focus by including the more recently developed imaging technologies. In other words, ISAC would concentrate on the technical development of new devices, while the role of fine-tuning and managing existing and new devices as actual or potential platform peripherals would be left to clinically oriented members in other settings.

Slide-Based Immunophenotyping

Let us now turn to slide-based IPT. David Y. Mason's work, mentioned in chapter 4, offers a convenient starting point. As briefly noted in chapter 3, funded by the U.K. Leukaemia Research Fund (LRF), Mason—an M.D. by training—spent time at the beginning of his career in the early 1970s in Seligmann's laboratory in Paris. While there, he worked on the analysis of cell-surface molecules on blood smears, i.e., thin layers of blood cells spread on a microscope slide. Back in Oxford, he concentrated on developing new "immunocytochemical" methods—i.e., methods of staining tissue and cell preparations on slides with immunological reagents[144]—quickly jumping on the monoclonal antibody bandwagon. Between 1976 and 1986, Mason received twelve separate grants from the LRF until eventually, in 1986, the fund decided to "rationalize" the situation by creating the LRF Applied Diagnostic Laboratory at Oxford's John Radcliffe Hospital, with the stated goal of developing new monoclonal antibodies for the diagnosis of human leukemia and lymphoma. In 1990, the LRF transformed the laboratory into a full-fledged unit, devoted to the task of developing immunocytochemical reagents.

The LRF justified its support, saying that Mason and coworkers had clearly shown "that immunocytochemistry was of practical value," in a series of papers in *The Lancet* in the early 1980s.[145] In a 1985 article, for example, the Oxford group had claimed that, using immunocytochemical methods, they had succeeded in classifying all but 8 of 120 biopsy specimens, "all of which had been referred by histopathologists because of diagnostic difficulties." Of these, 24 cases had previously been considered unclassifiable. In particular, the team had recategorized as lymphomas 29 cases previously described as "probable carcinomas." The authors triumphantly concluded that their new methods could "now resolve the majority of difficulties arising over the histological diagnosis of malignant tumours, and these methods should therefore be used on a wide scale by diagnostic histopathology laboratories."[146] The LRF further noted that, as an additional bonus, almost all of the antibodies used by the Oxford unit were homegrown, and, once made commercially available, they had been dispatched worldwide, generating much-needed royalties for the LRF.[147]

Mason's unit can thus be described as a center for the production of slide-based instantiations of the IPT platform. Later in this chapter, we analyze the conditions of possibility of this and related work.

Representational Continuity

IPT on slides, as opposed to IPT by flow, had the major advantage of maintaining a degree of continuity with previous pathological practices. Terms like "immunocytochemistry" and "immunohistochemistry" evoked a laboratory environment characterized by the presence of conventional light microscopes (although, in less routine settings, one would also occasionally run into an electron microscope), microscope slides, a standard set of stains to give contrast to specific features of cells and tissues, and equipment to cut, prepare, and preserve thin slices of tissue.[148] At first sight, the novelty introduced by IPT would appear to concern only a minor aspect of the overall procedure, namely the staining of specimens. Conventional cytology and histology used time-honored, eponymous combinations of chemical dyes (e.g., May-Grünwald-Giemsa, Papanicolaou, etc.) that selectively stained the various components of cells or tissues.[149] The new approach used antibodies targeting the structures of interest, which would subsequently be visualized using fluorescent molecules or, more often (in pathology, for reasons discussed later), enzymes, such as immunoperoxidase, coupled to the antibodies. Compared to the new, electronic representational space created by flow cytometry that translated cells into pixels, immunocytochemical preparations preserved the established representational order, allowing for the witnessing and observation of familiar cellular structures and tissue architectures.[150] The application of immunological tools to cytological and histological preparations created, however, a number of "translational" problems with wide-ranging consequences.

Consider Mason's own account of his early visit to Seligmann's Paris laboratory, where he met Jean-Louis Preud'homme, who had been working on the development of techniques for locating antibodies on the surface of B lymphocytes.[151] To Mason, trained in hematology, the application of immunological methods to slide preparations seemed an obvious thing to try, but this was apparently not the conventional wisdom of the time:

> When I was in Paris, I just followed up on something which I had seen before I went to Paris, which is that when you stain cell smears you can see a peripheral staining pattern, which I thought must be surface immunoglobulin, if you stain for immunoglobulin. Everybody at that stage would say you can't stain surface molecules on cell smears, it just doesn't work, because everybody was focused towards living cells in suspension. . . . So then with Jean-Louis Preud'homme, we just showed that really we were staining surface immunoglobulin, and so I was

in a way sort of mentally prepared for applying any antibodies that were available to hematological preparations, to cell smears with the idea that probably surface molecules would be visible and with the advantage that you can see the cells, because this was done with a conventional microscope.[152]

The issues raised by blood smears were significantly overshadowed by the problems posed by the standard preparations used by tissue pathologists, namely formalin-fixed, paraffin-embedded specimens. Here, the biological material had undergone extensive chemical treatment, raising significant doubts as to whether its molecular components had been sufficiently preserved for antibodies to react with them. One could, of course, search for alternative, immunochemistry-friendly ways of fixing and preserving tissues. But this would have bucked a long-standing series of traditions and conventions: the history of formalin fixation went back to 1893, and its continued use reflected its superior preservation of morphological detail that made it the right tool for morphology-oriented pathologists. As noted by a 1998 observer, "in the diagnostic pathology laboratory, sections of formalin-fixed, paraffin-embedded material have been the morphological gold standard for more than 100 years; there is little reason to believe that another general tissue preservation method will be introduced in the near future."[153] As a result, most of the criteria for pathological diagnosis had been established through morphology and thus a change in technique would also mean a change in diagnostic criteria. A 1997 review of the field restated this point, when it noted that in spite of several attempts to develop new methods

no ideal fixative has been found that can be used universally in [immunohistochemistry]. In addition, the modified fixatives do not closely reproduce the preservation of morphology achieved by formalin fixation. A change of fixative, therefore, may also mean changing the histopathological criteria employed for diagnosis. A direct consequence would be loss of the benefit of the rich collection of archival paraffin tissues the world over.[154]

Note here the reference to the collective nature of pathologists' activities. It deserves further attention. Lymph node pathology, for instance, involves more than a solitary confrontation between a pathologist, a microscope, and a few slides. Microscopic observations require an institutional infrastructure. Historically speaking, and even today for that matter, due to the relative rarity of diseases of the lymph nodes, they necessitate the centralization and collection of pathological material. In the United States, the American Association of Pathologists and

Bacteriologists created an American Lymph Node Registry in 1925. In the 1930s, the registry became the Lymphatic Tumor Division of the American Registry of Pathology. Sustained by funds from the National Research Council and housed at the Army Medical Museum, in its first seven years of operation it managed to amass 380 cases of lymphoma. The collection grew considerably once the American Armed Forces Institute of Pathology entered into a cooperative agreement with the American registry following the recognition that there was a delayed effect of mustard gas on the production of lymphomas.[155] By the mid-1950s, the combined collection had grown to over 5500 specimens.[156]

Data collected and analyzed in this and similar registries first appeared in the postwar era and, because of their large number, set new standards for the study of lymphomas and their classification.[157] Sometimes the standards were too high. The Oxford Lymph Node Registry, for example, founded in 1937, published the results of its first 1000 cases (which included clinical follow-up) in 1947. Commenting on the classification generated by the registry, Videbaek pointed out that in order to apply the, by then, fifteen different categories, one needed "a routine, experience and insight attainable only by a few."[158] Nonetheless, by the 1960s, the classifications produced by the various registries had come to dominate the field.[159] The chief pathologist of the U.S. Army developed his own system, the Rappaport classification, revised in 1966.[160] The Lymphoma Pathology Panel for Clinical Trial Studies of the NCI adopted Rappaport's system two years later making the classification the official system for chemotherapy trials in the United States and a number of other countries.[161] Robert J. Lukes, who gave his name to yet another of the major classificatory schemes of the lymphomas, grounded his proposal in his "experience as Chief of the Hematopathology Section of the Armed Forces Institute of Pathology from 1954–1962."[162] The European alternative to the "American concept" was similarly based on a German registry.[163] This is why the task facing immunochemistry by the mid-1970s was not so much the development of new cytological and histological preservation techniques but, rather, the development of techniques to make immunochemistry compatible with traditional methods of handling the specimens.[164]

A researcher trained in the old school, but living and working in the new school, Clive R. Taylor, took up the challenge. A pathologist by training, Taylor completed a doctoral dissertation in 1974 on the use of immunoperoxidase techniques in the study of the lymphomas, working under the supervision of a specialist in lymphoma studies and director of the Oxford Lymphoma Data Bank, A.T.H. Robb-Smith.[165] When, following his Parisian interlude, Mason returned to Oxford, he collaborated with Taylor, publishing a series of papers on the application of immunohistochemistry techniques to routine paraffin sections.[166] Summing up this and related work, Taylor enthusiastically claimed in 1978 that "we stand at the threshold of a new era in the histological diagnosis of [cancer]."[167] Soon, other researchers would develop additional methods and antibody reagents to make formalin-fixed antigens accessible to immunochemical analysis.[168] Yet, the "new era" heralded by Taylor was defined not by the availability of innovative techniques as such, but, simultaneously, by a profound transformation of the sociotechnical network of cancer diagnosis and treatment, as embodied in the IPT platform.

Taylor considered himself part and part victim of the "new immunological approach" to the study of the lymphomas. On the one hand, he freely borrowed both concepts and techniques from immunology, hoping, as noted by a Norwegian pathologist, that a "functionally-oriented methodology" could resurrect pathology from its status as a "'dead' science concerned mainly with descriptive morphology."[169] On the other hand, however, Taylor knew that those same concepts and techniques made the pathologist dependent upon the immunologist. Commenting on these matters in 1980, Taylor noted that

> It is much too early to evaluate whether or not the new generation of lymphocyte markers has any clinical value, but clearly such an evaluation must precede the decision as to whether or not clinicians and pathologists should take account of these new immunologic markers in attempting to assess the nature of a lymphocytic proliferation in a particular patient. The present time is perhaps best viewed as a time of waiting, a time for reevaluation of what we have learned in the light of new information and new techniques that are becoming available. How important will histology be, and how important immunological markers? How will we diagnose a lymphoma in 1984? Clearly, whatever the pathologist does, it now cannot escape the scrutiny of the immunologist. Big Brother is watching you.—George Orwell, *1984*.[170]

The remarks just quoted terminated the fourth volume in a series of annual reviews of the literature on the lymphomas. Wading through the twelve monthly volumes of *Index Medicus* and culling over one thousand papers a year, Taylor had attempted to bring some order to the ongoing revolution. For a pathologist it had looked like this:

> In the beginning there were pathologists; immunologists had not been invented, and the methods of the morphologist defined, and confined, the extent of our

knowledge concerning the nature and origin of [lymphomas]. In the past decade the traditional beliefs and time-honored methods of the surgical pathologist have been questioned, and found wanting in the face of a wealth of new information derived from the application of immunological methods to the study of normal and neoplastic lymphocytes. Histological concepts have, as a result, undergone radical revision, and the limitations of routine histological methods have been revealed. The morphologist's eye is not all-seeing.[171]

The Lymphomas before Immunophenotyping

The events that lay behind Taylor's somewhat dramatic statement have been analyzed in part in chapter 3, focusing mostly on the leukemias. Here we would like to add several remarks concerning the lymphomas. As noted, Preud'homme and Seligmann were among the first to use cell-surface markers in the study of the lymphomas. They chose to work on a nosographical entity well-known to Seligmann and one that transcended the anatomical distinction that separated the leukemias (a "liquid" cancer present in the bloodstream or peripheral blood) from the lymphomas (a "solid" cancer present in other organs of the lymphatic system). Unlike diseases in the previous two categories, the symptoms of Waldenström's macroglobulinemia could be found both in the bone marrow, one of the major organs of the lymphatic system, and in the bloodstream.[172] In 1972, using cell-surface markers, Preud'homme and Seligmann redefined the disease as a "B cell disease," thus introducing the first functional immunological cell into the description and classification of the lymphomas.[173]

To understand some of the problems in creating such an alternative, recall that for "cell-surface" immunologists of the 1970s, the description of the immune system remained largely separated from human anatomy in the sense that it coordinated a variety of experimental results, often obtained in the mouse, without necessarily localizing the events and the participants in normal or diseased human cells or tissues. At the same time, pathologists and, more precisely, pathologists who dealt with diseases of the immune system that expressed themselves as solid tumors diagnosed these disturbances in terms of histological lesions. They did so by looking at stained biopsy material taken from the lymph nodes of patients and describing deranged tissues and abnormally sized or shaped cells. Yet, standard morphology appeared to have just about run out of steam. By 1967 the German pathologist Karl Lennert, one of the major figures in the field, readily admitted that "We may deepen our morphological knowledge by tissue smears. We will not improve, however, our knowledge by this method in any further essential aspects."[174] Moreover, the booming biology of lymphocytes had created a somewhat hostile environment for morphologists: "Anyone who tries to identify these cells by morphological criteria is accused of sophistry and hairsplitting, whereas it is accounted scientifically correct and unbiased to speak of 'lymphoid cells,' 'blast cells,' etc."[175] But, hairsplitting notwithstanding, Lennert himself had a lymph node registry that collected all cases of lymphoma in Germany. He had too many smears and sections to become an immunologist and start raising rabbits. Given these advantages and constraints, the future seemed to lay in what he termed "subtle histological analysis" using an electron microscope.[176]

Ultramorphology, i.e., morphology using various kinds of electron microscopy (transmission or scanning electron microscopy, with or without cytochemical techniques at the ultramicroscopic level), did find its way into clinical research laboratories. Yet, it remained morphology and, as we have seen, following the redefinition of the structure and function of the immune system in terms of "cell-surface immunology," an alternative immunological description of cancer cells had emerged. Between 1972 and 1974, then, cell-surface immunology moved to the forefront of pathologists' preoccupations as they created a network of technical and personal relations that would allow them to map the T-B distinction onto the lymph nodes in a variety of overlapping ways.

Anatomically speaking, pathologists generally localized B cells in the follicles or germinal centers of the lymph nodes. T cells lay in the paracortex surrounding the centers. Like all generalizations, however, no simple correlation existed between anatomical structure and cellular function, and when disease had altered those same structures or functions, there seemed to be no correlation at all. The individual cells of the immune system, as defined by immunological function, did not correspond in name or description to the cells defined by pathologists according to morphological and staining criteria. The pathologist's "histiocyte," for example, had no equivalent in the cells identified through cell-surface markers. Furthermore, the developmental sequence of hematopoietic cells leading from the bone marrow to the final product in the blood described by morphological techniques no longer held. Consequently, the new cells meant new diagnostic categories and, ultimately, new classifications of the lymphomas. As a sign of the disarray wrought by the cells, between 1974 and 1977 pathologists developed over fifteen new classifications of the lymphomas.[177] So, although the immunological revolution and cell-surface immunology did not go unnoticed by pathologists, the modalities of its application to pathology were far from self-evident.

The advantages of Preud'homme and Seligmann's innovation can be more easily appreciated when compared to previous and concurrent attempts to use morphology rather than cell-surface antigens to introduce the immunological distinction between B cells and T cells into the diagnosis and classification of the lymphomas. In 1973, at the First International Symposium on the Non-Hodgkin's Lymphomata held in London, Robert J. Lukes and Karl Lennert,[178] two of the world's leading pathologists specializing in the diagnosis and classification of the lymphomas, both presented new, immunology-inspired yet morphology-based reformulations of previous morphological classifications. Both attempted to skirt IPT and to define immunological function in terms of morphology.[179] Indeed, despite their endorsement of a functional-immunological approach to the classification and hence to the understanding of the lymphomas, the subdivisions of the main categories and thus the bottom (empirical) line in both the Lennert and Lukes-Collins classifications remained morphological.[180]

For example, while admitting that "most of the malignant lymphomata investigated seemed to be derived from the B lymphocyte system,"[181] Lennert's group defined the B cells in terms of their appearance under an electron microscope or in Giemsa stains. Similarly, the Lukes-Collins scheme divided B-cell types of lymphoma into small and large-cleaved and small and large noncleaved cells. The identification of a category thus required the use of a microscope and the description of a size and a shape, not a function.[182] Not all pathologists viewed these "functional" classifications with enthusiasm. They clearly did not conform to recent WHO proposals that suggested that reporting and thus classification of the leukemias and lymphomas should avoid the use of morphological terms "based on as yet debatable functional interpretations."[183]

Even when researchers complemented the morphological interpretation of function with functional tests, critics decried the results as "difficult to interpret" and subject to the production of artifacts.[184] Despite the technical problems, the development of the new immunohistological techniques in the mid-1970s resulted in a partial fusion of the previously independent sociotechnical networks of pathology and immunology. After many years of battle between morphology-based classifications that had accommodated immunological considerations, this fusion led in 1994 to a radical reformulation of the classification of lymphoproliferative diseases. Known as the REAL (revised European-American lymphoma) classification, it was produced by an international consortium known collectively as the International Lymphoma Study Group (ILSG), of which Mason was a member.[185] The WHO stepped in a few years later, proposing yet another classification that adopted, by and large, the REAL classification.[186] Defined by a combination of morphology, immunophenotype, genetic features, and clinical syndromes, the categories of the REAL classification constituted more than a classification. Bordering on a nomenclature, REAL listed an extended number of lymphoid cancers with their corresponding features. Contrary to previous classifications, however, which accommodated immunology by reducing it to morphological variables, REAL and the classifications of the 1990s were children of the IPT (and genetic) work performed during the 1980s. They thus fully integrated IPT as an equal partner. We return to the REAL classification in the next chapter when we discuss the regulatory issues that were part of its development. Before closing this chapter, however, a few additional remarks concerning IPT on slides are warranted.

Immunocytochemical Methods

Lymphomas played a leading-edge role in the development of immunocytochemistry in diagnostic pathology, insofar as other neoplasms like breast cancer, soft tissue tumors, and bone tumors later adopted some of the technologies developed for lymphomas.[187] The development of immunocytochemical techniques, however, predated their application to cancer and can be tracked back to the early 1940s, when Albert H. Coons (Harvard Medical School) and coworkers introduced the indirect immunofluorescence methods.[188] Subsequent developments, however, were more or less contemporaneous with the events discussed in this book. For instance, the introduction of enzymes, as opposed to fluorescent molecules, as antibody labels followed about twenty years after immunofluorescence, with the development in the mid-1960s of methods using immunoperoxidase.[189] Further developments in the 1970s included unlabeled-antibody methods such as the peroxidase–anti-peroxidase (PAP) technique (1970) and the avidin–biotin complex (ABC) technique (1974),[190] both direct ancestors of the technique developed by Mason and colleagues in 1984, and the alkaline phosphatase–anti-alkaline phosphatase (APAAP) procedure.[191] These latter methods became "especially popular among pathologists" precisely because they allowed one to simultaneously assess the localization of antigens *and* tissue morphology.[192] Here, however, a number of important distinctions should be introduced.

Lymphoid cancers reach the diagnostic laboratory in various forms.[193] For instance, they do so as cell suspensions, which can be analyzed both by flow cytometry IPT or by slide IPT on blood smears. As we have seen, Greaves and Janossy performed much of their IPT work on this kind of material. In the case of leukemic blood samples this was not a problem, but in the case of solid samples, cell suspensions had first to be prepared, and this had several drawbacks, including a selective loss of cell types and, more important, a loss of the tissue architecture that was so important to pathologists. To work around this problem, one had to find ways of applying IPT to tissue samples. Tissue slides could be analyzed by resorting to either fluorescence or enzyme-based immunostaining methods. In addition to the staining method, however, the handling of the tissue specimen played a crucial role. Tissue slides came in two different forms: as frozen tissue sections, produced using a piece of equipment known as a cryostat,[194] and, as previously mentioned, as formalin-fixed, paraffin-embedded specimens. These two modalities (staining methods and specimen-handling techniques) interacted in complex ways.

Starting in the mid-1970s, researchers began using immunofluorescent antibodies that "worked" with frozen sections insofar as the latter preserved the internal and external cell antigens. In addition to the unpleasant fact that technicians had to spend hours with their hands in the −20°C environment of the cryostat,[195] however, the "precise morphologic detail of neoplastic cells [was] often lost in cryostat sections."[196] Pathologists recognized numerous other limits to the immunofluorescence techniques for the identification of B cells and T cells in lymphomas in addition to those just described. To begin with, pathologists did not normally have the specialized fluorescent microscopes needed to scrutinize the results. In addition, the immunofluorescent preparations themselves could not be stored, as they tended to fade. In a world where the collection of the relatively rare lymphoma samples in lymphoma banks constituted a major preoccupation of research pathologists, this was a problem. Retrospective studies set up to search for prognostic signs or to evaluate therapies, for example, could only be carried out on such stored samples. Furthermore, surgical routine created a scarcity of material for functional or immunological studies.

As a solid tumor, material for study came from biopsies. Surgical pathologists in charge of the initial collection of the material routinely fixed most of the biopsy material in formalin to ensure that there would be sufficient tissue for morphological studies. As fixed tissues could not be used in immunofluorescent antibody studies and, conversely, as material treated with the immunofluorescent antibody had relatively poor morphology, the two techniques, were, from a practical point of view, incompatible. Let us listen, once again, to Taylor:

> The advent of fluorescein-labeled antibody procedures, offering the prospect of identifying cells according to their antigenic characteristics, promised to provide a degree of specificity and versatility lacking in the usual histochemical techniques. However, the potential of this method in diagnostic pathology, though enormous, has not been realized because of several problems inherent in the technique. Firstly, akin to many . . . cytochemical methods . . . fresh or specially processed tissues are required. This constitutes a severe limitation, for often the pathologist has only fixed embedded material available to him when the need for special diagnostic procedures becomes apparent. Secondly, specialized ultraviolet microscopy is required for examination of specimens labeled by immunofluorescence, and the resulting resolution of morphological features is extremely poor.[197]

Thus, starting in the late 1970s, immunoenzyme staining methods became increasingly popular, especially in the diagnostic laboratory. In addition to being more economical, the resulting slides could be observed by conventional light microscopy, which allowed for an immediate correlation with morphological features. Harald Stein's Institute of Pathology in Berlin, famous for its work on lymphomas, worked almost exclusively with APAAP. In Oslo, the Laboratory for Immunohistochemistry and Immunopathology established by the Institute of Pathology in 1965, began offering diagnostic pathology services in 1979; confronted with its rising popularity—a twentyfold increase in clinician demand over the subsequent ten years—the head of the laboratory spent six weeks in 1985 in Mason's laboratory to receive training in the APAAP method, on both paraffin-embedded and frozen material.[198]

Numerous advantages resulted from the ability to display immunoglobulins in fixed, paraffin-embedded tissue samples. In addition to overcoming the obstacles posed by surgical routine mentioned by Taylor,[199] observation of specific patterns of immunoglobulin staining provided evidence of the neoplastic nature of the biopsy material.[200] Moreover, the technique permitted "the direct visualization of some functional aspect of a cell population (e.g., immunoglobulin or steroid hormone production) without sacrificing cytologic and histologic detail,"[201] in a word, superior morphology. Pathologists could then follow function and morphology without being forced to deduce function from morphology. Although initially intended to work around the problem of the morphological identity of functional differences, once identified the differences could be isolated on a biopsy slide. One could then work backward and spot previously unnoticed morphological differences on similar slides.[202] The immunoperoxidase method thus served as a bridge between immunological functions and morphological features, a role that became even more prominent as soon as monoclonal antibodies became available that could be used in conjunction with that method.

Here, however, another problem emerged. As recalled by Mason, "In those days [late 1970s], pathologists were getting the 'crumbs from the rich man's table.' They were using monoclonals made by immunologists which occasionally worked on paraffin sections, but which usually did not." Mason saw the task that awaited him, namely to develop the "right" monoclonals for that job: "many cellular molecules, which it had been assumed would never be detectable on paraffin sections, could be revealed if you had antibodies to the right epitopes." Accordingly, Mason had first to confront those who, for various reasons, believed that monoclonals "will never be of any use for immunocytochemistry."[203] With the support of the Leukemia Research Fund (LRF), he managed to transform his Oxford laboratory in to a leading institution for the production of CD monoclonal antibodies and related immunostaining techniques.

As with flow-based IPT, the years since have been filled with numerous improvements and extensions that have allowed clinicians and researchers to apply IPT to the study of specific diseases and, at the same time, deepen their understanding of the biology of the processes at work. As suggested earlier, our point here has been to describe the motives attendant upon and the kind of work necessary to make the immunological turn in the area of solid tumors. We therefore will not detail the numerous technical developments in slide-based IPT that have emerged since the beginning of the 1980s. Nonetheless, a final point should be added, namely, that in addition to institutions such as Mason's LRF unit, commercial institutions have played an important role in creating the possibility of a routine performance of slide-based IPT. In addition to previously mentioned companies mainly involved in the flow-based IPT commerce, the DAKO company has focused particularly on the area of immunohistochemistry.

Founded in 1966 in Denmark under the name DAKOPATTS (shortened in 1990 to DAKO)[204] by Niels M. G. Harboe, a research scientist at the protein laboratory of the health science faculty of the University of Copenhagen, DAKO was initially created to produce antibodies that were beyond the budget of Harboe's laboratory. In 1979, DAKO established a U.S. arm. The company presently supplies reagents (over two thousand monoclonal and polyclonal antibodies) and staining systems, including many immunohistochemical staining kits designed for routine clinical use and research. In the early 1980s, for instance, DAKO commercialized the first ready-to-use immunostaining (peroxidase–antiperoxidase) kit. In addition to DAKO, other companies, such as the Leiden-based Molecular Probes, market a steadily increasing number of fluorescent probes: a 1996 review of this domain found more than four hundred products.[205] Finally, insofar as the performance of immunocytochemistry involves complex, time-consuming sequences of immunostaining procedures, several companies have emerged to lighten the load. In the mid-1990s, for example, Ventana Medical Systems, Tucson, Arizona, began selling semiautomatic staining machines, which are marketed simultaneously as timesaving and standardizing devices that further entrench immunohistochemistry in the diagnostic pathology routine.

Conclusion

Chapters 4 and 5 were devoted to a detailed historical analysis of the initial development of the IPT platform. Chapters 6 and 7 have espoused a more synchronic approach, analyzing the various components of the platform which we divided into core and peripheral components. In particular, we saw how the introduction of monoclonal antibodies and the institution of the CD workshops facilitated the installation of the platform in a growing number of clinical and research laboratories. The process did not follow a single path: different "peripherals," adapted to different tasks, made the multiform process possible. Practitioners sometimes claim that IPT has moved along a one-way street from the laboratory to the clinic and that "[as IPT] has moved from research laboratories to clinical laboratories, the need for standardization has increased."[206] As we have seen, however, there has been considerably more interaction between "research" and the "clinic" in the development of the platform than the previous evaluation implies. Given the strategic role assigned to immune cells by contemporary biomedicine, the advent of IPT has subverted the traditional, unidirectional model of the laboratory-clinic relationship. In turn, design and regulatory practices on and around the platform have created norms and guidelines that have changed the very conditions of existence of immune cells. We now turn to these regulatory practices.

8

Regulating Immunophenotyping

Although none of the preceding chapters focused specifically on regulation, we have already discussed some of the practices that fall under this broad category. Recall the establishment of the CD (clusters of differentiation) nomenclature, analyzed at length in chapter 6. The latter clearly constitutes a form of regulation, as do the various workshops organized by George Janossy to ensure standardized immunophenotyping analyses throughout the United Kingdom which were described in chapter 5. The unregulated proliferation of reagents (in the first case) and of practices (in the second case) threatened to destabilize the growth of the IPT platform. Their regulation thus became a condition of possibility for further work on the platform. Moreover, these regulatory activities intersected since the workshops aimed at standardizing practices, for example, involved discussions of the reagents that ought to be used. In anticipation of one of our key conclusions, we may say that regulation does not target isolated parts of a platform, but parts as components of a platform and thus as interactive parts of a whole. In this respect, our previous discussions of regulation concern the core of the notion of platform. The goal of this chapter and of chapter 9 is to explain how and why this is so.

First, some terminological clarification is in order. Readers are justified in wondering what counts as "regulation." Generally speaking, the term refers to state intervention through various regulatory agencies; typical examples involve the setting of thresholds for the detection of toxic elements in the environment and of criteria that must be fulfilled by a drug before it can be marketed. In the previously mentioned examples of platform regulation, however, we offered no instance of state intervention. Moreover, French readers may wonder what happened to the distinction—not present in English—between *réglementation* (the enactment of specific rules and guidelines) and *régulation* (the more abstract process of mutually adjusting the various elements of a given socioeconomic formation).[1] Finally, one might ask whether the heterogeneous assembly of activities evoked in previous chapters, such as the setting of standards, guidelines, and nomenclatures, and the organization of educational workshops all deserve to be described as "regulation."

We have obviously broadened our use of the term to include, in addition to state intervention, de facto, informal, and even tacit agreements, standards, and guidelines. This is not an unwarranted extension; these informal modes of regulation underpin or act as conditions of possibility for the more formal, state-based regulations. We are not alone in opting for such a broad understanding of regulation. For instance, Georges Canguilhem's definition of the term reads as follows: ". . . the adjustment, according to some rule or norm, of a manifold of movements or actions and of their effects or products that, because of their heterogeneity or temporal separation, are initially foreign to each other."[2] Broad use of the term is also consistent with usages we found in the field and thus with our strategy, as outlined in chapter 2, of using those "perspicuous phenomena" that are recognized and defined by the actors' own language as a starting point of our inquiries.

Biomedical platforms require regulation in order to produce common measures and this is why it is possible to think of regulations as constitutive of platforms. Moreover, if, as we argued, platforms are one of the bases of biomedical innovation, then we need to understand how practitioners articulate older, established practices such as morphological pathology with a newcomer like IPT, a problem plainly outlined in the debate we analyzed in chapter 1. Clearly, then, relations between platforms and practices, just as relations within a single platform, require a multitude of implicit and explicit regulations and conventions. We must now specify the regulations and measures that constitute these relations and how they became part of the IPT platform. In what follows, we thus focus on the regulation of the IPT platform by describing how practitioners created common IPT measures within the laboratory, between laboratories, and across national boundaries. We also show how, in turn, they connected these measures to clinical information in order to endow them with commonly accepted diagnostic, prognostic, and classificatory meanings.

By opting for a broad definition of the term *regulation*, we have multiplied the examples that can be examined as part of our analysis. Our goal, however, is not to be empirically comprehensive but, rather, to present selected case studies that shed light on the various facets of platform regulation. With this in mind, we have opted for a close analysis of the regulation of the flow cytometry instantiation of the IPT platform. Regulation has been particularly visible in this domain because of the complexities and novelty of the equipment used and the rather dramatic context of one of its major uses, namely the emerging AIDS pandemic. Indeed, even though the initial regulation of the IPT platform focused on leukemia in the United Kingdom and preceded the AIDS epidemic in the United States, much of its subsequent regulation has been caught up in the IPT of blood from AIDS patients.

We begin our discussion with the regulation of equipment, reagents, and operators. These are common targets for regulatory measures. We subsequently single out for extended discussion the regulation of the novel images produced by IPT through flow cytometry. Because these images have no equivalent either in traditional morphological studies of cells or in the slide-based form of IPT, their production and regulation raises special problems of how to articulate the two. The contrast between flow-generated images and those produced by conventional slide-based IPT set the stage for a final discussion of how clinicians treating the same diseases arrive at a common diagnosis and definition of a biopathological entity. Here, we concentrate on two classes of diseases, the leukemias and the lymphomas. The first offers a concrete example of the clinical problems attendant upon the new kind of imagery offered by flow IPT. Our discussion of the lymphomas allows us to explore the diagnostic use of the platform against the larger background of the classifications and institutions that are the preconditions of medical diagnosis.

Although our analysis ends in the clinic, we do not wish to imply that IPT has traveled a one-way street from the laboratory to the clinic and that regulation is exclusively concerned with the clinical use of IPT.[3] As we have seen, there has been considerable interaction between "research" and the "clinic" in the development of IPT.[4] How has this been so? Certainly, the redefinition of clinical entities such as the leukemias and the lymphomas along biological lines counts as a prime instance. A less obvious manifestation of the interaction between clinical practice and biomedical research made possible by the IPT platform, however, can also be found in the circulation of standards, be they standardized reagents, procedures, images, or nomenclature. For not only does the platform require standards in order to function, once it functions, it creates further standards. Generated mainly within clinical settings,[5] these standards are fed back into the research system where they serve as guidelines for acceptable laboratory practices. Indeed, regulators who create guidelines for clinical diagnostic laboratories expect their rules to become the norm in basic research.[6] Standards and guidelines, in other words, are not always set at the research front; they often emerge, so to speak, from below.[7] In fact, in the field of IPT, as elsewhere in the biomedical sciences, one does not simply set standards for clinical purposes as if parallel and independent standards existed for research. Standards are not imposed on research and clinical practices: they emerge from that other form of scientific activity that we call regulation. In other words, setting local or universal standards is itself a form of research; standards and values are not always known in advance.

This situation is not unusual. It applies, for instance, to most hematological tests. We suggest, then, that the stabilization of laboratory practices in the clinic ultimately informs laboratory research and is not merely some downstream, applied activity of dubious import for the production of knowledge. Consequently, we propose that instead of conceptualizing standardization and, more generally, regulation, as one of the consequences of a technology transfer from one sector to another, we should look at regulation as one of the vehicles through which sectors are instituted and redefined. One might object that "official" regulations presuppose this distinction between the pure and the applied when, for instance, regulators label reagents and software for specific IPT instruments "for research only" or "approved for clinical use." As we shall see, however, those labels represent merely temporary outcomes of more complex processes to which we now turn.

A Short History of IPT Regulation

Reiser traces concerns with the accuracy and reliability of laboratory tests in the United States back to the first decades of the twentieth century, when physicians' growing reliance on these tests raised questions about possible misdiagnoses due to technical flaws or human error.[8] Moreover, as responsibility for test performance gradually shifted into the hands of technicians having no direct contact with the patient, fears emerged that this new category of health professionals, alienated from the clinical context of their work and exposed to repetitive routines, might well misjudge the results they produced. A pioneering study of laboratory accuracy carried out in 1919 by Boston Health Department officials confirmed these fears and, in 1923, led the American Medical

Association, supported by a number of professional healthcare organizations, to establish a first set of laboratory standards.

Studies performed at the end of the 1940s showed that faulty or inaccurate results were still quite common, as did major surveys carried out during the 1960s by government agencies such as the Centers for Disease Control and Prevention (CDC) and major professional organizations such as the College of American Pathologists (CAP). The complaints reached the ear of legislators and, in 1967, U.S. Congress passed the Clinical Laboratory Improvement Act (CLIA) which gave to the CDC regulatory power over laboratories doing interstate business. As most laboratories operated within a single state, however, by the mid-1970s yet another study by the CDC demonstrated continuing accuracy problems. According to Reiser, the debate on how to improve the situation centered on two major proposals—to broaden and sharpen federal regulation, and to increase laboratory automation. Observers at the time noted that automation could only ever be a partial solution, since it inevitably created further problems. In the absence of quality-control procedures, for instance, automated instruments delivered precise, yet faulty results. Eventually, in 1988, Congress passed the Clinical Laboratory Improvement Amendments (CLIA, same acronym) establishing quality standards for all laboratory testing. With regulations published in 1992, CLIA, as implemented by an interagency agreement implicating the Health Care Financing Administration (HCFA), the CDC, and the Food and Drug Administration (FDA), now covers approximately 170,000 laboratories. We will not explore the intricacies of CLIA, except to note that the debate that emerged in the 1970s surrounding the initial federal law established a strategic link between regulation and automation. It did so not by defining automation as an alternative to regulation but, rather, by establishing regulation as a condition of possibility of automation (whose development, in turn, modified the nature of regulatory activities). Correlatively, the debate brought to the fore a theme that has since dominated discussions in the field, namely "quality assurance."

"Quality assurance" refers to regulatory activities lying along a continuum running from "internal quality control" (IQC) to "external quality assessment" (EQA).[9] The former includes, for example, the procedures instituted by a single laboratory to monitor its own internal variability by setting fixed values for calibration or by using control materials, thus ensuring day-to-day consistency of measurements. The latter includes the retrospective comparison of results carried out by external organizations (such as CAP in the United States) in an attempt to establish between-laboratory and between-instrument comparability. As clearly stated by the World Health Organization (WHO), "the main object of [EQA] is not to bring about day-to-day consistency but to establish between-laboratory comparability."[10] In other words, if IQC tests the reproducibility of results within the same laboratory, EQA concerns first and foremost the comparability of results, an issue of growing importance in the age of multicenter clinical trials. In between the two lie a number of commercial and public programs conducted either on an ad hoc or continuing basis.

At this point, readers may wonder why the regulation of clinical activities requires such complex schemes. Why, in other words, do clinical laboratories not simply adhere to some absolute standard, as with physical quantities? The truth is that not only are such absolutes rare in the physical world[11] but, in the case of blood and its components, they are nonexistent. Standards here are produced in the course of interaction between laboratories, and thus are essentially self-referential. As explained by two biomedical regulators:

> A genuine assessment of accuracy is not possible without true reference standards which do not exist for any of the formed elements [cells] of the blood. The only available indicator of accuracy is therefore the degree of consensus on samples analyzed in different laboratories.[12]

Or, as noted by yet another regulator, openly contrasting biomedicine with international physical measurement standards:

> We don't have the obvious. We don't have absolute standards. We don't have a special unique vial of golden CD4s that is stored in the vaults of Paris and we all get our own special edition. So, right from the start, we were always comparing relative precision rather than absolute accuracy.[13]

Thus, even though quality assurance and standardization pursue quintessentially normative objectives, there are no preset standards. Normalization does not presuppose a norm; norms are the result of normalization.[14]

Since blood and bone marrow are major targets of the IPT platform, a closer look at the regulation of hematological practices is in order. Let us begin with international standardization which, in the contemporary sense of the word, first hit the hematology field in 1963 with the creation of the International Committee for Standardization in Hematology (ICSH) to deal with the measurement of hemoglobin. Following the establishment of a WHO international standard in this domain,[15] the ICSH established expert panels on other hematological topics, including cytometry, cytochemistry, stains and staining methods, and, more recently, leukemia and lymphoma IPT, with the purpose of obtaining "precision, accuracy, specificity, and harmonization between different laboratories in all countries and also between different instruments or methods in the same laboratory."[16] Throughout these endeavors, the ICSH continually confronted the vagaries of biomedical methods and materials. In the struggle against biological variation, the tool of choice has remained the production of "international reference standards," i.e., of "substances of defined value which have been characterized by chemical or physical means and established by an international authority such as (for hematology) ICSH or WHO."[17] Handling unstable, biological materials such as blood, however, generally alters their properties and thus affects their behavior. As a consequence, regulation in this field has focused on a category of materials known as "controls," i.e., substances that are "stable enough for use in sequential checking or reproducibility,"[18] such as the circulation of samples to the laboratories taking part in EQA schemes (more on this below).

As far as "methods" are concerned, the ICSH has recognized four categories, whose definition is worth quoting at length:

> A definitive method is one which has no known source of inaccuracy or ambiguity. A reference method is less certain than a definitive method but it is a clearly and exactly described technique which provides sufficiently accurate and precise laboratory data for it to be used to assess the validity of other laboratory methods. A selected method is one which is recommended for routine use having been shown to be sufficiently accurate and precise for its intended purpose and to be practical enough on the grounds of economy of labour and materials and ease of operation. Unfortunately even the selected method may be impractical under certain circumstances so that a simple routine method may be used albeit not recommended by ICSH.[19]

Clearly, in addition to having indiscernible boundaries, these definitions leave ample room for interpretation. Witness the use of terms such as "sufficiently accurate," "practical enough," and so on. Not only do the "sufficient" and the "practical" depend on the situation, they evolve. Consider, for example, the following claims that emerged in the course of an evaluation of automated blood counters: "Clearly the traditional 'reference method' using a haemocytometer counting chamber is totally outmoded," or "It might indeed be argued that optical microscopy of stained blood films is no longer valid for reference despite that Romanowsky stained films have been used as a basis for haematological diagnosis for almost 100 years."[20] The availability of new, automated instruments obviously redefined practices, and the ICSH has consequently represented itself as an interface between instrument manufacturers and clinical laboratory users.[21] Regulation, here, does not create a burden on industry but functions as a condition of possibility for bioindustrial activities.[22]

The activities of an international organization such as the ICSH and the WHO overlap with those of national organizations, both in Europe and in North America.[23] Beginning with clinical chemistry, for instance, external quality assessment schemes have been established in most Western European countries. Extension of these schemes to hematology has suffered some delay, in part because of professional hematologists' reluctance to undergo an audit, given hematology's "dual role as a clinical discipline as well as a laboratory science."[24] Delays have been further occasioned by the aforementioned problem of "obtaining trials material that is sufficiently stable and comparable in function to fresh human blood in the surveys to have meaning in practical terms."[25] Some countries have established compulsory schemes managed by the government or professional authorities, while others have opted for voluntary, profession-run schemes. France's compulsory, government-sponsored hematology scheme, which began in 1970, recruited 1600 laboratories by 1975 and over 4000 during the 1980s.[26] In comparison, the West German and the Dutch schemes, both voluntary and profession-sponsored, recruited, respectively, 350 and 200 laboratories in the mid-1980s.[27]

Regulating IPT in Europe

Unsurprisingly, given the role played by British researchers in the field of leukemia, the British began regulating IPT by surveying laboratories that used the platform to diagnose the disease. Nationwide hematology regulations had first emerged in the United Kingdom in 1969, when the British Committee for Standardization in Haematology, prompted by prior Dutch and ICSH initiatives, as well as by the widespread introduction of internal quality-control procedures during the 1960s, initiated an interlaboratory quality assessment scheme, limited at first to hemoglobin and red blood cell counts.[28] As with similar programs, the lack of suitable standards and reference preparations created serious problems. In spite of these difficulties, the performance and results of the initial trials furnished evidence for the need to conduct further interlaboratory trials on a regular basis, this need "becoming even more important in automated systems."[29] The establishment of government-supported, nonprofit national quality-control schemes for clinical chemistry and for hematology in the late 1960s led eventually to the development of a set of interconnected programs known as the UK National External Quality Assessment Schemes (UK NEQAS).[30] During the next two decades, these schemes expanded from hematology and clinical chemistry to cover all major disciplines of pathology (including microbiology, immunology, and anatomic pathology), so that by the late 1990s they constituted a network of over thirty-five schemes and sub-schemes, operating from twenty organizing centers and covering quantitative, qualitative, and interpretive investigations.

The scheme for leukocyte IPT began in the mid-1980s when David Barnett, a Sheffield medical laboratory scientist specializing in hematology with a focus on leukemia IPT, initiated a regional scheme that eventually gained national recognition. As readers will recall (see chapter 5), leukemia IPT had been initially centralized in Greaves's laboratory in London. Barnett saw the subsequent decentralization of the operation as an opportunity to increase the visibility of his laboratory and, in 1982, began performing the technique at a regional level using monoclonal antibodies. Initially, the Sheffield laboratory could not afford a flow cytometer and Barnett resorted to fluorescence microscopy using the APAAP (alkaline phosphatase—anti-alkaline phosphatase) immunocytochemistry technique developed by Mason at Oxford (see chapter 7). In 1988, with benchtop flow cytometers widely available, he switched to flow-based IPT. In the meantime, in 1986, prompted by the development of an EQA scheme for histochemistry laboratories, he had teamed up with a colleague to develop a program specifically designed for leukemia IPT, quickly enrolling twenty U.K. laboratories. The scheme encompassed two distinct branches of IPT: immunocytochemistry (under the microscope) and immunofluorescence by flow. Note that British IPT regulation began with leukemia, rather than AIDS, for several reasons. First, Greaves's and Janossy's work had given leukemia IPT considerable visibility in the United Kingdom. Second, before the late 1980s AIDS was not a problem of comparable magnitude in the United Kingdom as in the United States or Africa. Finally, we cannot neglect Barnett's personal motivations and initiatives.

Following up on a request by the Medical Research Council (MRC), Barnett and coworkers expanded the IPT regulatory scheme in 1989 to include CD4 counts as part of the well-known Concorde clinical trial (1988–90) designed to test the efficacy of azidothymidine (AZT) in AIDS and that involved thirty specialist laboratories.[31] In 1991, what had been until then an interregional EQA operation gained official recognition as a national UK NEQAS scheme. At that point 150 laboratories, no longer confined to the United Kingdom, were enrolled in the scheme. In 1996, in addition to leukemia immunocytochemistry, leukemia immunofluorescence, and AIDS CD4 counts, the IPT NEQAS added a fourth branch, a CD34 stem cell quantitation scheme, to the roster of programs.[32] By the end of the 1990s, 534 laboratories worldwide participated in the four IPT schemes.[33]

Here is how the UK NEQAS for leukocyte IPT work. Samples are sent out every two months to the participating laboratories which then return results and receive reports featuring their performance as compared to the average results, referred to as "the consensus." It will be noted here (we return to this issue below) that accuracy and precision are assessed self-referentially, i.e., without reference to an external yardstick. If a given laboratory's performance is consistently below average, regulators contact the laboratory and the two groups work out the reasons for the poor performance together. Confidentiality is the rule, since UK NEQAS are defined as "educational" as opposed to "repressive" or "punitive." Laboratories that continue to perform badly do, however, suffer the sanction of having their file sent to an advisory panel which may revoke the laboratory's accreditation. Interestingly enough, the regulators (redefined as "EQA providers") are themselves regulated, since they are accredited by Clinical Pathology Accreditation (UK) Ltd. (CPA), a nonprofit company established in 1992 as a joint venture between the Royal College of Pathologists, the Association of Clinical Pathologists, and several other professional groups.

The UK NEQAS IPT schemes assess the technical performance of the laboratories. They do not officially produce or dictate guidelines concerning the proper procedures and reagents for, say, leukemia or CD34 stem cell IPT. Other institutions, such as the ad hoc committees of the British Society of Haematology, draft official guidelines.[34] Nonetheless, the reports sent by the UK NEQAS leukocyte IPT scheme on an ongoing basis to each participating laboratory lead slowly but surely to guidelines, insofar as they show which technique "works better" (in the sense of being closer to the average performance or "consensus") and which reagents should be chosen or avoided (as a result, industrial producers of monoclonal antibodies maintain close contact with UK NEQAS).[35] In other words, the guidelines formalize practices that have already been normalized.[36]

The British approach, in this respect, differs from the strategy adopted by the Dutch Cooperative Study Group on Immunophenotyping of Haematological Malignancies (SIHON). The latter initiated quality assessments in 1985, at about the same time as its British counterpart, and has since grown to include thirty-eight Dutch and several Belgian laboratories.[37] Unlike the British, SIHON's scheme included an assessment of clinical immunohematologists' contribution to the diagnostic process. Arguing that IPT did not provide "numerical results carrying direct diagnostic information" and that "the various methodological steps, the interpretation of the data and the clinical significance of the results require[d] substantial participation and critical judgment by the laboratory professionals involved,"[38] SIHON formulated guidelines for the composition of antibody panels and the interpretation of results. Above and beyond the usual concerns with accuracy and precision, SIHON set out to evaluate the quality of the final immunological diagnoses by distinguishing between the quality of the experimental data generated by the technique and the quality of data interpretation. SIHON's approach proved fruitful when it turned out that a majority of misdiagnoses were caused not by technical problems but, upstream, by faulty antibody selection or, downstream, by the erroneous interpretation of results, or by a combination of both.[39] These differences between the British and Dutch approaches correspond to different ways of coming to terms with the interdependence of the different components of the platform. The Dutch explicitly confronted the problem of the continuity of the parts in their EQA scheme, whereas the British dealt with this issue through informal arrangements buried within an official division of the regulatory labor.

In addition to and following national regulations, several coordinated European regulatory investigations and initiatives have been launched and are likely to become more common given the growing integration of the European Union and the resulting need for common policies and common standards. The first European initiative in the field of flow cytometry IPT[40] grew out of a French experience conducted in the late 1980s that attracted participants from Belgium, Italy, and Switzerland.[41] Unlike previous efforts, user groups, flow cytometry societies, and manufacturers had all helped in the recruitment of participants in an attempt to develop a standard protocol for the larger task of regulating IPT in general but, "due to the magnitude of the subject," organizers abandoned that project.[42] A further restriction in objectives followed the restraint in scope when project organizers decided to send out standardized (fixed and stained) preparations instead of fresh blood samples, reasoning that the European postal system would not be up to the task of rapid delivery. As a result, the study examined only variables relating to instrument performance. As the organizers admitted in their final report, "The aim of the study was to establish uniformity in the application of flow cytometry in clinical and research laboratories. This, however, proved to be impossible due to the heterogeneity of machines and mode of operation."[43]

An unusual feature of this first European initiative was the division of the laboratories assessed into "research," "clinical," and "both." Although the evaluators left this last category unanalyzed as too "heterogeneous,"[44] data analyzed along the research-clinical axis gave unexpected results. In particular, clinical laboratories tended to be more "normal" than research laboratories. For example, in the CD3 sample, 30% of research laboratories posted results that lay outside the normal range (as defined by all laboratories in the study), whereas only 6% of clinical laboratory results lay outside the normal distribution. Organizers suggested that this "incomprehensible" result was perhaps the product of "ethical pressure on the clinical laboratory to double check results, which is absent in the research environment."[45]

Additional European initiatives have since taken shape. For instance, EQALM (European Committee for External Quality Assessment Programmes in Laboratory Medicine), a European network of organizations involved in the EQA of laboratory medicine, was created in 1997.[46] As far as IPT is concerned, the European Working Group on Clinical Cell Analysis has obtained funding from the European Community's program for research, technological development, and demonstration in the field of biomedicine and health, nicknamed BIOMED 2. Involving sixteen laboratories in thirteen European countries, the project formally separates technical issues such as instrument setup and calibration, sample preparation, and quantitation of antigen expression from clinical issues such as lymphocyte subset enumeration and function assays, leukemia and lymphoma IPT, and CD34/stem cells IPT, although, as we will see, the two are closely interconnected.[47]

The AIDS Pandemic and Regulation of IPT in the United States

As with many European countries, formal regulation in the field of hematology in the United States began during the 1960s. In addition to governmental agencies such as the CDC, professional organizations such as CAP played a key role in establishing EQA surveys and programs.[48] In marked contrast to the British situation, however, the emerging AIDS pandemic provoked the early regulation of the IPT platform in the United States. There are important technical consequences to this change of regulatory venue. Unlike leukemia phenotyping which deals in relative percentages of T- and B-lymphocyte subclasses, the diagnosis and monitoring of AIDS through IPT consists of the calculation of the absolute numbers of a subclass of T lymphocytes known as CD4+. Clinicians use these numbers as prognostic indicators to guide therapy. Normal subjects have around 1200 to 1400 CD4 cells per milliliter in the peripheral blood, and treatment for HIV-positive patients usually begins when their CD4 count has dropped to around 400 to 600/mm^3, with possibly fatal conditions setting in at under 200/mm^3. In the absence of an external biological and physical standard, standardizing absolute numbers is a difficult task. Indeed, in the mid-1990s, even after ten years of standardization, nontrivial variations persisted.[49] Finally, the introduction of triple therapy has not reduced the sense of urgency insofar as some national health systems base access to therapy on the absolute number of CD4+ cells.[50]

When U.S. regulators conducted their initial comparisons of how CD4 counts varied between laboratories in the mid-1980s, they described the results as "scary." For example, the chairman of an early National Institutes of Health (NIH) standardization committee who sent out his own blood as a control "got values on his CD4 cells from 200 to 1400. . . . There were at least as many people down at the bottom as at the top. It was all over the place."[51] Similarly, an early CDC study implicating forty-one laboratories using paired sample sets found that 25% of the laboratories could not identify two abnormal samples as abnormal.[52] Patients also knew about the variability of CD4 counts. At the beginning of the 1990s, informants told us that

> CD4 shopping goes on commonly in New York and other places where a patient wants to be entered into a [clinical] trial [for new anti-HIV drugs] and again it leads to the question of how variable are these results because what will happen is that if they have to be at a level of 500 [CD4 cells] or below to get in, they go to one place and get 600, they go to another place, 550, next place 490, bingo, they found their place, then you can go and get entered into the trial.[53]

In addition to this clinical urgency, the novelty of the IPT platform created yet another problem for regulators. Not only did the data vary unexpectedly, nobody knew what degree of reproducibility one could reasonably expect.

However pressing the problem, it would nonetheless be a gross simplification to see the regulation of IPT as simply a response to the AIDS crisis. The need for common scales and standards of measurement clearly preceded the epidemic. The regulation of IPT relies, moreover, on more than crisis intervention and calls upon a number of tried-and-true methods of quality control that, as we have seen, have been developed for other laboratory procedures since World War II. Proficiency testing, for example, involves sending out identical samples for analysis to laboratories throughout the country and comparing the results. CAP,[54] which inspects and certifies laboratories, is one of the leaders in this area. Participation in a recognized proficiency-testing program is more than an option for most laboratories as it is a sine qua non for laboratory certification. In turn, insurance carriers reimburse tests performed only in laboratories certified by a recognized organization such as CAP.[55]

Proficiency tests and quality control often have outside criteria such as guidelines that serve as methodological standards. Between 1988 and 1994, five different organizations published guidelines for IPT. The first was the American Society for Histocompatibility and Immunogenetics (ASHI). Developed for matching tissue transplants, the ASHI guidelines remained the only ones to stipulate training and education requirements for laboratory personnel.[56] A second player was the National Committee on Clinical Laboratory Standards (NCCLS). Created in 1968, the NCCLS defines itself as an interdisciplinary, nonprofit organization that promotes the development and use of voluntary consensus standards within the clinical laboratory community. NCCLS membership comprises medical laboratory professional associations, agencies of federal and state governments, manufacturers of laboratory equipment and products, and individual laboratories and healthcare institutions. In the case of AIDS IPT, the NCCLS developed guidelines after the chairman of the quality control and standards committee of ISAC (the International Society for Analytical Cytology, the professional organization of flow cytometrists; see chapter 4) approached the national committee in the early 1980s.[57] While AIDS may have been the trigger, participants recognized that all applications of the IPT platform would ultimately be implicated in the regulatory process. Thus, although the NCCLS subcommittee on flow cytometry decided to deal first with AIDS, other areas, such as leukemia and reticulocyte counts, soon followed.[58]

The scope of diseases covered by IPT forced the subcommittee to include individuals from medical centers countrywide as well as representatives of a variety of professional organizations. These included CAP, the American Society of Clinical Pathology (ASCP), the Society of Analytical Cytology, the American Society of Hematology, and other interested biomedical associations. In addition, the subcommittee included representatives from industry (Coulter, Becton Dickinson, and Ortho Diagnostic Systems) and from governmental groups, namely the FDA, the CDC, the NIH, and the HCFA.

The NIH also issued guidelines (often borrowing directly from the NCCLS guidelines) for centers involved in clinical trials on HIV-positive individuals, as did the CDC.[59] Similarly, the Walter Reed Army Institute has performed quality-control studies for the Department of Defense. When IPT uses a flow cytometer, as is usually the case in AIDS, the training of flow cytometry operators offers yet another means of creating and enforcing standards. The ASCP, through the efforts of ISAC and other groups, offers a certification examination in flow cytometry, and the American Medical Association holds yearly courses. Lastly, commercial enterprises participate in the standardization effort. Flow Cytometry Standards Corporation tells us that they are "the corporation that sets the Standards" and the manufacturers of flow cytometers and producers of CDs have conducted numerous studies to ensure reproducibility of results across laboratories.

Despite appearances, one cannot always fit institutions and individuals participating in the regulatory process into categories such as public and private. For example, most of the laboratories doing IPT in the United States are hospital laboratories. To a Canadian or European observer, this makes regulation a public affair. In the United States, however, many of the hospitals in this category are privately owned.[60] Moreover, NCCLS predicates its regulatory activities on the principle of involving professional, public, and private actors in a common initiative. The overall picture thus displays a variety of (often coordinated) initiatives coalescing into a movement to regulate the production and dissemination of the images and numbers produced by the IPT platform.[61] Let us therefore turn to the origins and development of this movement in the United States whose standards often set the standards for other countries.

Prior to the discovery of the etiologic agent of AIDS, the enumeration of lymphocyte subsets and the finding of a reduced CD4+ subset was the cardinal laboratory sign of AIDS and, thus, for a brief period, IPT stood as the only means of monitoring the AIDS epidemic. In 1983, for example, the National Heart, Lung, and Blood Institute developed a request for proposals to study the immunological consequences of blood transfusion in the hopes that tracking lymphocyte subset abnormalities would serve as "an index of 'pre-AIDS' in areas of high AIDS prevalence."[62] While the AIDS antibody test reduced the need for IPT to diagnose patients and to monitor the epidemic, the CD4+ count and IPT of other subsets remain key components in the development of therapeutic strategies; hence, their continued importance.

Conducted in 1984, the earliest regulatory study of AIDS IPT in the United States involved a comparison between three laboratories: one NIH laboratory and two private laboratories, including one run by the pharmaceutical multinational Smith, Kline & French. Using blood from "normal" donors, researchers restricted the study to one brand of flow cytometer (EPICS V by Coulter) and analyzed the results using the manufacturer's data packages.[63] The group attributed the finding of "no significant difference" between the laboratories to "the availability of quality reagents, precision instrumentation and a standard lymphocyte preparation."[64] The author responsible for the study, Gerald E. Marti, subsequently extended the program and, in February of 1986, began offering "quarterly flow cytometry leukocyte phenotyping proficiency-testing samples and monthly quality assurance programs to over 60 sites."[65] Carried out in "anticipation of certification and licensing requirements,"[66] the scheme devised by Marti's group now collected data on the basis of two commercial variables: make and model of flow cytometer and brand of monoclonal antibody used to recognize the cell-surface markers. Marti's program collected further data on a "methodological" variable, namely the means of specimen preparation.[67] At that date, only "small differences" arose on the basis of commercial make. These small differences turned out to be short-lived.

In the meantime, the articulation of IPT with other laboratory practices was of more immediate concern. To understand why, note that, at the time, most flow cytometers gave results in terms of the relative number of cells. Clinicians obtained the absolute numbers needed for diagnosis by combining those relative percentages of T-cell subsets with the absolute number of lymphocytes per cubic milliliter of peripheral blood as determined by other kinds of hematology equipment readily available in the clinical laboratory. This procedure thus required "a chain of multiplications"[68] that greatly magnified initial, minor variations. As noted by one respondent, "when you take a number generated by one instrument system and you add that to a number generated by another instrument system, you have at the very least two sources of error if not a synergistic result of combining errors. Because you do some multiplications, you can actually multiply your error through."[69]

More than just a problem of messy mathematics, standardizing at one point in the process engendered standardization effects both up and down the production line. As the authors of one study pointed out, "Although this report does not address the issue of standardization of absolute lymphocyte counts, it seems obvious that this will have to be done in order to generate reproducible values."[70] Three years after the original study, the reproducible values seemed even more remote given the now evident "intrinsic differences among hematology instruments produced by different manufacturers."[71] Since then, the further possibility of making the same kind of calculation now using flow cytometry instrumentation rather than the standard hematology equipment further complicated the problem of absolute counts. How to articulate the two remained contentious. Early 1990 NCCLS recommendations, for example, stated quite bluntly that "The performance of a differential by flow cytometry has not been standardized to the accepted methodologies of hematology instrumentation and therefore should not be used."[72]

Other groups and institutions quickly followed Marti's group at the NIH into the field of IPT regulation. CAP began their standardization efforts in 1986 when they began interlaboratory proficiency testing in clinical IPT.[73] The program did not directly undertake proficiency testing (hence the notion of *interlaboratory* proficiency),[74] but sought that end through indirect means. Sending out pretested samples yearly to participating laboratories, the survey provided data to laboratories using similar analytical systems, enabling them to compare their performance with other laboratories and to produce data that would give a general picture of clinical IPT. Curiously, in the course of the survey, rather than a movement of general improvement, researchers observed the opposite tendency. In particular, even though in the period 1986–91, "no differences were apparent,"[75] analysis of data gathered from over one hundred laboratories in 1991 and divided, once again, according to the two most common commercial instruments and protocols then in use showed that the participating laboratories had generated "systematically different results."[76] Reporting on the survey in 1993, CAP commented that "The reasons for these differences are not known."[77]

The CDC began their monitoring program the same year as CAP.[78] Known as the Model Performance Evaluation Program (MPEP), it started as a voluntary program. Initially restricted to HIV antibody testing, the CDC expanded the program in 1990 to include T-lymphocyte IPT, sending samples to 293 laboratories in October of that year. The conclusion: "Most testing laboratories experienced no difficulties in testing sample panels and most performed [IPT] within reference limits."[79] Despite the optimism, however, the aforementioned "reference limits" had no pretense of universality. As the NCCLS tentative guideline issued in May of 1992 explicitly recognized, "[a]t present there are no universally accepted standards for precision, accuracy and interlaboratory comparability in lymphocyte typing by flow cytometry."[80]

By the end of 1988, the U.S. Department of Defense (DOD) had screened over 4 million people for HIV and found 2000 cases of infection. The need for IPT here emerged when the DOD decided that infected persons should be categorized and monitored according to the Walter Reed Army Institute of Research classification for HIV infection that divided the various stages of the disease according to CD4 levels. The DOD further categorized the seven Walter Reed stages (WR0–WR6) into two therapeutic groups: WR0–WR2 designated patients with a CD4+ count of more than 400/mm^3 CD4, whereas less than 400[81] signified that the patient had advanced to clinical level WR3 and beyond.[82] Given the status of absolute CD4 counts in this system, some form of control was deemed necessary. So, like CAP, the army instituted training programs that it farmed out to the private sector. FAST Systems Inc., for example, handled training programs from 1986 to 1988. However, the army went further than CAP in the commercialization of the process by contracting FAST to undertake a proficiency-testing program. Symptomatic of the need to control for variation created by different commercial suppliers, FAST distributed the reagents used in the program according to market share (at the time, 60% Coulter, 40% Becton Dickinson). Similarly, the instrument standardization part of the study sought comparability between EPICS-C and EPICS-V (Coulter) and FACS (Becton Dickinson). FAST, itself, provided fluorescent intensity standard beads (key beads) for purposes of calibration.[83]

While the proficiency survey initially targeted the eight U.S. Army Medical Center laboratories, by the end of 1988 over fifty-six other laboratories had joined the program.[84] By the army's own assessment, the operation was a success: "Interlaboratory variabilities in the white blood cell count (WBC) were reduced approximately 50%, whereas the cv's [coefficients of variation] for the lymphocyte differential were reduced almost 75%." This translated into an improvement in absolute terms: the coefficient of variation of the absolute lymphocyte count dropped from 21.1% to 7.0%.[85] The very success of the operation served as proof of its original need.

Note, here, the "industrial" components of the regulation of IPT. Public regulators first delegated regulation to the private sector. The latter, in turn, devised a process that would incorporate variability arising from the existence of multiple manufacturers. For although the army had initially set out to "develop a standardized instrument set-up protocol and a simple straightforward sample preparation procedure," this operation presumed that "these protocols had to be compatible with instruments and monoclonal antibodies from multiple commercial sources."[86] Finally, industry (viz. Coulter) successfully patented part of the regulatory process by describing a procedure for "statistically evaluating the performance . . . of at least one analytical instrument in a pool of like or substantially like instruments by comparing the performance of the one instrument located in one laboratory with the performance of like instruments in other laboratories."[87]

Let us now take a closer look at the individual targets of platform regulation. In contrast to chapter 4 where we introduced an analytical distinction between the core of the platform (the CD markers) and its peripheral elements, we will now break down the various functional components of the platform into the items that have been subject to rules, regulations, and standards. In so doing, we will be in a position to follow more closely the activities of regulators.

Regulating IPT Equipment, Reagents, and Operators

Following the initial interventions, efforts to regulate IPT have intensified, not abated. This is partly because of the ever-increasing use of the platform, partly due to the evolution of the techniques bundled onto platform components, and finally, as we mentioned in the beginning, partly because hitherto unknown forms of variation are constantly produced. In other words, it is still possible for things to go wrong, and, when they do, as Katherine Muirhead of Zynaxis Cell Science puts it, "those who prepare the samples will always suspect instrument performance problems and those who operate the machine will always suspect sample problems: about 50% of the time, each will be right."[88] In addition to the sample preparation and the instruments,[89] regulators have continually scrutinized a third party, blood, for its ability to travel, to withstand different temperatures, to hang around in post offices without thawing, and, most important, to react consistently with fluorescent reagents. Above and beyond these intrinsic properties, as a sample blood represents a population. What therefore emerges from its continual testing is a norm for individuals in that population. Note that like any norm, this norm is the internally generated outcome of normalization practices, to which we now turn.

Regulating Practices

The idea of a norm resulting from normalization may seem counter-intuitive. After all, one could reasonably assume that the periodic survey of laboratories is supposed to be a way of finding out how they are doing vis-à-vis some external standard and, if needed, of discarding bad apples. The regulation of laboratory practices such as IPT, however, consists of a series of mutual adjustments between the regulators and the laboratories being regulated. Consider, for instance, the Canadian system for surveying laboratories involved in AIDS IPT which, in its workings, resembles the previously described scheme devised by UK NEQAS.[90] Initiating a step-by-step learning process, regulators initially sent out commercially produced polystyrene beads containing different levels of fluorescence to be used to demonstrate proficiency in setting up the instrument correctly. They then distributed "normal" blood (in this case, the blood of the head of the regulatory center), to see if laboratories could handle normal samples. A third step involved the shipment of normal samples artificially depleted of CD4 cells to mimic pathological blood. Lastly, regulators sent blood samples taken from infected individuals to the laboratories on a regular basis. To make sense of this procedure one must remember that, as previously noted, there is no absolute or gold standard that can be used to assess performance. Results are assessed in relation to each other, a task that involves the mutual acceptance of what should count as an acceptable result.[91] Thus, the process can be equated to a pedagogical process for both the center charged with the monitoring and the laboratories being monitored. Little wonder then, that an international survey of external quality assessment programs has described the Canadian program as the "most didactic of all."[92]

The Canadian system projects further interaction in cases of faulty or substandard performance. The surveyors first contact the director, and the reasons for the faulty performance are jointly investigated to decide if there is a problem with the sample itself, an occasional lapse in otherwise sound procedures, or questionable practices. The (relative) norm is the result of these interactions during which responsibility for error is distributed among reagents, equipment, and humans. A yearly meeting in Ottawa allows representatives of each laboratory, including the technicians, to negotiate with the federal authorities about procedures and regulations and to meet with each other during unsupervised workshops to compare and adapt their practices ("do the laundry"). There are, of course, national differences in the performance of laboratory surveys. Different procedures, however, do share the aforementioned fact of not being based on the a priori existence of an external norm.[93]

Regulating Reagents

IPT uses a variety of reagents in collecting, transporting, and storing fresh, frozen, and paraffin-embedded specimens; in lysing blood in preparation for a flow cytometric run or a microscope slide; and in "tagging" the cells with the appropriate antibody-fluorochrome conjugates. While each of these reagents, no matter how humble, has or can become the target of regulation, in keeping with the core position of the CD markers on the IPT platform, monoclonal CD reagents occupy the regulatory center stage and are also subject to FDA regulation. A controversy concerning the reagents used in the slide-based instantiation of the IPT platform illustrates this point.

The FDA classifies the monoclonal antibody (CD) reagents used as immunohistochemical (IHC) products as class I, II, or III devices.[94] Class III devices in the IHC category are subject to the strictest regulation, including premarket approval involving an expensive (up to $200,000) and long (180 days) scientific and technical review of the product. Class I and II devices are subject to more lenient regulation: either a premarket notification completed in 90 days at a cost of $23,000 to $40,000 or even, for class I devices presenting no risk for patients, no premarket notification at all.[95] As standard practice, the FDA classified new devices put on the clinical market after May 1976 automatically in the class III category, pending further classification.

In 1991, the FDA realized that monoclonal antibody reagents designated for research use only were being marketed to clinicians for diagnostic use without having gone through the controls required for class III devices. As a consequence, the FDA threatened to remove all unapproved monoclonal antibody reagents from the market. The threat triggered a panic attack not only among the manufacturers of these products but also among pathologists.[96] CAP teamed up with the ASCP, the Association of Pathology Chairs, the Biological Stain Commission, and the Association of Directors of Anatomic and Surgical Pathology to petition the FDA to classify IHC reagents as class II devices.[97] This infuriated the IHC manufacturers who had hoped to see their products reclassified as class I devices, thus significantly lowering regulatory costs. Concerns about FDA activities led to the creation of a new trade association, the Joint Council of Immunohistochemical Manufacturers (JCIM).[98]

In the ensuing debate the IHC manufacturers proposed an equivalence between their products and another class of products—biological stains—used by pathologists as diagnostic tools and classified as class I devices.[99] CAP countered that "IHC reagents have a potentially greater degree of interlaboratory variability than do biologic stains."[100] JCIM spokespersons responded that the variability in question arose mainly during fixation processes and did not reflect upon the quality of the antibody.[101] Even with this secondary variability, the manufacturers claimed to be seeking more appropriate alternative solutions. They had, for example, solicited "the Human Tissue Network to establish a common tissue bank to standardize the samples used by individual companies." They had also been working "hand in hand with the FDA on further developing the product insert template previously drafted by the [Biological Stains Commission], to include clearly defined characteristics for each reagent."[102] The final regulations issued in 1998 by the FDA placed the vast majority of IHCs into class I, using as a criterion for distinguishing between class I and class II IHCs whether the latter provided pathologists with adjunctive diagnostic information that was not reported to the clinician as an independent finding, or whether, to the contrary, they provided independent prognostic data. Moreover, the FDA exempted IHCs labeled for research use from marketing applications, the manufacturer's intent (as stated on the label), rather than actual laboratory practices, standing as the criterion of use.[103] Independently of the adversarial nature of the process and an outcome that favored the JCIM, we note that while both groups disagreed on the amount of regulation to be imposed on IHCs, both CAP and the manufacturers not only sought to ensure the continued availability of monoclonal antibody reagents but also clearly recognized that their clinical usefulness would be compromised without some sort of interlaboratory control.

Regulating the Instruments

From the point of view of instrument performance, there are a number of factors that enter into the production of an immunophenotypic cell count using flow cytometry. Roughly speaking, these include the flow cytometric instrumentation (the tubes, lenses, filters, and lasers that make up the hardware) and its calibration; the substance it operates upon (blood) software; reagents for the suspension, lysis; and tagging of cells; protocols; and nomenclature. Each of these items is subject to some form of regulation ranging from the most obvious, the registration of the flow cytometer as a medical device, to the development of implicit norms of practice. In what follows, we review the interlocking set of standards that allow a flow cytometer to function with a foreseeable degree of success.

From a legal point of view, flow cytometers are classified as medical devices and, as such, are regulated in the United States by the FDA which gained regulatory control over medical devices in the late 1930s.[104] Following major legislative revisions in 1976, two distinct regulatory paths emerged for manufacturers wishing to put new devices on the market: premarket approval and premarket notification, also known as 510K notification.[105] These two routes are significantly different in terms of travel time: the first requires approximately 2000 hours of FDA study, while, in the second, the workload is reduced to approximately 20 hours. Considerations of time and the attendant legal costs make the less scenic route more attractive to manufacturers. What determines when the shortest path will be followed, and it almost always is, is whether or not the manufacturer can show that the new device is not substantially different in what it does from devices already on the market. As a diagnostic device, flow cytometer manufacturers had to show that they produced substantially the same diagnostic information as prior techniques involving the enumeration of T cells. In this, the first manufacturer to seek FDA approval, Becton Dickinson, successfully claimed that their device replicated diagnostic information already available from fluorescent microscopes.

Once on the medical market, flow cytometers are subject to further legal regulations in the United States. For the purposes of Medicare reimbursement, a diagnostic procedure must be approved by the HCFA of the Department of Health and Human Services. Most private insurance carriers follow the Medicare guidelines so that the latter are to some extent a national norm. Because they require some "interpretation," flow cytometry tests do not count as "clinical laboratory tests," but as "physician services" according to the terminology of the HCFA. Although this means that they are not automatically reimbursed as part of a Diagnosis Related Group (DRG) procedure, it does not mean that reimbursement is free from diagnostic constraint. Disease groups for which Medicare reimbursement have been approved by the HCFA include the aforementioned leukemia, lymphoma, AIDS, and transplants.[106]

As already noted, in the absence of a gold standard for the formed blood elements, precision in flow cytometry seeks accuracy through consistency. Although many roads lead to consistency, calibration has attracted much attention.[107] To understand why, recall that, by definition, a flow cytometer does not measure exactly how many of a particular kind of cell there may be in a sample nor how much fluorescence is attached to those cells through the mediation of antibodies. Rather, flow cytometric measurement determines whether sufficient fluorochrome is present on the cell surface to distinguish a given cell from others. In other words, the flow cytometer is not, strictly speaking, a measuring device but a device that counts the results of a comparison.[108] As with all comparative questions, one may ask: compared to what? In the absence of an external standard, the answer to the question depends upon some kind of calibration.

A simple yet indirect form of calibration is the mutual adjustment of instrument settings in different laboratories (or the same instrument at different times) to produce the same or similar result when applied to material that has the status of being the same or similar. One might call this strategy "qualitative calibration." A second strategy has sought a more direct means of calibration through the quantitation of fluorescence on the antibody and the number of antibodies attached to the cell. Since fluorochromes do not have the variability of biological material, it is believed that they provide a relatively inert standard upon which to base calculations and, indeed, a number of commercial products are presently available. Flow cytometrists also use fluorescent microspheres[109] to evaluate fluorescence readings, and beads[110] to monitor the day-to-day fluorescence sensitivity of the instrument. Finally, cell analog mimic patterns of cellular fluorescent absorption and light scatter. While beads and cell analog have been traditionally used prior to a sample run to adjust the instrument, some laboratories resort to what Vogt and his colleagues call "internal calibrators." In this maneuver, operators mix standard microbeads with the sample and calibrate the apparatus *during* a sample run.[111] One of the claimed advantages of this procedure is that "internal calibrator values remain a permanent part of the raw data for each analysis,"[112] thus transforming calibration into one of the intrinsic properties of a given sample.

A number of calibration systems coexist but, to date, nobody has found an "ideal method."[113] As far as the future is concerned, we are told that

> The ideal system would include a "key bead" with a highly stable fluorochrome, a set of standardized calibration beads with measured amounts of the same fluorochrome as the stained cells and a stabilized cellular material (such as fixed calf-thymocyte nuclei) also stained with the same fluorochrome. The key bead provides the best indicator of instrument consistency, the calibration beads provide a standard curve that can [function as an indicator of antigen density], and the cellular material provides the best indicator of the consistency for light scatter and fluorescence intensity of stained leukocytes.[114]

Note, first of all, that the standard sought consists of a (relatively) stable system rather than a single entity and includes both biological and nonbiological material that attempts to mimic instrument performance.[115] Note, furthermore, that the "beads" (key and calibration) are not laboratory artifacts; they are also tools whose calibration qualities are industrially produced and maintained. This follows indirectly from the fact that there is more than one machine to be calibrated, for, while in the case of a single instrument, putting a measured amount of fluorochrome on a single bead might be an interesting experiment, in order for more than one instrument to be calibrated there must be a second level of standardization involving the production of the beads themselves. Consequently, the production of a series of beads, all containing the same amount of fluorochrome, requires an investment in form—what measures and what limits will be used to determine what counts as the same in the series?—that, in this case, separates the experimental from the industrial. While it would not be impossible for a laboratory to devote itself to such a task, it should not surprise the reader that only commercial suppliers have emerged to develop the standards of purity that the beads represent.

Regulating Blood

In the regulation of IPT there is a second level of calibration and it consists in setting the dial for "normal." The normal functions as a means of calibration in the following way. As a normal number of T or B cells lies, so to speak, outside the instrument, expressed, according to a commercial study, in healthy white adults, and serving as it does as a standard for the measurement of the pathological, it becomes itself a standard for instrument values.[116] The normal in question is not the kind that follows from a gaussian distribution. Instead, as a recent manual tells us, "[m]edian values are provided as a measure of central tendency, since lymphocyte subset values have a non-gaussian distribution. Values between the 5th and 95th percentiles are considered 'normal.' "[117] Nonetheless, the use of median values tends to represent/become the normal. Once the preceding semantic step has been taken, it is a simple matter to remove the scare quotes surrounding "normal." The same paragraph just quoted tells us, for example, that "[m]ost lymphocyte subset values in healthy children approach normal adult levels by age 5." Even "normal" adult levels, however, admit of enormous variation depending on the subset involved. For example, "Published values for the percentage of normal adult, $CD5^+$ B cells vary from 1 to 50%."[118] Further variations emerge from the numerous studies on the degree of circadian ($CD4^+$ cells, so it seems, are low in the morning and high in the evening) and weekly fluctuations of lymphocyte subsets within individuals.[119]

As noted above, biological (and as yet unexplained) variations aside,[120] some of the variation can be explained by the instrument and some by sample preparation. Regulatory studies abound measuring variables from the types of anticoagulants used to the effects of storage temperature on blood samples.[121] One study, for example, compared four new whole-blood lysing agents used to prepare lymphocytes for flow cytometry.[122] Given that the lysing agents were all commercial products (Immuno-lyse, Q-Prep, FACS Lyse, and Gen Trak Lysis), the study had the look of a consumer report. As the study uncovered no major differences—negative facts are equally as important as positive findings in the process of standardization—the study issued no recommendations.[123] Nonetheless, since the study inter alia established the superiority of the whole-blood lysis method over previous methods, it clearly entrenched the position of the owner of the general method, Ortho Diagnostic Systems. Indeed, as the NCCLS demurely points out in the inside cover stating its proposed guideline: "The attention of users is called to the possibility that adherence to this guideline may require use of an invention covered by patent rights held by Ortho Diagnostic Systems, Inc., Route 202, Raritan, NJ 08869."[124]

Regulators clearly recognize that, here, biological values confront industrial standards. They recommend, for example, that "No single commercial material should be used to verify the overall system. Fluorescent microspheres are useful for alignment and compensation *but they are not cells*. . . . Cells from healthy donors should be used to verify instrument performance."[125] Still, recommendations are not rules.

When it comes to internal calibration, some practitioners believe the "commercial" to be more reliable than the "biological"[126] and several options are open to manufacturers. Becton Dickinson has sought patent protection on a method (LeucoGate) using commercial antibodies to provide standardized representations of blood samples.[127] Coulter, on the other hand, has done the same for standardized cells (CYTO-TROL Control Cells). They allow for "a consistent biologic control to evaluate system performance," once again extending the commercial to the biological.[128]

Regulating Operators

As pointed out earlier, IPT involves the manipulation of several parameters at each stage of the process. Regulating the operators of the equipment used to produce the readout opens one of the doors to the regulation of practices. We will see further on how pathologists attempt to regulate slide-reading practices. For the moment, however, consider the following exchange that took place between November 1994 and February 1995 on a flow cytometry electronic discussion list as an example of the kinds of issues involved in this form of regulation.

The discussion began with a query from a group of investigators asking which machine would be best for a group of investigators planning to do their own sorting experiments. Reacting to this request for information, the codirector of a flow facility posted the following comment:

> Are these people NUTS??? . . . Without a single operator to monitor changes in the behavior of the instrument, numerous problems will likely go undetected. Furthermore, troubleshooting will be almost impossible. And that is not to mention the variability in the quality of instrument care that the various operators will take to the sorter. I see fist-fights in your future if you have anything to do with such a facility. I would advise the proponents of this idea to SERIOUSLY RECONSIDER![129]

A self-described "seasoned operator" sharply criticized this advice saying that one best let individuals operate the sorters for themselves, as this allowed the regular operators to work on other machines and obliged the users to understand what they were doing. He added, however, that successful self-operation required skilled operators to ensure that machines were "constantly fine-tuned and maintained at very high level," and to define "stable sort conditions on each machine."[130] Subsequent contributors to the debate pointed out how the success of the seasoned operator's facility ("one of the great flow laboratories in the world") resulted precisely from the constant presence of a chief operator able to "pick up the pieces if anything isn't right."[131] The manager of another flow cytometry core facility added that only 10% to 15% of managers questioned at a recent international flow cytometry conference allowed users to self-operate.[132] A minisurvey among list members confirmed that a "highly trained operator" who would align and calibrate daily, perform all troubleshooting, and be "VERY close by all the time" was essential for facilities that allowed sorters to be operated by nonfacility personnel.[133]

Obviously, access to the machine by those whose practices have been, if not streamlined, at least stabilized is one way of regulating practices. But how are these "regular operators" trained? As noted by one contributor to the discussion list, some "highly trained operators" practice "bootstraps flow cytometry," that is, they learn by doing.[134] More formal training avenues exist. Although simpler equipment and a larger pool of local resources have curtailed the practice,[135] manufacturers of flow cytometers used to train buyers on company premises. The decline in company training has been offset by the growing number of "workshops for a fee" offered by sundry associations and universities and by the creation of local "users groups." All function as vehicles for the stabilization of practices.[136]

Gaining access to training is one thing; being recognized as trained is another. In the United States, operators' certification is the result of a co-operative project—described as "useful in standardizing practice and validating technologists"—between ISAC and ASCP, "one of the largest certifying agencies of clinical laboratory practitioners in the United States."[137] The project encountered a variety of foreseen and unforeseen obstacles. Before complying with ISAC's request to offer a cytometry qualification examination,[138] for example, ASCP had first to be convinced that flow cytometry constituted a "distinct laboratory practice." Following that, an additional difficulty emerged. The variability of commercial equipment and software introduced "vendor bias" into the traditional examination format of 100 objective questions, prompting the demand for a change in examination format. ASCP responded by appointing judges to examine the candidates' "practice and proficiency." The judges were themselves "'calibrated' for severity."[139] Nonetheless, opinion as to how much training is required to become proficient at flow cytometry varies and evolves. The CDC has repeatedly asked participants in its Model Performance Evaluation Program how long training should take. In 1989, nearly 20% believed that training could be conducted in less than a month. In 1992, less than 5% thought so.[140]

Another way of regulating operators is to shift the burden of technical proficiency from the operator to the machine. In the case of flow IPT, as we have seen, manufacturers market highly dedicated pieces of instrumentation for performing, for instance, CD4 counts on AIDS patients. While these "black-boxed" instruments do not require any major fine-tuning, thus reducing the need for trained operators and providing for more reproducible measurements,[141] they do not have the flexibility of more complex equipment and perform a limited spectrum of measurements.[142] The development of these black boxes, which, from an engineering point of view, involve a high degree of sophistication, has not always met with success in the market. Regardless of the economic variables, such as the cost of the equipment in relation to its more or less limited capabilities, the demand for various diagnostic tests, and the availability of skilled operators able to handle more flexible machines, commercial failures tend to indicate that regulation operates at a crossroads characterized by a division of labor implicating not only different categories of scientific and technical operators but also, and more importantly, human and nonhuman actors on a given platform.

Regulating Imagery

The previous section discussed the regulation of reagents, blood, operators, and instruments. We could have added imagery, but this topic deserves special treatment, due to the fact that flow cytometric imagery raises unique issues and questions because it introduces a new space of representation that is incommensurable with previous representations of the spatial organization of cells and tissues. This is true of IPT in general, insofar as even on microscope slides displaying traditional histological and cytological structures, CD markers make visible previously invisible elements. The process, however, has had its most striking expression in flow IPT. In chapter 7, we gave some indication of the workings of a flow cytometer and presented some examples of the different kinds of visual displays that it generates (see figure 7.7). In this section, we address this issue again by focusing, this time, on the regulation of imagery, and by describing a procedure known as "gating" that lies at the operational core of a flow cytometer. Before doing that, however, we describe the new space of representation created by flow IPT.

Hematology without a Microscope

Bessis: That is actually what has been called hematology without a microscope!

Thorell: I should say that it is astonishing that the machine can see things quite differently from human eyes, and that the computer can treat what the machine tells it, quite differently from the human brain.

Bessis: Better?

Thorell: That, I do not know.[143]

One way of conveying the novelty of flow cytometric imagery is to relate our own experience with it. We first encountered the new imagery when we attended a meeting on "Clinical Flow Cytometry," held in Baltimore in 1992.[144] On the opening morning of the conference, the lights of the meeting room dimmed almost immediately as the first speaker uttered the ritual words, "May I have the first slide, please?"[145] As expected, color slides flashed across the screen and continued to do so for the next two days. The slides surprised us as they looked unfamiliar. Conference participants spoke of cell populations, but their laser-pointers picked out splashes of colored dots on what looked like topographic and relief maps. (see chapter 5, figure 5.4 and chapter 7, figure 7.7.) The populations were all inscribed within variously labeled, square, cubic, or even more elaborate geometrical constructions.[146] The imagery was surely not entirely new, even for those, such as ourselves, only vaguely familiar with oscilloscopic "scatterplots" (see chapter 4, figure 4.5) or illustrations in statistical textbooks on cluster analysis[147] from which, we learned, the imagery originated. The novelty lay in the transfer of images from electrical engineering and statistics to clinical and research immunology and the use of these images as representations of cell populations.

While the conference participants were familiar with the images, the latter were obviously a recent addition to the arsenal of biomedical data representation techniques. How had editors, referees, and readers of biomedical journals, or, for that matter, health professionals confronted with that imagery in their daily work, learned to tell "good" from "bad" images (provided this had happened)? How did one make the critical translation from a configuration of pixels (by 1992, computers generated flow cytometric imagery) to biologically relevant cell populations and immunophenotypes? How, in other words, had the production of those images been regulated and how did those images participate in the operations of the flow IPT platform?

On the IPT platform, cell populations are defined by the presence of markers on the surface of the cells made visible by fluorescence-labeled monoclonal antibodies. Accordingly, the entities targeted by IPT cannot, even from a scientist's point of view, be equated with an intrinsic property of the cells examined.[148] Rather, they are simultaneously structure and signal, morphological-chemical hybrids constructed for the specific purpose of being detected by the equipment used on the platform. This applies to both flow-based and slide-based IPT. There are, however, significant differences between these two instantiations of the platform. As mentioned in chapter 4, when microscopists immunophenotype, they see fluorescent signals against a morphological background of cells and tissues. In contrast, a flow cytometer measures the fluorescence intensity of particles and translates those measurements into dots or pixels on a cathode-ray screen.[149] The lack of a fixed anatomical referent sets flow cytometry images apart not only from slide-based IPT but also from the imagery of other clinical instruments that reconstitute in vivo anatomical structures—such as magnetic resonance imaging (MRI) and computed tomography (CT) scanners[150]—or metabolic processes—such as position emission tomography (PET) scanners.[151] While these instruments also transform complex measurements into digital images, users nonetheless start with the assumption that the structures under investigation are either anatomical or, as with PET, correspond to processes confined to distinct anatomical structures. As a consequence, the instrument measurements are not only transformed into images but, more important, are designed to mimic or to be mapped onto anatomical pictures. Thus, from a semiotic point of view, and disregarding technical niceties, it can be argued that computed medical images such as those provided by MRI and CT scanners, or even by ultrasound equipment, represent an extension of previous anatomical investigations.[152]

Not so with flow-generated immunophenotypes. These do not correspond to anatomical structures because, depending on the antibodies and the dyes used to tag the cells, the flow cytometer generates a virtual visual space where variously defined "cell populations" meet and are defined in relation to each other. Unlike the stained cell and tissue specimens that are used in slide-based IPT, no original topographic referent can be found for such visual arrangements. In other words, the representational order is better defined as "similitude" rather than "resemblance."[153] Flow-generated diagrams do not borrow the conventions of anatomical or morphological representations. They can be juxtaposed with histopathological tissue sections, they can be printed side by side,[154] or even "triangulated,"[155] but they do not mimic each other.[156] Flow IPT transduces an instrumental passage from the nonoptical to the optical domain and thereby creates a new representational order with no correspondence to the anatomical or morphological organization of the biological entities under investigation. Users of a flow cytometer reason and argue in terms of fluorescence signals and frequency distributions, not in terms of cells and shapes.[157]

There is a further sense in which IPT introduces a novel space of representation: immunophenotypic images allow one to visualize what literally cannot be seen, namely cell *populations*.[158] This is true of both slide-based and flow-based IPT. The former displays cells, albeit cells that have been treated in order to become visible, but what appears on the slide are groups of cells, not "populations." The screen of a flow cytometer shows pixels or dots, and the identification of dots with cells can only be made after extensive manipulation of the image. As a presenter at a talk on flow cytometry repeatedly insisted, "a dot on a dot plot is an event, not a cell," meaning that only after extensive manipulation of the image with the purpose of eliminating "artifacts" could one confidently assume that each dot could count as a cell.[159] But even if we allow for this translation, what appear on the screen are, for all intents and purposes, clusters of cells, and clusters are not populations. An additional translation is necessary for cell populations to become visible qua cell populations. This transformation combines IPT imagery with the other diagnostic and prognostic conventions that, as we saw in chapter 3, have become part of and are reproduced by the platform.[160]

As noted, this is true of both slide-based and flow-based IPT, but there is, in this respect, an important difference between the two. For reasons that will become clear below, flow cytometry, as used on the IPT platform, does more than simply display populations: it manipulates them. Using high-end cytometry equipment one can, for instance, sort cell populations, but even for the more modest purpose of counting them one has necessarily to intervene through a procedure known as "gating." The images act simultaneously as a tool for handling the apparatus, analyzing the data, and representing them. Each of these functions interacts with the others. This process involves, in other words, a condensation of data and evidence. The digital imaging produced by flow IPT consequently collapses the epistemic distinction between intervening and representing,[161] thus raising distinctive regulatory problems.

Gating and the Regulation of IPT Imagery

Here is a simplified description of a typical IPT "run" on a flow cytometer. The operator first pretreats the blood sample to eliminate cells of no interest such as red blood cells and to bind fluorescent-antibody molecules to the relevant cells. The sample then flows through the apparatus and a screen on the equipment displays a preliminary dot plot that positions cells according to their light-scattering properties (so-called forward/side scatter or FSC/SSC dot plot). The operator interprets the plot as a representation of the different cell populations in the sample as defined by their morphological characteristics. Cell size and granularity create different patterns of light scatter. The operator then isolates the population of interest (e.g., lymphocytes as opposed to granulocytes and monocytes) on the screen. This is known as "setting the acquisition gates." A central and very delicate procedure, gating is often described as an "art as well as a science."[162] Gates can be set, for instance, by drawing a parallelogram or a polygon around the selected population or by moving two cursors across the screen, which will, as a result, be divided into quarters containing different clusters/cell populations (see chapter 7, figure 7.7b).[163] Once a gate is set, the target population will be "gated in," while other cells will be "gated out," meaning that the apparatus will take and store measurements only on the cells falling within the chosen gates.

The selected population, lymphocytes for example, can then once again be represented on a dot plot. This time the screen displays, for instance, red and green fluorescence parameters that will allow one to discriminate between red-positive/green-negative and red-negative/green-positive cells. Translated into biological terms, these may be lymphocytes bearing a CD4 receptor (depleted in AIDS) and those bearing a CD8 receptor (increased in AIDS). Once again, one can "gate in" one of these subpopulations and make further discriminations within it. As a result of these sequential gating operations (see figure 8.1), measurements can be performed on specific cell subpopulations and stored for further (visual) treatment. Depending on the kind of apparatus used, purified samples of a given cell subpopulation can also be physically sorted and collected for further experimentation. As a real-time, interactive operation performed on data displayed in a constructed visual space, gating merges imagery as representation and imagery as a tool, transforming the former into the latter.[164]

With the development of more powerful computers, the actual physical sorting of the cells has, in many cases, been made redundant by multiparameter analysis, i.e., the performance of many measurements during a single run. Cells no longer have to be sorted for a wide range of analyses to be conducted.[165] The distinction between

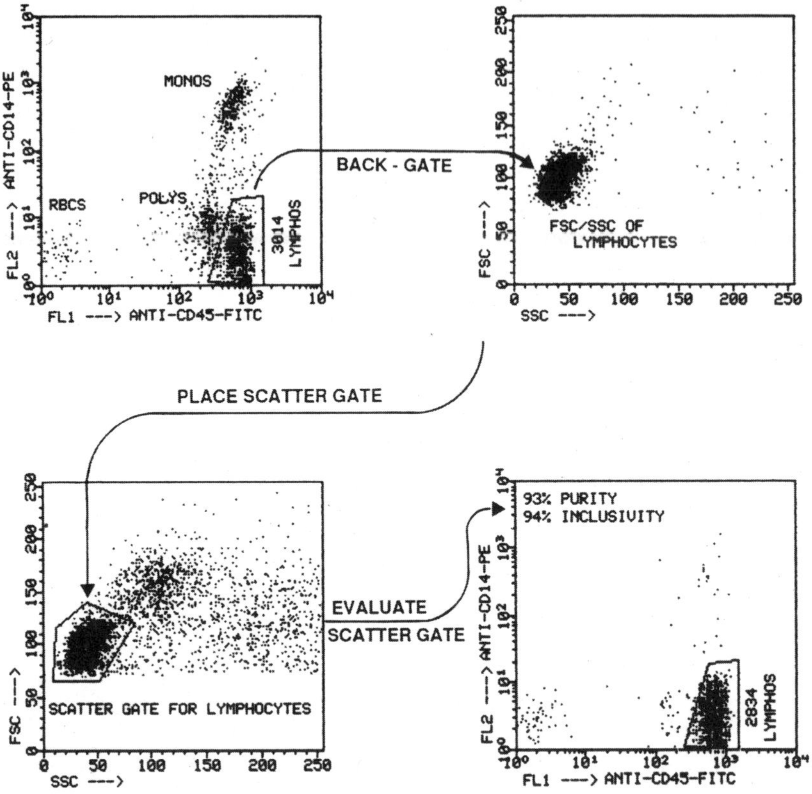

Figure 8.1
A sequential gating operation known as "back-gating." The original caption reads, in part: "Back-gating from CD14/CD45 fluorescence to determine the scatter characteristics of lymphocytes." (From Givan, *Flow Cytometry: First Principles*, 96. Copyright 1992 by John Wiley & Sons, Inc. Reprinted by permission of John Wiley & Sons, Inc.)

instrument-handling procedures such as setting the acquisition gates and data analysis has, consequently, been erased. For instance, a software package (CELLQuest) claims to have created "a seamless interface" that leaves no perceptible boundary between acquisition and analysis. CELLQuest produces "smart plots" that act as acquisition plots and then automatically transform themselves into analysis plots.[166]

Because of its central role in the production of data, gating attracts special regulatory interest. Final results of a flow cytometric run depend on gating decisions, since the inclusion or exclusion of certain measurements modifies the data sets that undergo analysis.[167] Yet scientific articles rarely, if ever, publish images of the initial gating decisions; they only publish pictures of the final results. In other words, readers must trust that operators performed the initial phases of the procedure "correctly" (a judgment that, even under favorable circumstances, is often open to interpretation). As pointed out by an interviewee, this, in principle, allows scientists to "play around" with gates until they get the picture they want.[168] While editors of scientific periodicals do not seem either to be aware of or concerned by these issues,[169] at least some practicing cytometrists have become increasingly uneasy with unregulated images. Their professional organization (ISAC) has established a committee to examine "how flow cytometry data are displayed (correctly and incorrectly)" with the goal of drawing up guidelines to be distributed to publishers.[170]

Flow cytometrists will argue that clusters of pixels can be equated with a given cell population only if measurements are performed on a reasonably "pure" (only the relevant cell type was selected) and "inclusive" (all the relevant cell types were selected) cell population. Gating should provide these conditions. Gating, however, is problematic because the boundaries between clusters of dots or contour-defined clusters are very often hard to define. Pathological blood samples or cells that have undergone laboratory manipulations present acute instances of the problem. In these cases, instrument operators are often confronted with images characterized by what one of our interviewees termed "a loss of distinct [light-scattering] characteristics."[171] Flow cytometry and IPT manuals acknowledge that gating involves a great deal of "subjectivity": a subjectivity "based on training, skill, and practices."[172]

The subjectivity of gating is not only a problem for researchers; it is also an embarrassment for manufacturers of flow cytometers who now aim at "walk-away, back-end automation" that would eliminate any (visual) intervention by operators and ensure "objectivity" and "consistency." Practitioners tend to resist this loss of control over the production of flow cytometric runs, claiming, among other things, that the quality of results is endangered.[173] Regulators try to strike a balance between these two extremes. [174]

Attempts to provide statistical algorithms for the automatic identification of cell populations have been part of the development of IPT since its beginnings and have taken different forms and affected imagery in different ways.[175] A procedure called "back-gating" (see figure 8.1), while still accompanied by the production of (dot plot) imagery, leads to the automatic setting of acquisition gates. Developed for use in routine clinical-diagnostic situations involving lymphocytes,[176] and prescribed as mandatory in the National Institute of Allergy and Infectious Diseases guideline,[177] "back-gating" takes advantage of the development of standardized reagents recognizing specific lymphocyte subpopulations. It draws on a recursive procedure whereby cell populations as defined by immunofluorescence are projected back onto light-scatter dot plots. The resulting populations are then assessed for purity and inclusivity with immunofluorescence, a procedure that can be iterated.[178] One of the striking visual aspects of back-gating is that it capitalizes on the redefinition of cells from morphological entities (and thus, in principle, optical entities) to phenotypic entities.[179]

The situation has become increasingly problematic, however, in light of the further development of the previously mentioned multiparameter analysis.[180] Increasing the number of parameters measured creates a problem of visual representation. For, while one can mathematically conceive of and work with an N-dimensional space, graphic representation is limited to two- or three-dimensional displays. As pointed out by Sychra and colleagues, "[t]here can be no doubt . . . that for most biomedical researchers and certainly also for many data analysts there is simply no substitute for graphic displays in two, or at most three, dimensions to provide for an immediate understanding of what is happening in the data set."[181] Another researcher has nicknamed this problem "the curse of dimensionality"[182]: while visual inspection "is one of the important steps involved in any data analysis," multidimensional data "cannot be easily displayed any more."[183]

In spite of these developments, it is certainly too early to sound the death knell for "manual" gating. For, as previously noted, the practice of gating involves learning visual patterns implicated in the assessment of both instrument quality (e.g., has the pattern I see been produced by a correctly aligned instrument?) and biological quality (e.g., does the pattern I see correspond to a correctly handled sample?). Pattern recognition, in turn, has to be learned by apprenticeship in a laboratory. For instance, Kidd and Vogt note that "Emphasis [for certification of flow cytometry operators] should be placed on education, laboratory experience and skills, and a high degree of cognitive judgment, much of which comes only through experience."[184] While such skills cannot be easily automated, regulators are loath to leave such matters under the sway of tacit or experiential knowledge. Given a health emergency such as AIDS, they have called for more explicit regulations.

The guidelines published by the CDC for performing CD4 counts in HIV-infected persons contain figures illustrating the proper light-scatter and fluorescence gating techniques for determining lymphocyte recovery and purity.[185] Similarly, the NCCLS tentative guideline for the IPT of peripheral blood lymphocytes features several prescriptive images designed to define the production of trustworthy representations of cell populations and, by the same token, to show how such representations should look. Figure 8.2 for instance, reproduces one of these illustrations, showing the effect of various factors on the resolution of various blood cell types (lymphocytes, monocytes, and granulocytes), and similar illustrations are used to present, for example, the effect of optical configuration and alignment on the definition of lymphocytes. The outcome of these kinds of regulations is "normative images" in the sense

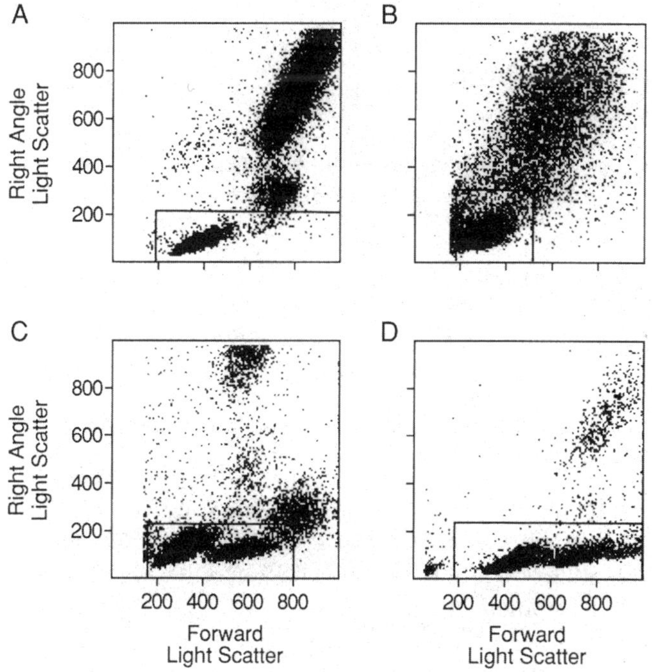

Figure 8.2
Regulation of visuals: imagery from an NCCLS guideline depicting the effect of various factors on "resolution between lymphocytes, monocytes and granulocytes. . . . (*A*) Well-resolved normal blood sample. . . . (*B*) Sample held 24 h before processing. . . . (*C*) Sample with improper erythrocyte lysing and subsequent fixation. . . . (*D*) Sample containing leukemic blasts." (From H42-T, *Clinical Applications of Flow Cytometry: Quality Assurance and Immunophenotyping of Peripheral Blood Lymphocytes; Tentative Guideline,* NCCLS, 940 West Valley Road, Suite 1400, Wayne, PA 19087. Reprinted by permission.)

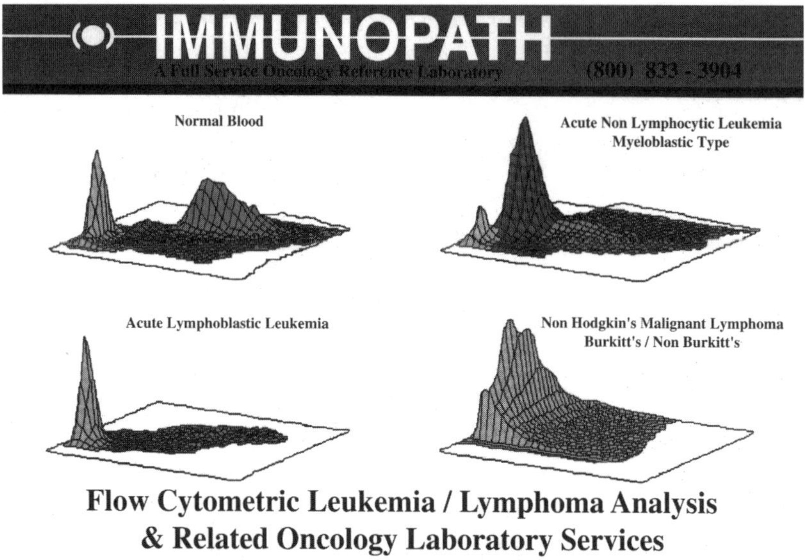

Figure 8.3
Perspective plots as icons of normal and pathological conditions. (Source: Immunopath advertisement, n.d.; original in color. Reprinted by permission of Immunopath, Oncology and Immunology Laboratories, Hialeah, Fla.).

that the images set the norm against which the successful production of the "right" images has to be judged and these same images become the ideal-typical representation of what normal (or pathological) blood should look like.

As hinted in the last sentence of the previous paragraph, IPT images, in their simplest expression, are tools for visualizing relations among different parameters. They can, however, also become icons or representative pictures of a given pathology, in a way similar to, say, histopathological slides. A multipage advertisement by Coulter for its EPICS PROFILE, a cytometer targeting the clinical market, featured a series of histograms of pathological blood samples and argued that the apparatus provided "a concise, complete and accurate immunology patient profile as easy as pushing a button." An advertisement for IMMUNOPATH, a "full service oncology reference laboratory" specializing in IPT, featured four color perspective plots with no external identification other than the label "normal blood" on the first of the diagrams and the name of specific kinds of leukemia and lymphoma on the other three (see figure 8.3).

Specific diagnostic entities were thus redefined in terms of immunophenotypic imagery, so that the latter stood for the former. While the clinical literature remains in general more circumspect, arguing that immunophenotypic imagery alone cannot define a pathological condition,[186] a similar trend has emerged.[187] The director of the Flow Cytometry Laboratory of the Roswell Park Cancer Institute in Buffalo has developed a set of pictures corresponding to the many patterns obtained with different antibodies for normal and leukemic samples. Residents rotating through the laboratory are expected to learn those patterns and thus to recognize the presence of a specific diagnostic entity by looking at the images.[188] Regulations targeting imagery, far from confining themselves to the technical aspects of the handling of the instrument, also target iconic, disease-defining images. In the diagnostic domain, however, the focus on imagery, as opposed to, say, numerical data (such as percentage values of positive markers), is by no means universally shared. A key regulatory issue in this respect concerns the definition of the proper use of the platform in relation to other platforms and to the various kinds of clinical activities. To investigate this matter further, it is thus necessary to turn, in the next chapter, to the regulation of the clinical uses of IPT results.

9

Regulating Diseases on the Platform

Just as the immunophenotyping platform functions across the entire laboratory–clinic spectrum, so, too, do regulations concerning the platform. In the previous chapter, we discussed the regulation of procedures close to the laboratory pole. As made clear by the activities of groups such as SIHON (the Dutch Cooperative Study Group on Immunophenotyping of Haematological Malignancies), however, even if one attempts to isolate the "technical" from the "clinical," the two will merge sooner or later. For instance, the IPT images (and the data that constitute them) are images of (and data on) something: in keeping with the ontological foundations of modern medicine they are images of specific clinical entities, diseases whose existence and natural history are defined independently of the individual patients who happen to suffer from them.[1] It is thus time to turn to the regulation of the activities by which a platform creates or redefines diagnostic entities.

We have singled out two classes of diseases for particular attention: the leukemias and the lymphomas. As neoplasms that target cells of the immune system, both are obvious candidates for IPT and, as we have seen in the case of the leukemias, the IPT platform has been instrumental in their reclassification. By regulating the relations between diseases, the production and organization of classifications creates yet another regulatory layer that intervenes between a "sample" and its immunophenotypic characterization and thus between an individual and his or her categorization as a patient suffering from a given disease. While, to the modern mind, "classification" may evoke some nineteenth-century form of butterfly collecting of secondary scientific import, we alert readers to the salient fact that the clinical significance of classifications can be easily gathered from the amount of criticism generated by the proposal of new classificatory schemes.

Therapeutic decisions (e.g., the timing and content of chemotherapy) depend on how a patient is categorized in an accepted classification. In addition, standards of care and clinical guidelines depend upon the equivalencies made possible by shared classifications. This is particularly true during periods of diagnostic and therapeutic innovation. As noted by an interviewee,

> Lymphomas are very heterogeneous . . . so early on there was a necessity for looking at these tumors a little bit more closely than other tumors and classify them, not only for predicting the outcome of that patient but also to develop better therapies. . . . In the late '60s when people were classifying these tumors all over the world, classifications were extremely complicated, with different names, and clinicians were fairly unhappy about the situation because they couldn't try new protocols, it was difficult to compare from one institution to another the results of their therapy because the pathologists were not really agreeing on what to call what and so on. And that was important—now this is the beginning to the mid-70s—when the new therapies began to appear, new, very important therapies, both in the area of radiotherapy as well as in the area of chemotherapy.[2]

In this respect, medical classifications are less a finished product than an active exploration of patients and their diseases. One might wish to reserve the term "classification" for the finished product or for the establishment of a classificatory system, and save the term "categorization" for the act of applying categories drawn from the general classification to individual patients. Practice conflates these terminological distinctions. Classification runs the entire gamut of activities, from the staining of slides and their observation under the microscope, to the flowing of blood through sophisticated equipment and the inspection of the resulting imagery, the discussions surrounding these activities, and the decision to inscribe a specific disease category in a patient's file.

These activities do not develop in a linear fashion, from diagnosis and classification to therapy. In late-twentieth-century medicine, classification coincided with diagnosis, and the constitution and transformation of both diagnosis and classification followed from and led to changes in the modalities of clinical management of the entities diagnosed and classified. Medical classification involves causal claims: etiologic, anatomical or histopathological, clinical, and prognostic claims. Any or all of these categories may figure in a particular diagnosis. Most biomedical researchers favor the etiologic principle (if and when available) as the gold standard, but a comprehensive understanding or description of any class of disease entails the mobilization of all four categories of cause.

Classification, as an ongoing clinical activity, thus occurs at the intersection of individual patients and abstract disease entities. Even though individual patients are diagnosed within local settings, diagnostic decisions transcend local events, since treating patients requires continuity across time and space.

Dagognet notes that while classifications do not passively register reality, the history of classifications can be read as an attempt to get at the principle that corresponds to the ontological truth (the essential elements) of the entities being classified.[3] Classifications, from this point of view, are less the ordering of what we already know than a tool leading to the development of new knowledge.[4] In this respect, although ontological claims may not be very popular in sociological or cultural studies, they do indeed constitute one of the driving forces behind classification. As we shall see in both leukemia and lymphoma classifications, one of the central questions raised concerns whether the clinical constructs classified are mere conventions or whether they rise to the status of thoroughgoing biological entities. Far from being a philosophical afterthought divorced from practice, this is, as we will see, a question of considerable practical import.

The development and transformation of medical classifications thus lie at the heart of the biomedical endeavor. Platforms, in turn, play a crucial role in the development and transformation of classifications. In chapter 5 we briefly discussed the French-American-British (FAB) classification of the leukemias, noting how it could be qualified as both an embodiment and a product of a morphological platform. In chapter 7 we discussed the development of slide-based IPT in relation to the classification of the lymphomas. In what follows, we revisit these two classificatory domains, with a focus on the regulatory aspects.

Regulation by Classification I: IPT and the Leukemias

In 1995, the European Group for the Immunological Characterization of Leukemias (EGIL)[5] published "Proposals for the Immunological Classification of Acute Leukemias." The EGIL proposals provoked a series of critical replies that focused on the proper clinical use of the IPT platform and the dual-purpose nature of the platform. At the most general level, proponents and critics raised the following questions. Should IPT be used for the routinization and objectification of diagnosis or should it be used for the study of biology? In other words, should quantification lead to research or to standardization and automation?

The answers to these questions are, as we shall see, dependent upon the organization of clinical work in relation to the platform.

Formed only a year before publication of the proposals, EGIL had emerged out of several national organizations devoted to similar purposes, the oldest of which was the French Groupe d'Étude Immunologique des Leucémies (GEIL), which had been created in 1983 and by the late 1990s included members of forty-three French hospital centers. Similar groups have been created since the mid-1980s in other European countries. The extent to which EGIL's proposals represent a Europe-wide consensus is, however, open to debate. For instance, while GEIL openly supported the French representative of EGIL, Dutch and German colleagues garnered more ambiguous support. Indeed, one year after publication of EGIL's proposals, *Leukemia* published a different consensus document signed mainly by German clinicians and which included two of the signatories of EGIL's proposals.[6]

EGIL's proposals did not seek to replace other classifications based on morphology or cytogenetics. As an ancillary to the FAB classification, EGIL assumed that its system would be used only in conjunction with the morphological classification. Moreover, EGIL made no attempt to integrate morphology, immunology, cytogenetics, and molecular biology into a unified, synthetic classification. Previous attempts by the Morphologic, Immunologic, and Cytogenetic (MIC) Cooperative Group in the second half of the 1980s had met with only limited success.[7] The EGIL proposals shared with morphological endeavors the common ground of being a classification based exclusively on a single parameter (in this case, immunological). For a renewed attempt to create a classification combining morphological, immunological, and genetic features one would have to wait until the late 1990s, when a group of 100 hematopathologists and clinicians crafted a new proposal patterned on a system that had emerged in the adjacent field of the lymphomas and which we discuss below.[8]

As previously mentioned, the EGIL system raised issues internal to the IPT endeavor. The markers detected by flow cytometry, quantitative though they may be, do not always give the clinician an all-or-nothing proposition. The numbers are based on fluorescence intensities that, in turn, must be assessed as markers. If, for example, you tag a sample with an antibody, what do you do if 25% of the cells in the sample turn up positive to, say, a B-cell marker? Can you then consider that sample as positive? And can you then use that positive finding to assign the patient sample to a given class of leukemia?

In the EGIL system, medical biologists, hematologists, or pathologists (depending on national conventions) examine the sample to determine the presence or absence of predetermined markers: in practical terms, this means that the sample is examined with a flow cytometer after treatment with a predetermined set of antibody reagents (a so-called antibody panel). EGIL conventions set the cutoff point for a positive marker at 20% of cells stained with the antibody.[9] This obviously arbitrary limit has been harshly criticized. To avoid misunderstanding, note that the threshold does not determine whether a patient has leukemia or not. According to EGIL stipulations, previous morphological examination has classified all samples as leukemic. The cutoff point determines the subtype of leukemia. The question then remains whether one should fix cutoff points or report results as continuous variables. As we will see below, some researchers frame this issue as a contrast between a will to standardize as a way to achieve a common language and a will to preserve the interpretative freedom of clinicians.

Once a sample is deemed positive for a given marker, the expression of the marker itself may then be classified as major (2 points), minor (a half-point), or intermediate (1 point). Adding the scores, one can assign a patient to one of the various types and subtypes of a preestablished classification. The latter is, of course, based on immunological criteria. In fact, an objective of national groups such as GEIL is to analyze large cohorts of patients in order to produce and periodically revise an immunological classification of acute leukemias. Large multicenter studies establish the clinical relevance of these classifications, that is, their prognostic value, and thus the resulting therapeutic strategy.

As with the cutoff point, the scoring has come under fire. Indeed, the EGIL scoring system contrasts sharply with North American approaches that favor visual evaluation. To understand the difference, note that one can perform flow cytometric analysis using either single markers or a combination of different markers (a so-called multiparametric approach). In the first case, one obtains a number that can be used to determine whether the sample is positive or negative for a given marker. In the second case, one obtains complex two-dimensional or three-dimensional figures that one can assess visually.

This is easier to see than to say and can best be expressed through illustrations. Figure 9.1 shows a laboratory report produced by a Texas hospital. The first page contains a summary of the tests performed on the patient, including a list of the immunological markers and the interpretation of the results. On the second page one finds, at the top of the

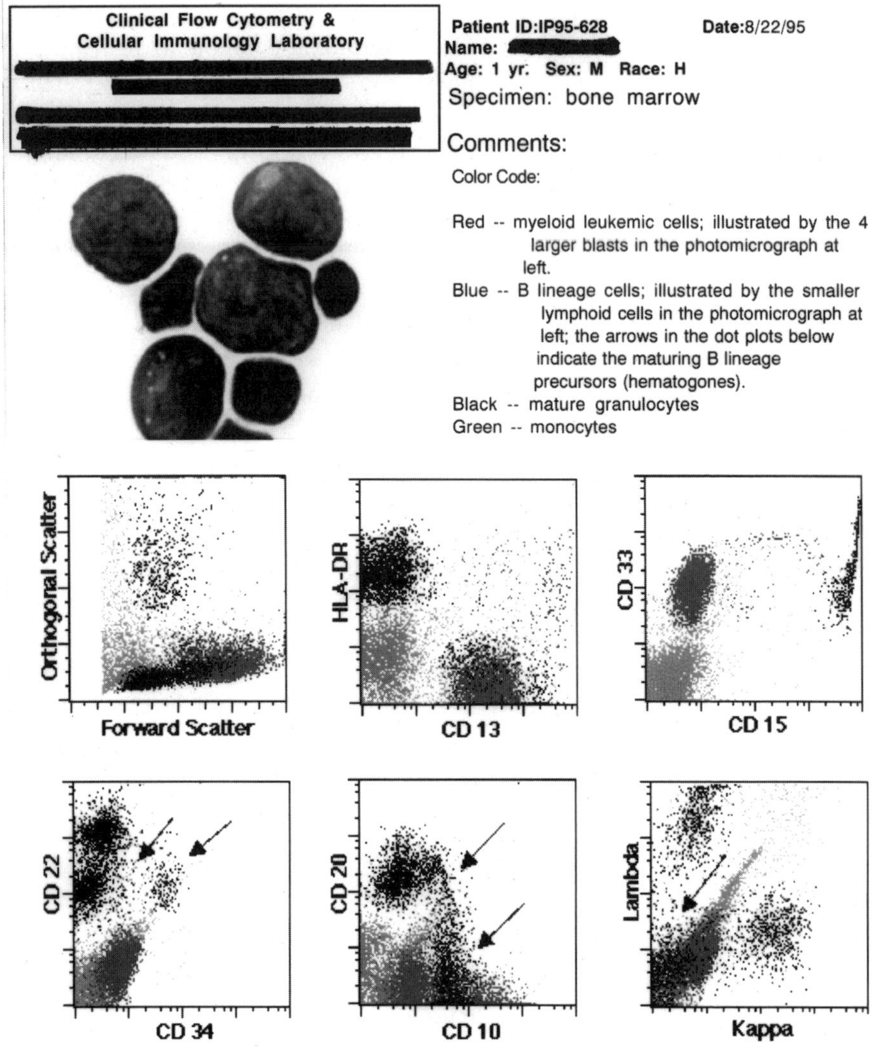

Figure 9.1
Laboratory report produced by the flow cytometry laboratory of a Texas hospital.

page, a microscope picture showing the cell morphology and, at the bottom, a series of two-dimensional flow cytometric images. A skilled analyst can interpret the visual patterns as pointing in the direction of a given type and subtype of leukemia. In other words, the name of the game here is to identify the abnormal cell population on a visual display, a skill that, as noted toward the end of chapter 8, is taught to residents rotating through selected American IPT laboratories. Figure 9.2 shows a report from a French hospital corresponding to the EGIL proposals. No images here. Instead, we have percentages and the resulting interpretation.

When asked to explain these differences, the practitioners we interviewed resorted to arguments ranging from economics (a multiparametric approach is expensive in terms of equipment and reagents), to questions of skills and standards (the difficulty of regulating laboratory practices increases with the complexity of the techniques used), to issues of professional training. French practitioners explain the last-named difference as follows: in most cases, North American laboratories are directed by pathologists, i.e., by individuals who have been trained in pattern recognition by spending years scrutinizing tissue slides. These individuals are presently transforming immunological approaches by hybridizing them with their established practice.

North Americans offer a symmetrical explanation. They observe that medical biologists rather than pathologists control flow cytometry in France and accuse the former of replacing clinical understanding with algorithms. Interestingly enough, the French scientists we interviewed also acknowledged the significance of clinical understanding and consequently concurred with their North American hematopathology colleagues in criticizing flow cytometry laboratories directed by PhDs. Such laboratories, they suggested, were technology-driven, as opposed to clinically driven. At the same time, and somewhat ironically, they saw an undue focus on technology as one of the leading forces behind the trend toward increasingly sophisticated multiparametric analyses.

These reciprocal characterizations hide important organizational and epistemic differences. The contrast between algorithmic vs. inspired clinical analyses has been formulated, in an epistemic form, by one of the American critics of the EGIL proposals. According to Elisabeth Paietta, scoring systems, or, more generally, any scheme using a preestablished classification based on a list of markers, has little clinical significance: in the leukemias, division into subgroups will only rarely give relevant prognostic information.[10] In her opinion, the a priori definition

NOM : [redacted]
Prenom : [redacted]
No d'inscription : 3339
Service demandeur : MED A2

Date de l'examen : 10/ 2/1997
Caracteristiques:
Sang=1 moelle=2 autre=3 2
Cellules atypiques % 97

PANEL D'ORIENTATION

LIGNEE B	LIGNEE T	MYELOIDES	AUTRES
Membrane (%)			
sIg : 0	CD2 : 95	CD13: 93	Classe II: 0
CD19: 0	CD5 : 0	CD33: 93	CD10 : 0
CD20: 0	CD7 : 0	CD14: 0	CD34 : 0
CD24: 0		CD15: 0	CD41 : 0
Cytoplasme (%)			
c-mu: 0	cCD3: 0	Lysozyme: ..	TdT : 0
cCD22: 0			

PANEL DE VALIDATION

LIGNEE B	LIGNEE T	MYELOIDES	AUTRES
CD21: 0	CD1 : 0	CD11b 0	CD9 : 0
CD22: 0	CD3 : 0	CD16: 0	CD11a 0
CD23: 0	CD4 : 0	CD35: 0	CD18: 0
Isotype sIg: 00	CD6 : 0	CD36: 0	CD38: 0
Isotype cIg: 00	CD8 : 0	CD65: 0	CD71: 90
	CD25: 9		CD54: 0
	CD26: 0		CD44: 99
	WT31: 0		CD45Ro: ..
			CD30: 0
			CD11c 0
			CD42: 0
			Facteur VIII 0
			Glycophorine 0

Nom autre: cCD79 % 0
Nom autre: cCD13 % 70

Nom autre: MPO % 90
Nom autre: BCL2 % 0

NOMENCLATURE GEIL: MYELOIDE

Pr [redacted] Dr [redacted] Pr [redacted]
IMMUNOPHENOTYPAGE REALISE APRES ENRICHISSEMENT SUR FICOLL SELON LES TECHNIQUES DE REFERENCE. SCORING ET SOUS-TYPAGE SELON LES RECOMMANDATIONS GEIL ET EGIL.

Figure 9.2
Laboratory report produced by a French hospital according to the EGIL guidelines.

of theoretically expected phenotypes should be replaced by the retrospective analysis of actually observed phenotypes with respect to their clinical relevance. Individual antigens, rather than a list of marker profiles, should be the focus of immunological analysis. From this point of view, standardization is not a meaningful goal, and the analysis of clinical data, rather than arbitrary thresholds, should establish the relevance of a degree of antigen expression:

> The objections raised to the proposal by [EGIL] must not be interpreted as dismissing their efforts to improve the uniformity and reproducibility of immunophenotyping in the setting of multicenter trials. However, it is doubtful that standardization alone is the answer to improved leukemia immunophenotyping. Antigen expression must be considered an independent (especially independent from morphology) biologic parameter. The degree of antigen expression that determines clinical relevance must be established by experience rather than convenience.[11]

Supporters of EGIL's approach counter by arguing that the routine use of immunological tools in the diagnosis and therapy of leukemia presupposes an immunological framework establishing, for instance, the significance of a given marker or set of markers. Such a framework requires the analysis of large cohorts of patients. A single center has only a limited number of patients, and only some of its patients can be included in a research scheme, because, for instance, certain patient samples provide only a small number of cells.[12] Only by pooling cases from different centers can one achieve a statistically relevant collection of cases of leukemia covering the entire spectrum of disease manifestations. In collecting cases, one can either centralize the samples in a collection or collate the results of the analyses performed on patients in a database. Thus, one needs to be sure that the same kinds of data are being collected (a problem that can be solved by using a standard form), and that the data collected are reliable, i.e., that the methods, reagents, and instruments used in laboratories are comparable. Standardization, from this point of view, no longer counts as antithetical to research but, rather, as one of its conditions of possibility.

GEIL's program, for example, aims at providing methods for achieving interlaboratory equivalence and involves both technical schemes—such as periodically circulating frozen, coded cells in a blind fashion to all members of the network to test intercenter agreement—and organizational schemes that adopt, for instance, a loose network structure without formal administration.[13] Economic initiatives, such as the negotiation of lower prices for the bulk supply of reagents so that every center can literally use the same antibodies complement these methods.[14] In order for a group like GEIL to function, then, two related, yet analytically distinct sets of practices must be instituted. The first, and most traditional, leads to the standardization of local routines, by allowing even small, marginal centers to align their practices with the protocols and reagents used in the more advanced centers. The second results in a new approach to the conduct of research, namely the creation of a collective, multicenter authorship that ensures, de facto, the intercenter robustness of results. Setting cutoff points in IPT participates in this process of standardization of immunological diagnosis and classification of the leukemias. Less the endpoint of research, standardization is seen as a precondition for the discovery of new or rare subtypes of leukemia. As Bené and Faure put it: "The EGIL consensus is a practical consensus, it amounts to building a unified language in order to identify rare kinds of leukemia in Europe."[15]

Despite appearances, things differ in the United States. In the field of oncology, clinical trials and thus diagnosis are organized under the Clinical Trials Cooperative Group Program run by the National Cancer Institute (NCI). Set up in 1955 following an initiative led by Sidney Farber, by 1958 seventeen groups had been organized to test new anticancer drugs. Centralization and reorganization along geographic lines has since whittled the number of groups down to twelve. Each year, about 20,000 new patients enter trials organized by these groups. This is where the large numbers lie.[16]

As far as leukemia is concerned, the "big three" are the Eastern Cooperative Oncology Group (ECOG), the Southwest Cooperative Oncology Group (SCOG), and the Cancer and Leukemia Group B (CALGB). Although they usually work independently, for rare cancers or limited supplies of experimental therapeutic agents, they form intergroup trials. Since these groups have existed since the 1950s, the immunological turn in oncology has had different organizational consequences. In particular, the advent of IPT in the leukemias has not led to the development of groups specifically devoted to this undertaking, like EGIL. Instead, the groups have generally incorporated IPT into already existing regimens. Let us consider one of those incorporations.

In 1985, ECOG, one of the original cooperative groups, wrote a protocol (E-1485) for leukemia that stipulated, for the first time, that all cases collected for clinical study would automatically be submitted for laboratory analysis that consisted essentially of IPT.[17] They thus created two parallel protocols, one for the clinical trial and one for a laboratory trial. Two immediate results followed from this decision. Rather than centralizing data, like EGIL, ECOG centralized samples, giving greater scope to the treatment of those samples and less emphasis to their standardization, as the group treated all samples in the same laboratory. Second, ECOG transformed leukemia diagnosis from the result of informed judgment to an ongoing problem. ECOG pursued the protocol until 1998 when the NCI terminated open-ended protocols.[18]

Today, as throughout the E-1485 regimen, protocol collaborators send IPT samples to Elisabeth Paietta's laboratory at Our Lady of Mercy Cancer Center in the Bronx in New York city. Trained in biochemistry at the University of Graz (Austria), Paietta had worked on biochemical indicators of leukemia. In the early 1980s she began combining the study of biochemical characteristics and phenotypic characteristics in the typing of leukemic cells by collaborating with Walter Knapp who, in the late 1970s, had created the first myeloid-specific antibodies (now known as CD15 and still in use). By 1982, she and her Austrian colleagues had "discovered" one of Greaves's bugbears, a biphenotypic leukemic cell—one that displayed both myeloid and lymphoid markers.[19] Like the other reports, this, too, went away. Nonetheless, Paietta had been sufficiently smitten by IPT to say yes to Peter Wiernik, a noted American oncologist and a member of ECOG's hematology steering committee, when, in 1982, he asked her to open an IPT laboratory at Montefiore.[20]

In 1985, ECOG designated the Montefiore IPT laboratory its reference laboratory. Overnight, Paietta's caseload rose into the thousands. Still using Walter Knapp's antibodies, Paietta carried out IPT using a fluorescence microscope and did not acquire a flow cytometer until 1991. Because of the lack of gating mechanisms on a microscope, and because of the fact that the latter could do no more than two-color IPT, data collected between 1985 and 1991 subsequently became unusable. Once converted to flow, Paietta had the choice of large or small antibody panels: the latter implied diagnosis, the former implied (clinical) research. Paietta chose relatively large panels, arguing that "to make the diagnosis [was] no longer the challenge. The challenge [was] to find new subtypes which require[d] different treatment because they [had] different prognoses."[21]

Cooperative oncology groups offer all those advantages that come from having a large number of patients following standardized treatments in standardized hands. They also tend to centralize statistics. As previously mentioned, the groups had opted for a complete separation of the laboratory studies from the clinical studies, in a sort of epistemic and organizational "double-blind" strategy designed to ensure the impersonal "objectivity" similar to that sought by clinical trial design.[22] Unsurprisingly, then, the analysis of phenotypic data, and in particular the setting of significance levels, was not entrusted to a consensus group, but, rather, to a multivariate statistical package.[23] The use of these statistical methods required, in turn, that the degree of antigen expression be expressed as a continuous quantitative variable rather than as a qualitative (presence/absence) one. Furthermore, statisticians asked for large numbers (400 to 500 cases) in all instances and ECOG has consequently centralized statistical analysis at Harvard University.

As we can see, there are two different ways of doing clinical research. One is first to standardize, then see what turns up as significant (the EGIL approach). The second is to "let the data do the talking." Individual antigens thus oppose antigen panels because, in the case of leukemia IPT, the latter presuppose the FAB category. If one uses a panel with fixed settings, the meaning of the panel has already been set and an individual antigen becomes a mere marker for a FAB category. Without a preexisting disease category, the panel makes no sense. But, according to Paietta, phenotypic data do not confirm morphological data although this has been the traditional view as far as the FAB classification has been concerned. One should thus treat the phenotypic data separately. Furthermore, as far as prognosis is concerned, they may even be superior data: "antigen expression may be useful in predicting clinical outcome, while the FAB classification has only limited value in that regard."[24] And indeed, the most recent proposal, at the time of this writing, for an integrated classification of the leukemias has eliminated "purely morphologic subtypes that have no current clinical relevance."[25]

Regulation by Classification II: IPT and the Lymphomas

The problems that we have just encountered in the leukemias recur in a different form in the diagnosis and classification of the lymphomas. Clinical management of the latter raises even more explicitly the problem of the articulation of IPT with the older, morphological platform. In fact, the mobilization of the IPT platform has created divisions within lymphoma pathology itself and, in the absence of successful therapies, has pitted an ontological view of the various forms of lymphoma against a more pragmatic approach centered on therapy. An appreciation of these competing demands, as well as the mechanisms for the formation of consensus, requires yet another detour through the history of lymphoma classifications, albeit with a different itinerary from the tour conducted in chapter 7.

Let us begin by stating the problem as it appeared to practitioners when an informal international network of nineteen influential pathologists known collectively as the International Lymphoma Study Group (ILSG) produced the latest classification of the lymphomas known as the REAL (*r*evised *E*uropean-*A*merican *l*ymphoma) classification. When first announced in 1994, the REAL classification was deemed so momentous that it was published more or less simultaneously in four different journals (*Blood, The American Journal of Clinical Pathology, Histopathology, Important Advances in Oncology*).[26] Initial reactions were mixed: some pathologists welcomed the initiative; others criticized it, as shown by the unusual titles of articles on this topic: "Here We Go Again," "America, You Deserve Better," "A Missed Opportunity?," and "Not Another Lymphoma Classification!"[27]

In an editorial accompanying the publication of the REAL article in *Blood,* Saul Rosenberg, a prominent American oncologist, voiced objections that, taken together, offer an introduction to the problems of instituting a classificatory scheme with all its regulatory implications.[28] First, he questioned the existence of a real consensus. True, nineteen pathologists, many of them leaders in this field, had cosigned the REAL classification. But what about the other major hematopathologists? Rosenberg further objected that the technical skills needed to institute the REAL classification were simply unavailable in many medical centers. Third, he cited established, routine practices (such as the fixing of tissues) as obstacles to the performance of the detailed examinations required by the REAL classification. The gap between clinical practice and the pathology laboratory constituted a fourth criticism: the new classification highlighted biological variables of interest to the pathologist but lacked or was meager or anecdotal with regard to clinical course, prognosis, or curability. In other words, clinical data did not (yet) support the classification. Finally, and consistent with the perceived pathology/clinic gap, the classification of various types of tumors (e.g., the inclusion of Hodgkin's disease with non-Hodgkin's lymphomas) ran counter to traditional clinical understanding. Social consensus, the distribution of skills, the weight of established practice, the division of labor, differences between thought styles—in short, the usual social, technical, cognitive, and institutional arguments!

ILSG's rebuttal did not deny the relevance of the issues raised by critics.[30] Rather, the study group claimed that despite their importance the concerns were unwarranted. There was, in fact, consensus, they argued (this was the largest group of pathologists ever to agree on a lymphoma classification). Sophisticated techniques (IPT and genetic studies) were available (at least in the United States and Europe) to most practicing pathologists. These techniques could also be applied to fixed tissues, thus meshing with established practice. Distinctive clinical features had been described for most of the disease entities in the new classification. And, last but not least, simplicity, namely the respect of simple clinical groupings, lost its (clinical) virtue if it overlooked distinct clinical entities. As Harris put it:

> This formulation includes a number of disease entities which may alarm those who believe that a lymphoma classification must be simple. The fact remains that these are the tumors that pathologists are seeing and diagnosing, and oncologists must be prepared to deal with them.[31]

The REAL classification had grown out of a series of classifications initiated in the 1970s by the new cell-surface immunology. The development of these immunology-based classifications had engendered yet another problem that plagued the classification of the lymphomas in the years to come: were the classifications mutually compatible? An early study carried out by the European Lymphoma Club[32] in the mid-1970s showed, paradoxically, that although the classifications were comparable, it was mainly because pathologists had equal difficulty in reproducing them. According to the study protocol, Club members had classified fifty cases of lymphoma according to each of the three classification schemes then competing for pathologists' attention (Rappaport, Lukes-Collins, and Kiel). Three independent observers had then reclassified the same cases. The degree of agreement between the two groups of classifiers had not advanced beyond random (50%) in the case of the Rappaport classification and had reached an unimpressive 60% in the case of the Kiel classification.[33]

Some contemporary observers felt that the differences between the systems were merely linguistic. Researchers at the World Health Organization affirmed, somewhat optimistically, that

> Despite what appears to be continuing and unresolvable controversy over the classification of malignant lymphomas, it should be emphasized that this is largely a matter of terminology. . . . If the natural history of specific disease entities is appreciated, the actual terms assume less importance, as does the method of classification, be it according to architectural pattern, cell type, behavior or function.[34]

In keeping with this view, the WHO researchers proposed their own system along with a conversion table that would, in principle, allow one to simply "translate" from one system to the other and thus "facilitate international comparisons."[35] As the quotation marks indicate, the translation was more metaphorical than substantive. In particular, since the entities from one scheme were redistributed in another scheme and not just renamed, as the previous quote implied, it was impossible to line up the three classes of entities in a table in anything like a one-to-one correspondence.

WHO's attempt to translate between systems had followed upon a series of conferences organized to iron out the differences between classifications. Rappaport had organized the first meeting entitled "Workshop on Classification of Non-Hodgkin's Lymphomas" in Chicago in June of 1973. The major protagonists came together the next year at the first international conference on lymphoma classification held in London. Optimism ran high as Henry S. Kaplan wrote in the introduction to the published proceedings: "It may confidently be predicted that pathologists will soon acquire an exciting new armamentarium of differential tests based on surface membrane receptors and other distinctive cytochemical and immunological properties of these cells and that histopathological classifications firmly rooted in these fundamental biological attributes will emerge."[36] But that did not happen soon. What did happen was generally considered the Florence fiasco, or the International Cancer Conference held in Florence in 1974, where irreconcilable differences became evident.

So Kaplan convened yet another conference in 1975, with money from the NCI.[37] Organizers closed the "by invitation only" conference to outsiders in an attempt to keep the heat down. The meeting engendered no consensus.[38] Undaunted, the NCI organized a retrospective study of biopsies of over one thousand cases classified according to the competing systems. Between September 1976 and June 1980, the NCI played the six different classification systems off against each other. The originators of the six systems (termed "experts") and six control pathologists classified 1175 cases according to each system, the experts classifying according to their own system and the control pathologists according to all six.[39]

The results of the showdown were discussed at conferences held at Stanford in 1979–80, and the participants agreed that no fundamental differences had surfaced with regard to reproducibility or prognostic value. In the absence of clinical features distinguishing the systems, the investigators developed a "working formulation." Drawing histological terminology from the Rappaport and Lukes-Collins classifications, the group offered the formulation not as a new classification, "but as a means of translation among all systems."[40] Published in 1982, the working formulation went on to become the classification of choice in North America. A 1988 study of pathologists showed that over 97% used the working formulation whereas only 5% were "familiar" with the Kiel system. Intended primarily for clinical use, the working formulation had a morphological base (pace the pathologists) with a prognostic superstructure (pace the clinicians): "high grade", "intermediate grade", and "low grade" based "primarily upon differences in survival."[41]

Not all the experts found the working formulation to their liking. The German pathologist Karl Lennert offered two reservations that ultimately led to the demise of the formulation: "Firstly, within this Formulation lymphoma entities which are biologically closely related are separated and entities biologically unrelated are grouped together. Secondly, all considerations regarding immunologic identities of lymphomas have been excluded."[42] Robert Lukes concurred.[43] Nonetheless, even though biology and immunology had not been included, Rappaport noted that they had not been precluded, adding, somewhat demurely, that they could be "readily added when future research establishes their clinical value above and beyond that of the histologic classification."[44]

With the advent of monoclonal antibodies and the CD nomenclature, a number of studies emerged suggesting that, contrary to Rappaport, immunology could not simply be added to histology. As early as 1982 researchers at the NCI using monoclonal antibodies concluded: "This histopathologic subclassification correctly predicted immunologic phenotype in only 61% of cases, suggesting that in diffuse non-Hodgkin's lymphomas, histologic appearances alone may not be a reliable indicator of immunologic surface markers."[45] Furthermore, despite its prognostic significance at the statistical level, the nodular/diffuse distinction did not always apply at the level of the individual patient.[46]

Systematic comparison of the ten morphological categories of the working formulation revealed further problems. A review of work carried out in the period 1982–88 put it as follows: ". . . many immunologic subtypes exist within certain WF [working formulation] categories and these cannot always be predicted by morphologic classification."[47] In the short term, however, since the new technology ("e.g., monoclonal antibodies, flow cytometry") sometimes produced "inexplicable results," it was felt that "the traditional histologic diagnosis [took] precedence over immunophenotyping."[48] In other words, IPT did not "suspend morphologic or medical judgement; it enhance[d] it at the level of additional adjunctive chemical detail."[49]

With the spread of immunohistochemical techniques as discussed in chapter 7, studies of T-cell and B-cell lymphomas proliferated throughout the 1980s even though the working formulation did not recognize the immunological division. Researchers in pathology learned how to subdivide histological subclasses of well-known B-cell lymphomas into different immunophenotypes and studied how the different phenotypes correlated with different stages of B-cell development. Clinical researchers found consistent correlations between the various working formulation categories and the maturation stages of normal lymphocytes as defined by immunophenotype.[50] These correlations reinforced the emerging model for the lymphomas, one that we have already seen in the case of the leukemias. In particular, the consistent correlation between pathological entities and stages of B-cell development led the researchers to speculate: "The unique array of immunologic markers within each group is evidence that these are not only morphologic variants of B-cell lymphomas but may represent distinct biologic entities as well."[51]

Alongside the experimental and clinical findings, calls for a new classification emerged: "In conclusion, new classification systems based on immunophenotype are needed to encompass the various [non-Hodgkin's lymphomas] and improve the predictability of prognosis."[52] Nonetheless, the working formulation remained the system of choice in the United States: in 1988, a follow-up study of the patients included in the initial study concluded that "the Working Formulation for non-Hodgkin's lymphomas is a simple and useful nomenclature for selecting treatment and reporting results."[53] But there is more to medicine than selecting treatment and reporting results. In yet another lymphoma classification proposal published in 1987, Nancy Lee Harris pointed out the obvious problem: since the 1970s, lymphomas had become tumors of the immune system and in that respect the working formulation was clearly outdated. Moreover, the model for a scientifically accurate classification was clear: pathological cells should be aligned with the various stages of development of the cells of the immune system. But knowledge of the immune system evolved independently of pathology and although progress had been made, that knowledge was still incomplete. As Harris put it, "We know too much to be satisfied with the old ways, but not enough to perfect a new one."[54]

In 1987, caught between the old and the new, Harris proposed "simply to list the lymphomas that can be recognized at present, giving synonyms where appropriate to place them in the various classifications."[55] Behind the pragmatic appearances, however, lay more than a simple list, for Harris had made several crucial choices. First of all, she had divided the list of entities into two parts: B-cell lymphomas and T-cell lymphomas, thus endorsing an immunology-based division. Second, she had chosen a vocabulary to name the entities that was consistent with the immunological orientation. Rather than using a histological description of cell types (cleaved, noncleaved, follicular center cell), she had borrowed Lennert's hematological terminology that offered a more ontogenic spin. Moreover, unlike previous classifications, no prognosis was built into the system. In making these choices, Harris brought together the European and the American traditions within a single list whose unstated principle was not simply "wait and see" as the previous quotation implies.

As already mentioned, the ILSG came together in 1991. In 1994, following "more than three years of intensive discussions and exchange of opinions among expert pathologists," the group produced the REAL classification soon hailed by enthusiastic supporters as "a most comprehensive summary of known entities and an important next step toward a more biologically oriented grouping of the malignant lymphomas."[56] Indeed, the REAL classification, following Harris's initiative, had divested itself of the prognostic criteria that structured the Kiel classification, retaining only its immunological basis, splitting some categories of previous classifications, lumping others, and turning the classification into a list. Lennert had recognized that much and had protested that the REAL classification was, in fact, only a list. The ILSG replied: "Rightly so." Choosing the list mode, in effect, created a more direct alignment with immunology by making prognosis an afterthought rather than the foundation:

> This approach to classification is based on the principle that a classification is a list of "real" disease entities, which are defined by a combination of morphology, immunophenotype, genetic features, and clinical features. The relative importance of each of these features varies among diseases, and there is no one "gold standard."[57]

The presentation of the REAL classification in the form of a list was not a sign of defeat. It was a challenge. As clinical oncologists and hematologists—the treating physicians—came to recognize:

The newer lymphoma classifications do not generally indicate the grade of a lymphoma subtype. Rather, the REAL and WHO[58] proposals are lists of disease entities, and they challenge both the clinician and the pathologists to recognize that clinical trials and treatment need to be designed not around broad groups, or grades, of lymphoma, but around specific biologic disorders.[59]

What does it mean to claim that REAL's horizon is a biological classification? Members of the ILSG knew full well that the listing of entities had no intrinsic prognostic value. Some members thought that their work ended there. In a letter published in the appropriately titled *Current Opinion in Oncology*, Belgian members of the group concluded that the "main objection of clinicians remains the lack of grouping of lymphoma entities according to their clinical behavior, which we as pathologists believe to be the clinician's task."[60] Nonetheless, on that road to biology, one still had to satisfy clinicians. Consequently, a series of formal and informal meetings between clinicians and pathologists have been held since 1994 to translate the REAL system into clinical terms.

Between 1995 and 1996, the NCI carried out the clinical validation process in hospitals around the world.[61] In addition to comparing classifications, the validation project sought to define the geographic distribution of the various types of lymphomas, determine the actual diagnostic impact of the clinical information and the immunophenotype, define the clinical relevance of the latter, and verify the inter- and intrapersonal reproducibility in the diagnosis of all entities. Research pathologists analyzed the medical files and samples of approximately 1400 previously untreated cases registered between 1988 and 1990 at the nine participating sites, focusing on clinical data, tissue biopsies, and IPT results.[62] Five expert "hematopathologists," only one of whom was a member of ILSG, visited each site and classified the specimens according to the REAL classification, the working formulation, and a revised version of the Kiel classification. In 1997, the REAL system was declared the winner, with reproducibility rates between the five experts ranging from 85% to 95% depending on the category.[63] This prompted observers to claim that the REAL classification defined "'real' clinical entities that [could] be diagnosed by expert hematopathologists."[64]

Meanwhile, WHO had entered the fray. Working with the European Association of Pathologists and the Society for Hematopathology since 1995 on the development of a new classification of hematological malignancies, WHO adopted the REAL classification. This time, the ILSG members acting from within WHO took care to construct closely monitored bridges[65] with the clinic by establishing a clinical advisory committee "to ensure that the classification [would] be useful to clinicians," and, in particular, to establish a series of consensual statements around a series of clinical questions that included the claim that a "clinical grouping of lymphoid neoplasms was neither necessary nor desirable."[66] What mattered was the specific type of lymphoma, to which one could add clinical prognostic factors derived from a standardized tool known as the International Prognostic Index.[67] Regulation by classification had finally managed, so it seems, to bring the clinic and the laboratory together, but this was, so to speak, an instance of self-vindication,[68] insofar as it was only through the emergence of a *biomedical* platform that this task had become both urgent and doable.

Technologies of Consensus

In the previous section, we presented the somewhat ethereal picture of self-appointed groups of pathologists, constructing classifications, debating nosological principles, and conducting studies designed to validate new classifications through comparison with existing systems. Grounded in the seemingly mundane work of drawing samples, reviewing slides, and examining computerized representations of phenotypes, the results of these activities attained the status of generality through the interlaboratory work we analyzed in chapter 8. A third kind of regulation, one we refer to as "technologies of consensus," mediates these regulatory layers.

The term "consensus" frequently occurs in the biomedical literature. Here, "consensus" designates a set of methodologies leading to a written statement about whether and how a given biomedical procedure should be performed. It refers both to process and results. As such, "consensus-making" or "consensus development" might be more appropriate terms. The latter has indeed come to define, in the United States, a National Institutes of Health (NIH) program initiated in 1977 to produce consensus statements on controversial biomedical issues.[69] The scheme consists of a "consensus conference" where, following presentations by investigators working in areas relevant to the issue under scrutiny and questions by conference attendees, a panel of experts drafts a consensus statement following closed deliberations. Consensus conferences of this kind are part of the more general field of health technology assessment,[70] and, accordingly, they target medical procedures that are either the topic of public controversy or have important policy or financial implications, or both. Many biomedical issues, and, in fact, most of those discussed in this chapter, do not qualify as candidates for this kind of public policy mechanism, but are nonetheless the object of various kinds of consensus exercises.

In order to learn more about consensus formation in biomedicine, we attended a 1995 consensus conference held at the NIH on the "immunophenotypic analysis of hematologic neoplasia by flow cytometry." The conference of experts had been called to set guidelines for the use of IPT in the diagnosis of the leukemias and the lymphomas and had been organized by pathologists who used IPT and who had published extensively in the field. One of the central questions addressed at the conference was how much IPT was truly necessary for the diagnosis, prognosis, and therapeutic monitoring of the leukemias and the lymphomas. Here the problem of classification loomed large since, as the conference organizers noted, the assessment of the value of IPT depended upon the definition of a given disease and, hence, the classificatory scheme in use. In particular, if IPT participates in a disease definition, then its relative value for the diagnosis of the disease, as compared to, say, morphology, is accordingly increased.[71] In turn, in order to make that diagnosis consistently, the performance of the technical tasks must also be consistent, and this requires a definition of the appropriate skills and procedures. Thus, given the range of issues involved, consensus discussions covered the spectrum of regulatory issues we have discussed in this and the previous chapter, ranging, in addition to medical indications,[72] from the selection of antibody combinations for IPT,[73] to data analysis and interpretation,[74] standardization and validation of laboratory procedures,[75] and data reporting.[76]

The consensus-building methodology rested on the so-called Delphi method for group decision-making.[77] The committee chairman circulated a series of general statements, usually framed in the strongest manner possible, to members of the committee who scored their agreement with the statements on a scale from 1 to 7 and provided comments. The chairman also provided references to the secondary literature for the statements. The working document for the session resulted from a second round of consultation conducted along the same lines and included the comments made by committee members. Statements used to produce consensus concerning the medical indications of IPT consisted, for example, of one-paragraph sentences such as "Flow cytometric immunophenotypic analysis of hairy cell leukemia increases diagnostic accuracy and provides essential information for clinical management of such patients," or "Flow cytometric immunophenotyping in acute lymphoblastic leukemia provides prognostic information in selected cases," or "Immunophenotypic flow cytometric analysis is recommended in case of suspected blast crisis of chronic myelogenous leukemia." In the case of data reporting, participants were confronted with a list of the data that might appear on a laboratory report. Here, the discussion centered on which data should be always, occasionally, or never reported. This seemingly mundane discussion led to more "philosophical" (their term) debates about the audience for these kinds of reports and about the degree to which the report should feature a medical interpretation of the IPT data. "Consensus" resulted from 80% agreement, although during the course of the meeting, statements were often watered down in order to attain unanimous or quasi-unanimous consent.

The legal and professional consequences of issuing guidelines constrain the formulation of consensus statements. In the United States, publishing a strong statement (i.e., "should be used") can be construed as a statement of "standard practice" that leaves clinicians open to malpractice litigation. A weak statement (i.e., "can be used") would have left the use of IPT optional, exposing clinicians that used IPT in contexts covered by that statement to the risk of nonreimbursement by insurance carriers. Consensus statements also sought to link IPT to the clinical and morphological skills of the pathologists and treating physicians to avoid giving the platform the status of a stand-alone technology. Conference participants thus sought to frame statements so as to set clinical judgment as the final arbiter of immunophenotypic data, and, at the same time, to cast IPT as a key element of an informed (or "evidence-based") clinical judgment.

Consensus or lack thereof showed the variety of ways IPT had been integrated into daily routine and the kinds of problems that arose from the coexistence of the morphological and IPT platforms. For the sake of brevity, consider the discussion surrounding a single disease. Conference participants asked, for example, whether IPT should be carried out in all cases of chronic lymphocytic leukemia (CLL). Down south, some did not think so: "I object to the statement that flow should be done in every case of CLL. In New Mexico, in day-to-day practice, the morphology is evident."[78] Other pathologists felt otherwise: "80 to 85% of the time with a microscope and the right stain I can diagnose CLL; but with flow we can get it 100% of the time." Why the divergence? Here is one answer: "The factor is the skill level of the people. It depends on the institution." But skill without opportunity is empty and in some cases, established routines favored the morphological platform: "If they [the surgical pathologists] dump everything into formalin, you won't be able to do anything [viz. IPT] with it. We should make some recommendations about sample collection." Routine also breeds routine. At the Mayo Clinic, for example, the slide remained the norm: "They are stuck in their ways and want to see a slide. I could name names."

Differential diagnosis—eliminating possibilities as opposed to identifying entities—raised yet another problem. Perhaps, for example, IPT in the right hands in the right place could recognize CLL. But when the clinical picture was clouded with related disorders collectively known as chronic lymphoproliferative disorders (CLPDs), then 100% was no longer possible: "In my opinion it is the integration of morphology plus flow cytometric immunophenotyping that is critical in the distinction between CLL and other types of CLPD." Finally, the preceding discussion presupposed that the patients were adults: "With children you should look for a virus. Forget about flow. In kids it's a problem. Kids are full of viruses."

And what about prognosis? Which platform predicted outcomes better: morphology or IPT? Once again, both at the conference and in the literature, opinions varied even among those who relied exclusively on IPT. The temporary reason for the quandary seemed to be the surfeit of surface markers which, in turn, had stymied the standardization of the prognostic value of the markers: "Which phenotypic markers are prognostically significant? The literature is a mess. Every paper gives a different marker."

The consensus conference participants recognized that the IPT platform functioned in most Western hospitals as an adjunct to morphological diagnosis, although in light of the evolution of classification systems, it would probably be more accurate to argue that the two platforms entertained complex relations of coexistence, cooperation, and mutual dependence. Unlike the morphological platform, however, the IPT platform and, in particular, the automated nature of its components had opened the additional and problematic possibility of routinely "screening" blood and marrow that had been diagnosed as leukemic or lymphomiatous. At the conference, opposition to screening—seen as a mixed blessing—was in part economic (cost-benefit analysis did not favor the option): "If bone marrow shows clear-cut non-Hodgkin's lymphoma, performing flow is redundant and expensive. The decision to perform flow should always be based on morphologic and clinical issues, not just a 'do flow on everything' mentality." Similarly with the leukemias: "If it is an obvious M2, M3 or M4, why do it?" "I am 100% confident than I'm not going to miss an obvious M2. Purely diagnostic, you don't miss it."[79] But "clear-cut" and "100%" are relative terms. They presuppose a degree of certitude that is not necessarily present in all practitioners and all institutions. Screening advocates believed that the expertise entailed in the previous quotes was a scarce resource. When questioned as to how the "little hospitals" could afford to conform with guidelines implying that all suspected cases of leukemia be immunophenotyped, they replied: "I think they will be forced to as it is getting harder and harder to find a morphologist. It is a vanishing species." Comparing the morphological and the immunophenotypic platforms might indeed become moot.

The views aired during the consensus conference broached a variety of topics ranging from the epistemological—Is morphological information equivalent to immunological information?—to the pragmatic—What sort of information enhances therapeutics? In view of the existence of different platforms and of their variable adaptation to local circumstances and needs, the pursuit of consensus has itself become a goal. In other words, consensus is not an "external" variable the presence or absence of which can be assessed by epistemologically privileged analysts; rather, it is part and parcel of the regulatory practices pursued by actors on a given platform: no more, no less.

10

Conclusion: Platform Sociology

Marco Polo describes a bridge, stone by stone.

"But which is the stone that supports the bridge?" Kublai Khan asks.

"The bridge is not supported by one stone or another," Marco answers, "but by the line of the arch that they form."

Kublai Khan remains silent, reflecting. Then he adds: "Why do you speak to me of the stones? It is only the arch that matters to me."

Polo answers: "Without stones there is no arch."[1]

This book opened with a description of a visit to a tertiary care hospital. In the course of research for this book we visited many other institutions: universities, public and private research centers, biotech startups, established biomedical instrumentation companies, regulatory agencies, and other hospitals. The thread connecting these sites is, of course, the notion of a platform: these institutions lay along the path of our search for the components of a biomedical platform that established the nucleus of our description of medical routines and innovation.

The title and topic of this book came to us as a sort of epiphany. Following up on previous work on innovation in the field of immunology and antibody reagents,[2] we developed an interest in the scientific instruments that used those reagents and, in particular, in their role in the production, maintenance, and regulation of clinical and laboratory practices. Among these instruments, flow cytometry, often presented as a complementary tool for antibodies, but also as a bridge between biology and medicine,[3] seemed to offer an interesting case study. To take it as the focal point of our endeavor, so we thought, would provide us with a solid beginning, something tangible around which biomedical practitioners organized their activities. At one point, we even believed that the instrument functioned as a "trading zone" between clinicians and researchers.[4] By following the instrument around, however, we were led in two different directions that seemed to absorb the object of our inquiry. The first was history: every part of the instrument offered yet another genealogy. The cytometer's lasers grew out of post-World War II military research strategies, its vibrating nozzle out of computer technologies, and the very idea of particle sizing went back to interwar Chicago pea-canning factories. The software for the instrument raised a whole new series of contexts and questions. Here, then, the instrument vanished into fragmenting genealogies. The second direction was practice: by following the instrument into its multiple uses (exobiology, radioactive fallout monitoring, cervical cancer screening, etc.), we came across zones of activity where the instrument competed with ongoing and similar practices that, ultimately, could not be defined by the use of the instrument; the instrument, in other words, disappeared into a multitude of practices. Our "materialist" strategy consequently lost its focus and its object.

Profiting from a sabbatical to mull over this conclusion in a nondescript Paris café, we reviewed the themes that had emerged in the course of our research on the instrument: the relationship of the normal and the pathological, the problem of standards, the transformation of clinical practices, and so on. Relating the themes to the instrument seemed forced and fruitless. Then, suddenly, a casual comment made a year or so before by the director of marketing of an American instrument manufacturer took on renewed meaning. We had visited the manufacturer's R&D complex in Florida to interview researchers who had worked on an early flow cytometer. Walking through the factory floor on our way to the interview, the marketing director suddenly gestured to the left saying, "That's where we make our platforms." At the time, we did not pay much attention to the remark, and we realized later, moreover, that neither of us had actually seen what the marketing director had been pointing to when he mentioned the company's platforms. Although we did not know it at the time, the marketing director had provided us with a key to the organization of our material: the idea that one could build something like a medical platform. We immediately knew we had something. We had seen bits and pieces of it over the years. The stories we had been following cohered, but it was not around the instrument, as we realized, but within the larger category used by the instrument manufacturer to describe his enterprise; he built platforms, not instruments. And, as we came to understand in the course of our discussion, from his point of view he built two kinds of platform: medical platforms and research platforms. From our point of view, however, he participated in the construction (literally!) of biomedical platforms. We finally had our object of investigation, and this time it could not disappear; it was already invisible insofar as it was part practice and part object.

There is, of course, another way of describing what we have done. In the simplest terms, our book describes a biomedical innovation and the translation of that innovation into a variety of medical practices. We have, however, offered more than a case study in an attempt to break down the dichotomy presupposed in the previous sentence between innovation and translation. In addition to the case study, we have proposed a means of describing that case that brings together innovations and routine within a single *dispositif*,[5] namely a biomedical platform. We have done so by articulating two closely related themes: a historical one, the emergence of modern biomedicine; and a sociological one, the regulation of biomedical practices.

In this concluding chapter, we would like, first, to add a few theoretical and empirical specifications to our proposal and, second, revisit the main themes of the book and discuss how the notion of biomedical platforms elucidates our understanding of the development of biomedicine.

Platforms, Networks, Medical Technologies, Infrastructure, and Experimental Systems

The notion of platform was not snatched out of thin air. We have already noted (chapter 2) that it derives, in part, from "native" terminology in medicine and elsewhere. It is also connected to theoretical proposals developed by the growing number of historians and sociologists who study the development of the biomedical sciences. In what follows, we review some of these complementary and sometimes competing notions and confront the empirical limits of our study.

Although biomedical platforms coordinate action, they are not the only means of doing so. Social and technical networks are often instanced as a major form of coordination and their constitution and maintenance have become the centerpiece of scientific and medical innovation policy programs such as those sponsored by the European Union.[6] In a different guise, they are a key notion of the sociological approach known as "actor-network theory" that has been widely applied to the analysis of science, technology, and medicine.[7] In some respects, networks are a ubiquitous feature of the scientific world. In our discussion of the CD system (chapter 6), for example, we examined the operations of a distinctive network of laboratories.[8] We can, however, distinguish networks from platforms. Insofar as they embody regulations and conventions of equivalence, exchange, and circulation (see chapters 8 and 9), platforms are not simply one among many forms of coordination that include networks; rather, they account for the generation of networks or, at the very least, they are a condition of possibility for the very existence and transformation of networks. The intermediaries that stabilize networks are produced and reproduced on the platform. Platforms supply networks with conventions, generate novel entities, and entrench them in clinical routines.

Much of the phenomena that we have described could be classified under the head of medical technology. Why not simply say that we have described yet another "medical technology" such as those examined in Stanley Reiser's seminal overview of clinical instruments and machines.[9] Although, as we will see, biomedical platforms are more than medical technology, there is no doubt that Reiser's book raised a number of themes that have since become standard and thus form something like a tradition. We have, however, already implicitly distanced ourselves from that tradition. It is generally held, for example, that medical technologies tend to remove the patient from the clinical picture and redirect the clinicians' attention from the bedside to the laboratory. In addition, it is maintained that medical technologies have downgraded or eliminated skills embodied in what is termed "clinical judgment," forcing diagnosing physicians to become increasingly subservient to technologies whose development they cannot control. The theme of technology overtaking medical practice also surfaces, in less normative terms, in Joel D. Howell's book on the turn-of-the-century introduction of diagnostic equipment and scientific management methods in U.S. hospitals.[10] As we have seen, whether it is deskilling, "objectification," or "fragmentation," none of these themes offer much to the understanding of the development of biomedical technologies or of the evolution of modern biomedicine. We thus feel that unlike the trope of "technology out of control," platforms have more to offer than the usual denunciations.

Similar limitations can be observed in approaches that take a more interactive view of the relation between technology and medicine. Consider, for example, Keith Wailoo's discussion of how medical technologies modified disease definitions (or, in trendier terms, disease "identities") in twentieth-century America.[11] Using hematology as a case study, Wailoo purports to show how the technologies implicated in the development of the field participated in the construction and transformation of the various diseases (chlorosis, pernicious anemia, sickle cell anemia, leukemia, etc.), the patients that were the target of diagnostic and therapeutic interventions, and, finally, the very practitioners (e.g., oncologists vs. hematologists) who intervened. In turn, Wailoo claims, social, political, and cultural forces shaped these technologies in the sense that the latter acquired as much of their meaning and power from the cultural context of their use as from their use per se.

This is not the place to examine Wailoo's thesis in detail, except to note that his use of the term "technology" makes no difference between kinds of technology and therefore lacks analytical specificity.[12] As mentioned earlier (chapter 3), even medical reformers such as Lewis Thomas distinguished different *kinds* of technology. While the actors categories clearly cannot be taken at face value, they do, however, suggest that the technologies used in medicine are considerably more complex than Wailoo allows. At the very least, they suggest that there is no such thing as a "technology" that confronts "medicine" but, rather, many kinds of technologies that participate in different ways in the articulation of biology and medicine and thus in the establishment of new configurations of *biomedicine.* In other words, despite traditional usage, the notion of technology is too generic and, at the same time (even when stretched to include social and political actions and events) too narrow to capture the dynamics of biomedical innovation.

Describing the relevant divisions of this process in appropriate terms is a problem not only for historians and sociologists; it also preoccupies practitioners. Consider, for example, the notion of clinical research. The content of this category has generated a great deal of soul-searching on the part of U.S. biomedical practitioners and administrators. Numerous authors and institutions have proposed taxonomies of this activity, including such hybrid, finely tuned designations as "basic patient-oriented research" and "applied oriented research." Yet other contributors have redefined the entire field as a continuum without categorical distinctions.[13] While policy clearly inspires these classificatory endeavors, given the increasing complexity and diversity of biomedical practices the taxonomies necessarily call upon a variety of epistemological, material, and discursive traits of biomedical research for their formulation. Because of their static nature, however, taxonomic categories (rigid or porous) are ill-suited to capture complexity: dynamic notions are needed, that is, notions that are able to account for processes rather than list traits.[14]

In this spirit, the authors in a recent collection of historical essays on twentieth-century medicine have coined the term "molecularizing" in an attempt to capture biomedicine's distinctiveness and dynamics.[15] The term does not, as one might assume, refer to molecular biology. Rather, it refers to the broader historical processes that led researchers and clinicians in biology and medicine to focus on molecules as the solution to their problems. From this point of view, molecular biology represents only the latest incarnation of a transformation with deeper historical roots insofar as molecularizing approaches were prominent in the interwar period. While we are sympathetic to this approach, we consider that, in the end, it fails for reasons quite similar to those mentioned for the medical technology tradition. Borrowing a useful distinction from French historical epistemology, one could say that "molecularizing" is a label, rather than a notion. As such, it merely isolates a set of practices and objects without showing what holds them together and qualifies them as a set. As such, it cannot be used as an analytical resource.

In addition to these historical approaches, researchers in the sociology of science have advanced a number of analytical categories that resemble platforms. Showing how our notion differs from theirs allows us one final series of theoretical specifications. Consider, first, Star and Ruhleder's notion of infrastructure, a sophisticated reworking of the notion of technology.[16] Embedded in material and discursive structures, infrastructures, according to Star and Ruhleder, become visible only upon breakdown (viz. normally, they are transparent). More than inert pieces of machinery, infrastructures incorporate heuristics and are learned as a part and sine qua non of membership in a collective activity, thus being shaped by and shaping conventions of practice. While, as we have seen, biomedical platforms incorporate the infrastructure necessary for the pursuit of biomedicine, they are not reducible to infrastructure. Moreover, although platforms contain infrastructural components, these components are visible. Unlike Star and Ruhleder's passive and transparent infrastructure, platforms are active, generative, and opaque. Indeed, we have seen that even though platforms extend beyond the walls of the clinical or diagnostic laboratory, they are more than technology or infrastructure. In fact, we have shown that biomedical platforms are neither science nor technology but a way of articulating the two. If a definition is needed, even at this late date, then we can define them as the bench upon which conventions concerning the biological or normal are articulated with or connected to conventions concerning the medical or pathological. As such they define the standards according to which biomedical actions are evaluated.

Biomedical platforms may also be usefully contrasted with Joan Fujimura's notion of standardized packages, which she defines as a "theory-methods package" whose description shows "how tools, practices, and theories circulate through and across worlds of practice . . . and both change and are changed by their circulation."[17] In practice, Fujimura's application of her concept results in the recapitulation of the actors' narratives, insofar as it tells the story of how biomedical innovations (in her case, oncogene theory and related techniques) emerged from within a few elite biology laboratories and spread, as a prepackaged technique, to lower-level clinical laboratories.[18] In other words, Fujimura's theory-methods package, because it adheres so closely to the actors' accounts, becomes little more than a description of a linear process of innovation leading from the laboratory to the clinic. Such a narrative omits all mention of clinical work in the innovation process itself; the clinic and clinical research are represented as merely the endpoints of biology. In this sense, standardized packages do not so much "circulate" as "drive" the teleological accounts offered by participants.

Attentive readers will have noted that we have used the term "experimental system" several times in this book. We owe our use of the term to Hans-Jörg Rheinberger who has developed the notion in a series of books and articles.[19] Rheinberger's notion avoids the pitfall just mentioned insofar as it takes into account the fact that, for instance, an experimental system instituted for the study of cancer can easily become a system for the study of protein synthesis. In this sense, it crosses the biology-medicine divide. Similarly, it straddles the topic-resource divide and functions as an analytical category for both analysts and actors since, unlike Fujimura's notion of standardized packages, it is widely used by scientists to describe the problems they study and the techniques they use to study them. Defined in an admittedly compressed way as "a machine for the production of difference," the notion of an experimental system describes a fundamental unit of scientific activity.

Experimental systems also cross the science-technology divide. In particular, according to Rheinberger, the difference between science (epistemic things) and technology is generated within an experimental system. Thus, in the latter, as opposed to a technological system where differences are reduced to enable production of the same, the reproduction of the same is subordinated to the production of differences. It will be noted that the previously criticized use of generic notions such as science and technology is here subordinated to and specified by a given experimental system: as such, it loses much of its indeterminacy and acquires analytical specificity. For our present purpose, we will note, however, that while experimental systems enter into the description of biomedical research, they do not cover the whole range of biomedical practices that stretch from the clinic to the research laboratory. Rheinberger himself is aware of the need for a notion that would go beyond individual research laboratories and encompass a broader range of activities such as those described in this book.[20] He has thus proposed—we assume somewhat half-heartedly—the notion of experimental cultures, somewhat reminiscent of Karin Knorr Cetina's notion of epistemic cultures.[21] We believe this notion is a nonstarter, because it signals a return to the culturalist, humanist assumptions that the notion of experimental systems was designed to avoid and that we have already criticized at the end of chapter 1.

Thus, while we have used Rheinberger's notion of experimental systems when discussing biomedical platforms, the two notions should not be confused. As we saw, the immunophenotyping (IPT) platform grew out of experimental systems set up in clinical and nonclinical immunology. Once in place, IPT reproduced the entities and distinctions generated by those systems in daily clinical and research practices. Generalizing, we can say that historically, an experimental system precedes a platform; yet, experimental systems presuppose the existence of platforms. Platforms are neither infrastructures nor experimental systems, but another configuration of the biomedical process. While both experimental systems and platforms create spaces of representation, the notion of platform allows us to focus on the regulation of the objects generated, rather than on the production of epistemic things.[22]

Within a larger time frame, platforms signal the transformation of medicine into biomedicine, a process that we have located in the postwar era. It can thus only be applied recursively to past events in the special sense that a present platform creates a common perception of the past. From a platform, the past is seen as caught up in a previous platform, for instance, as having been constrained by some technical problem. History recounted from the platform tells us that there is some consensus about what counts as technology in the present. To return to our example of morphology vs. IPT, it is doubtful that morphology would have been understood as a platform at, say, the turn of the century. Yet, practitioners can retrospectively view morphology as a platform once the IPT platform is in place. In this sense, platforms must be understood as historicized, or, rather, historialized.[23]

Turning now to the empirical limits of our study, one might easily object (as, in fact, some of our readers have) that we have unduly generalized from a single case study and that while the notion of platform may be an appropriate rendering of the emergence of IPT, it does not go much beyond that. While it is true that most of our discussion is based on hematology, immunology, and pathology (which, by themselves, it should be admitted, cover considerable territory), there are two ways our argument can be easily extended. First, although we restricted our examples of the application of IPT to the earliest and, therefore, most easily accessible fields, the platform has not been restricted in its use to the aforementioned disciplines. Where there are white blood cells implicated in the disease process, IPT is a potential player. Second, our platform analysis does not rely on the existence of a single "immunological" platform. Numerous others arise whenever there is an attempt to articulate problems of biology with problems of pathology. Consider, for simplicity's sake, the outpouring of technologies from molecular biology over the last quarter of a century. For these technologies and the problems that they raise to find purchase within medicine, they must become platforms in the sense that we have given the term. Even as we write, a platform composed of molecular biological techniques known as reverse transcriptase and the polymerase chain reaction bundled onto a diagnostic platform in a variety of configurations is rearranging the classification of the lymphomas (once again) and other cancers.[24]

A second empirical limit to our investigation can be framed in terms of a question: to what extent does the platform we have analyzed affect clinical outcomes? Clearly, the answer here depends upon a number of considerations. Most AIDS patients in the Western world have access to CD4 counts. Note, first of all, the important qualifier "Western world." For countries lacking effective public health systems, many of the practices discussed previously are meaningless. Even when there is easy access to something like CD4 counts, it is next to impossible to know exactly how such numbers enter into clinical decision-making on a daily basis other than at an ideal-typical level. Practitioners may develop their own rules of thumb, ignore guidelines, or have their advice fall on deaf ears. As readers will by now have gathered, variation is the rule and much the regulation that goes into the maintenance of a platform consists in discovering just how much variation there is. We cannot here substitute ourselves for regulators and say with any assurance exactly how IPT has changed the lives of patients and practitioners. Unlike therapies for life-threatening disease, there is no quick and easy body count with which we can make our case. Suffice it say that it is part and parcel of our argument that whether or not there is an immediate impact on patient care is less relevant in the era of biomedicine than it once was. As we saw in the debate between clinicians and pathologists in the case of the REAL (revised European-American lymphoma) classification, having the "right" biological categories was held by some to be more important in the long run than having the more "useful" clinical categories.

There is one other potential oversight in our treatment of biomedical platforms. While we have discussed the consistent failure to redefine pathological lesions in terms of the continuous function of a biological variable, as in the case of diabetes and the Pap test, we did not discuss the rise of "risk factors" (high blood pressure, high blood sugar, etc.) that precede the formation of lesions, and their relation to biomedical platforms. Unlike the reductionism criticized by Canguilhem, the construction of biological risk factors and their use in clinical trials, epidemiology, and clinical medicine has met with considerable success.[25] Note that while risk factors do not replace symptoms, just as prognosis does not replace diagnosis, there is a prevailing tendency to construe correlation as cause. There is no doubt that by making biological variables more readily available to the clinic, biomedical platforms contribute to the production of risk factors and the spread of statistical thinking. The new genetics and the associated biomedical platforms, moreover, will accentuate this tendency.

A Final Review of the Main Themes

In conclusion, let us briefly review the main themes examined in this book and discuss how the notion of biomedical platforms elucidates our understanding of the development of biomedicine.

Let us begin with the first theme, the emergence of a new way of conducting research in biology and medicine since World War II. We have described how, in the case of IPT, and in a manner consistent with trends since the war, biology and medicine came together, both institutionally and intellectually, to create a hybrid practice that is neither syncretic nor synthetic. Rather, in analyzing the constitution of this practice, we described the creation of a *problematic* space of scientific representation in which truly biomedical entities—cell-surface markers—exist as both normal biological entities and as pathological signs. We showed that markers are, in other words, *biomedical* substances with regard to their origins, their uses, and their meanings.

This particular alignment of the normal and the pathological is just that, an alignment, not a fusion. As our discussion of Canguilhem and the related discussions concerning, for example, the evolving status of tumor antigens or normal and pathological experimental systems show, not only has the division between the normal and the pathological been constitutive of modern medicine, it has remained so. Despite the continuing redescription of pathological processes in biological terms, the notion of a pathological event resulting in a lesion remains central to the understanding of disease. We saw, for example, that Greaves's critique of the pathologist's notion of "dedifferentiation" resulted in the equally pathological construct of "uncoupling." This point is not always immediately evident as the rise of cellular and molecular medicine has tended to obscure this fact. Indeed, in the era of "molecular pathology" one might be tempted to say that biology has supplanted pathology as the form of explanation of disease.

Our second theme, the importance of regulation in the conduct of biomedical research, has highlighted a category of scientific activity that has too often been dismissed as "routine" or "applied" in the negative senses of these terms. In our description of the regulatory activities related to IPT, we have tried to point out how such work is necessary for the effective functioning of the platform; how, in a sense, regulation is a constitutive component of the platform. Rather than treating regulation as some dreary bureaucratic ritual, we have tried to describe and recapture the work, and indeed the innovative work, that lies behind such enterprises and show how such work relates to the construction and maintenance of an effective platform. The CD workshops, for example, did not merely assign conventional names to cell-surface markers; without the international collaboration, the markers could not have attained their international, independent status and been freed from the contingencies of the individual laboratories that produced them.

The notion of platform enlarges the connotation of regulation which, when viewed in terms of platforms, no longer appears as an obstacle to fruitful work or innovation, targeting mainly routine activities. Regulation now appears as a condition for the production, circulation, and interchangeability of novel entities and practices. We are tempted to add a more epochal twist to our claim. Daston and Galison have convincingly argued that scientific objectivity, far from being a logical category, is a historical construct: there are many kinds of objectivity, and their emergence can be dated.[26] Thus, a form of objectivity grounded in the expertise of the skilled practitioner, or in the judgment of a group of experts, can be contrasted with the mechanical objectivity of inscription devices or recording instruments. Platforms embody a new form of objectivity, a regulatory one, grounded in the procedures of internal quality control and, especially, external quality assessment.

We defined biomedical platforms as material and discursive arrangements that act as the bench upon which conventions concerning the biological or normal are connected with conventions concerning the medical or pathological. We have used this category to describe a range of activities in contemporary biomedicine running from laboratory research to clinical trials and routine diagnosis. Has it been worth it? By looking at post-World War II biomedicine in terms of platforms, we believe that one can rethink a number of assumptions that have been nagging the science studies scholars for some time now. First of all, medical sociology and the sociology of biomedical research generally presuppose a division between mundane or routine medical activities and the more exceptional work of biomedical discovery and innovation. Thinking in terms of platforms allows one to see and analyze the continuities between these apparently distinct activities. Biomedical innovation, in other words, is as continuous as it is undirected and surprising. Going beyond the innovation/routine dichotomy, platform sociology thus opens up the field for the investigation of those activities that, borrowing a term from evolutionary economics, can be termed "innovating routines."[27]

The notion of platform draws together actors—physicians, researchers, industrialists, patients—as well as objects—research materials, specimens, standards, contracts, high-tech and low-tech equipment—that were previously thought to inhabit separate social worlds, although, empirically speaking, they are often found in the same room. Analyzing the different constituents of biomedical platforms shows cooperation and interdependence—between the various components of a platform and the related actors, as well as between platforms—to be equally as important as, if not more important than, segmentation and conflict. As an additional bonus, the dichotomy between science and technology that has dominated the analysis of technoscientific and medical activities can now be overcome without being discarded. Whereas "technoscience" points to a problem without providing a solution or, in other words, raises an issue that still begs for analysis, a focus on the platform allows one to move from one contingent embodiment of the division to the other, without overlooking the continuities or denying the differences. In addition to articulating the normal and the pathological, biomedical platforms articulate the scientific and the technological.

As developed in this book, the notion of the biomedical platform allows for historical contingencies in the sense that the platform we have described is not a structural constraint on action; our description of IPT has no recourse to technological determinism. As we saw, researchers instantiated IPT in a variety of ways using components that articulated previous practices, as in slide-based IPT. A word of caution, however, is necessary here. Although they do not determine practices, platforms are not "social constructions" open to endless negotiation, leading to malleable natural and social arrangements. While the list of CDs is not fixed in advance, for instance, the scientific and cultural meaning of CD4 cannot be reduced to social variables. As an "entrenched" convention, it cannot be defined away. From this point of view, platforms are neither trivial conventions nor transcendental machines or concepts. We did not "see" the platform even when it was pointed out to us by the marketing director in the instrument factory. Nonetheless, manufacturers build platform components.

One final comment about the nature of the IPT platform: following our description of this category of practice and analysis one might easily conclude that the essential component of the platform, the cell-surface markers, is *somewhat* immaterial. Recall that we defined platforms as arrangements of things rather than the things themselves. In this sense, the core of the IPT platform is indeed less the cell-surface molecules than the arrangement and consequent understanding of those proteins as markers. In that sense, they are immaterial. This arrangement, however, is less ephemeral than might be imagined and we have underlined "somewhat" to call to the reader's attention the fact that because the markers have acquired standard meanings through regulation, they can be bottled and sold on the open market. In turn, their practical and theoretical meaning depended upon their being bottled and exchanged.

Where do we go from here? Their heterogeneity and their contingent, local nature often characterize biomedical practices. The same pathology is treated differently in different institutional or geographic locations; indeed, what counts as the same pathology can also vary, along with the material practices used to define a given disease entity.[28] Yet, while individual patients are diagnosed within local settings, diagnostic decisions transcend local events, since treating patients requires continuity across time and space. The development of biomedicine coincides with a sharp increase in specialization, and, as we have seen, critics have complained that both medical knowledge and the patient's body have accordingly become fragmented. Yet these fragments are fragments of some body, and treating individual bodies requires relations of consult, rather than divisions of labor. Different styles of reasoning—statistical for epidemiologists, experiential for clinicians, and experimental for laboratory scientists, to which one could add lay reasoning for patient groups—define the various branches of the biomedical enterprise, yet there is a sense in which both promoters and critics of the latter perceive it as a coordinated whole.[29]

How is this possible? Standardization and new forms of collaboration between biomedical practitioners are part of the answer, but beyond standardization and cooperation, formal and informal regulations that allow for the continued existence of heterogeneities have become part and parcel of the biomedical enterprise. To understand biomedicine is to understand its regulation. Yet regulation does not target single objects or practices; rather, as we have argued, it targets the heterogeneous array of items and activities brought together by a given platform. Thus, the notion of platform should prove to be essential to further investigations of this process.

"I have a question. Say I want to use your platform sociology to analyze my own material, for instance, the application of molecular genetic approaches to schizophrenia. How should I go about it? Where should I begin? In other words, do you have a checklist of steps for performing platform analysis?"

"Well, we do not really like checklists and methodological algorithms, but here are a few indications. Start right in the middle of the game, with regulation. Look, for instance, to quality-control procedures, the meetings and discussions surrounding their development and enforcement, the formal and informal agreements in which they are grounded; from there, move up and down along the regulatory continuum, letting your investigation range from matters of equipment to clinical matters such as those discussed during consensus conferences. Then, investigate the debates and practices surrounding the redefinition of the lesion that defines the disease. Do so with a view toward specifying biomedical (i.e., normal and pathological) entities that are both the input into and the outcome of this process. Finally, look for alignments with other forms of work. You can ask yourself, for instance, how the new entities generated by the platform have been articulated with previous ones, for instance, with prior diagnostic and prognostic classifications. Does this answer your question?"

Appendix: List of Interviewees

What follows is a list of the persons interviewed for this book, with the date and location of the interview. In the few cases in which the interview did not take place at the interviewee's working place, we have added this information in brackets.

AUER, Robert, Hialeah, Fla., 7 May 1996.

BACH, Marie Anne, Paris, 11 December 1996.

BARNETT, David, Sheffield, U.K., 24 April 1999.

BÉNÉ, Marie-Christine, Nancy, France, 13 February 1997.

BERNARD, Alain, Nice, France, 26 September 2001.

BIGOS, Martin, Stanford, Calif., 17 February 1993.

BISCONTE, Jean-Claude, Les Ulis, France, 10 March 1997.

BOILEAU, Jacques, Montreal, 16 April 1996.

BOUMSELL, Laurence, Paris, 18 December 1990.

BRAYLAN, Raul C., Bethesda, Md., 18 November 1995 and Gainesville, Fla., 11 May 1996.

BRUGAL, Gérard, Grenoble, France, 7 July 1997.

BURKE, Bohdana, Boston, 22 July 1996.

CANTOR, Harvey, Cambridge, Mass., 1 May 1992.

CATOWSKY, Daniel, London, 1 June 1999.

CHESSELS, Judith, London, 25 May 1999.

CORNELISSE, Cees, Leiden, The Netherlands, 13 May 1997.

CREWS, Harold, Hialeah, Fla., 7 May 1996.

DEAN, Phillip N., Los Alamos, N.M., 8 September 1997.

DELAAGE, Michel, Marseilles, 24 February 1997.

DEVILDER Renaud, Nantes, France, 4 July 1997.

DE VITA, Raffaele, Casaccia, (Rome), Italy, 7 April 1997.

D'HAUTCOURT, Jean-Luc, Paris, 24 April 1997.

DIGHIERO, Guillaume, Paris, 23 December 1996.

FAURE, Gilbert, Nancy, France, 13 February 1997.

FLANDRIN, Georges, Paris, 7 November 1996.

FRELAT, Gérard , Fontenay-aux-Roses, France, 17 March 1997.

FULWYLER, Mack J., San Francisco, 3 May 1990.

GAUCHER, Jean-Claude, Saclay, France, June 1997.

GIORGI, Janis V., long-distance interview, Los Angeles, 20 March 1997.

GOGUEI, Alain F., Paris, 25 May 1994.

GÖHDE, Wolfgang, Münster, Germany, 24–27 June 1997.

GOLDBERG, Michel, Paris, 21 November 1996.

GREAVES, Melvyn F., London, 2 July 1996.

GUTIERREZ, William, Hialeah, Fla., 7 May 1996.

GUTTMAN, Ronald D., Montreal, 27 June 1991 and 9 July 1991.

HEDLEY, David, Toronto, 1 May 1996.

HERZENBERG, Leonard, A., Stanford, Calif., 27 March 1988, 29 April 1990, and 2 May 1990.

HERZENBERG, Leonore A., Stanford, Calif., 27 March 1988 and 29 April 1990.

HILL, Catherine, Villejuif, France, 19 December 1990.

HIRN, Michel, Marseilles, 24 February 1997.

JANOSSY, George, London, 27 April 1999 and 6 May 1999.

JULIUS, Michael, Montreal, 24 June 1993.

KAMENTSKY, Louis A., Cambridge, Mass., 29 April 1992.

KAMOUN Pierre, Paris, 27 June 1997.

KOMAROVER, Bernard Henri, Marseilles, 24 February 1997.

KUNG, Patrick C., Cambridge, Mass., 15 July 1993.

LANDAY, Allan, Chicago, 21 November 1991.

MANDY, Frank, Ottawa, 16 December 1994.

MARTI, Gerald E., Bethesda, Md., 15 February 1995.

MASON, David Y., Oxford, 20 May 1997.

MAURO, Francesco, Casaccia (Rome), Italy, 7 April 1997.

MAWAS, Claude, Marseilles, 22 October 2001.

MAYALL, Brian, Oslo, 28 May 1997.

MELAMED, Myron, Valhalla, N.Y., 17 June 1997.

MENDELSOHN, Mortimer, Livermore, Calif., 6 September 1997.

MÉTÉZEAU, Philippe, Paris, 7 January 1997.

MILLER, Keith, London, 5 May 1999.

MISHAL, Zohar, Villejuif, France, 17 January 1997.

MITCHISON, Nicholas A., London, 20 May 1999.

OI, Vernon, Palo Alto, Calif., 2 May 1990.

PAIETTA, Elisabeth, New York, 30 May 1999.

PEDROSO, Paul, Hialeah, Fla., 7 May 1996.

PLOEM, Johan S., Paris [Leiden, The Netherlands], 12 May 1997.

PRAT, Jean-Jacques, Paris, 13 March 1997.

PREFFER, Francis I., Boston, 27 August 1996.

RAFF, Martin, London, 2 June 1999.

RATCLIFFE, Michael, Montreal, 10 May 1995.

ROBILLARD, Nelly, Nantes, France, 7 July 1997.

ROITT, Ivan M., London, 24 May 1999.

ROSENFELD, Claude, Paris, 10 January 1997.

ROTHE, Gregor, Oslo [Regensburg, Germany], 27 May 1997.

SCHLOSSMAN, Stuart F., Cambridge, Mass., 20 September 1988 and 30 April 1992.

SEIGNEUR, Alain, Saclay, France, June 1997.

SHAPIRO, Howard, Cambridge, Mass., 29 April 1992.

SHOOR, Bernard, San José, Calif., 6 September 1997.

SHUSTIK, Chaim, Montreal, 18 July 1996.

SIMPSON, Mary Ann, Boston, 13 August 1996.

SPANÒ, Marcello, Casaccia (Rome), Italy, 7 April 1997.

STARACE, Giuseppe, Rome, 9 April 1997.

STEINKAMP, John, Los Alamos, N.M., 12 September 1997.

STEWART, Carleton C., Bethesda, Md. [Buffalo, N.Y.], 17 November 1995.

SWEET, Richard D., Palo Alto, Calif., 3 May 1990.

TAFURI, Agostino, Rome, 15 April 1997.

TANAKA, Noboru, Tokyo, 6 January 1998.

TANKE, Hans, Leiden, The Netherlands, 14 May 1997.

TIRINDELLI, Donatella, Casaccia (Rome), Italy, 7 April 1997.

TRIADOU, Patrick, Paris, 2 October 1996 and 23 October 1996.

VALENSI, Françoise, Paris, 18 December 1997.

VAN AGHTOVEN, Andreas, Marseilles, 27 November 2001.

VAN DILLA, Marvin, Santa Fe, (N.M.), USA, 12 September 1997.

VEIZADES, Nicholas, Palo Alto, Calif., 30 April 1990.

Notes

Chapter 1

1. Foucault, "Pierre Boulez: L'écran traversé," 1039.

2. See, e.g., Ashmore, *The Reflexive Thesis.*

3. Rheinberger, *Toward a History of Epistemic Things.*

4. In October 1988, a giant quilt produced by the Names Project AIDS Quilt was displayed on the Mall in Washington, D.C.; see Steven Epstein, *Impure Science,* 225. The Holocaust Museum in Washington also features a "tile-quilt" with drawings by children.

5. For a discussion of drawings by children in relation to cancer, see Williams and Bendelow, "'Recalcitrant Bodies'?"

6. On the voice of the lifeworld/voice of medicine distinction, see Mishler, *The Discourse of Medicine.*

7. Medical sociology is full of denunciations of "medical reductionism" and of a largely mythological construct referred to as "the biomedical model," the two terms being used interchangeably. There is no such thing as *the* biomedical model. For a critique of this "sociology of accusation," see Boltanski, *L'amour et la justice comme compétences.*

8. Cure rates in childhood leukemia have increased dramatically in recent times. This is unfortunately not (yet) the case for many adult leukemias. On the development of childhood leukemia therapies, see Laszlo, *The Cure of Childhood Leukemia.*

9. See Daston, *Biographies of Scientific Objects.*

10. Silverman, *Communication and Medical Practice,* 198. One could also mention, in this respect, Foucault's concluding chapter in *The Birth of the Clinic,* according to which the deployment of the clinical gaze forms an integral part of our individual experience and identity.

11. See, e.g., Tomes, *The Gospel of Germs*; Latour, "Give Me a Laboratory."

12. A disclosure: both of us have manipulated and inspected microbes as part of our initial training as biologists.

13. Porter, "The Enemy Within." This is not to deny that there are empirical grounds for acting so (or that microbes exist!). After all, even without a microscope and a bacteriology kit, one could have experienced, directly or indirectly, a wound infection resulting from a lack of hygienic precautions. But the relevant issue is that these empirically derived precautions are now justified and explained by reference to the invisible world of "microbes."

14. Gajewska, "Sida: la trithérapie entre la vie et la mort," 11 (our translation). While this example is particularly striking, similar examples can be found elsewhere. For instance, as noted on the Website of the Childhood Leukemia Center, citing material from Keene, *Childhood Leukemia*, "keeping track of their child's blood counts becomes a way of life for parents of children with leukemia."

15. On this mode of circulation of biomedical tests, see Crespin and Lascoumes, "Régulation de la carrière d'un instrument de santé."

16. OTA [Office of Technology Assessment], *The CDC's Case Definition of AIDS*; Osmond, "Classification and Staging of HIV Disease." See also Chang, Kate, and Hernandez, "The New AIDS Case Definition;" Ryder and Mugerwa, "The Clinical Definition and Diagnosis of AIDS in African Adults." Recourse to a laboratory definition created problems in Africa because of a lack of available facilities. Furthermore, because of a different spectrum of clinical conditions in Africa, the clinical definition was also problematic.

17. CDC/HIV/AIDS Prevention, *Meeting on the Expansion of the AIDS Surveillance Case Definition.*

18. Steven Epstein, *Impure Science.*

19. Steven Epstein, "Activism, Drug Regulation, and the Politics of Therapeutic Evaluation in the AIDS Era." For criticism of Epstein's analysis of the role of lay activism, see Löwy, "Trustworthy Knowledge and Desperate Patients."

20. See Canguilhem, "Le statut épistémologique de la médecine."

21. Although this and following messages were posted to a public discussion forum, we have decided to keep them anonymous by simply indicating the date the message was posted as well as the institution from which it was sent. In the present case: 3 January 1997—Lenox Hill Hospital, New York City.

22. Discourse analysts may be interested in the textual features of this excerpt which displays some of the linguistic properties of a typical medical case report; see Atkinson, *Medical Talk and Medical Work*; Hunter, *Doctor's Stories.*

23. Figure 1.5 nicely illustrates Atkinson's account of morphological inspection as a linguistically (and, we would add, materially) organized activity that

combines looking, seeing, and describing as collective accomplishments; see Atkinson, *Medical Talk and Medical Work*, esp. chapter 4, 60–89.

24. Follicles are distinctive morphological features of lymph nodes. This is tissue morphology as opposed to cellular morphology.

25. 6 January 1997—City of Hope, Duarte, Calif.

26. 7 January 1997—British Columbia Cancer Agency, Vancouver.

27. 8 January 1997—Maine Medical Center, Portland.

28. 9 January 1997—Laboratory of Pathology, National Cancer Institute, National Institutes of Health (NIH), Bethesda, Md.

29. See chapter 5 for a discussion of the so-called REAL (revised European-American lymphoma) classification of lymphomas.

30. On the notion of triangulation, see Star, "Triangulating Clinical and Basic Research."

31. 8 January 1997—Maine Medical Center, Portland.

32. 13 January 1997—City of Hope, Duarte, Calif.

33. 9 January 1997—Pathology, Mayo Clinic Scottsdale, Ariz.

34. 9 July 1998—Michigan State University, East Lansing.

35. 10 July 1998—Laboratory of Pathology, National Cancer Institute, NIH, Bethesda, Md.

36. 11 July 1998—William Beaumont Hospital, Royal Oak, Mich. It will be noted that our opening example of an electronic message spoke precisely of an "atypical lymphoid infiltrate."

37. Bucher and Strauss, "Professions in Process"; Bucher, "Pathology."

38. Strauss, "A Social World Perspective"; Strauss, "Social Worlds and Their Segmentation Processes."

39. Clarke, "A Social Worlds Research Adventure"; for an extended treatment, see Clarke, *Disciplining Reproduction*; Clarke and Casper, "From Simple Technology to Complex Arena." Fujimura's work, originally embedded in a social world perspective, has progressively integrated insights from different approaches, namely actor-network theory; for an example of early work, see Fujimura, "The Molecular Biological Cancer Research Bandwagon." For an example of more recent work, see Fujimura, "Crafting Science."

40. Conein, Dodier, and Thévenot, *Les objets dans l'action.*

41. For recent work on specialization, see Weisz, "The Emergence of Medical Specialization"; Weisz, "Regulating Medical Specialties in France"; Weisz, "Medical Directories and Medical Specialization."

42. Atkinson, *Medical Talk and Medical Work,* 61.

43. The situation admittedly differs in predictive medicine (e.g., genetic screening) where the body becomes a statistical construct and the individual patient (now a member of a population) is replaced by the extended family; see, e.g., Nukaga and Cambrosio, "Medical Pedigrees and the Visual Production of Family Disease."

44. On the role of medical records, see Berg, "Practices of Reading and Writing."

45. See Hacking, *Representing and Intervening.*

46. Many thanks to Armand Hatchuel (École des Mines, Paris) for taking the time to discuss with one of us (A.C.) the issues raised in the next paragraph; see Hatchuel and Weil, *Experts in Organizations.* For a pioneering study of "task interdependencies" among physicians, i.e., physicians' "interactions across departmental boundaries for sharing knowledge, information, resources and clientele" following advances in medical technologies, see Gosselin, "Probing into Task Interdependencies."

47. We are, of course, not alone in rejecting this dualism. Social constructionism and, more generally, sociological reductionism have recently come under fire from many quarters, for reasons quite different from the early "realist" criticisms (for an example of those "early" debates in the field of medical sociology, see Bury, "Social Constructionism and the Development of Medical Sociology"; Nicolson and McLaughlin, "Social Constructionism and Medical Sociology"; Bury, "Social Constructionism and Medical Sociology.") On this topic, see also Hacking, *The Social Construction of What?* Avoiding the marked tendency of social scientists to engage in "ontological gerrymandering" (Woolgar and Pawluch, "Ontological Gerrymandering"), and drawing on the field of science and technology studies, several scholars have devoted themselves to the task of examining the coproduction of nature *and* society, thus questioning the rigid dichotomy between humans and things. "Actor-network theory" and the "mangle of practice" immediately come to mind; see Latour, *Science in Action*; Pickering, *The Mangle of Practice.* Other proposals include Peter Galison's "trading zone," although in this latter case, and in spite of the detailed attention paid to instruments and techniques, one cannot overlook a resurrection of social world theory; see Galison, *Image and Logic.* Galison's proposal is indebted to the notion of "boundary objects" developed within a symbolic-interactionist framework; see Star and Griesemer, "Institutional Ecology, 'Translations' and Boundary Objects."

48. This remark is based on an exchange with Nicolas Dodier, whom we thank for commenting on an earlier published version of our argument. A "pragmatics of action" leads to the discovery of social regularities, less the result of a priori dispositions than of an accumulation of previous choices in similar situations. For an example of Dodier's approach, see Dodier and Barbot, "Le temps des tensions épistémiques." See also Baszanger and Dodier, "Totalisation et altérité dans l'enquête ethnographique."

49. In an important sense, our argument also confirms the presence of an "endogenous critical inquiry" deployed by scientific and medical actors in the course of their daily activities and leading to the construction of the various "sides" of a debate or controversy (see Lynch, "Technical Work and Critical Inquiry"); we would add, however, that in the biomedical field this kind of "endogenous inquiry" is platform dependent.

Chapter 2

1. This is sometimes referred to as the topic/resource distinction. See Lynch, "The Discursive Production of Uncertainty," 867 n. 88.

2. Lynch, personal communication, 26 November 1997. See also Lynch, *Scientific Practice and Ordinary Action,* 300. In a different tradition, Hatchuel has spoken of "axiomatic notions," i.e., a language that can work simultaneously for an observer as a language of description and for the actors as a language for action; see Hatchuel, "Les axiomatiques de la production."

3. Claude Simon quoting Marcel Proust in Simon, *Le jardin des plantes,* 196.

4. Robert, *Dictionnaire alphabétique et analogique de la langue française,* 390; Centre National de la Recherche Scientifique, *Trésor de la langue française,* 538–9; Rey, *Dictionnaire historique de la langue française,* 1545; *Oxford English Dictionary* (1970), 966–7; *Webster's Third New International Dictionary of the English Language,* 1735; Craigie, *A Dictionary of American English on Historical Principles,* 1764.

5. Example given in Robert, *Dictionnaire alphabétique.*

6. This meaning may have originated from the now obsolete use of the term platform to refer to a topographical plan, chart, or map. This could have led to the emergence of the early figurative sense of a plan, a pattern, or a model.

7. In English, but not in French, one also finds the verb "to platform," the meanings of which range from "to plan or draw up a scheme" to "to speak on a platform."

8. See Bergeron et al., "Comparison of Single versus Double Platform," 255; Tillemans, "The Netherlands AIDS Platforms," 303.

9. For a verbatim transcription of an extremely adversarial meeting on the implications of the changing definition of AIDS, see CDC/HIV/AIDS Prevention, *Meeting on the Expansion of the AIDS Surveillance Case Definition.* This and similar meetings were characterized by the presence and intervention of lay activist groups such as ACT UP. Steven Epstein has chronicled and analyzed the role and activities of these groups; see Steven Epstein, *Impure Science.* One could ask whether and how patient groups have had any input on the development of a given biomedical platform. In the case, for instance, of AIDS, the answer is none, since patient groups worked on the platform, taking CD4 for granted.

10. Steven Epstein, "Activism, Drug Regulation, and the Politics of Therapeutic Evaluation."

11. For a similar argument concerning objectivism and foundationalism in legal practice, see Barbara Herrnstein Smith, *Belief and Resistance*, 1–22.

12. Many thanks to Hank Van Cleef (an electronic engineer with 40 years of experience in the field), for discussing with us via e-mail the historical use of the term platform in the American computer industry.

13. *McGraw-Hill Dictionary of Scientific and Technical Terms*, 1525.

14. Bresnahan and Greenstein, "Technological Competition and the Structure of the Computer Industry," 1. According to these authors, the development of the personal computer market has been characterized by a "fast reduction in the number of platforms available to buyers," a fact accounted for by the "social costs of maintaining a standard bundle." Thanks to Abdel-Kérim Ousman for this reference.

15. Interview with Bernard Henri Kormarever, Immunotech, Marseilles, 24 February 1997.

16. See Yorkton Securities Inc., "Valuation," 32.

17. Orsi, *Droits de propriété intellectuelle et marchés financiers*, 246–8.

18. See, e.g., Schena et al., "Microarrays."

19. Bréchot, "Les enjeux pour l'INSERM."

20. Ciborra, "The Platform Organization"; Gerstein, "From Machine Bureaucracies to Networked Organizations." Thanks to Pascale Bourret for the Ciborra reference.

21. Many thanks to Armand Hatchuel (École Nationale Supérieure des Mines de Paris) for discussing this issue with one of us.

22. Ciborra, "The Platform Organization," 113.

23. Both Ciborra, "The Platform Organization" and Gerstein, "From Machine Bureaucracies" explicitly contrast the notions of platform organization and network organization. A similar contrast can be drawn between platforms and networks as described by actor-network theorists. Instances of this flexible and adaptive behavior without central planning or management can also be found in the world of insects; see Carl Anderson and John J. Bartholdi, "Centralized versus Decentralized Control in Manufacturing."

24. Kuhn, "Second Thoughts on Paradigms."

25. See Deschamps, "Paris: L'Hôpital Saint-Louis."

26. We feel warranted in translating "plateau" as "platform" since not only are these terms also used as synonyms in other expressions (e.g., continental plateau

or platform), but because this is how our French informants tended to translate the term.

27. Maillard, *Histoire de l'hôpital de 1940 à nos jours.*

28. Sournia, *Histoire du diagnostic en médecine,* 173.

29. *Architecture et conception hospitalière.*

30. Duval, "L'Hôpital moderne: 1920–1980."

31. Binet, *Les architectes de la médecine,* 13 and 138.

32. *L'architecture hospitalière au XIXe siècle: L'exemple parisien.* As such, pavilion medicine is now retrospectively presented as the antithesis to the project of a modern "synthetic" medicine, one that would replace isolated specialists with multidisciplinary teams; see Binet, *Les architectes de la médecine,* 132.

33. On the adoption of the so-called pavilion (or Nightingale) plan in France, see *L'architecture hospitalière au XIXe siècle.*

34. Physicians were requested to work full-time in hospitals as officials of the ministries of health and of education, while research teams, previously located in the faculty of medicine, moved to hospital locations, closer to the patients. For a detailed sociological analysis of the 1957 healthcare reform, see Jamous and Peloille, "Professions or Self-Perpetuating Systems? Changes in the French University-Hospital System;" Jamous, *Sociologie de la décision*; see also Picard, "Poussée scientifique ou demande des médecins?" On the Caen hospital, see the twentieth anniversary issue of the hospital's journal *TransVersal* (October–November 1995). On the role of the "Centre de lutte contre le cancer," the network of French institutions devoted to cancer research and treatment, in providing a model for the transformation of French public hospitals, see Ménoret, *Le temps du cancer,* 21–30.

35. French architecture has produced an even more whimsical, iconographic metaphor with the Gonesse Hospital Center (1967–70) which, seen from above, is shaped like a human body; see Verderber and Fine, *Healthcare Architecture in an Era of Radical Transformation,* 48 and 50.

36. Binet, *Les architectes de la médecine,* 130–2.

37. Thanks to Annmarie Adams and David Theodore of McGill University (Montreal) for introducing us to the literature on hospital architecture.

38. Verderber and Fine, *Healthcare Architecture,* 17.

39. On the U.S. situation, see James and Noakes, *Hospital Architecture,* 11–4 and Verderber and Fine, *Healthcare Architecture,* passim.

40. See, e.g., the discussion of the "complex maze of buildings" making up the Massachusetts General Hospital (Boston), in Brandt and Sloane, "Of Beds and Benches." In the early 1970s, a new kind of provider organization, large-scale

investor-owned hospital chains, entered the game (Verderber and Fine, *Healthcare Architecture*, 83).

41. Verderber and Fine, *Healthcare Architecture*, 48.

42. On the "tower-on-podium" form, see James and Noakes, *Hospital Architecture*, 11–4, and Hughes, "The 'Matchbox on a Muffin.'" The term "matchbox on a muffin," according to Goldin and Thompson, *The Hospital: A Social and Architectural History*, should be restricted to square wards on a round podium. The term "brutalist hospitals" is used in Verderber and Fine, *Healthcare Architecture*, 50–2, in reference to the U.K. hospital architecture of the 1960s, a grim "distinct variant of the International Style."

43. Binet, *Les architectes de la médecine*, 124–5. See also Pallez, "Une politique architecturale pour l'Assistance publique," 2–7.

44. Verderber and Fine, *Healthcare Architecture*, 48; Murken, *Vom Armenhospital zum Grossklinikum*, 234–67.

45. Thanks to David Theodore for calling these points to our attention.

46. Foucault et al., *Les machines à guérir.*

47. Prior, "The Architecture of the Hospital;" Prior, "The Local Space of Medical Discourse." For a blander version of this approach, insisting primarily on the symbolic dimension, see Brandt and Sloane, "Of Beds and Benches." For an intriguing look at (domestic) architecture and medical knowledge, see Adams, *Architecture in the Family Way.*

48. Moreover, the debate, as framed by Prior, turns on the question of whether architectural artifacts should be viewed as merely reflecting or embodying developments in medical knowledge, or whether they should be seen as prescribing medical practices. This kind of question rests on a dubious operation that consists in positing the existence of two abstract, discrete entities ("architecture" and "medical knowledge") whose relation (or lack thereof) one can then set out to explore. The alternative consists in examining empirically the long chain of intermediaries into which abstractions such as "architecture," "knowledge," "theory," and "experiment" can be dissolved. See Hacking, "The Self-Vindication of the Laboratory Sciences," as well as Bruno Latour, "The 'Pédofil' of Boa Vista."

49. Verderber and Fine, *Healthcare Architecture*, 63–76.

50. See, e.g., the special issue "Le plateau technique hospitalier." *Technologie et santé* is published by CNEH, a professional, nonprofit association established in 1974 that does consulting, training, information, and communication for public hospitals, clinics, health industrials, governmental bodies, etc. About 280 healthcare centers are members of CNEH, whose team of consultants consists of hospital directors, physicians, pharmacists, biologists, administrators, engineers, lawyers, and economists.

51. Interview with Françoise Valensi, Saint-Louis Hospital, Paris, 18 December 1997.

52. Thévenot, "Les investissements de forme," 63 (our translation). For a shorter English version, see Thévenot, "Rules and Implements."

53. The French *Nomenclature* contains detailed descriptions of each test, and can thus be used as a rough measure of the expansion and diversification of diagnostic tests; this can be contrasted with the tools used in other Medicare systems that use more general categories that are rarely modified (new tests are included under older headings).

54. For a similar preoccupation with juxtaposing architectural and organizational diagrams in German publications, see Murken, *Vom Armenhospital zum Grossklinikum*, 235.

55. Michel, *L'informatique dans les laboratoires centraux d'hématologie.*

56. Madec, "La biologie hospitalière."

57. Cazaubiel, "Une nécessité: le plateau technique de biologie;" Devilder, "Une nouvelle logistique pour les laboratoires hospitaliers."

58. Interview with Jean-Jacques Prat, Hôpital Lariboisière, Paris, 13 March 1997; see also Sournia, "La place actuelle de la biologie dans la pratique médicale et dans les dépenses de santé," 214.

59. Hôpitaux de Toulouse, *Programme général.* Vol. 1. *Institut Fédératif de Biologie. Hôpital Purpan* (Toulouse: unpublished document, 1996). The platform of the new Pompidou hospital (also known as "the hospital of the twenty-first century"), had a planned surface of almost 20,000 m^2, corresponding to more than 35% of the hospital; see the folder entitled *L'Hôpital du XV*[e]. Box D-1493, archives of the "Assistance Publique-Hôpitaux de Paris (AP-HP), Paris. See also Laedlein-Greilsammer, "Place de l'Anatomo-Cyto-Pathologie dans le plateau technique hospitalier."

60. Gouget et al., "La dynamique de la biologie au sein du plateau technique hospitalier." For a discussion of the ways molecular biology is changing medicine, see Rheinberger, "Beyond Nature and Culture."

61. Interview with Renaud Devilder, C.H.U. Nantes, 4 July 1997. On automation as leading to the performance of different activities, see below; see also Keating, Limoges, and Cambrosio, "The Automated Laboratory." Devilder's claim, far from being the expression of an exaggerated faith in the capabilities of the Nantes platform—of which he is the technical director—does correspond to the kinds of questions that key French clinicians have raised following the spread of automation. For instance, two eminent hematologists noted back in 1980 that automated equipment was producing "a perception of the state of health or illness of the patient very different from that which we derived and still derive by our eyes, hands, ears, in association with our memories, emotions, and our

clinical intuition." See Jean Bernard and Marcel Bessis, "The Impact of Automation on the Future of Hematology."

62. Interview with Renaud Devilder, C.H.U. Nantes, 4 July 1997; see also Gouget et al., "La dynamique de la biologie au sein du plateau technique hospitalier."

63. See Sournia, "La place actuelle de la biologie." Similar increases have generated calls for limiting the use of diagnostic technologies, a recurring theme being that they are often used for no medically justifiable purpose; for the United Kingdom, see, e.g., Fowkes, "Containing the Use of Diagnostic Tests."

64. Reiser, *Medicine and the Reign of Technology*, 158–60.

65. Sournia, *Histoire du diagnostic*, 155–200. Sournia's criticism can be put in perspective by noting how it is part of a long French clinical tradition of hostility to scientific innovation; see, e.g., Jamous and Peloille, "Professions or Self-Perpetuating Systems?" esp. 131–2.

66. The French epistemologist Dagognet similarly spoke of the "contamination" of medical semiology by the basic sciences. Arguing that a diagnostic sign only made sense as part of a set of signs and symptoms, he rejected any understanding of diseases as a collection of individual signs and as fully formed, a priori defined entities; clinical investigations should thus follow a strategy of differential diagnosis rather than obey a logic of screening (*dépistage*); see Dagognet, "La nature de la pensée médicale." Of course, Dagognet fought a losing battle, as shown by the present-day development of screening procedures. For a discussion of periodic screening in asymptomatic (note the term "asymptomatic" rather than healthy) adults, a notion backed by major institutional groups, including a "Canadian Task Force on the Periodic Health Examination," and key medical organizations such as the American Cancer Society, the American College of Physicians, and the American Medical Association, see Oboler and LaForce, "The Periodic Physical Examination in Asymptomatic Adults." For a discussion of the pros and cons of mass screening, see Mant and Fowler, "Mass Screening: Theory and Ethics."

67. 11 September 1998—Pathology, Karolinska Hospital, Stockholm.

68. 11 September 1998—Pathology, National Cancer Institute, NIH.

69. 15 September 1998—Pathology, Karolinska Hospital, Stockholm.

70. 16 September 1998—Mount Sinai School of Medicine, New York City.

71. 17 September 1998—FDA/NIH.

72. Interview with Renaud Devilder, C.H.U. Nantes, 4 July 1997.

73. Roussel, *Une nouvelle fonction à l'étude*; Hagenmuller, "Projet du plateau technique et enjeux de la gestion des ressources humaines."

74. Centre de recherche bioclinique de Grenoble. Dossier de présentation (Université scientifique technologique et médicale de Grenoble, Faculté de

Médecine de Grenoble, La Tronche, 20 March 1987). Institut Albert Bonniot. Schéma Directeur. Équipes Fondatrices (Université Joseph Fourier Grenoble I, 15 May 1992). Institut Albert Bonniot, Université Joseph Fourier, Grenoble I. Présentation générale (10 January 1994). Thanks to Gérard Brugal for supplying us with various IAB documents as well as with a collection of press clippings.

75. According to the architects, the IAB design was meant to simultaneously convey the sense of an entry pavilion to the hospital, of a monastery-like research site built around a cloister, and of modern technology, thanks to the building materials.

76. Gouget et al., "La dynamique de la biologie." See the figure on p. 456 showing that the specialization of bioclinical interfaces increases gradually when one leaves the zone of routine activities.

77. We generated a sample of forty-five articles explicitly devoted to "translational research" that appeared between 1993 and 1999 using MEDLINE and subsequently added references found in the initial batch of articles. More than 70% of the articles in the sample originated from the United States, and a majority of these articles came from major medical centers in Houston, Bethesda, Boston, New York, and Gainesville, Fla. Over two thirds of the articles are related to cancer, a field where the notion seems to have been developed before spreading to other biomedical domains. Among the agencies funding "translational research," the National Cancer Institute has played a major role. Many thanks to our research assistant Jean-François Auger (CIRST-UQAM) who collected this information.

78. "Physician-Scientists Receive $7.5 Million in Awards," 1.

79. This is clearly the case, e.g., in an article by Smit, "'Translational Research,' the 'Linker Laboratory' or a Paradigm Shift in Cancer Care?," 388, according to which, "to get these new ideas [molecular research] and methods from the research laboratory to the patient, on a clinically useful scale, will require the mediation of the basic laboratory specialist medical scientist. Hence research findings > laboratory preparation > physician > patient."

80. Coleman and Harris, "Current Scientific Issues Related to Clinical Radiation Oncology," 132. See also Friedman, Bigner, and Bigner "Cyclophosphamide Therapy of Medulloblastoma: From the Laboratory to the Clinic and Back Again (and Again and Again);" Bowler, "Review: Translational Research: Bench to Bedside and Back Again."

81. Pollak, "Peptide Growth Factors and Breast Cancer Treatment,"43.

82. Chabner, Boral, and Multani, "Translational Research: Walking the Bridge between Idea and Cure," 4211.

Chapter 3

1. See Thomson, *Half a Century of Medical Research*, vol. 2. Funding for medical research in the form of grants in aid (as opposed to public health projects) rose 46 times, from £500,000 to £23 million in the period 1946–71. Thomson, *Half a Century of Medical Research*, vol. 1, 197.

2. Geiger, "Science and the University." The National Institute (singular) of Health preceded the NIH; see Harden, *Inventing the NIH*. For an overview of American medical research before World War II, see Shryock, *American Medical Research*.

3. Rothstein, *American Medical Schools and the Practice of Medicine*, 238. Between 1970 and 1984, funding rose to over $6 billion a year (ibid., 238). The budget proposed by President George W. Bush would give the NIH $23.1 billion for the budget year 2002. See Toner, "Who Gets What Slice of the President's First Federal Budget Pie."

4. For an overview of the history of clinical research, see Booth, "Clinical Research"; Lawrence, "Clinical Research."

5. Rothstein, *American Medical Schools*, 251.

6. On the Hippocratic authors, see, e.g., Jouanna, *Hippocrate*; Joly, *Hippocrate médecin grec*; on Sydenham, see, e.g., Dewhurst, *Dr. Thomas Sydenham*; Duchesneau, "La philosophie médicale de Sydenham"; Cook, "The New Philosophy and Medicine in Seventeenth-Century England"; Cain, "Thomas Sydenham, John Ray, and Some Contemporaries on Species."

7. See Cunningham and Williams, *The Laboratory Revolution in Medicine*.

8. See, e.g., Ackerknecht, *Rudolf Virchow*.

9. According to linguists, the adjectival form of a word generally follows the emergence of the substantive. Because of the prior existence of both "medicine" and "biology," this is probably not the case for "biomedicine." It is, nonetheless, worth noting that in some languages, the term "biomedical" has had a career independent of the substantive "biomedicine." French dictionaries, such as the *Larousse*, have the adjective but not the noun. Moreover, in the 1960s the neologism "bio-medical" (with the hyphen) existed in English independent of the noun. One of the earliest journals to use "biomedical" in its title was the British journal *Bio-medical Engineering* which first appeared in 1965. The journal intended to review "engineering techniques applied to Medicine. In other words, everything involved in analysis, measurement, computing and control applied to diagnosis and therapy" ("Bridging the Gap," 3). The first (French-British) journal bearing the title *Biomedicine* appeared in 1973 as a continuation of the *European Journal of Clinical and Biological Research*.

10. "Colloque politique scientifique et recherche médicale," CIOMS, UNESCO, 26–9 February 1968 (archives DGRST). Thanks to Jean-François Picard for this

document. See also Picard, "De la médecine expérimentale (1865) à l'INSERM (1964)," 342.

11. Dill, "Strengthening Biomedicine's Roots."

12. Schechter, "Medicine and Biology Are More Than Biomedicine," 424.

13. *Ibid.* Schecter's view of the centrality of clinical research at the NIH and how clinical research has recently been marginalized can be found in Schechter, "The Crisis in Clinical Research."

14. Feinstein, "The Crisis in Clinical Research."

15. Guralnik, *Webster's New World Dictionary*, 142.

16. See, e.g., Gordon, "Tenacious Assumptions in Western Medicine."

17. Barnhart, Steinmetz, and Barnhart, *The Barnhart Dictionary of New English Since 1963*, 62. The citation is to *Science News*, (10 January 1970), 37.

18. Rey, *Dictionnaire historique de la langue française*, 1212 (biomédecine) and 1214 (biomédical); Gilbert, *Dictionnaire des mots nouveaux*, 59.

19. *Merriam-Webster's Collegiate Dictionary*, 115. The dating is based on a short passage in Fosdick, *The Rockefeller Foundation. A Review for 1947*, 17, where the word appears only in passing in a short reference to Soviet "biomedicine" (Joanne M. Despres, Etymology Editor, Merriam Webster, personal communications, 4 October 1999 and 12 April 2000). According to Ahrens, *The Crisis in Clinical Research*, 34, "another 1947 occurrence, this time of the adjectival form 'biomedical,' is to be found in a foreword written by Arno B. Luckhard to a book on the evolution of scientific English by Edmund Andrews in 1947 (but the word itself did not appear in the text of the book)."

20. Flexner, *Random House Unabridged Dictionary*, 210.

21. Proffitt, *Oxford English Dictionary Additions Series*, 72. The citation is to Dorland, *The American Illustrated Medical Dictionary*, 172. The fact that, in spite of the 1923 dating, the term "biomedicine" did not figure in the revised 1989 second edition of *The Oxford English Dictionary*, but only in the 1997 volume of the *Additions Series*, is in itself quite revealing: absence sometimes tells as much as presence.

22. *The Oxford English Dictionary*, 2nd ed., 206. Flexner, *Random House Unabridged Dictionary*, 209. Kohler, "The Enzyme Theory and the Origins of Biochemistry."

23. Goodhart, "The Passing of Morbid Anatomy," 1130; cited in Reiser, *Medicine and the Reign of Technology*, 218.

24. "Biophysics," according to the *OED*, was coined in 1892 by Karl Pearson. The other neologisms were coined by researchers such as Detlev Bronk, who worked at the University of Pennsylvania before becoming president of Johns Hopkins and subsequently of Rockefeller University in the postwar period, and who is

credited for his contribution to the establishment of biophysics. Thanks to Harry Marks for sharing this information with us.

25. Franklin C. McLean, "A University Department of Psychiatry" (1931), cited in Kroker, *From Reflex to Rhythm,* 187 n. 8. On McLean's claim that medicine should be recognized as a biological science, and, more in general, on the University of Chicago's distinctive biological approach to medicine, see Blustein, "Medicine as Biology," and Urist, "Phoenix of Physiology and Medicine."

26. "Partie de la médecine qui étudie les médications propres à conserver la vie, les fonctions vitales." *Robert Électronique* (1994); our translation.

27. Dorland, *The American Illustrated Medical Dictionary,* 172; Flexner, *Random House Unabridged Dictionary,* 209; *Webster's* (Web version, 10th ed.).

28. Proffitt, *Oxford English Dictionary Additions Series,* vol. 3, 72.

29. Flexner, *Random House,* 209. *Random House* lists both meanings. Barnhart, Steinmetz, and Barnhart, *Barnhart Dictionary,* 62; Stedman, *Medical Dictionary.* The *Robert Électronique* definition quoted above can also be brought back to this second meaning.

30. Hewlitt and Duncan, *A History of the United States Atomic Energy Commission,* chapter 8. On medical work during the Manhattan Project and subsequent plans to establish health physics, biophysics, and nuclear medicine, see Lenoir and Hays, "The Manhattan Project for Biomedicine."

31. Although the group was alternatively known as the "Biological and Medical Research Group," the first annual report (1949) of the Health Division used the term "Biomedical Research Group" and would routinely do so in subsequent reports (Los Alamos Scientific Laboratory, *Health Division Annual Report 1949*). Initial reports of the Biomedical Research Group were included in the *Health Division Annual Report.* The title of the 1959 as well as subsequent reports used the name "Biological and Medical Research Group," but in the text one also finds the term "Biomedical Research Group." A first semiannual report was issued by the Biological and Medical Research Group in 1959: see Los Alamos Scientific Laboratory, *Biological and Medical Research Group (H-4) of the Health Division—Semiannual Report July through December 1959.* Ahrens, *The Crisis in Clinical Research,* also stresses the link between the term biomedical and atomic bomb testing, although he focuses on the Pacific instead of Los Alamos. According to him (p. 34, his emphasis), the term biomedical "seems to have come into common usage after World War II in connection with atomic bomb testing in the Pacific, where biologists and physicians were deeply engaged in studies on the biological effects of radiation on experimental animals. The earliest *official* use of the term appears to have been the 1949 designation of George LeRoy as director of the Biomedical Division of Operation Greenhouse, the atomic bomb testing program in the Marshall Islands in 1951. 'Biomedical' does *not* appear in the records of early military and civilian groups engaged in radiation research: Operation Crossroads, The Joint Commission for Investigation of Effects of the Atomic Bomb in Japan, or the Manhattan Project."

32. Lenoir and Hays, "The Manhattan Project for Biomedicine." Already in the 1949 report of the Health Division one learns that "Nowhere else in the world has a mouse ever been placed *inside* a concentrated critical assembly!" and that therefore "Los Alamos can and should become a national and a world center of biomedical research." See Los Alamos Scientific Laboratory, *Health Division Annual Report 1949*, 7.

33. Systematic examination of the American powdered milk supply began in 1956 and measurements in cyclotron workers and hamburgers followed two years later. See, e.g., Van Dilla and Anderson, "Personnel Monitoring with Large Liquid Scintillation Counters."

34. Los Alamos Scientific Laboratory, *Annual Report of the Biomedical and Environmental Research Program of the LASL Health Division. January through December 1973*, vii. Pp. xvii–xix of this report contain a short history of the biomedical research program.

35. Many thanks to Harry Marks for first calling our attention to the NASA connection. On biomedicine at NASA, see Pitts, *The Human Factor*; see also Engel and Lott, *Man in Flight*. The history of biological and medical research at NASA involved many administrative reorganizations following debates and controversies on such topics as the subordination of life sciences to engineering, lack of independent links to academic scientists, research corporations and industries, the lack of real basic research, and so on. Pitts's contribution contains a detailed analysis of all these controversies up to 1980.

36. Pitts, *The Human Factor*, 4.

37. Hugh L. Dryden to Roy W. Johnson, 17 November 1958, NASA Archives. We thank Mark Kahn and Roger Launius at the NASA history office for having uncovered this early use of the word for us.

38. Pitts, *The Human Factor*, 16–17.

39. Ibid., 25.

40. Reiser, *Medicine and the Reign of Technology*, 200.

41. Pitts, *The Human Factor*, 179.

42. Work on this topic was well under way at Stanford in the 1960s: see, e.g., Levinthal, Hundley, and Lederberg, "Multivator. A Biochemical Laboratory for Martian Experiments."

43. Wooldridge, *Biomedical Science and Its Administration.*

44. The manuscript of the proceedings is to be found in the Archives du Ministère de la Recherche, AN 77/321–323 liasse [file] 748. Thanks to Jean-François Picard for sharing these documents with us.

45. Ahrens, *The Crisis*, 34.

46. Thomas, *Aspects of Biomedical Science Policy*; thanks to Rainer Hohlfeld and Karl Peter Ohly for calling this text to our attention. On Thomas, see his autobiographical sketch, *The Youngest Science*.

47. "*L'automatisme en hématologie*"; "Automation: What to Measure and Why."

48. Jean Bernard, "Summing Up."

49. Howell, *Technology in the Hospital*.

50. Lorraine Daston has conclusively shown that the notion of objectivity must be historicized, insofar as different meanings have been assigned to this term: for instance, objectivity has been defined by the presence and judgment of expert subjects or, alternatively, by their replacement by automatic recording devices. See, e.g., Daston and Galison, "The Image of Objectivity," 84.

51. At least Georges Friedmann's work in the 1940s and Harry Braverman's very popular study in the 1970s. Braverman, *Labor and Monopoly Capital*.

52. Barley, "Technology, Power, and the Social Organization of Work," 53.

53. Collins, *Artificial Experts*.

54. Ibid., 9. Harry Collins and Hubert Dreyfus have presented opposing views as to the possibilities for the computerization or automation of a given area of human activity. In order for automation to happen, the activity to be automated must first be routinized to the extent that automation is at least remotely conceivable. At this point, however, Collins and Dreyfus part company. Whereas Collins believes that a form of life involving machine-like behavior can ultimately invade any activity, Dreyfus believes that this possibility is not equally present in human activities; it depends upon the kind of activity. Some activities, simple as they may appear, simply defy description in the sense that they cannot be described in terms of the rules or mechanical procedures that would be a necessary condition for their automation. We side with Collins in this instance. We do automate certain activities even in the absence of a complete reduction of the activity to a series of rules that would make the mechanical replication of the activity possible. A reasonable facsimile is often acceptable. Dreyfus, "Response to Collins' *Artificial Experts*"; Collins, "Hubert L. Dreyfus, Forms of Life, and a Simple Test for Machine Intelligence."

55. Collins, *Artificial Experts*, 216.

56. Collins's more recent work with Martin Kusch abandons this problem altogether. In the course of developing a theoretical description of human action, Collins and Kusch admit that they have nothing to say about the role of tools and innovation in the division of labor. See Collins and Kusch, *The Shape of Actions*, 125.

57. Banda-Gamboa et al., "Automation in Cervical Cytology," 41.

58. The history of the Pap smear has recently attracted the attention of several authors. Our purpose here is not to provide an alternative account of that

complex process, but to focus on a single element: automation and its relation to the normal/pathological dichotomy. See Casper and Clarke, "Making the Pap Smear into the 'Right Tool' for the Job"; Clarke and Casper, "From Simple Technology to Complex Arena"; Singleton and Michael, "Actor-Networks and Ambivalence"; Kaufert, "Screening the Body"; Vayena, *Cancer Detectors.*

59. On the program, see Herman and Bunnag, "Goals of the Cytology Automation Program of the National Cancer Institute."

60. Recent work on the influence of large science-based funding institutions and cancer research policy (Rushefsky, *Making Cancer Policy*) on biomedical research has described a number of "crusades" (Rettig, *Cancer Crusade*; Panem, *The Interferon Crusade*), "bandwagons" (Fujimura, *Crafting Science*), "missions" (Studer and Chubin, *The Cancer Mission*), and "wars" (Proctor, *Cancer Wars*). Here, political factors have been privileged over the content of the changes described.

61. "Committee on Cytology Automation," *Annual Report*, 15 August 1981, Federal Records Center, Washington, D.C., RG-443-97-0019, 3–4.

62. Cytology Automation Contract Program: Annual Report Summary, 1 July 1973 to 30 June 1974. *NCI Annual Report*, 1974, Vol. 2, S-1.

63. The Cancer Biology Branch of the National Cancer Institute was reorganized in 1978. Renamed Cancer Biology and Diagnosis, it consisted of the two divisions indicated in the title. The first contained five sections: Basic Cancer Biology, Tumor Biology, Clinical Immunology, Cellular Immunology, and Molecular Immunology. The second contained three sections: General Diagnosis, Diagnostic Radiology, and Cytology Automation ("Minutes of the Committee on Cytology Automation," (29 June 1978), 2).

64. It should be noted that even though the Cytology Automation Program was shut down in 1980, funding for a number of these grants, notably Mullaney (in 1980–81, but who appears to have dropped out in 1982) and Mayall (funds granted for 1980–82), continued under the new Cancer Diagnosis Research Program. At the final meeting of the Cytology Automation Committee, the longtime chairman of the committee, Chester Herman, claimed that the closure boiled down to a mere question of macroeconomics: the political commitment to national screening programs had evaporated with the advent of the economic downturn (U.S. Department of Health and Human Services, *Committee on Cytology Automation: Annual Report*, 15 August 1981, 3).

65. Kendall Preston and John A. Zecca, "Research Conference Proposal." New York: *Archives of the Engineering Foundation* (1971), 2.

66. When the Bethesda system supplanted the Papanicolaou classification in 1988, among the four reasons cited for abandoning the classification was: "2. The Papanicolaou classes have no equivalent in diagnostic histopathologic terminology." The point, of course, is that while it never did have an equivalent, there was always hope that it would (Schneider, "The Bethesda System: The European Perspective," 114).

67. Grunze and Spriggs, *History of Clinical Cytology*, 89–90.

68. See Casper and Clarke, "Making the Pap Smear," 261–2.

69. Koss, "The Papanicolaou Test for Cervical Cancer Detection," 737. Note that the test continues to be controversial for a number of reasons. According to Koss, "The efficiency of the cervical smear has never been tested in a prospective blinded study" (ibid.; 737). This is not a comment on the biological validity of the test. The key word is "efficiency" whose meaning is dependent upon the variable "compared to what?"

70. Quoted in Ross, *Crusade*, 87.

71. Memorandum to director, NCI, 7 July 1958.

72. Erickson et al., "Preliminary Report of 20,000 Women Studied by the Vaginal Smear Technic in a General Population Cancer Screening Project"; John E, Dunn, "The Use of Vaginal Cytology for Uterine Cancer Case-Finding in Memphis and Shelby County, Tennessee," *NCI Archives*, AR-5407-001780.

73. By 1958, in the course of these research projects, over 300,000 of a projected 1.3 million slides had been examined. In 1961, 30 out of every 100 women reported having had at least one Pap test. By 1966, this number had risen to 67 out of every 100 (or at least 43 million tests). This latter number was based on a survey of women. A survey of pathologists (all the members of the College of American Pathologists) carried out by the Cancer Control Program the same year estimated the number of women tested at 15.7 million. In any event, millions of tests were being done which meant that thousands of cytotechnicians had to be trained. As of 1971, there were 110 approved schools of cytotechnology. See "Memorandum" by Carl Baker, Director of the National Cancer Institute for the Assistant Secretary for Health and Scientific Affairs, 9 July 1971 (NCI Archives). In 1966, the American Cancer Society published a pamphlet advertising for trainees for cytotechnology. The cytotechnology course for a person with two years of college was twelve months. The career was deemed particularly suitable for "wives and mothers" because of its part-time nature. People with "impaired hearing" were also considered particularly apt. See Cameron, *Cytology—Best Early Detector of Cancer*, 17.

74. Dr. John Roderick Heller, "Evaluation of the Validity of Uterine Cytology." Speech to the International Cancer Cytology Congress, Chicago, 8 October 1956; *NCI Archives*, AR-5610-003862.

75. See Commission on Chronic Illness. *Chronic Illness in the United States.* More generally, see Wilson and Jungner, *Principles and Practice of Screening for Disease.*

76. Press Release, National Cancer Institute, 20 January 1955, National Cancer Institute Archives: AR-5501-003191.

77. Medical and Biological Physics, Company Brochure c. 1963; courtesy of M. Mendelsohn.

78. Tolles and Bostrom, "Automatic Screening of Cytologic Smears for Cancer: Instrumentation."

79. Tolles, "The Cytoanalyzer," 251.

80. Ibid., 191.

81. This capacity, however, was based on a failure rate of 10% (10% of the smears classified as normal were not). (NCI, Annual Report, 1960, vol. 1, 109); Courtney et al., "Field Trial of the Cytoanalyzer; 1,184 Specimens Analyzed." The machine was also tested on sputum samples taken from uranium miners in Colorado, but in this instance there were no final results as the entire uranium miner sputum study was transferred to the Bureau of State Services (ibid., 110).

82. Sort of. In 1962–63, Sandritter and his colleagues in Germany developed a hand-operated cytophotometer explicitly modeled on the cytoanalyzer. Following a field trial with approximately 9% false positives, they recommended that "an automatic prescreening with a cytophotometer is advisable." Sandritter, Lobel, and Kiefer, "Photometric Cytodiagnosis of Vaginal Smears," 1221.

83. Koss, "Analytical and Quantitative Cytology," 254.

84. Nadel, "Computer Analysis of Cytophotometric Fields by CYDAC and Its Historical Evolution from the Cytoanalyzer," 203.

85. Kenneth M. Endicott to Deputy Surgeon General, U.S. Public Health Service, through director, NIH and director, NCI. 19 September 1961 (NCI Archives, unprocessed).

86. Ibid.

87. The work was done at the Airborne Instruments laboratory at Deer Park Long Island, New York.

88. For a description of the apparatus, see Bostrom and Holcomb, "CYDAC: A Digital Scanning Cytophotometer." On the connections between the cytoanalyzer and CYDAC, see Nadel, "Computer Analysis."

89. After initial development, NCI handed CYDAC over to researchers at the Department of Radiology of the University of Pennsylvania headed by Mortimer Mendelsohn. The problem was: what was it good for? Mendelsohn's career was almost immediately taken over by the apparatus, its management, and the search for some clinical activity it could automate: "All of a sudden I had engineers, physicists, I had a mathematician, and programmers and biologists all working for me in the radiology department. Big operation. But well funded and we did well with it" (interview with Mortimer Mendelsohn, Livermore, Calif., 6 September 1997). Indeed, within a year, the group had published the first computer-generated images of leukocytes (Mendelsohn, Kolman, and Bostrum, "Initial Approaches to the Computer Analysis of Cytophotometric Fields"). Although the automation of the Pap smear receded into the background, the more general objective of clinical automation remained prominent. Given his

background in DNA microscopy, Mendelsohn turned to the digital analysis of chromosomes. By early 1965, Mendelsohn's group was able to generate images of chromosomes, thus opening the realm of karyotyping, the display and analysis of the 46 human chromosomes, to possible automation (Mendelsohn et al., "Morphological Analysis of Cells and Chromosomes by Digital Computer," and Mendelsohn et al., "Computer-Oriented Analysis of Human Chromosomes I. Photometric Estimation of DNA Content." They were neither the first nor alone in that field; in 1969, Mendelsohn estimated his competition at "at least seven other groups" (Mendelsohn, Mayall, and Prewitt, "Approaches to the Automation of Chromosome Analysis," 123). By 1974, there were, again according to Mendelsohn's estimation, about 17 laboratories involved in the field (Mendelsohn and Mayall, "Chromosome Identification by Image Analysis and Quantitative Cytochemistry," 317). But by then, the good times were over. For all intents and purposes, the field had been rendered obsolete through the development of chromosome banding by Caspersson. Rather than working on DNA content (as in the automation strategy) or on size and shape (as traditional cytogeneticists did), Caspersson had worked on stains, fluorescent (biological) stains to be more precise. This had allowed the chromosomes to sort themselves, so to speak, through distinctive banding patterns specific to each chromosome. The effect on human cytogenetics was almost immediate. Within a year of publication, Caspersson's banding method became standard among cytogeneticists. Reviewing the automation scene in 1975 during a conference that brought all the different karyotype automation laboratories together in California, Mendelsohn commented: "This discovery made many automated systems obsolete overnight, opened an enormous new frontier to every practicing cytogeneticist, and obliterated any dependency of the cytogeneticist on comprehensive machines for diagnostic precision" (Mendelsohn, "Introduction," 2).

90. The hospital was, by the way, equipped with a cytoanalyzer that was not working interview with Myron Melamed, Valhalla, NY, 17 June 1997.

91. Their first article together was Kamentsky, Derman, and Melamed, " Ultraviolet Absorption in Epidermoid Cancer Cells." The following year, they published their first flow cytometry paper: Kamentsky, Melamed, and Derman, "Spectrophotometer: New Instrument for Ultrarapid Cell Analysis."

92. Kamentsky, Derman, and Melamed, "Ultraviolet Absorption." Citing this paper in 1969, Melamed and Kamentsky summarized its conclusions as follows: "It has been shown that at least some of the cancer cells from epidermoid carcinomas of the human uterine cervix are relatively rich in nucleic acids" (Melamed and Kamentsky, "An Assessment of the Potential Role of Automatic Devices in Cytology Screening," 921).

93. Louis A. Kamentsky, *Devices and Applications*, Report submitted to IBM Watson Laboratory, February 1967, 3 (personal archives of Louis A. Kamentsky).

94. See Wied, "History of Clinical Cytology and Outlook for the Future," 2. Direct government funding for the schools ended in the 1970s at which point the number of schools fell to forty.

95. Wied, "Automated Cell Screening," 43.

96. Ibid., 45.

97. Kamentsky and Melamed, "Instrumentation for Automated Examinations of Cellular Specimens." The editorial board of the journal had decided that a special issue on technology and health services was in order. They formed an editorial committee to invite papers on the topic. The topic, they admitted, overlapped with other institute journals (namely the *IEEE Transactions on Biomedical Engineering* and the *IEEE Transactions on Computers*) that also published papers "relevant to automated health services" ("Scanning the Issue," 1799). Note that the byword is automation; the relationship between medicine and technology is seen as one in which medical work is somehow independent of technology and can be speeded up and made more accessible through automation. Specifically, we are told that "Technology can . . . give more people access to health care." In general, "Devices, equipment, and systems for improved medical testing, diagnosis, treatment, communications, and transportation are needed." The transformation envisioned is thus quantitative as opposed to qualitative; medical judgment remains the same. Speed, accuracy, and the volume of service are to be amplified through electronics.

98. Ibid., 2007.

99. Kamentsky, "Photoelectric Particle Separator Using Time Delay," 1.

100. For a description and review, see Banda-Gamboa et al., "Automation in Cervical Cytology."

101. Concerted Action Automated Analytical Cytometry (CAAC), *Final Report* 1983–87, European Community, 18.

102. Ibid., 26.

103. Ibid., 34.

104. See, e.g., Tucker and Stenkvist, "Whatever Happened to Cervical Cytology Automation?"

105. Although this de facto standard was announced in 1986, it had been promoted and tacitly accepted by cytopathologists for a number of years. For the 1986 announcement, see International Academy of Cytology, "Specifications for Automated Cytodiagnostic Systems Proposed by the International Academy of Cytology," 146.

106. See Bogdanich, "Lax Laboratories," and "False Negative." Bogdanich received a Pulitzer Prize for this series of reports. Further fallout from these articles can be found in Grady, "Going Overboard on Medical Tests."

107. Linder, "Automation in Cytopathology."

108. Grohs, "Impact of Automated Technology on the Cervical Cytologic Smear."

109. Baffert et al., "Évaluation médicale et économique d'un système d'analyse des frottis cervico-utérines (FCU) assistée par ordinateur."

110. Cioran, *Syllogismes de l'amertume*, 52.

111. Claude Bernard, *Introduction à l'étude de la médecine expérimentale*, 34–5.

112. It should be noted that Bernard was not utterly dogmatic in this respect insofar as he recognized that a biological explanation remained the ideal explanation. The following proviso places clinical observation (the "disease") at the center of experimental procedure: "Given the present state of biology, however, nobody can claim to have completely explained pathology by physiology; this is the direction to be taken because it is the way of science; nonetheless, it is illusory to believe that the problem has been solved. Consequently, it is at present both reasonable and prudent to explain what we can of disease through physiology, leaving what cannot be explained for the future progress of biology" (ibid., 280) (our translation).

113. Canguilhem, *The Normal and the Pathological*, 26.

114 The idea here is fairly obvious to students of natural selection. If a trait or characteristic has a negative selective value, then it will, by definition, be eliminated in the course of evolution.

115. This is sometimes interpreted to mean that Canguilhem is asserting the "primacy of the patient." Stuart Spicker seems to believe that one of the consequences of Canguilhem's work should be to "stress the uniqueness of each patient (organism) and the implications of this thesis in producing and prescribing complex, yet individualized, drug regimens" (Spicker, "An Introduction to the Medical Epistemology of Georges Canguilhem," 407).

116. Canguilhem, *The Normal and the Pathological*, 151. It is sometimes suggested that Canguilhem ends up in a kind of relativism. But a relativity about norms does not necessarily imply a relativity about disease, just as a relativity in the division between the normal and the pathological does not entail cultural determination. Nevertheless, this is one of the readings offered. Dagognet, for example, begins a commentary on Canguilhem by pointing out that it is difficult to "evaluate" a scar (Dagognet, "Le normal et le pathologique: Prolégomènes"). Whether and to what extent a scar is unwanted depends on a number of factors, including where it is and whether or not it was the product of ritual scarification and therefore wanted (at least initially). Dagognet goes on to tell us that pathology is not objective because what is taken as illness depends on the context. Both examples that he offers come from the field of mental diseases. An easy target. It would seem to us that death by smallpox would stand out in any cultural context one could imagine as definitely unwanted.

117. The classic history of the natural history approach in clinical medicine is Faber, *Nosography in Modern International Medicine.* See also Temkin, "The Scientific Approach to Disease," and Hannaway and La Berge, *Constructing Paris Medicine.*

118. This does not mean that once recognized as a tumor, parts of the morbid structure cannot be described using the vocabulary of the normal. Here is Müller himself on the differences and similarities between normal and morbid appearances in the case of normal and pathological cartilage. "For particulars on the growth of normal cartilage, I must refer the reader to Schwann's studies. Pathological cartilage formation differs from the normal mainly in that embryonic cell formation persists. In many other tumors there is opportunity to make the same observation. It is not the form of the elementary constituents that is distinctive in morbid structures. The defect lies partly in the formation of ordinary primitive structures where they do not fit in with the purpose of the whole, partly also in incomplete tissue development, which often advances no further than to a stage that is transient under normal conditions, This is characteristic of morbid growth" (Müller, *On the Finer Structure and the Forms of Morbid Tumors,* 116).

119. On the clinical origins of tissue pathology, see Keel, *La généalogie de l'histopathologie, une révision déchirante,* and Keel, "La pathologie tissulaire de John Hunter."

120. Rather, "Johannes Müller, Theodor Schwann," 27.

121. Virchow, *Cellular Pathology,* 89.

122. As in "many attempts had indeed been made even before this to refer the apparently so irregular forms of new formations to physiological paradigms, and herein essential service has been rendered by natural philosophers" (ibid.; 89–90).

123. Rudolf Virchow, "Cellular Pathology". In Virchow, *Disease, Life, and Man.*

124. Rather, "The Place of Virchow in Medical Thought," xv. Virchow's 'transformations' remain difficult to pin down. "In theory, transformation is defined as a stable, heritable alteration in the growth control of cells in culture. In practice . . . no set of characteristics invariably distinguishes transformed cells from their normal counterparts" (Escobar, "Oncogenic Viruses").

125. Rather, "The Place of Virchow," xv.

126. Ibid., xxi. As Benaroyo ("La renaissance de la pensée biologique de Rudolf Virchow dans l'oeuvre de Ludwig Aschoff") has recently shown, Aschoff attempted to resuscitate Virchow's biology in the form of Kantian teleology. Again, a philosophical project, not a biomedical practice. See also Bonah, "Pathological Anatomy versus Pathological Physiology."

127. Rössle, "Eröffnungsansprache," 1. Quoted in Kajita, "Rudolf Virchow and His Successors," 170.

128. Kajita, "Rudolf Virchow," 170.

129. Lenoir, "Science for the Clinic," 149. Lenoir, by the way, uses the term biomedicine anachronistically throughout the paper to describe various forms of

'physiological medicine' in nineteenth-century Germany. For a similar example of "physiological medicine," see Tuchman's description of Jakob Henle's theory of the 'deviation' of types as the production of disease (Tuchman, "From the Lecture to the Laboratory").

130. A classic example is the Reed-Sternberg cell described at the turn of the century by pathologists as distinctive of Hodgkin's disease. The biological origin of this cell has yet to be found. See, e.g., Pinkus et al., "Fascin, A Sensitive New Marker for Reed-Sternberg Cells of Hodgkin's Disease."

131. Much of the prewar interaction between basic science and the clinical consisted in attempts to apply physics and chemistry to medical problems. See, e.g., Amsterdamska's recent study of Donald Van Slyke: "Chemistry in the Clinic."

132. See, e.g., Amsterdamska, "Stabilizing Instability." In this respect, Clifford Albright and his clinical endocrinology can serve as an example of an intermediary figure, halfway between the projections of a Virchow or a Wunderlich and the present-day situation. On Albright, see Sinding, "Basic Science and Clinical Research," and Sinding, *Le clinicien et le chercheur.* Similarly, as Delaporte and Pinell point out in their study of muscular dystrophy and associated disorders: "Curiously, the first theoretical rearrangement of what until then had constituted the homogeneous domain of the paralyses was not the result of the integration of normal and pathological neurology but of the early efforts to define a pathology of muscle action" (Delaporte and Pinell, *Histoire des myopathies,* 46).

133. Cole, "Hospital and Laboratory," 549–50.

134. He said: "In the department of medicine, the student should never forget that he is studying disease. . . . Otherwise he would probably be better working in the laboratory of physics or chemistry or physiology" (ibid., 550).

135. Thomas, *The Youngest Science,* 120. See Petersdorf, "The Evolution of Departments of Medicine."

136. Wooldridge Report, 1965, quoted in Rothstein, *American Medical Schools,* 240.

137. See Picard, "De la médecine expérimentale," and Gaudillière, "Les biochimistes français entre légitimité médicale et légitimité biologique."

138. Gaudillière, "Biochimistes et biomédecine dans l'après-guerre," 109 (our translation); see also Gaudillière, *Inventer la biomédecine.*

139. The question was raised, e.g., with respect to molecular biology in the 1970s. Since the discovery of the structure of DNA in the early 1950s, there had been little direct medical application of molecular biology. For a defense at the time, see Perutz, "Fundamental Research in Molecular Biology."

140. Wooldridge Report, quoted in Rothstein, *American Medical Schools,* 244.

141. Readers can learn much more in the journals devoted to these issues in France. See *Revue française des laboratoires, Annales de biologie clinique,* and *Le*

biopathologiste. The last is the official organ of the French Union of Medical Biologists which includes mainly medical biologists working in private medical biology laboratories.

142. Lesec, "Exercice en anatomocytopathologie dans le cadre de la loi sur la biologie de 1975."

143. Ibid.

144. Guy Lesec, vice president of the French Anatomocytopathology Union, to Jean-Paul Donzel, president of the French Anatomocytopathology Union, 21 November 1994. Reproduced in *Bulletin d'information et de liaison du syndicat des médecins anatomo-cyto-pathologistes Français*, no.43 (1995), 9.

145. See Büttner, "Clinical Chemistry."

146. See Ibid. See also Büttner and Habrich, *Roots of Clinical Chemistry*, and Kohler, *From Medical Chemistry to Biochemistry*.

147. For a review of training requirements for directors of medical laboratories on a country-by-country basis, see Rubin and Lous, *Education and Training for Clinical Chemistry*.

148. See Purdy and Melville, "The Manpower Crisis in Clinical Chemistry."

149. The journal itself was founded in 1901 under the name *The Journal of Medical Research*. In 1925, following the merger of the American Society for Experimental Pathology and the American Association of Pathologists and Bacteriologists, it became *The American Journal of Pathology*. See Fausto, "What's in a Name?" 1.

150. In this respect, in addition to the funding mechanisms previously mentioned that make such interaction possible, there are other less formal undertakings that have brought biology and medicine together. Leaving aside the numerous journal clubs to be found in laboratories throughout the world (according to Rall, the first 'Journal Club' was organized by Milton Rosenau at the NIH in 1902; see Rall, "Epilogue"), unofficial societies such as the "Antibody Club" organized in the early 1960s in Britain by clinicians interested in immunology and wishing to promote the use of immunology in clinical practice served as an efficient conduit of ideas and techniques prior to the establishment of the more official routes prescribed by translational research. See, e.g., "Clinical Immunology: Report on the Joint Meeting of the Antibody Club and the Dutch Society of Immunology, Leiden, 13 June 1970." Similarly, in France in the same period, hospital laboratory directors organized the first of what were to become "Biological Sundays," seminars organized to keep hospital physicians up-to-date with the latest biological techniques. See Rousselet et al., *Dimanches biologiques de Lariboisière, 1960–1990*.

Chapter 4

1. The transfer of a procedure from the laboratory to the clinic is not the issue here since even when the IPT platform was subsequently implemented on a routine basis, the diagnostic work still took place in a laboratory (although, admittedly, often in a clinical, as opposed to an experimental, one). Conversely, when IPT was still an experimental procedure, it drew blood from clinical settings.

2. No single path led from one event to the other, nor did we uncover parallel paths somehow converging into some sort of general synthesis. In fact, it is only retrospectively, from the point of view of the IPT platform, that the items figuring in our account appear to be connected.

3. Greaves, *Immunodiagnosis of Human Leukaemia*, Application for an MRC Project Grant (MRC75/1141). We thank Philip Toms, MRC Records Manager, for providing us with a copy of the grant application.

4. Not so short-lived, in fact, since it has recently been used in an address by the president of the European Society of Analytical Cellular Pathology; see Valet, "Analytical Cellular Pathology and Biology."

5. Vogel, "The Leukemias." Additional information on the (early) history of leukemia can be found in Freireich and Lemak, *Milestones in Leukemia Research and Therapy*; Piller, *The History and Presentation of Leukaemia*; Piller, *John Hughes Bennett and the Discovery of Leukaemia*; Gunz, "The Dread Leukemias and the Lymphomas."

6. Gunz, "The Dread Leukemias."

7. Vogel, "The Leukemias," 68; Cecil, *A Text-Book of Medicine*, 977.

8. Gralnick et al., "Classification of Acute Leukemia," 741. These days, however, acute and chronic leukemias are defined according to cell maturity. Acute leukemia implicates immature cells referred to as stem cells, blasts, or "pro" cells, whereas chronic leukemia is diagnosed when more mature cells are involved. Textbooks now tell us that "in general, these two groups correspond to a rapid (acute) or slow (chronic) clinical course"; see, e.g., Perkins, Odell, and Braziel, "Introduction to Leukemia and the Acute Leukemias," 295. Presently, then, cellular diagnosis takes precedence over clinical phenomena. This reversal of fortune is part of what concerns us here.

9. Largely neglected in the United Kingdom, leukemia had no national charity until 1960 when the parents of a young leukemia victim, appalled by the prevailing treatment and the lack of medical research into the disease, launched the campaign that led to the foundation of the Leukaemia Research Fund; see Piller, *Rays of Hope*. The LRF officially incorporated in 1962. The first leukemia unit to be established in the United Kingdom was set up with LRF money at London's Hospital for Sick Children. Although the initiative came from lay parents, medical professionals quickly took the further development of the LRF into their own hands.

10. Galton and Kay, *U.K. Leukaemia Clinical Trials for Children and Adults.* Treatment of children with ALL had by 1977 already met with spectacular success. The same could not, unfortunately, be said of adult AML. On chemotherapy's success story in the case of ALL, see Laszlo, *The Cure of Childhood Leukemia.*

11. J. Peto, *Draft Review of MRC Trials* (November 1984), MRC Head Office Archives (henceforth MRC/HOA), FD23/4074 S1101/108 Committee on Leukaemia, Working Party on Leukaemia in Childhood Meeting, 26 November 1984. The UKALL VIII trial (1980) derived from an identical study in the United States that examined the value of adding a fourth chemotherapeutic agent (daunorubicin) to the previous cocktail of three agents (vincristine, prednisolone, asparaginase) during remission induction. UKALL X (1984) explored a West German proposal for early intensification of induction therapy (*UKALL X Trial. For All Cases of Newly Diagnosed Acute Lymphoblastic Leukaemia under the Age of 15 Years* (November 1984), MRC/HOA, ibid).

12. Galton and Kay, *U.K. Leukaemia Clinical Trials,* 3.

13. For a discussion of the social, ethical, and political dimensions of clinical trials, see Marks, *The Progress of Experiments.*

14. Galton and Kay, *U.K. Leukaemia Clinical Trials,* 30.

15. Treatment monitoring provided yet another "equally valuable" application of the new immunological techniques; see Smith, "Cancers of Childhood," *ICRF Annual Report* 1977–78, 10–3. By 1984, the UKALL X protocol included a pretreatment assessment based on the examination of the patient's bone marrow using the following three techniques: morphology/cytochemistry, cell typing (immunodiagnosis), and chromosome analysis (*UKALL X Trial. For All Cases of Newly Diagnosed Acute Lymphoblastic Leukaemia under the Age of 15 Years* (November 1984), MRC/HOA, FD23/4074 S1101/108 Committee on Leukaemia, Working Party on Leukaemia in Childhood Meeting, 26 November 1984).

16. Zuckerman, *Cancer Research,* 2.

17. See Stoker, "Limits to Oncology," 547–8, in which cell-surface research is presented as an example of strategic research, and Stoker, "New Medicine and New Biology," in which the term "ruthless reductionism" signifies the use of simple model organisms (such as viruses) and a set of new technologies mainly concerned with purification (of populations of cells, molecules, etc.).

18. As stated in a 1971 report from the coordinating committee of the three major U.K. cancer research organizations. The coordinating committee was created in 1970 and their 1971 assessment summarized in the Zuckerman report; see Zuckerman, *Cancer Research,* 7.

19. Seligmann, *Lymphocyte Membrane Markers in Human Leukaemias and Lymphomas.* The LRF had already invited Seligmann to London shortly before in April 1975 at the first international research symposium organized by the LRF on "Characterization of Cells in Leukaemias and Lymphomas." His talk on "B and T Cell Membrane Markers in Human Leukaemias and Lymphomas" was

immediately followed by a paper by Greaves on "Surface Antigens of Leukaemic Cells."

20. Our emphasis; see Greaves, *Biology of Acute Lymphoblastic Leukaemia.* So many people asked for tickets to attend the lecture that the LRF had to move it to larger premises (LRF, *Minutes of the Meeting of the Medical and Scientific Advisory Panel* (henceforth *Minutes MSAP*), 30 October 1980). Furthermore, the LRF MSAP sought wide circulation for the lecture; a copy of the lecture was first sent to *Nature* (LRF, *Minutes MSAP,* 26 February 1981, 13 May 1981), and subsequently resubmitted in a redrafted, abbreviated version (LRF, *Minutes MSAP,* 19 October 1981, 8 February 1982).

21. Greaves, 1975 MRC proposal.

22. "Identification, Enumeration, and Isolation of B and T Lymphocytes from Human Peripheral Blood."

23. Ibid., 521.

24. Seligmann, *Lymphocyte Membrane Markers in Human Leukaemias and Lymphomas,* 5. For an analysis of a situation whereby regulation does not follow stabilization but, rather, is part of the latter, see Bourret and Eisinger, "Guidelines of 'Good Practices' in Cancer Genetic Clinics."

25. INSERM Archives, Box 9203-186, 1974–76 Scientific Report of Unité 108 (Prof. Maxime Seligmann); our translation.

26. Interview with George Janossy, Royal Free Hospital, London, 27 April 1999.

27. INSERM Archives, Box 9203-186, 1974–76 Scientific Report of Unité 108 (Prof. Maxime Seligmann); our translation.

28. Pinch, "Towards an Analysis of Scientific Observation." The notion of externality refers to the chain of interpretations involved in making an observation. Results expressed in terms that follow closely the procedural aspects of the experiment and the resulting traces are said to have a low degree of externality.

29. Cambrosio and Keating, *Exquisite Specificity.*

30. *ICRF Scientific Report* 1978, 117–8. *ICRF Scientific Report* 1978–79, 130–2. The British laboratories included two ICRF and an Oxford laboratory, the American laboratories were located at Stanford and the University of Pittsburgh.

31. Fujimura, "Crafting Science." We say "relatively" because, for instance, the extent to which commercially available antibody markers to be used with the FACS have been black-boxed is open to dispute; see Preud'homme, "Lymphocyte Markers."

32. Mitchison, "The Fund at University College London," *ICRF Scientific Report* 1990, xix–xxii.

33. Hall, *A Commotion in the Blood,* 265.

34. "Director's Introduction," *ICRF Annual Report* 1967–68, 31–4. Many of the "social" initiatives of the new director created major strains with the staff; see Austoker, *A History of the Imperial Cancer Research Fund.*

35. Stoker, "New Medicine and New Biology."

36. Stoker, Introduction, *ICRF Annual Report* 1969–70, 32–4.

37. Zuckerman, *Cancer Research*, 12.

38. Stoker, "A Proposal for Two ICRF Research Units for Work on Human Cancer," July 1970, containing G. Hamilton Farley, "An I. C. R. F. Medical Oncology Research Unit at St. Bartholomew's Hospital with an Additional Clinical Unit at the Hackney General Hospital. Research Programme," July 1970. ICRF Archives.

39. In fact this is not quite true, since other institutions, such as the MRC Working Party on Leukaemia, were carrying out clinical trials. The rationale given for the MOU was that the MRC trials involved a large number of centers, each with a small number of cases, while the MOU goal was to collect in a single center a large number of cases allowing for the quick testing of new chemotherapeutic combinations.

40. Wilson, *Body and Antibody*. The book is based on interviews and material from both the United States and United Kingdom.

41. For these numbers and others, see Humphrey, "The Growth of Immunology." For an overview of the development of immunology in terms of its professional organizations, conferences, and publications, see also Nicholas and Nicholas, *Immunology: An Information Profile*; Silverstein and Söderqvist, "The Structure and Dynamics of Immunology."

42. Silverstein, *A History of Immunology*; Moulin, *Le dernier langage de la médecine*, 199–200.

43. Nor did many people, especially pathologists, seem to care: "In those days pathologists spoke of lymphocytes and plasma cells as being similar to medical students—always there, never doing very much, but standing around looking on when important things were going on in medicine" (Good, "The Minnesota Scene," 112).

44. Gowans, "The Mysterious Lymphocyte."

45. See Moulin, "The Immune System: A Key Concept for the History of Immunology."

46. Calder, "Immunology: Research at Mill Hill Institute."

47. Stoker, "Proposed New Unit for Tumour Immunology" (1969), ICRF Archives; see also "Memorandum for the Director of Research on the Proposed Unit for Tumour Immunology" (1970), ICRF Archives.

48. Mitchison, "Tumour Immunology," *ICRF Annual Report* 1971–2, 41–8.

49. There had indeed been a history of 'miracle' cures based on immunotherapy. On the history of immunotherapy, see Löwy, *Between Bench and Bedside.* Mitchison's statement that "glimmers of success" had appeared in immunotherapy, namely thanks to the work of the French clinician Georges Mathé, were not fully shared by other observers; for instance, H. E. M. Kay noted in 1979, discussing clinical trials, that "in 1969 . . . we were aware of the claims of Georges Mathé. The weakness of the claim was evident at the time." Yet, Kay goes on to admit that "there was enough to stimulate the planning of a controlled trial" that failed to show any benefit. See Galton and Kay, *U.K. Leukaemia Clinical Trials,* 20.

50. Mitchison, "Tumour Immunology," 41.

51. Stoker, "Limits to Oncology," 547–8.

52. Stoker, "Introduction," *ICRF Annual Report* 1969–70, 32–4; Stoker, "Introduction," *ICRF Annual Report* 1970–71, 32–4. Stoker mentioned planned collaborations between the team headed by Dulbecco and both the MOU and the TIU.

53. National Cancer Institute, *Digest of Scientific Recommendations for the National Cancer Program Plan,* III.1–III.15.

54. Old and Boyse, "Current Enigmas in Cancer Research," 273.

55. Note the conflation of the normal and the pathological: "the *biological* behavior of *tumor* and *normal* cells"; see Berlin et al., "The Cell Surface," 515.

56. Doljanski, "A New Look at the Cell Surface," 251.

57. Weissmann, "Cell Biology and Medicine," 15.

58. Ibid. Obviously keen on Kuhnian vocabulary (revolutions, paradigms) Weissmann was professor of medicine and director of the Division of Rheumatology, New York University School of Medicine.

59. Gorter and Grendel at the University of Leiden in 1925. However, the model in its postwar (1952) formulation is attributed to Danielli and Davson in *The Permeability of Natural Membranes.*

60. For a critique of the first model, see Singer, "The Molecular Organization of Biological Membranes." For a presentation of the fluid mosaic, see Singer and Nicolson, "The Fluid Mosaic Model of the Structure of Cell Membranes."

61. Our emphasis. Zuckerman and Douglas, "The Lymphocyte Plasma Membrane," 120.

62. Old's name is not to be found in the indexes of Moulin, *Le dernier langage*; Gallagher et al., *Immunology: The Making*; Silverstein, *A History of Immunology*; or Podolsky and Tauber, *The Generation of Diversity.* Although mentioned by Löwy

in *Between Bench and Bedside*, it is only as one of the discoverers of the antitumor properties of bacilli Calmette-Guérin (BCG), not for the discovery of immune cell markers. Nor does he appear in the popular histories of Desowitz, *The Thorn in the Starfish*, or Clark, *The Double-Edged Sword of Immunity*. He is mentioned once in Brent, *A History of Transplantation Immunology* in connection with a skin graft antigen. See also Ford, "The Lymphocyte."

63. On the role of mice, see, e.g., Löwy and Gaudillière, "Disciplining Cancer."

64. For a review of Haldane's and Gorer's work, see Jan Klein, "Seeds of Time."

65. In this case it was sarcoma and leukemia cells transplanted from two American strains of inbred mice. There is some doubt as to the exact identity of the strains of mice used. Klein believes that both strains came from the Jackson Laboratory; see Jan Klein, "Seeds of Time."

66. Gorer, "Future Studies on Antigenic Differences in Mouse Erythrocytes."

67. Details of the dispute may be found in Brent, *A History of Transplantation Immunology*, 74–8. As it turned out, both were partly right; it depends on what is being transplanted. Single-cell suspensions, like leukemia, can provoke the production of antibodies leading to rejection, whereas tissues require the participation of lymphocytes.

68. Brent, *A History of Transplantation Immunology*, 77.

69. Old, Boyse, and Stockert, "Antigenic Properties of Experimental Leukemias I," 985.

70. Ibid.

71. Boyse et al., "Genetic Origin of Tumor Antigens."

72. "Conference on Tumor Specific Antigens."

73. "The Possible Role of Immunology in Cancer." This is not the place for a detailed review of the pre-1960 development of cancer immunology. Let us note, however, that at the 1961 conference Old and Boyse had performed a *coup de force* by calling for the enforcement of new rules of the game, i.e., for an exclusive focus on "those experimental systems in which antigenic differences between tumor and host have been most clearly defined," thus excluding the human domain. As noted by another observer, "The restoration of cancer immunology to a position of reasonable respectability was the result of improvement in methodology. The use of the inbred mouse was perhaps the single most important development. A high degree of genetic uniformity among the animals certainly minimizes the chances of nonspecific immunologic reactions" (Prehn, "Tumor-Specific Antigens of Putatively Nonviral Tumors," 1326). Work in the human domain had been characterized by crass empiricism involving, for instance, the subcutaneous injection of cancer cells into normal subjects ("volunteers" from Ohio State Prison) and cancer patients and comparing the resulting effects (local inflammation and quick regression in the former, sus-

tained growth and little or no inflammation in the latter) as an indicator of impaired immune response; see Southam and Moore, "Induced Immunity to Cancer Cell Homografts in Man." Whether this was due to "properties inherent in malignant cells" or, in other words, to tumor-specific antigens remained an open question; see Grace, "Discussion of the Paper," 651. As far as the therapeutic possibilities went, they did not seem very fruitful either. Chester Southam at Sloan-Kettering was especially critical of attempts to treat patients through active immunization, i.e., by injecting tumor cells into the patient in the hopes of generating an immune reaction, hopefully rejection. Reviewing sixty years of ad hoc injections of tumor extracts and the attendant "cures," he pointed out that "all hope of success through this approach hinges on the existence of antigenic differences between cancer cells and normal tissues which might allow selective or preferential action against the cancer cell. The very fact is, as amply demonstrated in this symposium, that there is no proof and only scanty data to suggest that cancer cells contain such unique antigens." Similarly, a review of sixty years of passive immunization—injecting patients with antibodies produced by injecting animals with cancer cells—made it "embarrassingly clear how little real advance there has been." The evaluation of various forms of immunological therapy involving "factors" of varying degrees of obscurity led to the following conclusion: "One can conclude—with no expectation of controversy, with no fear of prematurity, and without accusation of personal prejudice—that they have contributed nothing to applied immunology"; see Southam, "Application of Immunology to Clinical Cancer," 1311.

74. Boyse et al., "Genetic Origin of Tumor Antigens," 1280.

75. Ibid.

76. Boyse et al., "Ly-A and Ly-B: Two Systems of Lymphocyte Isoantigens in the Mouse."

77. For a review of all the work done on the Ly series, see Mackenzie and Potter, "Murine Lymphocyte Surface Antigens", 179–337; on Ly-1, see esp. 221–225.

78. Boyse et al., "Ly-A and Ly-B," 191.

79. Boyse et al., "Genetic Origin of Tumor Antigens," 1283.

80. Boyse and Old, "Some Aspects of Normal and Abnormal Cell Surface Genetics."

81. Ibid., 271. A note appended to the term "differentiation" explained that "In the sense in which Jacob & Monod have used the term, '. . . two cells are differentiated with respect to one another if, while they harbor the same genome, the pattern of proteins which they synthesize is different.' "

82. Ibid., 273.

83. Boyse, "The Invitation to Surveillance," 7.

84. Ibid., 19.

85. Ibid., 21.

86. The resulting maps were later shown to be artifacts induced by the binding of the antibodies. Martin Raff, personal communication, 4 March 2000.

87. Moulin, "The Immune System."

88. The term "experiment of nature" was used extensively by Robert Good (see n. 89), who attributed a key role to this kind of phenomenon in his research strategy. See, e.g., Good, "Experiments of Nature in Immunobiology" and Good, "The Minnesota Scene." An example of subsequent use of the term is provided by the title of chapter 6 ("A Crucial Experiment of Nature: Multiple Myeloma and the Structure of Antibodies") of Swazey and Reeds, *Today's Medicine, Tomorrow's Science.*

89. For an overview of the rise of cellular immunology and Good's contribution in this respect, see Silverstein, *A History of Immunology*, and Moulin, *Le dernier langage.* Personal accounts of these events are to be found in Mazumdar, *Immunology 1930–1980* and Gallagher et al., *Immunology: The Making.* Good is an extremely prolific writer (between 1945 and 1975 he cosigned 1245 articles) who has been presented as the quintessential American scientist; see Wilson, *Body and Antibody.* In 1973, Good left Minnesota where he had performed his seminal work on T and B cells, to become the director of the largest cancer facility in the world, the Sloan-Kettering Institute in New York City.

90. Good, "The Minnesota Scene," 113–5. Good emphasizes, in this respect, the importance of the long hours spent talking to patients, from whom he elicited histories about their susceptibility to infections. There is a long clinical history of the relationship between Hodgkin's disease and immunological deficiencies. Observations of immunological problems in Hodgkin's disease can be traced back to the 1930s. See DeVita and Hellman, "Hodgkin's Disease and the Non-Hodgkin's Lymphomas," 1358.

91. There are at least two different versions of this story. Clark (*The Double-Edged Sword of Immunity*, 65) says that one of Good's residents happened to be reading *Poultry Science* one day in 1959 and noticed the article, adding "what this resident might have been doing reading *Poultry Science* we may never know." Good's version ("Runestones in Immunology," 1420; "The Minnesota Scene," 126–7) is that the information about the *Poultry Science* article was relayed to him at a scientific meeting by an immunology colleague who had actually replicated the article's findings. Bibel (*Milestones in Immunology*, 129) reports this latter version, but changes the immunologist into a biochemist. Both Bibel and Good note that the *Poultry Science* article (Glick, Chang, and Jaap, "The Bursa of Fabricius and Antibody Production.") had first been sent to *Science* which had judged it to be of no general interest or significance.

92. Good, "Runestones in Immunology," 1420.

93. See, in this respect, Stillwell, "Thymectomy as an Experimental System in Immunology". Miller's recollection is to be found in Miller, "The Discovery of

Thymus Function." Other researchers, in addition to Miller and Good, played a role in the establishment of the T-B distinction. A fierce controversy developed between Good and Miller about who had discovered what and when. This perhaps explains why they never received a Nobel Prize, in spite of the fact that Medawar repeatedly suggested their names to the Nobel committee. In his letters to the committee, Medawar stressed that in his opinion, and in spite of the controversy, both had reached their conclusions independently through different routes, Good starting from clinical observations and Miller using experimental laboratory work. Medawar described Good as the most important clinical immunologist of his time (Medawar Papers, CAMC Archive, Wellcome Institute Library [henceforth MP], Box B 12, B 14).

94. A summary of the research program can be found in Cooper et al., "The Two-Component Concept of the Lymphoid System." As it turned out, it was not that simple. The lymphocytes—the T cells and the B cells—interacted. In order for the B cells to produce antibodies, they needed the help of the T cells or a subset thereof, later to be called helper T cells (Good, "Runestones in Immunology," 1421).

95. Interview with Martin C. Raff, London, 2 June 1999.

96. Interview with Melvin F. Greaves, London, 2 July 1996.

97. Roitt et al., "The Cellular Basis of Immunological Responses." It is sometimes claimed that the article introduced the T-B terminology. For instance, Moulin (*Le dernier langage*, 309) mentions the "legend" (her term) according to which Roitt, sitting in bed with the flu and nothing else to do, came up with the new terminology; the same account was given by Roitt (interview with Roitt, London, 24 May 1999); as for Greaves, he claims that he and Roitt jointly invented it: "sitting in a revolving coffee bar in Sweden we decided to call them T and B cells" (interview, 2 July 1996). A few years later, Greaves coauthored a book-length overview of the state of the art concerning T and B lymphocytes, that, he claims, was "something of a landmark publication, heralding in the era of clinical application of the [T-B distinction]" (Melvyn Greaves, personal communication, 6 March 2000).

98. Good, "Lymphocyte Surface Markers," 305.

99. Here is just a sample of the opening lines of three clinical papers: "Lymphoid cells of the immune system can be divided into two functional compartments" (Shevach et al., "Receptors for Complement and Immunoglobulin," 1933); "Lymphocytes are divided into two major groups according to their origin and function" (Aiuti et al., "Lymphocyte Surface Markers in Lymphoproliferative Diseases," 275); "Based on their origin and functions, normal lymphocytes have been classified in two main groups: bone marrow-derived (B) and thymus-dependent (T) lymphocytes" (Borella and Sen, "T- and B-Lymphocytes in Untreated Acute Lymphocytic Leukemia," 646).

100. We did not use the term "marker(s)" because a quick search showed that although 375 papers used it in their titles between 1966 and 1970 (as opposed

to only 4 papers with the previous, more precise set of terms), most of those papers did not discuss immunology but, rather, genetics (genetic markers, chromosome markers, etc.). From this we may infer that the term "marker" was probably borrowed by immunologists from genetics. Conversely, some of the papers that did refer to cell-surface markers were not retrieved by our procedure, since none of the three terms appeared in that title.

101. The sharp rise in 1975 is probably due to the fact that, starting that year, abstracts were added to the MEDLINE database. The trend is nonetheless clear.

102. Preud'homme, "Lymphocyte Markers." See also Cambrosio, Keating, and Guttman, "New Medical Technologies and Clinical Practice."

103. Reif and Allen, "Specificity of Isoantisera against Leukemic and Thymic Lymphocytes."

104. For a history of Thy-1 from Reif's point of view, see Reif, "The Discovery of Thy-1 and Its Development." As with Good and Miller, we are confronted with a priority dispute. Reif's account is an attempt to retrospectively claim priority for the discovery of Thy-1 as a T-cell marker, both on the basis of the argument (collapsing the normal and the pathological) that "after all, leukemia cells *are* lymphocytes," and by claiming to have repeatedly suggested an extension of his work to thymus-derived normal lymphocytes. Reif also admits that he "was unwilling to spend additional time working on this problem, since [he] believed that [his] primary mission was to do cancer research."

105. Why did they pick theta (Thy-1) instead of TL? According to Raff (personal communication, 22 July 1999) they were aware of the TL paper but apparently Mitchison had heard Reif speak about theta at a conference and got the idea there. See also Reif ("The Discovery of Thy-1 and Its Development"), who makes a similar claim.

106. Brent, *A History of Transplantation Immunology*, 22. Brent shared the Nobel Prize with Medawar for their work on skin grafting and cellular immunology. At the time, Raff wrote: "A revolution is taking place in immunology. It began with the recognition that there are two classes of lymphocytes involved in the immune response in birds, one thymus-dependent, and the other thymus-independent. . . . It gathered force as the dichotomy became apparent in mammals . . . and is now culminating as the fundamental importance of the two-cell concept to the immune response becomes generally appreciated. . . . The revolution has thus created an urgent need for methods that enable one to distinguish and separate the two lymphocyte classes" (Raff, "Surface Antigenic Markers for Distinguishing T and B Lymphocytes in Mice," 52).

107. As researchers at the Pasteur Institute pointed out, "Inevitably, investigators in this area seek simplifying approaches: (1) the search for a pathological phenomenon, e.g., a lymphocytes tumor, which might provide copious quantities of identical receptor immunoglobulins" (Wofsy, Truffa-Bachi, and Naor, "Chemical Approaches to the Cell Receptor Problem," 432).

108. Raff, "Theta Isoantigen as a Marker of Thymus-Derived Lymphocytes in Mice;" Schlesinger and Yron, "Antigenic Changes in Lymph-Node Cells after Administration of Antiserum to Thymus Cells." The citation count is to be found in Raff, "Citation Classic Commentary."

109. Schlesinger, "Antigens of the Thymus;" Raff, "Surface Antigenic Markers for Distinguishing T and B Lymphocytes in Mice."

110. Reif, "The Discovery of Thy-1 and Its Development," 24, 31; interview with Martin C. Raff, London, 2 June 1999.

111. Fujimura, *Crafting Science.*

112. Interview with Melvin F. Greaves, London, 2 July 1996.

113. Inspired by Medawar, Möller worked on histocompatibility antigens (H-2) in the mouse. In a 1961 paper that became a "citation classic" Möller showed the presence of immunoglobulin at the surface of lymphocytes. He claims, retrospectively, that he recognized that those molecules acted as receptors at the surface of lymphocytes and that his discovery was "rediscovered" nine years later by Raff. Raff disagrees with this interpretation, arguing that a close reading of the paper shows that Möller did not recognize at the time the implications of his work, namely that those immunoglobulins sitting at the surface were an intrinsic part of the cell, acting as cell receptors, as opposed to passively acquired molecules (Möller, "Citation Classic Commentary" interview with Martin C. Raff, London, 2 June 1999). See also Raff, *Cell Surface Immunology,* where he writes that Möller did "inadvertently" show the presence of immunoglobulin receptors. For Raff's work on immunoglobulins as markers of B cells, see Raff, "Two Distinct Populations of Peripheral Lymphocytes in Mice Distinguishable by Immunofluorescence," and Raff, Sternberg, and Taylor, "Immunoglobulin Determinants in the Surface of Mouse Lymphoid Cells."

114. This is reminiscent of the criteria, previously discussed, set out in 1961 by Old and Boyse. In the case of Mitchison, the four criteria were (1) the immune response must be strong and repeatable; (2) it must take place in animals whose immunological mechanisms are already well understood; (3) the antigens eliciting the response must be suited to characterization in molecular terms; and (4) the unit should be able to benefit from ICRF's expertise and facilities in tumor virology. Note the mixed social and technical nature of these criteria.

115. TIU Report, *ICRF Annual Report* 1971–2, 73–4. Mitchison added that in so doing "the Unit hope[d] to help write the ground rules of differential lymphocyte triggering."

116. *Rapport d'activité 1975—Maxime Seligmann,* INSERM Archives.

117. Möller, in whose laboratory Greaves spent a year of postdoctoral research, is, as previously noted, credited with having first detected the presence of immunoglobulins at the surface of lymphocytes. Greaves argued in two articles that the Ig on the surface was the result of active synthesis by the B cells, and

not of passive absorption of circulating Ig; see Greaves, "The Expression of Immunoglobulin Determinants on the Surface of Antigen-Binding Lymphoid Cells in Mice. I;" and Greaves, "The Expression of Immunoglobulin Determinants on the Surface of Antigen-Binding Lymphoid Cells in Mice. II."

118. Curiously, the reaction was specific to sheep; horse, ox, rabbit, guinea pig, and mouse blood didn't do it; see Lay et al., "Binding of Sheep Red Blood Cells to a Large Population of Human Lymphocytes," 531. Bach et al. ("Summary of Round-Table Discussion on the Technical Aspects of the Rosette Test") also noted that "The origin of the red blood cells (RBC) used as antigen is very important. The sheep RBC seem to occupy a special position."

119. For example, Greaves and Möller had already shown that, in the mouse, the rosette-forming cells could be inhibited by theta antibody indicating that they must be T cells; see Greaves and Möller, "Studies on Antigen-Binding Cells. I: The Origin of Reactive Cells." On humans, see Lay et al., "Binding of Sheep Red Blood Cells" 531.

120. Fröland, "Binding of Sheep Erythrocytes to Human Lymphocytes," 276. The most convincing evidence in this respect came from patients lacking B lymphocytes: they formed the same number of rosettes as normal individuals. Nonetheless, the phenomenon was highly variable. A study of fifty normal persons the same year showed that the number of rosette-forming cells in the peripheral blood varied from 4% to 40%. In 1976, Taylor reported variation in reports of normal T cells in peripheral blood ranging from 10% to 70%: (Taylor, *Hodgkin's Disease and the Lymphomas,* 11). Reviews of the pitfalls associated with E-rosette determinations at the time came be found in Preud'homme and Seligmann, "Critical Evaluation of B and T Cell Markers in Man," and Kunkel, "Surface Markers of Human Lymphocytes." But, once again, examination of *patients* with immunological disorders (in this case, lack of B cells) suggested that the cells must be thymus-derived (T cells). See Wybran, Carr, and Fudenberg, "The Human Rosette-Forming Cell as a Marker of a Population of Thymus-Derived Cells".

121. Borella and Sen, "T Cell Surface Markers on Lymphoblasts from Acute Lymphocytic Leukemia." In addition, the patient was clinically "different"; at the time of diagnosis, the T-cell patient had 7 to 20 times as many lymphocytes as the other patients (ibid., 1260).

122. Bach et al.; "Summary of Round-Table Discussion," 336–7.

123. Greaves and Hogg, "Inhibition of Rosette Formation by Antisera to Cell Surface Determinants," 355.

124. Brown and Greaves, "Cell Surface Markers for Human T and B Lymphocytes."

125. Incidentally, but significantly, the human material forming the basis of the paper had been supplied by colleagues at the Institute of Child Health (London's main center for childhood leukemia) and the medical oncology unit established by the ICRF at London's St. Bartholomew's Hospital.

126. *ICRF Scientific Report* 1973, 117–21.

127. Aiuti et al., "Lymphocyte Surface Markers in Lymphoproliferative Diseases."

128. In 1975, there were approximately seventeen methods reported for the separation of B cells and T cells. For a list, see Taylor, *Hodgkin's Disease and the Lymphomas,* 8.

129. LRF, *Minutes of the Meeting of the Medical Advisory Panel* (henceforth Minutes MAP), 8 June 1971.

130. The establishment of the fellowship followed negotiations between the LRF and INSERM initiated in the early 1970s (LRF, *Minutes MAP,* 8 June 1971, 16 March 1972, 15 June 1972). Early on, the LRF had looked at both the United States and France, but when the French went ahead securing funds for their part of the deal, the LRF decided to go ahead with them and suspend negotiations with the United States (LRF, *Minutes MAP,* 11 November 71). The first British fellow left for Saint-Louis Hospital in January 1973 (LRF, *Minutes MAP,* 31 October 1972). The scheme was upgraded in 1973 to include the possibility of short visits by senior researchers (LRF, *Minutes MAP,* 8 November 1973).

131. LRF, *Minutes MAP,* 15 June 1972.

132. Initially scheduled for 1974 under the title "Cell Biology and Cell Kinetics in Relation to Leukaemia" (LRF, *Minutes MAP,* 1 March 1973), the meeting was moved to 1975 and the theme changed to "The Biology of Leukaemic Cells," allegedly "in order to attract younger research workers as opposed to those already established in the field" (LRF, *Minutes MAP,* 8 November 73).

133. "Characterisation of cells in leukaemias and lymphomas" (April 1975): program and abstracts (LRF Archives).

134. Cline, *The White Cell,* 383–4. For a description of the various research topics addressed by Seligmann's group in the mid-1970s, see "Rapport d'activité 1975—Maxime Seligmann," and "Rapport d'Activité 1977—Maxime Seligmann," INSERM Archives, which contain a forty-page report on the 1974–8 period. For an overview of fifteen years of the unit's research activities, see "Candidature à une direction d'Unité 1987—Jean-Claude Brouet," INSERM Archives.

135. For an example of this kind of debate, see Catovsky, "Ph1-Positive Acute Leukaemia and Chronic Granulocytic Leukaemia: One or Two Diseases?"

136. For instance, a 1974 paper by Salmon and Seligmann ("B-Cell Neoplasia in Man," 1230) opens with the statement that the new immunological approach provides "the basis for a unifying view of the diverse human neoplastic disorders arising from cells of the B-cell series of immunocytes."

137. Picard, "Poussée scientifique ou demande des médecins?" 88–91. A few years later, in 1963, the center created a "laboratory for the immunology of leukemias," as part of a five-floor complex with the patients on the ground floor

and each successive floor characterized by the presence of increasingly fundamental sciences. Immunology occupied the fourth floor, which was divided between Jean Dausset and Maxime Seligmann (ibid. 94–5). For Seligmann's early work, see "Titres et travaux scientifiques du Pr. Maxime Seligmann (1971)," Archives INSERM; Association Claude Bernard pour le développement des recherches biologiques et médicales dans les hôpitaux de l'Assistance Publique à Paris, *Travaux scientifiques 1955–1965*. Paris: Association Claude Bernard, 1965, Archives AP-HP (Box C 4435).

138. Interview with Georges Flandrin, Paris, 7 November 1996.

139. Mathé et al., "De l'hématologie *avec* à l'hématologie *sans* microscope." A similar title (*L'hématologie sans microscope*) was used by Marcel Bessis (another of the leading neoclinicians) for a movie he produced on automatic equipment (Technicon).

140. This episode is mentioned in Moulin, "Un objet scientifique à la charnière des sciences biologiques et sociales," 308 n. 9. See also Maxime Seligmann, personal communication, 30 March 2000.

141. "Titres et travaux scientifiques du Docteur Maxime Seligmann, 1971," INSERM Archives.

142. *Rapport d'activité 1980–1983—Maxime Seligmann.* INSERM Archives.

143. Interviews with Georges Janossy, London, 27 April and 6 May 1999.

144. Maxime Seligmann, personal communication, 30 March 2000.

145. Interview with Georges Flandrin, Paris, 7 November 1996; interview with Françoise Valensi, Paris, 18 December 1997.

146. Interview with Georges Flandrin, Paris, 7 November 1996.

147. The first French researcher to ask for and obtain a FACS was Claude Rosenfeld, from the Institute for Cancer Research at Villejuif (on the outskirts of Paris), and not, as one might have expected, someone from Seligmann's group at Saint-Louis. Rosenfeld played a pioneering role in lymphocyte cell cultures and, as we will see below, collaborated with Greaves in testing surface markers on these cell lines. Rosenfeld had difficulty convincing authorities to provide him with a FACS and finally opted for private, American support to obtain his first machine around 1978 (interview with Claude Rosenfeld, Paris, 12 January 1997). French interest in flow cytometry emerged in the early spring of 1979, when two of France's leading biomedical researchers—the molecular geneticist and Nobel Prize winner François Jacob of the Pasteur Institute and the immunologist Jean-François Bach—showed up at a cocktail party that was also attended by Constant Burg, the then director of the main biomedical funding agency, INSERM, and by François Gros, director of the Pasteur Institute. Jacob and Bach used that occasion to point out to their administrative heads that a revolutionary technology, flow cytometry, had been developed in the United States and made available to researchers there, while no such instru-

ment was yet available in France (in fact, it was, in Rosenfeld's laboratory). Apparently, a decision was made on the spot to acquire a flow cytometer and to house it at the Pasteur Institute, where it would be made available to both the institute's and INSERM's researchers. Gros immediately asked Michel Goldberg, the scientific director at Pasteur, to set up the cytometry unit. Goldberg had no idea of what a cytometer was, and thus Gros suggested that he contact a young researcher at the Necker hospital, Patrick Niaudet, who had just returned from a stay in Greaves's laboratory in London, where he had become acquainted with the instrument (interview with Michel Goldberg, Paris, 21 November 1996).

148. Seligmann, *Lymphocyte Membrane Markers in Human Leukaemias and Lymphoma,* 7. The same argument appears in an overview of the subject presented at a 1976 symposium: "A classification which would appear relatively safe for the markers of normal B and T lymphocytes may not be valid when extrapolated to leukemic or lymphomatous cells. Neoplastic cells may undergo surface changes and express new markers or conversely lose some normal membrane properties, thus preventing their identification. Moreover leukemic cells may also express membrane antigens only at certain stages of the cell cycle and the presence of fetal antigens or tumor associated antigens may invalidate the results obtained with antisera to B or T fetal or neoplastic cells" (Seligmann, Brouet, and Preud'homme, "The Immunological Diagnosis of Human Leukemias and Lymphomas," 2).

149. Brouet et al., "Classification immunologique des leucémies aiguës lymphoblastiques," 148.

150. See, e.g., Boyse et al., "Modification of the Antigenic Structure of the Cell Membrane by Thymus-Leukemia (TL) Antigen."

151. Metzgar, Mohnanakumar, and Miller, "Antigens Specific for Human Lymphocytic and Myeloid Leukemia Cells;" Mohanakumar, Metzgar, and Miller, "Human Leukemia Cell Antigens;" Mann et al., "Detection of an Antigen Associated with Acute Leukemia;" Baker, Ramachandar, and Taub, "Specificity of Heteroantisera to Human Acute Leukemia–Associated Antigens;" Viza, Davies, and Harris, "Solubilization and Partial Purification of Human Leukemic Specific Antigens."

152. For a review of this work, see R. Harris, "Leukemia Antigens and Immunity in Man." Remember that, for clinicians, cancer antigens were a good thing. If they were leukemia-specific, then a therapeutic possibility opened up: "absorbed heteroantisera with defined specificity might be used for passive immunotherapy of acute leukemia with more success than past trials of less specific antisera" (Baker, Ramachandar, and Taub. "Specificity of Heteroantisera to Human Acute Leukemia–Associated Antigens," 1277). According to Pegrum ("Leukaemic Antigens," 1), "The identification and characterization of specific leukemia antigens is essential if any rational immunotherapeutic measures are to be instituted in the treatment of the condition."

153. Our emphasis. Greaves, *Biology of Acute Lymphoblastic Leukaemia,* 15.

154. Old, "Cancer Immunology," 193.

155. Salmon and Seligmann, "B-Cell Neoplasia in Man."

156. Greaves, "An Immunological Window on Leukemia," 57–8; Greaves, *Biology of Acute Lymphoblastic Leukaemia,* 15–16.

157. Greaves, "An Immunological Window on Leukemia," 59.

158. Seligmann, *Lymphocyte Membrane Markers in Human Leukaemias and Lymphoma,* 19.

159. Ibid., 5.

160. Greaves, Janossy, and Doenhoff, "Selective Triggering of Human T and B Lymphocytes in Vitro by Polyclonal Mitogens." On p. 2, one reads: "We have studied the response capacity of T and B lymphocytes to a variety of lectins and other polyclonal stimulants when cultured as purified cell populations or alternatively when cultured as mixed T-B lymphocyte populations. The identity of the 'starting'-cell populations and the activated lymphocytes has been carefully established using a panel of seven discriminatory cell surface markers."

161. Janossy and Greaves, "Lymphocyte Activation 1. Response of T and B Lymphocytes to Phytomitogens," 484.

162. Greaves, "Clinical Applications of Cell Surface Markers," 258.

163. Ibid.

164. Brown et al., "Expression of Human T and B Lymphocyte Cell-Surface Markers on Leukaemic Cells," 753.

165. Ibid., 755.

166. The panel also turned up biological anomalies; one patient with CLL lacked receptors for all seven markers. Was this indicative of the existence of a hitherto undetected normal stage in the development of B and T cells? The answer was, for now, unknown. Ibid.

167. Ibid., 753. For a summary of the pre-1975 Seligmann's results, see Seligmann, *Lymphocyte Membrane Markers in Human Leukaemias and Lymphoma.*

168. Ibid., 22.

169. Ibid., 21–2: "It is possible that these non-T non-B ALL cells do not involve the lymphoid differentiation pathway. However, the involvement of lymphoid stem cells devoid of markers of mature lymphocytes or the occurrence of surface changes preventing the identification of the blast cells are more likely."

170. Greaves, "An Immunological Window on Leukemia." The reason why the experiment should not have worked is that Greaves himself, while working in Sweden with Möller, had published an article showing the immunosuppressive effect of antibodies.

171. For instance, he could get access to frozen leukemia blood samples maintained at St. Bartholomew's Hospital in the other ICRF extramural units, the MOU concurrently established with the TIU. Not only did Greaves obtain frozen leukemia blood samples from the MOU, but, in return, he collaborated with them by mobilizing his marker technology in the clinical testing of a new classification of lymphomas. Another important source of patient blood, this time from children, was the Institute of Child Health at the London Children's Hospital, where the anti-ALL serum was used to follow patients through from presentation, remission, and relapse. *ICRF Scientific Report* 1973, 120–1.

172. Brown, Capellaro, and Greaves, "Leukemia-Associated Antigens in Man"; Brown, Hogg, and Greaves, "Candidate Leukemia-Specific Antigen in Man." In the 1973 *ICRF Scientific Report,* 120, the project is described as an "attempt to identify leukaemia-specific markers" and talk by Greaves of "cancer specific antigens" appears in a report as late as 1976 (1976 *ICRF Scientific Report,* 136). We would agree, however, that terminology in scientific reports tends to be more "sloppy" than in published articles; scientific reports, on the other hand, allow one to draw a close chronology, as opposed to articles, with their notorious publication delays.

173. Brown, Hogg, and Greaves, "Candidate Leukemia-Specific Antigen in Man", 454.

174. Brown, Capellaro, and Greaves, "Leukemia-Associated Antigens in Man," 1281.

175. "Identification, Enumeration, and Isolation of Band T Lymphocytes from Human Peripheral Blood"; Seligmann, *Lymphocyte Membrane Markers in Human Leukaemias and Lymphoma,* 7. There is no space in this chapter to report on the development of fluorescence microscopy as a tool. According to standard historical accounts, a new era in this field began in 1941 when Coons and colleagues in the United States pioneered the use of fluorescence-tagged antibodies to detect antigens, a technique leading to the subsequent development of immunohistology. See Missmahl, "Fluoreszenzmikroskopie," 63–79; for the original contributions, see Coons, Creech, and Jones, "Immunological Properties of an Antibody Containing a Fluorescent Group," 200; Coons, "Fluorescent Antibodies as Histochemical Tools," 558.

176. In recent times, there have been attempts to open microscope slide examination to collegial inspection by resorting to telemedicine, i.e., the electronic circulation of morphological images. The French hematologist Georges Flandrin, a member of the French-American-British (FAB) team who is involved in the development of such a system, explained that previous practices were often characterized by esoteric discussions without direct confrontation with morphological visual information, and that the latter was also of doubtful value in the absence of systematic and timely reviews of the visual evidence. Collegial inspection as made possible by telemedicine should result, in his view, in an increase in scientific credibility (interview with Georges Flandrin, Paris, 7 November 1996).

177. Interview with Martin C. Raff, London, 2 June 1999. Mitchison and Raff did not know what to do with it and felt guilty for not using such an expensive machine. Raff was relieved when Greaves left with it.

178. *ICRF Scientific Report* 1974, 146.

179. Interview with Melvyn F. Greaves, 2 July 1996.

180. Ibid.; see also Greaves, "An Immunological Window on Leukemia," 59–60. Schlossman, however, did claim he had used the microscope: "Whereas Greaves and Janossy et al. have reported that cALLA-positive cells are present in fetal and regenerating bone marrow, we have been unable to demonstrate similar reactivity with monoclonal J-5 *using both the FACS-1 and fluorescence microscopy*" (Ritz et al., "A Monoclonal Antibody to Human Acute Lymphoblastic Leukemia Antigen," 585; our emphasis). It should be noted that Greaves considered Schlossman's laboratory at the Dana Farber Cancer Center in Boston as the main player (and thus competitor) on the U.S. side for lymphocyte markers. The debate between the two laboratories encapsulated issues such as the concept of rare cell types and the cellular origins of leukemia, and continues today at the level of molecular genetics (Melvyn Greaves, personal communication, 6 March 2000).

181. Interview with Melvyn F. Greaves, 2 July 1996.

182. *ICRF Scientific Report* 1975, 144.

183. Interview with George Janossy, London, 6 May 1999.

184. *ICRF Scientific Report* 1976, 136.

Chapter 5

1. Austoker, *A History of the Imperial Cancer Research Fund*, 303–304. This is almost exactly the same formulation used by Greaves in the 1979–1980 *ICRF Scientific Report*, 143.

2. Fleisher, "Introduction to Diagnostic Laboratory Immunology," 1826. See also Lopez, Fleisher, and deShazo, "Use and Interpretation of Diagnostic Immunologic Laboratory Tests," 2976.

3. Janossy in Hungary was a member of a team that, under the pioneering lead of Dr. G. Petranyi at the University Radiology Clinic (Head: Prof. Z. Zsebok) and soon at the National Blood Centre (Head: Prof. Z. Hollan) in Budapest, had established the then novel branch of cellular and transplantation immunology under the inspiration of the famous Czech school of M. Hasek and his pupils, the Ivanyi brothers.

4. Janossy, *Polyclonal Activation of Murine and Human T and B Lymphocytes.*

5. Greaves, "An Immunological Window on Leukemia," 56.

6. Report on MRC grant G84178330 (grant holder: G. Janossy) (1994).

7. The network implicated hematology departments participating in the MRC UKALL chemotherapy trials, as well as a series of key London institutions. These included the Royal Marsden Hospital, the ICRF Medical Oncology Unit (MOU), and the hematology department at St. Bartholomew's Hospital, the Institute of Child Health (ICH), the University College Hospital, the Royal Free Hospital, and the Royal Postgraduate Medical School.

8. As already mentioned, the French collaborator in this endeavor was not Seligmann but Claude Rosenfeld from the Villejuif cancer research center.

9. For a history of the cell lines, see Drexler and Minowada, "History and Classification of Human Leukemia-Lymphoma Cell Lines."

10. Interview with Claude Rosenfeld, Paris, 12 January 1997.

11. Such as terminal deoxynucleotidyl transferase, myeloperoxidase and, subsequently, the rearrangements of immunoglobulin and T cell receptor genes.

12. While CML, and its blast transformations, involve the Philadelphia chromosome in their pathology, typical cases of ALL are Philadelphia negative.

13. Janossy et al., "Membrane Marker and Cell Separation Studies in Ph^1 Positive Leukemia."

14. On the growing role of prognosis, see Christakis, *Death Foretold.*

15. Brouet, "Marqueurs immunologiques des leucémies."

16. For the admittedly different, yet comparable case of graft survival curves, see Guttmann, "The Graft Survival Curve: Ideology and Rhetoric". On survival curves, see also Samet, "Concepts of Time in Clinical Research."

17. Brouet et al., "Immunological Classification of Acute Lymphoblastic Leukemias."

18. Chessels et al., "Acute Lymphoblastic Leukaemia in Children," 1309.

19. Ibid.

20. *ICRF Scientific Report* 1978, 117.

21. Greaves et al., "Immunologically Defined Subclasses of Acute Lymphocytic Leukaemia in Children," 194.

22. Ibid., 179.

23. Greaves, "Subtypes of Acute Lymphoblastic Leukemia: Implications for the Pathogenesis and Epidemiology of Leukemia," 130.

24. Greaves et al., "Immunologically Defined Subclasses," 194. Greaves presented this same argument at a conference organized by the National Cancer Institute in March of 1980 entitled "Cell Markers in Acute Leukemia." The con-

ference brought together a number of groups working on the IPT of leukemia. In the introduction to the papers presented at the conference, it is asserted that "It is now recognized that phenotypic description of cell populations can be correlated with clinical behavior, thereby aiding in the development of successful treatment strategies" (Ungeleider, "Introduction to the Conference on Cell Markers in Acute Leukemia," 4751).

25. All of this, of course, is intended to improve therapy for ALL in children. By 1987, long-term remission or probable cure was expected in 50% of cases (Pinkel, "Curing Children of Leukemia"). Presently, the probability of extended remission or cure is approximately 80%. Pinkel, along with Sidney Farber, was one of the initiators of the new chemotherapy for cancer in the 1950s. See Farber et al., "Advances in Chemotherapy of Cancer in Man." Reviewing the situation in 1987, Pinkel felt that IPT had improved therapy. Note, however, how the immunophenotypes are 'retranslated' into anatomy: "The significance of immunophenotypic classification of ALL was twofold. It confirmed the impression that childhood non-Hodgkin's lymphoma is a phase of ALL, most often T-cell ALL if the lymphoma is thoracic and most often B-cell ALL if the lymphoma is abdominal. As previously suspected, childhood non-Hodgkin's lymphoma is best treated by methods found successful for ALL. The other significance of immunophenotype for treatment of ALL was in the selection, combination, and dosage schedule of antileukemia drugs. Based on laboratory and clinical observations, both T-cell and B-cell ALL are now treated differently than early pre-B ALL" (Pinkel, "Curing Children of Leukemia," 1684).

26. Interview with Melvyn F. Greaves, London, 2 July 1996. An example of how one can maintain that IPT has prognostic implications, while admitting that more traditional parameters have higher prognostic value, can be seen in the statement by Gomez and colleagues that "multivariate analysis showed that [age], together with FAB morphology and WBC counts were the best combination of parameters for predicting survival. . . . although the immunophenotype helps us in understanding the biological heterogeneity of ALL, having also prognostic implications, there are other clinical and hematological features that yield stronger prognostic information." See Gomez et al., "The Value of the Immunological Subtypes and Individual Markers Compared to Classical Parameters in the Prognosis of Acute Lymphoblastic Leukemia," 33.

27. On the notion of "self-vindication," see Hacking, "The Self-Vindication of the Laboratory Sciences."

28. In spite of the official-sounding name, the formulation of the FAB classification was not the result of a high-level meeting between representatives of the three countries, but, rather, a spontaneous initiative of a small group of medical researchers from those countries. The acronym itself (FAB) was apparently chosen during a taxi ride when one of the researchers, in a moment of unrestricted enthusiasm at the end of the working day, exclaimed "It's fab!" (interview with Georges Flandrin, Paris, 7 November 1996). We mention this anecdote to point out that, far from there being a unique, bureaucratic path to the establishment of biomedical classifications, there can be several, ranging from the

formal to the informal. For the FAB proposal, see Bennett et al., "Proposals for the Classification of the Acute Leukaemias."

29. They were able to achieve 85% degree of uniformity in a final exchange of slides. This rate of agreement was not always to be reached by other users of the FAB classification. As with other morphological classifications, its application continued to be characterized by "observer subjectivity" and "interobserver variability"; see, e.g., Dick, Armitage, and Burns, "Diagnostic Concurrence in the Subclassification of ALL Using FAB Criteria"; Head et al., "Reproducibility of the FAB Classification of Acute Leukemia." The proposed classification was based on the classic characteristics. The two large groups ("lymphoblastic" and "myeloid") were respectively divided into three (L1–L3) and six (M1–M6) subgroups based on morphological and staining characteristics. Whether or not the lymphoblastic leukemias were indeed lymphoblasts was the subject of subsequent discussions. As the formulators of the classification admitted, it was more a matter of tradition than a matter of visibility: "Thus three broad divisions of undifferentiated non-myeloid blast-cell leukemias emerged. Because the majority fell into the first group of childhood leukemia, traditionally called lymphoblastic, this term was retained for the whole group, although in nearly three quarters of all patients specific evidence of lymphocytic characteristics was lacking" (Gralnick et al., "Classification of Acute Leukemia," 741). For a short discussion of the FAB classification, see Debru, *Philosophie de l'inconnu,* 283–6.

30. Bennett et al., "Proposals for the Classification of the Acute Leukemias."

31. See, e.g., Bennett et al., "Proposed Revised Criteria for the Classification of Acute Myeloid Leukemia." See also interview with Georges Flandrin, Paris, 7 November 1996: "We adapted FAB, we published eight or ten revisions, we permanently modulated, we kept the acronym and modulated." Members of the FAB group participated in a further classificatory endeavor aimed at combining morphological, immunological, and cytogenetic parameters and known as the MIC working classification. See First MIC Cooperative Study Group. "Morphologic, Immunologic, and Cytogenetic (MIC) Working Classification of Acute Lymphoblastic Leukemias"; Second MIC Cooperative Study Group. "Morphologic, Immunologic, and Cytogenetic (MIC) Working Classification of the Acute Myeloid Leukaemias."

32. Interviews with George Janossy, London, 27 April and May 6 1999.

33. These summary papers include Greaves, "Recent Progress in the Immunological Characterization of Leukemic Cells"; Greaves, "Clinical Applications of Cell Surface Markers"; Greaves, Brown, and Hayward, "A Panel of Markers for Human Lymphocyte Subpopulations."

34. Greaves et al., "Exploitation of Monoclonal Antibodies," 271.

35. Ibid.

36. *ICRF Scientific Report* 1974, 146.

37. *ICRF Scientific Report* 1978, 117.

38. W. E. Paul, *Membrane Immunology Laboratory* (29 September 1980). ICRF Archives.

39. For a detailed analysis of the development of monoclonal antibodies, including a discussion of their standardizing consequences, see Cambrosio and Keating, *Exquisite Specificity*.

40. Abbas, Lichtman, and Pober, *Cellular and Molecular Immunology*, 19.

41. Cambrosio and Keating, "A Matter of FACS."

42. G. Klein, *Quinquennial Review 1980. Report on Membrane Immunology Laboratory*, ICRF Archives.

43. W. E. Paul, *Membrane Immunology Laboratory* (29 September 1980), ICRF Archives.

44. The search for the elusive stem cell is a fascinating chapter in modern biomedical research, which cannot be explored here, but see Lajtha, *Stem Cells*.

45. According to Wintrobe, "Greaves has proposed, in the context of acute leukemias, that the normal cell surface phenotype of stem cells and progenitors is perfectly compatible with malignant behavior provided the neoplastic lesion results in a subtle uncoupling of proliferation and maturation" (*Wintrobe, Hematology: The Blossoming of a Science*, 481). As previously noted, the maturation perspective had also been proposed by Seligmann.

46. Janossy et al., "Use of the Fluorescence Activated Cell Sorter in Human Leukaemia," 111.

47. Greaves, "'Target' Cells, Cellular Phenotypes, and Lineage Fidelity in Human Leukaemia," 113.

48. Greaves et al., "Exploitation of Monoclonal Antibodies," 273.

49. Pinkel, "Curing Children of Leukemia," 1683.

50. Greaves et al., "Exploitation of Monoclonal Antibodies," 272.

51. Greaves et al., "Lineage Promiscuity in Hemopoietic Differentiation and Leukemia," 2–4.

52. Greaves, "An Immunological Window on Leukemia," 59.

53. This is not exactly what we were told in 1989: "Leukemic cells have composite immunophenotypes that are asynchronous with respect to normal developmental stages rather than identical, which is not surprising once it is appreciated that the disorder arises from the uncoupling of proliferation and differentiation rather than the imposition of a blunt ended maturation arrest or freezing" (Greaves, "An Immunological Window on Leukemia," 57–8). The latest consensus document produced by the National Committee for Clinical Laboratory Standards has decided that "aberrant" cells do exist: "The central concept that underlies leukemia immunophenotyping is that leukemic cells

express cell surface antigens that are related to normal cells of a particular lineage and that these antigens can be detected with appropriate antibodies. It is important to note, however, that leukemia cells may exhibit aberrant or unusual patterns of cell surface antigen expression that are different from those of normal circulating blood or bone marrow cells" (National Committee for Clinical Laboratory Standards, *Clinical Applications of Flow Cytometry: Immunophenotyping of Leukemic Cells; Proposed Guideline*, 23). The "may" does not, however, deny the fact that such cases are rare.

54. Interviews with George Janossy, London, 27 April and 6 May 1999; interview with Martin C. Raff, London, 2 June 1999.

55. Greaves, "Molecular Phenotypes," 37.

56. Catovsky et al., "Multiparameter Studies in Lymphoid Leukemias," 736.

57. Greaves et al., "Biological Diversity of Acute Lymphoblastic Leukemia," 107. The shift to molecular biology was, of course, not limited to leukemia research. In 1988, for instance, Gus Nossal reported: "Before the 1980s, cell signaling was conceived mainly in terms of cell surface ligands, membrane receptors and cellular differentiation. During the 1980s, a whole new literature has developed which goes more directly to the nucleus of the stimulated cell. . . . As a result, immunology now finds itself within the mainstream of classical molecular biology" (Nossal, "Triumphs and Trials of Immunology in the 1980s," 288). On the molecularization of immunology, see Podolsky and Tauber, *The Generation of Diversity*.

58. Greaves, "'Target' Cells," 115.

59. Greaves, "Regulation of Cell-Surface Structures in Malignancy, Differentiation and Proliferation," 532.

60. Greaves, Pegram, and Chan, "Collaborative Group Study of the Epidemiology of Acute Lymphoblastic Leukaemia Subtypes," 716.

61. Interview with Melvyn F. Greaves, 2 July 1996.

62. Ibid.

63. See Podolsky and Tauber, *The Generation of Diversity*.

64. W. F. Bodmer, "Introduction to the Scientific Report," *ICRF Scientific Report* 1979, 1–6, on p. 2. The reader will have noted Bodmer's mention of "specific tumour-associated cell surface changes" that conflates the two notions of tumour-associated and tumour-specific antigens.

65. Ibid., 5.

66. For an in-house history of the LRF, see Piller, *Rays of Hope*.

67. For instance, at the first meeting of the LRF executive committee in 1962, the president and chairman drew "attention to the fact that clause 7 of the memorandum of the Fund stated that if a cure for leukaemia were found and the

Fund was no longer necessary," any property of the LRF would be given to other charities. Similarly, when the LRF Chair of Haematological Medicine was established in 1968 at Cambridge, the university assured the LRF that "if a cure for leukemia were found before the termination of the [20-year] endowment," discussions between LRF and the university would take place to decide use of the unexpended endowment (Piller, *Rays of Hope*, 14, 21–2).

68. Ibid., 31.

69. For instance, at a 1979 meeting of the Medical Advisory Panel, "the Panel considered papers from Professor Williamson, Dr. Greaves and Dr. Janet containing proposals for the Fund's further involvement in basic scientific work." LRF, *Minutes MAP*, 24 May 1979.

70. LRF, *Minutes MSAP*, 16 October 1979.

71. Piller, "The Molecular and Cellular Basis of Human Leukaemias," Report to the LRF executive council, November 1982. The Leeds world summit meeting was co-organized by the LRF and the National Cancer Institute in October 1981. A verbatim transcription of the proceedings is to be found in the LRF Archives. The meeting was attended by Greaves who used this opportunity to energetically present and defend his etiologic understanding of leukemia.

72. Piller, *Rays of Hope*, 20; LRF, *Minutes MAP*: report on a meeting of a subcommittee of the MAP on "How to Further Leukaemia Research?" 24 October 1962.

73. LRF, *Minutes MSAP*, 3 June 1982, 11 November 1982, 21 February 1983, 13 June 1983, 17 October 1983, 5 June 1984; Piller, *Rays of Hope*, 61.

74. Piller, *Rays of Hope*, 60; *Minutes MSAP*, 26 February 1985.

75. LRF, *Minutes MSAP*, 11 November 1985.

76. LRF, *Minutes MSAP*, 3 March 1986, 3 November 1986.

77. *Quinquennial Review: 1980. Membrane Immunology Laboratory. Dr. M. F. Greaves.* ICRF Archives.

78. Melvyn Greaves, personal communication, 6 March 2000.

79. Greaves to Robin Weiss [day missing] December 1985, with copy sent to Piller asking for comments. LRF Archives. Loose documents in the folder box. An appendix on the above-mentioned collaborations included the following items: development of a computer program for the differential diagnosis of leukemia using immunological and molecular phenotypic data sets, application of multiparameter flow cytometry to leukemia diagnosis, with reagents and machine provided by Becton-Dickinson; international collaborative study group on the etiology of ALL.

80. Piller to Greaves, 11 December 1985, LRF Archives. The term "stamp collecting" refers to the mere collection of repetitive data or, in other words, data whose heuristic potential has been exhausted. Speaking in 1996 of IPT, Greaves

noted, "I think there still is a case clinically for knowing what sort of leukemia you've got in [IPT] terms because it can have an influence on the choice of therapy and so on. If you're saying I want to put a lot of effort into this and to refine the classification, then there's not a very good case and there's certainly a much stronger case for saying the real action is really going to be in the molecular genetics and the biochemistry of gene products, for sure, so, you know, stamp collecting—it's a bit unkind—but there's an element of truth in that. . . . The business of just classifying and subclassifying into finer and finer cell groups is just a few dotting the i's and crossing the t's. . . . There's plenty of people still doing that who have their meetings and so on and I think it's very boring" (interview with Melvyn F. Greaves, London, 2 July 1996).

81. Greaves to Piller, 13 December 1985. LRF Archives.

82. Greaves to Piller, 5 November 1986. LRF Archives (Folder: LRF Centre at the Institute of Cancer Research (ICR) pre-1988).

83. Chessels to Greaves, 6 November 1986. LRF Archives.

84. Report on the site visit to the LRF Centre at the ICR, University of London 1 February 1988, LRF Archives. The situation, as far as adult material was concerned, was improving. In 1988 at the ICR of the Royal Marsden Hospital (the same institution where Greaves's center was located), a new department was established, headed by Daniel Catovsky, who had been working previously at the Royal Postgraduate Medical School with David Galton, a major figure in leukemia clinical trials. The new department's main goal was cell characterization of acute and chronic leukemia by means of monoclonal antibodies, electron microscopy, chromosome studies, and DNA analyses, in order to define distinct disease entities showing different responses to specific kinds of treatment (Folder: LRF Centre at ICR, 1990–1; Annual Report 1989–90, ICR). Greaves was pleased by Catovsky's move, since he was hoping that the work of markers for leukemia diagnosis would be taken over by the new department (Folder: Mel [sic] site visit 1988. Report on the site visit to the LRF centre at the ICR, University of London, on 1 February 1988). In a 1989 letter discussing the recent addition to the ICR of the Royal Marsden Hospital of an academic unit of hematology under Catovsky, an observer commented that the latter was "doing a fine job and ha[d] already found his way to Mel Greaves's lab." McVie, director of the scientific department of the Cancer Research Campaign, to Piller, 5 February 1989. LRF Archives (Folder: LRF Centre at the ICR 1989–90).

85. Greaves to Piller, 3 March 1989 (Folder: LRF Centre at the ICR 1989–90).

86. G. Janossy, *The Immunological Diagnosis and Intraclonal Heterogeneity of Adult Lymphoblastic Leukaemia (ALL)* (application for a project grant, 1987), FD23/4088 S1101/119 *Committee on Leukaemia, TdT Antibodies,* MRC/HOA.

87. The 1984 steering committee of the Working Party on Leukaemia consisted of thirty-six members (including Greaves), plus two members from the leukaemia trials office and three members from the MRC head office; see *Com-*

mittee on Leukaemia, Working Party on Leukaemia in Childhood Meeting (6 February 1984), MRC/HOA, FD23/4068 S1101/103.

88. Committee on Leukaemia, Working Party on Leukaemia in Childhood Meeting (6 February 1984). *Minutes of the Meeting Held on Monday 6 February 1984,* MRC/HOA FD23/4068 S1101/103.

89. *Guide to Leukaemia Immunophenotyping with Monoclonal Antibodies. Compiled by Membrane Immunology Laboratory (ICRF London) in collaboration with Laboratory Impex (B-D)* (June 1984), MRC/HOA FD23/4068 S1101/103. The central section of the document focused on the B-D IPT panel (the set of seven antibodies then available from that company) but it also included a table listing the corresponding reagents from other sources that were defined as "comparable" and "similar." Interestingly enough, the table ended with the following warning: "For research only. Not for use in human diagnostic or therapeutic procedures," which, in a sense, shows the hybrid nature of clinical trials, since the reagents would be used for human diagnostic purposes albeit within a clinical research framework.

90. MRC, *Ad Hoc Meeting of the Working Group to Discuss Immunotyping in Childhood Leukaemia* (4 June 1986), FD23/4088 S1101/119, Committee on Leukaemia, TdT Antibodies, MRC/HOA.

91. MRC. Cell (October 1984). *Prof. G. Janossy. The Immunological Diagnosis and Intraclonal Heterogeneity of Adult Lymphoblastic Leaukaemia (ALL). Application for Extension of Special Project Grant Support*; MRC. Cell (October 1987); *Prof. G. Janossy. The Immunological Diagnosis and Intraclonal Heterogeneity of Adult Lymphoblastic Leukaemia (ALL). Application of Renewal of Special Project Grant Support*; FD23/4088 S1101/119 Committee on Leukaemia, TdT Antibodies; MRC/HOA.

92. See the letters exchanged in *Grants Prof. G. Janossy,* vol. 1, FD10/858 G84 17830; *Grants Prof. G. Janossy,* vol. 2, FD10/859 G84 17830, MRC/HOA. For an analysis of the rewriting strategies of scientists, see Myers, *Writing Biology.*

93. For details about these workshops, see *Practical Aspects of Leukaemia Typing for UKALL Trials* (1986), FD23/4088 S1101/119, Committee on Leukaemia, TdT Antibodies; MRC UKALL-X; *Technical Suggestions for Standardising Immuno-Diagnosis* (1987), FD23/4088 S1101/119, Committee on Leukaemia, TdT Antibodies; Committee on Leukaemia, *Immunophenotyping Workshops,* 3 October 1988 (re: UKALL XI Trial), FD23/4129 S1101/163, MRC/HOA.

94. *MRC UKALL-X. Technical Suggestions for Standardising Immunodiagnosis.* Immunology Department, Royal Free Hospital (1.10.1987), FD23/4088 S1101/119, Committee on Leukaemia, TdT Antibodies, MRC/HOA. An approach developed in Janossy's laboratory (the microplate assay) was presented as a method of choice for laboratories that did not have expertise in cell-marker analysis; see Campana and Janossy, "Leukemia Diagnosis and Testing of Complement-Fixing Antibodies for Bone Marrow Purging in Acute Lymphoid Leukemia."

95. Judith Chessels to Janossy (29 February 1988), Chessels to Jean Mossman (11 March 1988), Mossman to Chessels (21 March 1988), FD23/4088 S1101/119, Committee on Leukaemia, TdT Antibodies, MRC/HOA. Researchers not performing the assay or showing unreliable performance were further to be invited to attend one of the workshops and given the chance of performing the test at the bench.

96. Ibid. The Royal Free Hospital produced a whole range of monoclonal antibodies to T, B, and accessory cells. The distribution of reagents to laboratories involved in the MRC UKALL trials raised the question of whether this resulted in unfair competition to commercial companies. A solution to this problem was found in the use of an agreement form, stating that reagents provided by Janossy's laboratory were only to be used by nonprofit institutions for their own research work; see Janossy to Jean Mossman (4 February 1988) and Stephen D. Thornton to Janossy (5 January 1989), FD23/4088 S1101/119, Committee on Leukaemia, TdT Antibodies, MRC/HOA.

97. Interviews with George Janossy, London, 27 April and 6 May 1999; George Janossy, personal communication, 22 February 2000. Greaves's attitude was shared by other researchers involved in the MRC trials, who also felt that small individual units should not be encouraged to do their own assays, since this would result in problems of standardization and of interpretation of results; see C. S. Scott to Dianne Duston (25 March 1985), FD23/4088 S1101/119 *Committee on Leukaemia, TdT Antibodies,* MRC/HOA. The problem is still with us, judging from a recent article asking for additional standardization of technical procedures to ensure competent performance as well as standardization of data interpretation and reporting as a remedy for the problem of clinical sense. For, "in spite of the well-established utility of immunophenotyping for the diagnosis, classification, prognostic stratification, and monitoring of hematological malignancies, only a small part of the information on the immunophenotypic characteristics of pathological hemopoietic cells has been used routinely" (Orfao et al., "Clinically Useful Information Provided by the Flow Cytometric Immunophenotyping of Hematological Malignancies," 1708).

98. For instance, data from Africa showed that "common (pre-B) ALL but not T-ALL appears to be underrepresented in black Africans," a finding that was explained away by the selective underdiagnosis caused by preemptive death from infection in young Africans. Greaves and collaborators, in fact, favored the hypothesis that the true incidence of ALL worldwide would be remarkably independent of the ethnic or genetic background of the patients and of the environmental setting. See annual report of the LRF Centre, May 1986 (Folder: LRF Centre at the ICR pre-1988. See also annual report 1988–89, ICR, 18–9 (Folder: LRF Centre at the ICR, 1990–91).

99. See, e.g., Greaves to Dr. S. Issaragrisil, Bangkok (date missing); LRF Archives. (Folder: LRF Centre at the ICR pre-1988).

100. Interview with Melvyn F. Greaves, London, 2 July 1996.

101. The project seems to have been short-lived given the fact that Greaves had more pressing priorities. It nonetheless resulted in a few publications; see, e.g., Alvey and Greaves, "A Computer Program for Interpreting Immunophenotypic Data as an Aid to the Diagnosis of Leukemia."

102. For an article that explicitly claims that IPT as performed by flow cytometry "can yield valuable information on cell morphology in addition to cell surface antigen expression," see Terstappen et al., "Flow Cytometric Characterization of Acute Myeloid Leukemia. Part I."

103. Five-dimensional flow cytometry as used by Janossy was developed by Loken and Terstappen who have direct links with Becton Dickinson, the commercial producer of the FACS; see Terstappen and Loken, "Five-Dimensional Flow Cytometry as a New Approach for Blood and Bone Marrow Differentials."

104. Interview with William Gutierrez, Hialeah, Fla., 7 May 1996. And he added, "we don't see an end to the number of colors, the number of parameters, all we're seeing is that you're putting more and more capability in a smaller and smaller box and trying to keep costs down, and making it all more user friendly, more automated."

105. For a recent assessment of work conducted as part of the concerted action, see Lucio et al., "Flow Cytometric Analysis of Normal B Cell Differentiation."

106. See, e.g., Terstappen et al., "Flow Cytometric Characterization of Acute Myeloid Leukemia. Part II," 70.

107. A good example of this kind of work can be found in Dario Campana's research initiated in Janossy's laboratory and later transferred to St. Jude's in Memphis. See, e.g., Campana, Coustan-Smith, and Janossy, "The Immunologic Detection of Minimal Residual Disease in Acute Leukemia"; Campana and Pui, "Detection of Minimal Residual Disease in Acute Leukemia: Methodologic Advances and Clinical Significance."

108. See, e.g., Janossy et al., "Affordable CD4(+) T-Cell Counts on 'Single Platform' Flow Cytometers."

Chapter 6

1. Moulin, "The Immune System."

2. Claman, Chaperon, and Triplett, "Thymus-Marrow Cell Combinations." It is true that it is an anachronism to speak of T-B cooperation in 1966. Claman and coworkers, however, had just recently come across in the clinic what was to be named the T-B distinction. See Fulginiti et al., "Dissociation of Delayed-Hypersensitivity and Antibody Synthesizing Capacities in Man." For reasons we do not understand, Silverstein lists the work of Claman and colleagues under the heading of "T cell subsets." Under this same heading, he also places Mitchell

and Miller, "Cell to Cell Interaction in the Immune Response." From the title alone, it looks more like a paper on T-B cooperation in antibody production.

3. Gershon and Kondo, "Cell Interactions in the Induction of Tolerance."

4. It was, of course, possible to use both. In a paper describing the "recovery of helper cell function" through a particular assay, the authors go on to describe how to "assay for cooperators." See Julius, Simpson, and Herzenberg, "A Rapid Method for the Isolation of Functional Thymus-Derived Murine Lymphocytes," 648.

5. Interview with Stuart F. Schlossman, Boston, 20 September 1988.

6. Cantor and Boyse, "Functional Subclasses of T Lymphocytes Bearing Different Ly Antigens. I."

7. As Boyse put it: "Both their [the antigens'] presence and retention are difficult to explain because, in many experimental situations, and possibly also in nature, these antigens enable the immune surveillance mechanism to pick off small colonies before they can grow out" (Boyse, "The Invitation to Surveillance," 26–7).

8. Ibid., 27.

9. See the illustration in Raff, "Cell-Surface Immunology," 36.

10. Preud'homme and Seligmann, "Immunoglobulins on the Surface of Lymphoid Cells in Waldenström's Macroglobulinemia." Shortly after Raff's work and following directly from it, Eva Klein, Bo Johansson, and their associates at the Karolinska Institute in Stockholm claimed that "fluorescence staining showed an unevenly distributed pattern, so that the density of the immunoglobulin structures is probably different on different parts of the cell surface" (Eva Klein et al., "Surface Immunoglobulin-Moieties on Lymphoid Cells," 146–7).

11. Koo et al., "Topographical Location of H-Y Antigen on Mouse Spermatozoa by Immunoelectronmicroscopy," 1505. For further examples of attempts to correlate distribution of antibody on the cell surface and function, see Rabellino et al., "Immunoglobulins on the Surface of Lymphocytes I," and Grey, Rabellino, and Priofsky, "Immunoglobulins on the Surface of Lymphocytes IV."

12. Pernis, Forni, and Amante, "Immunoglobulins as Cell Receptors," 427.

13. Cantor, Asofsky, and Talal, "Synergy among Lymphoid Cells Mediating the Graft-versus-Host Response I."

14. Cantor and his associates concluded that old, sick cells "can be rendered immunologically more reactive in the presence of a normally reactive population" (ibid., 233).

15. Cantor and Asofsky, "Synergy among Lymphoid Cells Mediating the Graft-versus-Host Response II," 243: "The observations may be explained by postulating that at least two cell types are required to mediate GVH reactions."

16. Interview with Harvey Cantor, Boston, 1 May 1992.

17. Raff and Cantor, "Subpopulations of Thymus Cells and Thymus-Derived Lymphocytes," 86.

18. Ibid., 90.

19. See Raff, "Selective Removal of Lymphocyte Populations," 79. It should be noted that Raff generously described their relative roles in the work as follows: "The model that I want to tell you about is largely the work and ideas of Harvey Cantor. My contribution has been relatively minor."

20. Ibid., 84. There was, course, no T3 in the model presented by Raff. It had emerged in the course of the discussion when Benacerraf objected that, in the model, there was no reason for the process leading from T1 to T2 to stop there; therefore, why not T3? Raff replied: "Please don't ask questions like that" (ibid., 81).

21. Raff and Cantor, "Subpopulations of Thymus Cells," 92.

22. Ibid., 90. In the book on immunological intervention, there is an interesting diagram. The caption reads: "Fig. 21 Failure to remove 'helper' activity (T cells) from 'anti-BSA'-spleen cells by filtration through a column coated with anti-mouse Ig"; see Raff, "Selective Removal," 87.

23. Kisielow et al., "Ly Antigens as Markers for Functionally Distinct Subpopulations of Thymus-Derived Lymphocytes of the Mouse," 219.

24. Shiku et al., "Expression of T-Cell Differentiation Antigens on Effector Cells in Cell-Mediated Cytotoxicity in Vitro," 239.

25. Raff, "Selective Removal," 96.

26. For a review of work done by the Herzenberg group up to October 1973, see Julius et al., "Fluorescence-Activated Cell Sorting and Its Applications"; similarly, see Hulett et al., "Development and Application of a Rapid Cell Sorter." For a review of methods used to isolate lymphocyte subsets prior to the use of FACS and monoclonal antibodies, see Chess and Schlossman, "Methods for the Separation of Unique Human Lymphocyte Subpopulations."

27. Loken and Herzenberg, "Analysis of Cell Populations with a Fluorescence-Activated Cell Sorter,"163.

28. These experiments thus recapitulated research using conventional methods, for it was known that the antibody used (the Thy antibody), even though absorbed in differing amounts by different functional types of T cells, ultimately reacted with all T cells. Leonard A. Herzenberg, grant application to the Dept. of Health, Education, and Welfare, U.S. Public Health Service, GM 17367-07-11, (1975), 43.

29. Raff, "Selective Removal," 96–8; Julius et al., "Fluorescence-Activated Cell Sorting."

30. The new system gave this result: "Our findings indicate that separated subpopulations of splenic T cells interact synergistically in the *in vitro* generation of cytotoxicity" (Cantor et al., "Characterization of Subpopulations of T Lymphocytes I," 195). As findings, they did not differ greatly from Cantor and Asofsky's conclusions five years earlier.

31. Herzenberg laid out two lines of research in 1975 to improve the resolution of the FACS with regard to lymphocytes. First, following technology developments at Los Alamos, he decided to extend the use of the physical parameter known as light scatter as a cell marker in order to be able to "subfractionate the small lymphocytes [T cells] according to their refractive indices" (Herzenberg, grant application to the Dept. of Health, Education, and Welfare, U.S. Public Health Service, GM 17367-07-11, (1975), 38). This would have constituted cell separation according to physical characteristics as opposed to biological characteristics. The second approach called for the development of a larger number of fluorochromes. Herzenberg proposed, in effect, that a combination of these two techniques would lead to the "identification of various types of regulatory T cells and T cell subpopulations defined and separated by the FACS on the basis of immunofluorescence and light scattering characteristics" (Herzenberg, grant application, 44).

32. Cantor and Boyse, "Functional Subclasses of T Lymphocytes Bearing Different Ly Antigens," 1378.

33. As we made clear earlier, the mouse/human distinction is not synonymous with, and in fact cuts across, the normal/pathological distinction.

34. Interview with Stuart F. Schlossman, Cambridge, Mass., 30 April 1992.

35. On inbred mice as research material, see Löwy and Gaudillière, "Disciplining Cancer."

36. Interview with Stuart F. Schlossman, Cambridge, Mass., 30 April 1992. Pathologists sending samples would get, in return, antibodies; the situation changed when flow cytometry companies began selling machines and the related antibody reagents: pathologists could now perform their own analyses and charge for them; as a result, the flow of samples dried up.

37. In 1983 Emil T. Frei shared with Emil J. Freireich the General Motors Kettering Award for cancer research. According to the GM news release: "These researchers, working together for 17 years, developed the first treatment for leukemia that truly cured patients. In the process, they established nearly all the principles of scientific chemotherapy trials for cancers of all kinds" ("Frei, Freireich Share One GM Award," 5).

38. Stuart F. Schlossman, Cancer Center Support Grant (2P02 CA06516-12), Emil T. Frei III, principal investigator, submitted September 1973, 564.

39. Ibid., 580.

40. Ibid., 695.

41. Shevach, Green, and Ellman, "Heterologous Antiserum to Thymus-Derived Cells in the Guinea-Pig."

42. Stuart F. Schlossman, Cancer Center Support Grant (2P02 CA06516-12), Emil T. Frei III, principal investigator, submitted September 1973, 567.

43. Interview with Stuart F. Schlossman, Cambridge, Mass., 30 April 1992. It is interesting to note that the "mouse researcher" Harvey Cantor, while accepting that for human T-cell subsets "the combination of mono-specific (monoclonal) antibodies and FACS-assisted analysis represented an *essential* technical development," still maintains that "reliable serological definition of murine T-cell subsets was possible before the introduction of monoclonal antibodies/FACS technology because of the development of congenic inbred mouse strains that differed only at the relevant Ly locus" (Harvey Cantor, letter to the authors, 28 June 1993).

44. Interview with Stuart F. Schlossman, Boston, 20 September 1988. The number 006 was inscribed on the apparatus.

45. Interview with Stuart F. Schlossman, Cambridge, Mass., 30 April 1992.

46. See, e.g., Chess and Schlossman, "Anti-Immunoglobulin Columns and the Separation of T, B and Null Cells."

47. Interview with Stuart F. Schlossmann, Cambridge, Mass., 30 April 1992. Note that use of the terms "CD4" and "CD8" is anachronistic.

48. Evans et al., "Detection, Isolation and Functional Characterization of Two Human T-Cell Subclasses Bearing Unique Differentiation Antigens."

49. Evans et al., "Two Functionally Distinct Subpopulations of Human T Cells."

50. Interview with Stuart F. Schlossman, Cambridge, Mass., 20 September 1988.

51. Evans et al., "Two Functionally Distinct," 1426.

52. Even within a single application of the protocol. Indeed, "in a recent experiment only one of four rabbits immunized concurrently with equal numbers of T cells from the same donor raised significant titers of antibody to TH2 antigen" (ibid., 1427).

53. See, e.g., McCaffrey et al., "Terminal Deoxynucleotidyl Transferase in Normal and Neoplastic Hematopoietic Cells;" Kung et al., "Terminal Deoxynucleotidyl Transferase in the Diagnosis of Leukemia and Malignant Lymphoma."

54. See Cambrosio and Keating, *Exquisite Specificity*, where we analyze in detail the uncertainties initially surrounding the new technique and the work that reduced that uncertainty.

55. Ironically, Schlossman had originally signed up with Ortho, mistakenly believing Ortho to be in possession of a cell bank (interview with Stuart F. Schlossman, Cambridge, Mass., 20 September 1988).

56. Herzenberg, De Rosa, and Herzenberg, "Monoclonal Antibodies and the FACS," 385.

57. Reinherz et al., "Separation of Functional Subsets of Human T Cells by a Monoclonal Antibody"; Kung et al., "Monoclonal Antibodies Defining Distinctive Human T Cell Surface Antigens"; Reinherz et al., "A Monoclonal Antibody with Selective Reactivity with Functionally Mature Human Thymocytes and All Peripheral Human T Cells." As previously noted, the Ortho group used the Cytofluorograph, a flow cytometer marketed by Ortho, for their part of the work (involving the selection and growth of hybridomas), whereas the Dana Farber group worked with the FACS (e.g., to characterize OKT reactivity): the two instruments met in the materials and methods sections of the joint papers. Shapiro tells the following story: "In 1978, Stuart Schlossman, at the Farber, began a collaboration with Ortho Diagnostics which led to the development of the first of many monoclonal antibodies reactive with cell surface antigens on human lymphoid cells. He advised his then-colleagues at Ortho to purchase a B-D FACS, the same apparatus he used for immunofluorescence flow cytometry; this advice didn't exactly thrill Lou Kamentsky and his group, then manufacturing Ortho's own flow cytometers in the Boston area. A 'gunfight at the OKT corral' was arranged, with the same samples being run on the FACS, which used a water-cooled argon laser emitting 200 mW at 488 nm, and on an Ortho FC-200, which used an air-cooled laser emitting 20 mW at 488 nm. The sensitivities of the two instruments . . . were comparable, but the results of the test never found their way into either the scientific literature or Ortho's advertising" (Shapiro, *Practical Flow Cytometry,* 3rd ed., 66).

58. According to Ortho, by binding to all T cells, OKT3 effectively shut down only part of the immune system (the T-cell compartment and not the antibody-producing B-cell compartment) and thus prevented T cell–mediated graft rejection. In 1991, Kung received the Discoverers Award from the U.S. Pharmaceutical Research and Manufacturers Association for the development of OKT3. In 1986, the FDA had approved it as the first therapeutic monoclonal antibody to treat organ transplant rejection.

59. Rosnay, *Biotechnologies et bioindustries,* and Pelissolo, *La biotechnologie, demain?*; Advisory Council for Applied Research and Development, Advisory Board for the Research Councils, The Royal Society, *Biotechnology: Report of a Joint Working Party*; Committee for Scientific and Technological Policy, *Biotechnology and Government Policies*; Government of Canada, *Biotechnology: A Development Plan for Canada*; Gouvernement du Québec, *A l'heure des biotechnologies.* For an analysis of this kind of document, see Cambrosio, Limoges, and Pronovost, "Representing Biotechnology."

60. The story is, of course, more complex; on the development of the biotech industry, see, e.g., Bud, *The Uses of Life*; Kenney, *Biotechnology: The University-Industry Complex*; on rDNA technology, see Susan Wright, "Recombinant DNA Technology and Its Social Transformations;" on hybridoma technology, see Cambrosio and Keating, *Exquisite Specificity.*

61. Antabi and Fishlock, *Biotechnology: Strategies for Life,* 76.

62. U.S. Department of Commerce, International Trade Administration, *High Technology Industries: Profiles and Outlooks: Biotechnology.*

63. Office of Technology Assessment, *Commercial Biotechnology.*

64. Scott, "Monoclonal Antibodies: Approaching Adolescence in Diagnostic Immunoassays."

65. Löwy, *Between Bench and Bedside,* 161–3. The topic of university-industry relations in the biotech era is closely analyzed in Kenney, *Biotechnology.* For a discussion of older forms of university-industry relations, see Swann, *Academic Scientists and the Pharmaceutical Industry.* For the wider, social consequences, see, e.g., Brodwin, *Biotechnology and Culture.*

66. For a criticism of the "context" trope (also known as the "container metaphor"), see, e.g., Callon and Law, "On the Construction of Sociotechnical Networks."

67. Kung was reportedly told that only eleven of the people surveyed showed an interest in buying the product, and that they were "all [his] friends" (interview with Patrick C. Kung, Cambridge, Mass., 15 July 1993).

68. Interview with Patrick C. Kung, Cambridge, Mass., 15 July 1993. The circumstances surrounding the research carried out at Ortho have also been briefly described in Shorter, *The Health Century,* 254.

69. Pambianchi, "Biotechnology Marketing Strategies." The second strategy is linked to the emergence of a series of new biotech startups such as Hybritech, Monoclonal Antibodies, and Centocor and has thus attracted a lot of media attention; the first strategy, while less fashionable, is still with us: see Deyoung, "Many Factors Must Be Weighed in Decision to Purchase Antibodies," 18.

70. With respect to the second outcome, it is interesting to note that when, in 1979, Henry Weinert, the founder of Boston Biomedical Consultants—a consulting company created two years earlier—wrote an influential assessment of the monoclonal antibody market that was acquired by over forty companies and became a key guidance document for many of them, he had first heard about monoclonal antibodies at Dana Farber (Henry Weinert, personal communication, 4 January 2001).

71. Herzenberg, De Rosa, and Herzenberg, "Monoclonal Antibodies," 384.

72. Ibid. As noted in the article, while the human eyes looking through a microscope could make the difference between background (false-positive) fluorescence and true-positive fluorescence, a flow cytometer could not perform this task: specific, painstaking immunization strategies, absorption procedures (to eliminate unwanted antibodies and contaminants), and fluorochrome-coupling procedures were needed to produce acceptable reagents for flow cytometry, and they did of course not solve the problem of laboratories using different reagents and thus producing results that were difficult to compare.

73. On "art" and "science" in the production of monoclonal antibodies, see Cambrosio and Keating, *Exquisite Specificity*, chap. 2.

74. Milstein pointed out that "The possibility that the specificity of antisera was more the result of the heterogeneity of the polyclonal response than a specific molecular recognition was discussed many times, and was the subject of a major paper presented at a meeting held only 2 years earlier. . . . So it had to be demonstrated that [monoclonal antibodies] to differentiation antigens *could* be made and that when made they did not show signs of unexpected cross-reactions"; see Milstein, "Introductory Remarks," 3.

75. Interview with Stuart F. Schlossman, Cambridge, Mass., 20 September 1988.

76. Economists of innovation speak, in this respect, of "network externalities" and of "lock-in mechanisms." For a recent overview, see Shapiro and Varian, *Information Rules*; our thanks to Jean-Paul Moatti for this reference. For a discussion of these notions in relation to scientific activities, see Callon, "Is Science a Public Good?"

77. Interview with Patrick C. Kung, T-Cell Sciences, Cambridge, Mass., 15 July 1993.

78. "Antibodies Rescue 10 Grafts from Rejection," 3.

79. Cosimi et al., "Use of Monoclonal Antibodies to T-Cell Subsets for Immunologic Monitoring and Treatment in Recipients of Renal Allografts," 308; see also Colvin et al., "Circulating T-Cell Subsets in 72 Human Renal Allograft Recipients," 1166.

80. W. J. Smith, Burdick, and Williams, "Immunologic Monitoring of Renal Transplant Recipients," 1183.

81. Morris et al. "Role of T-Cell-Subset Monitoring in Renal Allograft Recipients;" Kerman, Van Buren, and Payne, "Monitoring of T-Cell Subsets in Renal Allograft Recipients."

82. Guttmann and Poulsen, "Fluorescence Activated Cell Sorter Analysis of Lymphocyte Subsets after Renal Transplantation"; Forsum et al., "Methods for Monitoring T-Lymphocyte Subsets in Renal Allografts"; Chatenoud et al., "Correlation between Immunoregulatory T-Cell Imbalances and Renal Allograft Outcome."

83. Our emphasis. Burton, "Lymphocyte Monitoring in Renal Transplantation," 983.

84. Hayes et al., "Correlation between Two-Color Flow Cytometry Quantitation of Activated T-Cells and Acute Allograft Rejection," 1605; Gross et al., "In vivo–in Vitro Correlates of Human Rejection," 1610; see also Brando et al., "The Leu-2+7+ Cell Subset as a Marker of Immune Activation in Renal Transplant Recipients."

85. J. B. Klein, "Immune Monitoring in the Monoclonal Era"; yet, see Baehr et al., "An Immune Monitoring Program for Controlling Immunosuppressive Therapy," who wrote of the "high sensitivity of immune monitoring."

86. For more details, see Cambrosio, Keating, and Guttmann, "New Medical Technologies and Clinical Practice."

87. These data do not involve, of course, the use of IPT for the monitoring of OKT3 antirejection therapy, where a "self-vindicatory" mechanism is at work. Immunosuppressive therapy is performed by administering OKT3 monoclonal antibodies, i.e., antibodies designed to selectively knock out lymphocytes bearing the CD3 marker. In order to control whether the therapy is effective, monoclonal antibodies measuring the CD3 subset have to be employed; in other words, the monitoring is embodied in the therapeutic procedure.

88. As biologists, the Herzenbergs did it first with mice; see Ledbetter et al., "Murine T Cell Differentiation Antigens Detected by Monoclonal Antibodies." The first study of human monoclonals by the laboratory reference, although it does not bear Herzenberg's name, is included in the list of Leonard A. Herzenberg laboratory publications. It is Engleman et al., "Functional Characteristics of Human T-Cell Subpopulations Distinguished by a Monoclonal Antibody."

89. Interview with Leonard Herzenberg, Stanford University, Stanford, Calif., 2 May 1990.

90. Herzenberg, De Rosa, and Herzenberg, "Monoclonal Antibodies," 384–5. This had also been the case for the FACS: Herzenberg's team had developed the machine and offered it to different companies before turning to Becton Dickinson who finally agreed to produce it commercially (interview with Bernie Shoor, San Jose, Calif., 6 September 1997).

91. Interview with Leonard A. Herzenberg and Leonore A. Herzenberg, Stanford University, Stanford, Calif., 27 March 1988.

92. On the de facto standards, see David, "Clio and the Economics of QWERTY;" David, "Path Dependence and Varieties of Learning in the Evolution of Technological Practice."

93. Interview with Robert Auer, Harold Crews, and Arthur Yang, Coulter Corporation, Hialeah, Fla., 7 May 1996.

94. The account according to which Coulter's acquisition of Immunotech can be explained by a strategic shift from an almost exclusive focus on hardware to an increased focus on reagents was provided by Michel Delaage (Immunotech, Marseille-Luminy, 24 February 1997). Another, not necessarily conflicting account was provided by a Coulter marketing official (interview with William Gutierrez, Hialeah, Fla., 7 May 1996):

> We created a market and then little companies went in and started really developing products very quickly for that market as it grew exponentially. So we

didn't have the resources to be able to move as quickly as somebody like Immunotech did. The Immunotech type mindset is very different from Coulter's. Where Coulter has to justify things, everything has to stand on its own financially. It's difficult to justify a CD123b, we don't even know what it's going to be used for and we don't know what the return on that is. The time that it takes to develop that is the same as it takes to develop CD4 which brings in millions of dollars. . . . We wanted a company that was focused on doing CD123b's and had no trouble justifying that, and that was Immunotech. They can really go out much further into the future. In this field you have to develop enough products that don't turn out to be big winners in order to find the ones that do. You may have 50 or 100 products of which one or two become real clinically relevant and highly profitable, but if you're not there, then just having the one that's the winner is not good enough.

95. The information on Immunotech is derived from the following sources: Stamatakis, *Immunotech*; interviews with Michel Delaage and Michel Hirn, Immunotech, Marseille-Luminy, 24 February 1997.

96. This is how it was defined in a special issue of *Science* on European science and technology; see Maurice, "Immunology Powerhouse in the Marseilles Hills."

97. As a comparison, the diagnostic kit market was estimated in 1984 at 250 million francs: about forty companies, however, competed for that market.

98. As we argued in another book, patenting has often been analyzed in terms of private appropriation of public science, thus neglecting the fact that so-called public science is in fact produced by and can in practice be accessed by a restricted number of workers; a lot of work is needed to make such a "private" science public; see Cambrosio and Keating, "Monoclonal Antibodies: From Local to Extended Networks."

99. Interviews with Patrick C. Kung, T-Cell Sciences, Cambridge, Mass., 15 July 1993, and Stuart F. Schlossman, Dana Farber Cancer Institute, Boston, 30 April 1992.

100. Interview with Leonard A. Herzenberg and Leonore A. Herzenberg, Stanford University, Stanford, Calif., 29 April 1990.

101. And even providing them for free after they went on sale to those institutions that could not afford them. Interview with Patrick C. Kung, T-Cell Sciences, Cambridge, Mass., 15 July 1993.

102. For a list of these patents, see Fox, "Encroaching on Research Freedom."

103. U.S. District Court of Delaware, *Ortho Diagnostic Systems v Becton Dickinson Inc*, Civil Action #8-1-519, 21 September 1984; "Battle Continues in Ortho v Becton Dickinson Patent Case;" "Deposit Case before CAFC."

104. As shown, e.g., by the sometimes acrimonious debates at a meeting between lawyers and scientists convened in 1981 to discuss these issues; see Plant, Reimers, and Zinder, eds. *Patenting Life Forms.* By 1986, 130 U.S. and 830 world-

wide patents relating to hybridoma technology and monoclonal antibodies had been granted. For further discussion of these issues, see Cambrosio and Keating, *Exquisite Specificity*, chap. 5; for a recent update on the patenting situation in the monoclonal antibody field, see Ansell, "Hybridoma Technology: A View from the Patent Arena."

105. On this issue, see Woodruff and Miller, "Patenting of Hybridomas and Genetically Engineered Microorganisms," as well as the discussion raised by Geoffrey Dellenbaugh's (Ortho's attorney) questions in Plant, Reimers, and Zinder, *Patenting Life Forms*, 24–6.

106. Interview with Michel Delaage, Immunotech, Marseille-Luminy, 24 February 1997.

107. See also Nenning and Bourcevet, "Zum Rechtsschutz monoklonaler Antikörper," 855; McGough and Burke, "The End of Monoclonal Patents?"

108. Interview with William Gutierrez, Hialeah, Fla., 7 May 1996.

109. Interview with Janis Giorgi, 20 March 1997; Giorgi et al., "Quality Control in the Flow Cytometric Measurement of T-Lymphocyte Subsets."

110. See Oi, Glazer, and Stryer, "Fluorescent Phycobiliprotein Conjugates for Analyses of Cells and Molecules."

111. Parker et al., "Leucocyte Immunophenotyping by Flow Cytometry in a Multisite Study."

112. "Coulter Corp. Is Sued by Stanford University on Patent Violation," 1; Katharine Ku (Office of Technology Licensing, Stanford University), personal communication, 17 January 2001. Cumulative royalties from the phycobiliprotein patent had by 2000 reached $25 million.

113. Herzenberg, De Rosa, and Herzenberg, "Monoclonal Antibodies," 385.

114. These and the following data were taken from a series of reports produced by Direction Resources Inc.: Sannes, *Sales of in Vitro Diagnostic Products to 2001*; Sannes, *Sales of in Vitro Diagnostic Products to 2002*; Sannes, *Sales of in Vitro Diagnostic Products to 2003*; Kadens, *Sales of in Vitro Diagnostic Products to 2004*; Block and Sannes, *Therapeutic and Diagnostic Monoclonal Antibodies for Cancer*. We thank Decision Resources, and in particular Frank Sama, for sending us excerpts of, and giving us permission to cite from, these reports and from the other Decision Resources reports cited below.

115. As mentioned in chapter 2, in France diagnostic tests reimbursed by the French Medicare are listed in an official nomenclature originally established in 1985 and periodically revised. CD4 and CD8 measurements by flow cytometry were added to the list in 1993 and leukemia and lymphoma IPT (or, to be more exact, "the phenotyping of abnormal blood and marrow cells following explicit medical prescription in cases of diagnosed pathologies of the blood, using flow cytometry or tissue slides and at least 8 monoclonal antibodies") in 1994. While

the listing of IPT in the French nomenclature is a clear sign of its routine use in hospitals, it is unfortunately impossible to obtain national statistical data concerning its actual use. Trends, however, can be extrapolated from the data available from single hospitals. Take, for instance, the Paoli-Calmettes Institute in Marseille, one of the twenty hospitals belonging to the National Federation of anticancer centers. After using, during the 1980s, various slide-based IPT methods (such as immunoperoxidase and APAAP (alkaline phosphatase–anti-alkaline phosphatase); see chapter 4), the hematology laboratory switched to flow cytometry in 1990.

116. We thank the staff of Quebec's "Régie de l'assurance médicale" for providing us with the data.

117. Data were collected directly from the person in charge of the IPT laboratory.

118. For example, the growth of both the incidence and prevalence of pediatric and adult ALL in the United States, Europe, and Japan is expected to be 0.1% in the 1998–2008 period, while the growth in the incidence and prevalence of AML is expected to be, respectively, 1.4% and 1.3% during that same period in the same geographic areas; see Block, *Acute Leukemias.* Data from one of the major pediatric oncohematology wards in southeastern France show, for instance, that between 1992 (the year flow cytometry replaced slide-based IPT) and 2000, the number of yearly tests for acute leukemia remained stable between 50 and 60 (average 52).

119. "Availability of Flow Cytometric Immunophenotyping of Lymphocytes to Hospital Patients—United States, 1990."

120. Herzenberg, De Rosa, and Herzenberg, "Monoclonal Antibodies," 386.

121. The example is taken from Zola, "The CD Nomenclature," 226.

122. Fortanier, Gérard-Varet, and Moatti, "Un cas de recherche et développement dans le champ biomédical," 297. This idea is borrowed from the "economy of conventions" school: see, e.g., Boltanski and Thévenot, *De la justification.*

123. See Boumsell et al., "Surface Antigens on Malignant Sézary and T-CLL Cells Correspond to Those of Mature T Cells," and Alain Bernard et al., "Cell Surface Characterization of Malignant T Cells from Lymphoblastic Lymphoma Using Monoclonal Antibodies." Jean Dausset had spent some time after World War II in the same Harvard Medical School institute where Schlossman was now located.

124. A description of the HLA workshops can be found in Dausset, *Clin d'œil à la vie,* 79–108, 119–41. We should add that, although Dausset was not to play a role in the subsequent unfolding of the CD enterprise, his junior Saint-Louis colleagues had clearly learned his lesson, for Dausset had from the very beginning placed himself at the interface of biology and medicine, both from a conceptual and an institutional point of view. A central figure in the so-called

neoclinicians' movement that aimed at reforming the French medical system (see chapter 2), Dausset, while continuing his laboratory and hospital work, had acted as an advisor to the ministry that carried out the 1958 reform of the hospital system. He also joined forces with another key figure of that time, Jean Bernard, in creating a research institute for blood diseases. His HLA system was conceived both as a biomedical working hypothesis and a material infrastructure ultimately leading to the establishment of transnational networks such as Eurotransplant. On the HLA system, see Löwy ("Tissue Groups and Cadaver Kidney Sharing"; "The Impact of Medical Practice on Biomedical Research;" "Variances in Meaning of Discovery Accounts") and Moulin (*Le dernier langage de la médecine*, 208–26). Interestingly enough, Dausset went on to found yet another innovative institution that was to play a key role in the recent saga of the Human Genome Project, namely the Centre d'études du polymorphisme humain (CEPH), whose activities were grounded, inter alia, in the construction of a network of reference families; see Rabinow, *French DNA*, 24–46.

125. Zola, "The CD Nomenclature," 226.

126. Abbas, Lichtman, and Pober, *Cellular and Molecular Immunology*, 19. The CD nomenclature is not restricted to lymphocytes but includes all leukocytes. It was originally used only for human leukocytes, but has more recently also been used for other species.

127. Roitt, Brostoff, and Male, *Immunology*, 2–4

128. Zola, "The CD Nomenclature," 228, paraphrasing David Mason, the chair of the seventh workshop, held in 2000.

129. Milstein, "With the Benefit of Hindsight," 359.

130. Milstein, "What Next?," 1. An expression of this trend may be found in recent work on CD14 which has transformed this molecule from a mere marker used to separate cell subclasses into a molecule with significant immunophysiological attributes; see Ziegler-Heitbrock, and Ulevitch, "CD14: Cell Surface Receptor and Differentiation Marker;" Grogan et al., "Immunologic Approaches to the Classification of Non-Hodgkin's Lymphomas."

131. Milstein, "What Next?," 2. Further trouble has emerged in the attempt to apply CD technology to clinical fields, such as lymphoma classification: "Our newly acquired technology (e.g., monoclonal antibodies, flow cytometry) sometimes produces as yet inexplicable results."

132. Milstein, "With the Benefit of Hindsight," 359.

133. Knapp et al., "Towards a Better Definition of Human Leucocyte Surface Molecules," 253.

134. Things are actually more complex, because a distinction has to be made between "functions" as laboratory immunologists understand them and "functions" in the clinical sense. We thank Dr. Alfred I. Tauber for bringing this to our attention.

135. Interview with Laurence Boumsell, Paris, 18 December 1990.

136. Kersey and LeBien, "What Happened to Lineage- and Leukemia-Specific Antigens?" An example of this reorientation can be found in a review article by Springer, "Adhesion Receptors of the Immune System," which by March 1993 had received 892 citations; see Veggeberg, "Immunology: Highlights from a Hot Biological Field," 14–15.

137. Zola, "The CD Nomenclature," 227. Zola further notes that "up to a third of antibodies submitted to workshops as being against known CDs turn out to be wrongly assigned by their submitters," wrongly, that is, as sanctioned by the workshop. The official blessing, however, does not eliminate possible problems with individual batches of a given antibody.

138. Each laboratory received a set of antibodies identified only by a number. Different numbers could, and indeed did, hide the same antibody, while some numbered vials contained negative controls.

139. Shaw, "Characterization of Human Leukocyte Differentiation Antigens."

140. Called Réseau-Lu, the software is produced and commercialized by the company Aguidel (*http://www.aguidel.com*). The results shown here are only a small part of the complete results, which have been reported in Cambrosio, Keating, and Mogoutov. "Mapping Collaborative Work and Innovation in Biomedicine."

141. Interview with Alain Bernard, Nice, 26 September 2001.

142. See Zola, "The CD Nomenclature," 227–8, and Mason, "HLDA Workshops: Past and Present."

143. Emphasis in original. "Nomenclature for Clusters of Differentiation (CD) of Antigens Defined on Human Leukocyte Populations," 809.

144. Interview with Dr. Laurence Boumsell, Saint-Louis Hospital, Paris, 18 December 1990. Actually, their collaboration had begun earlier, before the antibody panel was sent out to the workshop participants, and involved the drafting of standardized forms to collect the results. Interview with C. Hill, Institut Gustave-Roussy, Villejuif, 19 December 1992.

145. C. Hill, letter to the authors, 3 March 1992.

146. That the measurement of T-cell subsets is affected by the techniques used to perform it, not to speak of variations in the entities being measured, is a point explicitly acknowledged in the scientific literature. One reads, for instance, that "Technical factors, such as flow cytometry versus immunofluorescence microscopy, Ficoll-Hypaque versus buffy coat cells, and large versus small lymphocytes, may affect the results" (Colvin et al., "Circulating T-Cell Subsets in 72 Human Renal Allograft Recipients," 1168).

147. Alain Bernard et al., *Leucocyte Typing*, 15.

148. "Nomenclature for Clusters of Differentiation (CD) of Antigens Defined on Human Leukocyte Populations." For the role of the WHO in establishing and managing, e.g., the International Classification of Diseases, see Bowker and Star, *Sorting Things Out.*

149. "Note on Nomenclature," 660.

150. Zola, "The CD Nomenclature," 226–7. For instance, the chair of the eighth workshop stated that it would be a "retrograde step" to call the transferrin receptor CD71 in everyday discussion or in a paper, although it is still important to assign a CD number, both for the sake of "completeness" and to indicate that the antibody had been "through the rigorous process of Workshop analysis."

151. The new system was originally proposed in Morse, "Genetic Nomenclature for Loci Controlling Surface Antigens of Mouse Hemopoietic Cells."

152. CD nomenclatures have also been established for other animal species, such as dogs and swine; see Cobbold and Metcalfe, "Monoclonal Antibodies That Define Canine Homologues of Human CD Antigens"; Saalmuller et al., "Overview of the Second International Workshop to Define Swine Cluster of Differentiation (CD) Antigens."

Chapter 7

1. According to a study by the Institute of Scientific Information (ISI) of the most-cited U.K. scientists between 1981 and 1991, Mason and Janossy ranked, respectively, sixth and seventh with 7143 and 7059 citations. We thank David Mason and George Janossy for providing us with a copy of the ISI data.

2. Cordell et al., "Immunoenzymatic Labeling of Monoclonal Antibodies Using Immune Complexes of Alkaline Phosphatase and Monoclonal Anti–Alkalilne Phosphatase (APAAP Complexes)."

3. Erber, Mynheer, and Mason, "APAAP Labelling of Blood and Bone Marrow Samples for Immunophenotyping Leukaemia," 761.

4. Our thanks to Élaine Gauthier for performing the bibliometrical work. The years chosen were 1984 and 1991 for Janossy and 1986 and 1993 for Mason. We did not select the same years for the two authors since their careers were not synchronized and they thus published their highly cited contributions at slightly different periods.

5. We took into account all the papers published as first authors and as coauthors; we used the CD-ROM version of the *Science Citation Index*, downloading all the 1986 and 1993 references citing Mason's pre-1986 and pre-1993 publications, and the 1984 and 1991 references citing Janossy's pre-1984 and pre-1991 publications.

6. After discarding all the titles contributing less than 1% of the total number of citations for each year, the matrix contained the following number of

journals: 33 journals for Mason 1986, 24 for Mason 1993, 29 for Janossy 1984, and 27 for Janossy 1991. The number of "journal-to-journal" citations was obtained from the *ISI Citation Report.* We analyzed the matrix with the SPSS factor analysis routine, using principal components analysis as an extraction method.

7. An additional difference lies in the presence or absence of certain factors: dermatology (factor 6) only appears in Mason, whereas transplantation and gastroenterology (factors 5 and 6) only appear in Janossy. The contribution of these factors to the overall variance is, however, limited.

8. The presence of three pathology clusters could point to an internal differentiation of the pathology audience interested in Mason's work (thus confirming their growing importance), but a confirmation of this interpretation could only be provided by a closer examination of the content of the journals represented within each cluster.

9. We can also analyze the transformation in time, i.e., the passage from 1984–86 to 1991–93; the main result is to be found in the remarkable stability of Janossy's citational environment as compared to the relative transformation of Mason's citational environment. Except for the movement of gastroenterology from factor 6 to factor 3, replacing cancer, the cluster lists in Janossy 1984 and 1991 are identical. The disappearance of the cancer cluster does not necessarily mean that a cancer audience is no longer present; it could simply mean that cancer has been subsumed under hematology. The stability in Janossy's citational environment could (and does) hide changes in topic and in the audience for his work, for instance, in the case of immunology, a shift in focus from leukemia to AIDS research. At this aggregate level of analysis, however, we must content ourselves with the observation that, regardless of these changes in intradisciplinary focus, the broad disciplinary audience remains stable. As for Mason, we note the growing centrality of pathology, which now covers three clusters. The increasing centrality of pathology goes hand in hand with a decrease in the presence of immunology.

10. David Y. Mason, e-mail message to the authors, 24 February 2000. While, at first, staining a slide and peering at it might look like a far more simple task than operating a flow cytometer, the performance of immunocytochemical operations is a rather complex one that, in spite of the development of semiautomatic staining machines, requires a lot of expertise. As noted by another expert in the field, "despite being simple in principle, immunostaining methods can be difficult to perform and they pose many pitfalls. . . . It is important in the planning that all reagent sequences are carefully designed, and flow-charts must be prepared and studied in advance to avoid spurious results." The author goes on to argue that "immunological expertise" should "hopefully" provide a guarantee against the various pitfalls of these methods; see Brandtzaeg, "The Increasing Power of Immunohistochemistry and Immunocytochemistry," 51.

11. This quote has been reported independently by two different interviews: interview with Robert Auer, Coulter Corp., Miami, 7 May 1996.

12. Interview with Bernard Shoor, San José, Calif., 6 September 1997.

13. Herzenberg, De Rosa, and Herzenberg, "Monoclonal Antibodies," 385; Shapiro, *Practical Flow Cytometry*, 3rd ed., 29.

14. See n. 146, chapter 4.

15. See Ratinaud and Métézeau, "Cytomètres en flux: implantation en France et description des appareils commercialisés;" Métézeau and Ratinaud, "L'implantation et l'environnement de la cytométrie en flux;" Métézeau and Ratinaud, "Flow Cytometry: Technical Description and Some Applications in France."

16. Givan, *Flow Cytometry: First Principles*, 135–6. As we note in chapter 5, they are neither: they are somewhat in-between; and what places them there is collective disciplining or regulation (in the broadest sense of the term).

17. Givan, quoted in Krumm, "Flow Cytometry Expanding in Clinical and Research Labs," 17.

18. Shapiro, *Practical Flow Cytometry*, 3rd ed., 29.

19. Ratinaud and Métézeau, "Cytomètres en flux."

20. Shapiro, *Practical Flow Cytometry*, 2nd ed., 292.

21. Cambrosio, Keating, and Guttmann. "New Medical Technologies and Clinical Practice."

22. Noel Warner subsequently also left Albuquerque to assume the position of research director at Becton Dickinson in Mountain View, Calif.

23. Interview with Janis Giorgi, Los Angeles, 20 March 1997. Giorgi joined John Fahey, along with Michael Gottlieb and Andrew Saxon of the department of clinical immunology at UCLA in what later became known as the MultiCenter AIDS Cohort Study (MACS); Michael Gottlieb is the author of the now famous note in *Morbidity and Mortality Weekly Report* (5 June 1981) where physicians first learned of a health problem affecting mainly homosexuals. See Garrett, *The Coming Plague*, 283–5.

24. Givan, *Flow Cytometry: First Principles*, ix–x. Other authors go so far as to argue that, as happened to microscopy, cytometry, once a "methodology" or a "tool," has transited into a "discipline science," albeit a multidisciplinary one. "The common interests of biologists, hematologists, pathologists and engineers generated initially the *synchronized* effort of a small fraction of scientists in each of the disciplines to set out for the fast measurement of cellular parameters. The basis for a *pulsing* new body of intellectual and experimental knowledge was generated by this effort" (author's emphasis). See Valet, "Cytometry, a Biomedical Key Discipline."

25. We thank Gavin Svennson for performing these calculations.

26. Kling, "Flow Cytometry: It's Not Just for Immunologists Anymore," 14.

27. Herzenberg, Sweet, and Herzenberg, "Fluorescence-Activated Cell Sorting," 111.

28. Shapiro, *Practical Flow Cytometry*, 3rd ed., 1.

29. Parks, Herzenberg, and Herzenberg, "Flow Cytometry and Fluorescence-Activated Cell Sorting," 781.

30. For a discussion of whether peering into a microscope can be equated to seeing, see Hacking, *Representing and Intervening*, 186–209.

31. Cees J. Cornelisse, Department of Pathology, Leiden University, the Netherlands, letter to the authors, 8 September 1994.

32. For sure, continuities or discontinuities can be emphasized or played down, depending on whether one is trying to promote flow cytometry as a radical innovation, to familiarize potential customers with an esoteric technology, or to deal with regulatory requirements. Cf. Loken and Herzenberg, "Analysis of Cell Populations," 163; and Givan, *Flow Cytometry: First Principles*, 1–2, 90.

33. Coulter, "High Speed Automatic Blood Cell Counter and Size Analyzer."

34. For examples of historical reviews of flow cytometry published in various textbooks, see Shapiro, *Practical Flow Cytometry*, 3rd ed., 43–73; Givan, *Flow Cytometry: First Principles*; Melamed, Mullaney, and Shapiro, "An Historical Review of the Development of Flow Cytometers and Sorters."

35. For a history of the Pap test, see Vayena, *Cancer Detectors*.

36. Kamentsky had returned from Sweden, where he had worked at the Karolinska Institute with Bo Thorell, a student of Torbjörn Caspersson, and a pioneer, with the latter, of cytophotometric techniques (methods for the quantitative measurement of DNA using microscopes and photodetectors). This is one of the many bridges between European and American-based contributions. On Thorell's work, see Kohen, "In Memoriam: Bo Thorell." See below for information on the European work in this field.

37. Louis A. Kamentsky, undated curriculum vitae (c. 1987).

38. Interview with Myron Melamed, Valhalla, NY, 17 June 1997.

39. Ibid.

40. E. N. Adams, "A New Device for Detecting and Concentrating Abnormal Cells in Fluid," 3 September 1963. Thomas J. Watson Research Center, Engineering Science, Department 475 (Louis Kamentsky's personal papers).

41. Ibid. The possibilities enumerated in the footnote included: " 2. Detection of cancer cells in blood. 3. Research or clinical use for determination of the morphology and the distribution and amount of nucleic acid and protein of living or fixed cells. 4. Large volume studies for determining the statistical distributions of cell parameters."

42. Louis A. Kamentsky, "Photoelectric Particle Separator using Time Delay"; see also Kamentsky, Melamed, and Derman, "Spectrophotometer: New Instru-

ment for Ultrarapid Cell Analysis." One should distinguish, here, the issue of analyzing cells from the issue of physically sorting cells. Two systems of cell separation were developed: the first, demonstrated in December 1963, used an electrostatic field to deflect droplets containing cells of interest into separate containers. This, however, was abandoned as it was believed that the target cells were too large and being cancerous would have a tendency to clump, thus impeding the flow. Moreover, IBM had a new typewriter technology which involved a fluidic switching device etched on a molybdenum plate. Having established relations with H. Glattli at the IBM Zurich laboratory which had developed the technology, Kamentsky decided to apply the fluid switch technology to the sorting of cells. By 1963, a fluidic switch which drew targeted cells out of the flow was developed and subsequently patented; see Kamentsky, "Photoelectric Particle Separator Using Time Delay." The claimed utility of the invention was based on its ability to partly automate the Pap test and other diagnostic procedures based on the discrimination between normal and pathological cells; see also Kamentsky and Melamed, "Spectrophotometric Cell Sorter," 1364–5. When plans were then made to test false positive and false-negative rates of the screening machine, the separator itself was detached from the screener, for, as pointed out in an IBM Research Order, "[r]esults have come faster, thus far, by not using the cell separator." Research Order, Watson Laboratory, 20 July 1965, 6. Testing the first machines showed that detection rates of 95% entailed false positives of 40% (Louis A. Kamentsky, *Devices and Applications,* Watson Laboratory, February 1967). Even though this might have been a first step on the road to automation, the project ultimately failed. As Kamentsky later recounted, it was less a problem of pathology than a problem with pathologists. Back then, "pathologists were perfect, their labs were perfect, their error rates were one in thousands, they never missed anything, cytologists were very motivated, they didn't have to be highly paid. There was no need to automate" (interview with Louis A. Kamentsky, Cambridge, Mass., 29 April 1992).

43. Ibid.

44. "Introduction," 9.

45. Ibid., 11.

46. Los Alamos Scientific Laboratory, *Semiannual Report, July through December 1959,* 338. See Lushbaugh and Hale, "Clinical Applications of Whole Body Scintillometry. III," and Lushbaugh and Hale, "Iodine[131] Retention in Normal and Starved Rats."

47. Marvin A. Van Dilla, letter to the authors, 22 May 1992.

48. Ibid.

49. See Lushbaugh, Basmann, and Israel, "Electronically Determined Erythrocyte Volumes. III."

50. See Lushbaugh, Maddy, and Basmann, "Electronic Measurement of Cellular Volumes I"; Lushbaugh, Maddy, and Bamann, "Electronic Measurement of

Cellular Volumes II." Lushbaugh's claims were immediately contested; see Bahr and Zeitler, "Distribution of Erythrocyte Volumes [letter]," and Lushbaugh, "A Rejoinder."

51. Examined under a microscope in 1972, the spheres looked like golf balls.

52. Harlow and Van Dilla, "Flow of Particles Through a Coulter Aperture: Hydrodynamic Considerations."

53. Ibid., 111. The biophysics group pursued the issue further. A closer examination of events in the aperture showed that cells traveled at two different speeds through the aperture, resulting in two different readings on the pulse height analyzer. The technical reasons for this artifact were independently described by Kubitschek who had been working on the theory and practice of the Coulter counter since the beginning of the 1960s at the Argonne National Laboratory and with whom Van Dilla consulted. See, e.g., Kubitschek, "Apertures for Coulter Counters."

54. Interview with Mack Fulwyler, San Francisco, 3 May 1990; Sweet, "High Frequency Recording With Electrostatiscally Deflected Ink Jets." The *Review of Scientific Instruments* is considered the bible of those interested in scientific technology.

55. Fulwyler, "Electronic Separation of Biological Cells by Volume."

56. Ibid.; Fulwyler, *Particle Separator.* Fulwyler developed yet another cell sorter as part of a thesis entitled *Electronic Volume Analysis and Volume Fractionation Applied to Mammalian Cells,* which he presented to the University of Colorado's physics department. He left Los Alamos in 1971 to start a company called Particle Technology, funded by Coulter. He moved to Becton Dickinson in 1977 to become technical director of the FACS group. In 1982, he joined the faculty at the University of California at San Francisco.

57. Fulwyler, "An Electronic Particle Separator with Potential Biological Applications."

58. Fulwyler, "Further Development of the Cell Separator."

59. Establishing nuclear research institutes was a popular European activity at the time. The French, Italians, Belgians, and British set up similar institutes during the same period. The Italian nuclear research center at La Casaccia, near Rome, also harbored a core group of cytometrists (interview with Marcello Spanò, Donatella Tirindelli, Raffaele De Vita, and Francesco Mauro, Casaccia (Rome), 7 April 1997).

60. Göhde, *Zellzyklusanalysen mit dem Impulscytophotometer.* The original report of the apparatus appeared four years earlier. See Dittrich and Göhde, "Impulsfluorometrie bei Einzelzellen in Suspensionen."

61. Interview with Wolfgang Göhde, Münster, 24–27 June 1997.

62. On Caspersson's work, see Caspersson, "History of the Development of Cytophotometry from 1935 to Present." For a more general view, see Meijer et al., "Image Analysis in Clinical Pathology." In addition to Kamentsky, other American researchers involved in cytometry who visited Caspersson included M. Mendelson, B. Mayall, and S. Darzynkiewicz (New York). G. K. Valet, personal communication, 24 January 1997.

63. The terms refer to the measurement by the machine of the differing amounts of light absorbed by nucleic acids and proteins.

64. See, e.g., Sprenger et al., "Flow-Through-Cytophotometry."

65. Interview with Wolfgang Göhde, Münster, 24–27 June 1997. Italian researchers working in the same field with a Leitz microscope also complained about the many hours of tiresome work spent in collecting measurements on 100 to 300 cells (interview with Giuseppe Starace, Rome, 9 April 1997).

66. Interview with Wolfgang Göhde, Münster, 24–27 June 1997.

67. The reason for this is a concern for precise DNA measurements, inherited from previous work on cytophotometry; this design would enable one to focus on the nucleus (where the DNA is located) no matter where it was situated within the cell.

68. According to Göhde, he later found out that the Los Alamos group had tried, but failed, to use mercury arc lamps, the reason being that they used a standard photon counting device that did not efficiently integrate the signals coming from single photons. This mistake generated much debate over the relative merits of inexpensive arc lamps vs. costly lasers. Italian researchers claimed that mercury lamps perform better than lasers for DNA studies, and, given the European research tradition in this field (see below), this would explain why European instruments had a preference for this technique (interview with Giuseppe Starace, Rome, 9 April 1997).

69. The technique allows the simultaneous visualization of different fluorescent colors on tissue slides. For a discussion of the role of epi-illumination, see Brandtzaeg, "The Increasing Power." Ploem was awarded the 1998 Ernst Abbe Memorial Award by the New York Microscopical Society for his contributions to microscopy instrumentation.

70. J. S. Ploem, letter to the authors, 27 March 1998. Dr. Ploem's letter included a copy of the letter he received from Phywe in November 1970.

71. Haanen et al., *First International Symposium on Pulse-Cytophotometry.*

72. Hillen, Wessels, and Haanen, *Cell Proliferation Patterns in Acute Leukemia Monitored by Pulse-Cytophotometry.*

73. Göhde, Schumann, and Büchner, *Pulse-Cytophotometry: Application in Cancer Research and Hematology with Special Reference to Cell Kinetics*; Lutz, *Pulse-*

Cytophotometry. 3rd International Symposium on Pulse-Cytophotometry; Laerum, Lindmo, and Thorud, *Flow Cytometry IV.*

74. They include plant cell chromosome measurements for plant breeders, quality control in food production, biotechnology, or microplankton cells in seawater or freshwater.

75. Elliot C. Levinthal to Leonard A. Herzenberg, 21 May 1969, attachment to grant application, NIH, Automated Cell Sorting: Clinical and Biological Uses, Leonard A. Herzenberg, principal investigator.

76. Herzenberg wrote to Kamentsky in 1965 to ask about Fulwyler's cell separator which one of Herzenberg's colleagues had heard about at the National Academy of Sciences meeting that spring. Leonard Herzenberg to Louis A. Kamenstky, 28 October 1965. Lederberg visited the Columbia University IBM Watson Laboratory several weeks after Herzenberg's letter.

77. Henderson Cole to Louis A. Kamentsky, IBM Confidential, 5 November 1965.

78. W. P. Porter (research division controller, IBM) to D. B. Adams (business manager, Stanford University), 28 July 1967, 5.

79. Technical Report, Instrumentation Research Laboratory (Stanford University) to National Aeronautics and Space Administration, no. IRL 1076, 1 October 1967–31 March 1968, 39–41.

80. Technical Report, Instrumentation Research Laboratory (Stanford University), no. IRL 1082, 1 April 1968–30 September 1968, 48.

81. See, e.g., Van Dilla et al., "Cell Microfluorometry: A Method for Rapid Fluorescence Measurement." The Los Alamos work on laminar flow built on work performed in the early 1950s at the Middlesex Hospital in London; see Crosland-Taylor, "A Device for Counting Small Particles Suspended in a Fluid through a Tube."

82. Technical Report, Instrumentation Research Laboratory (Stanford University), no. IRL 1110, 1 July 1969–1 July 1970, 20.

83. Henry R. Hulett, "Status Report on IBM Rapid Cell Spectrophotometer," n.d. n.p. (Louis Kamentsky, personal papers).

84. A patent, filed in 1972, was granted in 1974; Bonner, Sweet, and Hulett, *Particle Sorting Method and Apparatus.*

85. Interview with Bernard Shoor, San José, Calif., 6 September 1997.

86. Salzman et al., "Development of Flow-Systems Instrumentation for Rapid Cell Analysis and Sorting," 106.

87. Price, Kollman, and Salzman, "Classification of Microalgal Species."

88. Julius, Masuda, and Herzenberg, "Demonstration That Antigen-Binding Cells Are Precursors of Antibody-Producing Cells after Purification with a Fluorescence-Activated Cell Sorter."

89. Steinkamp, "Flow Cytometry," 1384.

90. Work separating leukocytes with this apparatus was reported in Salzman et al., "Cell Classification by Laser Light Scattering." A review of light-scattering techniques and analysis can be found in Salzman, "Light Scattering Analysis of Single Cells."

91. Bartholdi, "A High-Sensitivity Flow Chamber," 165.

92. Bartholdi and Salzman, "A Light-Scattering Flow Photometer," 98–9.

93. Mullaney et al., *Automated Cancer-Cell Sorting and Analysis: Progress Report, June 1–November 30, 1977.*

94. The return to morphology was seen as a solution to the following problem. Cells are not symmetrical. Therefore, it is always possible to find "light-scattering differences which are not biologically significant." One way around this ambiguity would be to stop the flow and examine the "signatures" of individual cells in the hopes of obtaining a "direct correlation between the cell and its corresponding scattering pattern" (Mullaney, Burger, and Salzman, "An Instrument for Static Light-Scattering Measurements on Individual Cells," 168–9). To do so required comparisons between the numbers generated by the light scatter and an image of the cell obtained through 35-mm film. An instrument capable of such a comparison was available only at the Battelle Institute in Frankfurt, Germany. Thus began a series of experiments—ostensibly classified as studies in cytology automation—conducted throughout 1977 to pin down the meaning of light scatter. Once again, early results were promising. But further progress demanded further technology. If, for example, the problem of the orientation of the cells in flow was treated adequately, interactive video graphics would be needed. Similarly, a new nonparametric statistical approach would be necessary to treat the data. Mullaney et al., *Automated Cancer-Cell Sorting and Analysis: Progress Report, December 1, 1977–May 31, 1978*, 2. Moreover, because of program constraints, in 1978 the instrument became inaccessible. So it was time to build an instrument to understand the instrument that had been the center of the laboratory's activity for the previous decade.

95. Mullaney et al., *Automated Cancer-Cell Sorting* (LA-7412-PR), 1.

96. Rotman and Papermaster, "Membrane Properties of Living Mammalian Cells as Studied by Enzymatic Hydrolysis of Fluorogenic Esters," 134. In 1971, while associated with Associated Biomedic Systems Inc., Papermaster was looking for a "rapid screening technique for infectious mononucleosis." The technique didn't use fluorochromasia; it did, however use "the counter [Kamentsky's] plus specific antibody." I don't know if he found it. Ben Papermaster to Louis A. Kamentsky, 11 May 1971.

97. Marvin A. Van Dilla, letter to the authors, 22 May, 1992.

98. Technical Report, Instrumentation Research Laboratory (Stanford University) to National Aeronautics and Space Administration, no. IRL 1056, October 1966–April 1967, 32–40.

99. Interview with Leonard A. Herzenberg, Stanford, Calif., 2 May 1990; for a description of the assay, see Rotman and Papermaster, "Membrane Properties," Technical Report, Instrumentation Research Laboratory (Stanford University), no. IRL 1092, 1 July 1968–1 July 1969, 21. The technique was originally used at the Los Alamos Scientific Laboratory a year earlier by Van Dilla who had had the collaboration of the senior author, Boris Rotman. See Van Dilla, Mullaney, and Coulter, "The Fluorescent Cell Photometer: A New Method for the Rapid Measurement of Biological Cells Stained with Fluorescent Dyes."

100. In a 1968 technical report, three immunological uses were envisioned: "a. Isolation of antigen-processing cells by phagocytosis of fluorogenic substrate. b. Isolation of immunologically competent cells by size. c. Isolation of antibody-forming cells by size following adherence of large antigenic particles" (Technical Report, Instrumentation Research Laboratory (Stanford University), no. IRL 1076, 1 October 1967–31 March 1968, 38). It should be noted that the graft rejection ("fluorochromasia") studies were conducted on Kamentsky's apparatus. IBM lent the machine to Stanford for the period August 1967–August 1968. See Louis A. Kamentsky, "Installation of Cell Analyzer at Stanford University Medical Center," 11 September 1967 (Louis Kamentsky, personal papers).

101. As of 1968, the projects included G. Hahn, Department of Radiology, Stanford University: isolation of cells in mitosis using size criteria; H.S. Kaplan, Department of Radiology, Stanford University: detection and isolation of cancer cells determination of the cell type responsible for Hodgkin's disease; isolation and testing of "stem cells" in bone marrow for possible treatment of radiation exposure in space (funded by NASA and the Air Force). (Technical Report, Instrumentation Research Laboratory (Stanford University), no. IRL 1076, 1 October 1967–March 31 1968, 38).

102. Henry R. Hulett, "Status Report on IBM Rapid Cell Spectrophotometer," n.d. n.p. (Louis Kamentsky, personal papers).

103. Henry R. Hulett to Louis A. Kamentsky, 7 June 1968 (Louis Kamentsky, personal papers).

104. Laerum and Farsund, "Clinical Applications of Flow Cytometry: A Review."

105. Italy, like Germany, had a strong local tradition of work on solid tumor cell cycle research. Somewhat unsurprisingly, the first flow cytometers introduced in Italy were Phywe's IPC instruments. Given their connections to both Germany and the United States, Italian flow cytometrists have acted as a sort of bridge between Europe and North America in this domain. Italian cell kinetics studies have led to the demonstration of the clonal heterogeneity of solid tumors, a result later confirmed by Dutch researchers also working with DNA cytometry;

see interview with Giuseppe Starace, Rome, 9 April 1997; and interview with Cees Cornelisse, Leiden, 13 May 1997.

106. This led, indirectly, to the development of the chromosome banding technique which profoundly transformed cytogenetics: Caspersson developed this technique when he realized that changes in DNA content of tumor cells were too small to be observed by cell DNA measurements and that one thus needed subtler means to map transformations in gene-carrying portions of the DNA; see Caspersson, "History of the Development," 5.

107. In Europe during the 1970s, cancer treatment was influenced by the notion that one could achieve a better chemotherapeutic effect by synchronizing tumor cells in cycle phases different from normal cells; see Wilmanns, Wilms, and Rajewsky, "Biochemische Grundlagen der Behandlung von Leukosen." In general, cell cycle studies of the 1970s did little to improve cancer therapy. Consider, e.g., a recent assessment of prior cell cycle studies and therapy: "Classical studies on the cell cycle phase specificity of antitumor drugs have been done by exposing cultured cells, synchronized at particular phases of the cell cycle, to the drug and studying their subsequent viability or reproductive capacity, e.g., by analysis of their clonogenicity. While these studies provided valuable evidence of the cell cycle phase sensitivity of cells to different drugs, they were neither able to uncover the mode of cell death (e.g., apoptosis or necrosis) nor to reveal the actual phase of the cell cycle in which the cells were dying. It was not known, therefore, whether the treatment led to interphase cell death (i.e., occurring in the same cycle in which the cells were exposed to the drug) or whether it resulted in reproductive or mitotic cell death (i.e., occurring in the cycles following the one in which the cells were exposed to the drug)" (Halicka et al., "Cell Cycle Specificity of Apoptosis during Treatment of Leukemias," 26).

108. This assessment of the field is largely shared by participants. For instance, at the 1997 conference of the European Society for Analytical Cellular Pathology (ESACP, Oslo, 25–29 May, 1997), the keynote address ("Ploem Lecture") by Gérard Brugal was entitled "Cytometry of Tumor Cell Proliferation: Can the Tragedy Be Turned into a Success Story?" Brugal noted that half of the 3000 articles published between 1987 and 1989 on S-phase fractions claimed to have found a correlation between that biological variable and patient outcome, while the other half claimed that no such correlation existed (field notes, 25 May 1997). Recent attempts to resurrect the domain focus on the combination of flow cytometric techniques with new techniques derived from molecular biology. While it is outside the boundaries of this book, the field of DNA cytometry would make for a fascinating sociological study, especially in view of its ongoing controversial status and the repeated, only partially successful attempts at regulation.

109. Examples of the microscope-based systems included the Dutch-German Ploemopak, developed by J. S. Ploem in Leiden and commercialized by Leitz and the French SAMBA system, developed by Gérard Brugal in Grenoble. Various automated systems have also been developed in the United States; for a

short overview, see Meijer et al., "Image Analysis." The enormous increase in computer power of the last decades has made possible renewed attempts at image cytometry, and several companies have started commercializing new equipment in this field, including a company created by Kamentsky, CompuCyte.

110. Shapiro, *Practical Flow Cytometry*. Shapiro, whose book has gone through three editions, is a recognized technical leader in the field. With almost no exceptions, all the persons we interviewed told us that, to learn about the various aspects of flow cytometry, we should absolutely speak to Howard Shapiro, which, of course, we did.

111. In 1997, Beckman, one of the leaders in the fields of clinical chemistry and immunochemistry, acquired Coulter (a privately held, family corporation and the market leader in hematology with $700 million in sales at the time of acquisition), for $875 million in cash, assuming in addition $175 million in Coulter debt, thus creating a $1.7 billion company. On the history of Coulter, see Upbin, "What Have You Invented for Me Lately?"

112. Algeo, "Developing a Safe Way of Screening." An example of specific tasks for high-speed sorters is fetal cell screening of maternal blood.

113. The development of the machine was greeted in the 20 April 1984 issue of *Le nouvel observateur*, a popular French, left-leaning weekly, by an article entitled "The Machine for Exploring Cancer." The said machine, according to the article, was able to "sort cells, count anomalies, and verify the efficacy of remedies." Furthermore, it was said to be "unique in the world and—O miracle!—French made" (Gruhier, "La machine à explorer le cancer"). The article shows a particularly belligerent version of technoscientific nationalism or, rather, anti-Americanism: MIT, Stanford, and the University of California are accused of attempting to seduce French inventors into migrating to the United States, and the competing American cell-sorting machines are described as "a lot less performing and technologically obsolete."

114. Owing apparently to regional incompatibilities between Alsace and southern France, the attempt to integrate the ATC with the CD reagents produced by the Marseilles-based Immunotech was never realized (interview with Michel Delaage, Marseilles, 24 February 1997.) Immunotech, as we know, was subsequently acquired by Coulter.

115. A precious source of information on this topic is Shapiro, *Practical Flow Cytometry*. Our thanks to Gavin Svensson for his assistance on this topic.

116. "Presently . . . most of our products . . . are directed both towards the clinical and the research market and so the same product can be used by both markets, so that's why we're called the research platform but we're really focused in cytometry" (interview with William Gutierrez, Miami, 7 May 1996).

117. We use here Howard Shapiro's designation and, in part, his periodization; see Shapiro, *Practical Flow Cytometry*, 2nd ed., 199. As previously noted, the three editions of Shapiro's *Practical Flow Cytometry* are highly respected in the flow

cytometry community. An initial version, privately printed in 1984, went under the name *Building and Using Flow Cytometers.*

118. This led to a confrontation between manufacturers, the FDA, and the College of American Pathologists when the FDA discovered that reagents designated for research use were in fact being used for diagnostic purposes. On this episode, see Keating and Cambrosio, "Interlaboratory Life."

119. The considerable confusion of the early 1980s as to where the market for flow cytometers actually lay implied difficult design choices. As a biological research device, emphasis on sorting capacity and flexibility was clearly necessary. As a clinical diagnostic device, computer-controlled simplicity was the key. A partial solution to this fundamental design problem emerged in the mid-1980s when Ortho went modular with its Cytofluorograf 30/50 system. Rather than design an instrument that either sorted (research) or did not sort (clinic), Ortho decided to manufacture a "system" where the sorter could be treated as a "module" that could be added or subtracted from the system as a whole. Modularity has become a characteristic of recent instruments such as Becton Dickinson's FACSCalibur.

120. Leif, Leif, and Auer, "The EPICS C Analyzer"; Shapiro *Practical Flow Cytometry*, 2nd ed., 204 n. 873.

121. That the relation between manufacturers and users is particularly close in the biomedical field has long been noted; see, e.g., Narin and Noma, "Is Technology Becoming Science?" On breaking down the inside/outside dichotomy, see Latour, "Give Me a Laboratory."

122. Interview with William Gutierrez, Miami, 7 May 1996.

123. See, e.g., the debate that took place in 1997 on the "cytometry mailing list," managed by the Purdue University Cytometry Laboratories, comparing the FACSCalibur with the Coulter XL.

124. On Coulter's customer support strategies, see Gay, "How 'Team Learning' Raises Customer Service Levels," 9.

125. Interviews with Raul Pedroso and William Gutierrez, Miami, 7 May 1996.

126. Our thanks to Madeleine Akrich for making this point.

127. This point is nicely made in Dubuisson and Hennion, *Le design: l'objet dans l'usage.*

128. Interview with G. E. Marti, Bethesda, Md., 15 February, 1995.

129. Becton Dickinson, *Normal Values.*

130. Created in 1967 in the form of a central register of patients waiting for a donor organ (initially only kidneys, and later other organs), Eurotransplant mediates and coordinates organ donation procedures in Austria, Belgium, Germany, Luxemburg, and the Netherlands.

131. Interview with Hans J. Tanke, Leiden, 14 May 1997. See Tanke, *Cytochemical Staining of DNA and RNA for Analytical Cytology*; Van Es, *Immunological and Clinical Factors Influencing Rejection of Human Renal Allografts*; Gratama, *Immunological Studies in Allogeneic Marrow Grafting.* Asked to characterize the status of that kind of thesis, Dr. Tanke (interview, Leiden, 14 May 1997) replied: "It is fundamental research of biological applications. Human molecular genetics is very important for us for oncological applications, but at the end of the thesis it may indicate diagnostic applications and in that situation we have a good relationship with pathology and genetics."

132. Interview with Hans J. Tanke, Leiden, 14 May 1997.

133. For the purpose and scope of the conferences, see Metz and Viest, *The First 75 Years*, 229–34.

134. Engineering in Medicine—Multiphasic Health Screening, July 10–14, 1967, University School, Milwaukee; Engineering in Medicine, Physical Parameters in Multiphasic Screening, Proctor Academy, Andover, N.H., 5–9 August 1968.

135. On multiphasic screening, see Reiser, *Medicine and the Reign of Technology*, 217–8. The term "multiphasic," using statistics developed by Jerzy Neuman, had been popularized by M. F. Collen in a series of publications in the second half of the 1950s. For a review of this work, see Collen et al., "Automated Multiphasic Screening and Diagnosis." [This article was reprinted as a "classic article" in *M.D. Computing* 11 (1994), 170–7.] For Collen's work in the 1960s, see M. F. Collen, "Machine Diagnosis from a Multiphasic Screening Program," *5th IBM Medical Symposium*, Endicott, N.Y., 1963 (Archives Engineering Foundation); Collen, Rubin, and Davis, "Computers in Multiphasic Screening."

136. A MEDLINE search (keywords = multiphasic + health + screening) for the period 1974–89 shows a steady decline in the number of papers devoted to the issue: 1974–79 (26), 1980–84 (16), 1985–89 (11). Moreover, a closer inspection of the 15 multiphasic screening papers in the period 1994–97 shows them to be almost exclusively devoted to multiphasic screening of psychological parameters (as in the Minnesota Multiphasic Personality Inventory).

137. Interview with Mortimer Mendelsohn, Livermore Calif., 6 September 1997.

138. Kendall Preston, "Research Conference Proposal," The Engineering Foundation, New York, N.Y., 1971, 2.

139. Cytomation's previously mentioned high-speed flow cytometer, the MoFlo, was subsequenlty built using technology patented by the Lawrence Livermore National Laboratory.

140. Dean, "Membership Profile of the International Society for Analytical Cytology." Nonetheless, it is partly through the pursuit of technical standards that the society hopes to set the "scientific standards" for the discipline.

141. Mayall, "Technical Tutorial—A New Feature," 247.

142. Quotations in this paragraph come from an undated, unsigned capsule history of the Clinical Cytometry Society, posted on the society's Website in the late 1990s: http://www.cytometry.org.

143. Watson, "From the President: The State of the Society."

144. The "cyto" in immunocytochemical stands for cell, and the corresponding term for the examination of tissue ("histo") specimens is "immunohistochemical." The corresponding traditional disciplines are cytology and histology. To simplify things, we will sometimes use a single term even when the argument applies to both domains. This corresponds to usage in the field: "Immunohistochemistry is a collective term for various methods used to recognize constituents of tissues as antigens in situ by means of colour-tagged antibodies, usually (but not always) derived from another species. When applied to cell preparations, the same methods should be called immunocytochemistry, although some authors also use the latter term for immunological tracing of cellular antigens in tissue sections" (Brandtzaeg, "The Increasing Power," 50). Cell preparations on slides are prepared from cells in suspension (e.g., blood cells), e.g., in the simplest case, by putting a drop of blood on a slide and spreading it thin with the help of another slide (cells can also be concentrated by centrifugation before being spread on the slide, a procedure known as a cytospin); in the case of tissue preparations, thin layers of tissue are prepared, e.g., by sectioning frozen tissue (using a freezing chamber containing a microtome) or as formalin-fixed, plastic-embedded specimens. As we will see, each of these methods has its advantages and shortcomings.

145. *LRF Yearbook*, 1990, 8–9.

146. Gatter et al., "Clinical Importance of Analysing Malignant Tumours of Uncertain Origin with Immunohistological Techniques."

147. *LRF Yearbook*, 1990, 8–9. One of the antibodies (against bcl-2, a protein that blocks apoptosis) was particularly successful: it was dispatched to over 150 research groups around the world; *LRF Yearbook* 1992, 12; *LRF Yearbook* 1993, 15.

148. Although one could think of stains as a mundane matter, they were in fact a key development that allowed visualization of previously invisible features; on the role of stains in microscopy, see Collard, *The Development of Microbiology*, Chapter 2: "The Development of the Microscope, Staining Methods and Morphological Description." See also Bracegirdle, *A History of Microtechnique*.

149. Here again, a wide variety of methods are available, depending on both the staining compounds (nonspecific stains, enzymatic stains, radioactive compounds, etc.) and the microscope equipment (light, phase-contrast, fluorescent, or electron microscope).

150. The transformation of scientific specimens into "witnessable-observable" elements has been analyzed in ethnomethodological accounts of scientific visual practices; see, e.g., Lynch, "The Externalized Retina."

151. Preud'homme and Seligmann, "Surface Bound Immunoglobulins as a Cell Marker in Human Lymphoproliferative Diseases."

152. Interview with David Y. Mason, Oxford, 20 May, 1999. On the work with Preud'homme, see Mason, Labaume, and Preud'homme, "The Detection of Membrane and Cytoplasmic Immunoglobulins in Human Leucocytes by Immunoperoxidase Staining."

153. Brandtzaeg, "The Increasing Power," 63.

154. Shi, Cote, and Taylor, "Antigen Retrieval Immunohistochemistry: Past, Present, and Future," 328. On the notion of the "right tool," see the contributions in Clarke and Fujimura, eds., *The Right Tools for the Job.*

155. See Callendar, "Tumors and Tumor-like Conditions of the Lymphocyte, the Myelocyte, the Erythrocyte and the Reticulum Cell." On the role of nitrogen mustard gases in the development of leukemia therapy, see Rhoads, "The Sword and the Ploughshare."

156. Armed Forces Institute of Pathology, *Annual Report,* 1954, 19.

157. In the late 1950s, the Army itself offered the following rationale for the global collection of lymphatic tumor specimens: "Today with the world-wide commitments of the U.S. Government and the potentialities of military action by our Armed Services anywhere on the globe, information on disease processes on a global basis becomes of paramount importance" (Armed Forces Institute of Pathology, *Annual Report,* 1957, 40). In matters of microscopic diagnosis of tumors, the authority of the institute is still unparalleled. According to Majno and Joris, "To maximize the reliability of microscopic diagnosis there are specific guidelines for each type of tumor based on statistics and experience. The internationally recognized authority is represented by the U.S. Armed Forces Institute of Pathology (A.F.I.P.) which also functions as a diagnostic consulting service world-wide" (Majno and Joris, *Cells, Tissues and Disease,* 752).

158. Videbaek, "Do Malignant Lymphomas Represent Varying Differentiation of the Same Growth?," 202.

159. Sreenan and Tubbs, "The Influence of Immunology and Genetics on Lymphoma Classification."

160. Rappaport, "Tumors of the Hematopoietic System."

161. DeVita, Rappaport, and Frei, "Announcement of Formation of the Lymphoma Task Force and Pathology Reference Center."

162. Lukes, "A Review of the American Concept of Malignant Lymphoma."

163. Lennert, "Classification of Malignant Lymphomas (European Concept)."

164. Attempts were also made to make paraffin-embedded material amenable to flow cytometry, albeit for DNA rather than IPT; see Hedley et al., "Method for Analysis of Cellular DNA Content of Paraffin-Embedded Pathological

Material Using Flow Cytometry;" Hedley et al., "DNA Flow Cytometry of Paraffin-Embedded Tissue;" Hedley, "Flow Cytometry Using Paraffin-Embedded Tissue: Five Years On." The practical value of this method was immediately realized insofar as it allowed cytometrists to bypass the need for fresh pieces of tumor and to conduct retrospective studies, particularly on rare tumors where a paraffin-embedded "archive" is generally the only source of significant numbers of pathological specimens; see Coon, Landay, and Weinstein, "Flow Cytometric Analysis of Paraffin-Embedded Tumors."

165. Taylor, *An Immunohistological Study of Human and Murine Lymphomata.* As part of a postdoctoral fellowship, Taylor moved in the late 1970s to southern California to work with Robert J. Lukes. Taylor never returned to Britain, but retained ties with his thesis director with whom he published a book on the histopathology of diseases of the lymph nodes.

166. Taylor and Mason "The Immunohistological Detection of Intracellular Immunoglobulin in Formalin-Paraffin Sections from Multiple Myeloma and Related Conditions Using the Immunoperoxidase Technique;" Mason and Taylor, "The Distribution of Muramidase (Lysozyme) in Human Tissues;" Mason and Taylor, "Staining of the A Antigen Human Erythrocytes;" Mason, Farrell, and Taylor, "The Detection of Intracellular Antigens in Human Leucocytes by Immunoperoxidase Staining."

167. Taylor, "Immunohistologial Approach to Tumor Diagnosis," 196.

168. For a review, see Shi, Cote, and Taylor, "Antigen Retrieval Immunohistochemistry."

169. Olav Torgersen, cited in Brandtzaeg, "The Increasing Power," 52.

170. Taylor, *Hodgkin's Disease and the Lymphomas*, 263.

171. Ibid., "Foreword."

172. Preud'homme and Seligmann, "Surface Bound Immunoglobulins." First described in 1944, Waldenström's macroglobulinemia remains a bona fide nosological entity. Described at the morphological level as a proliferation of lymphoplasmacytoid cells that secrete IgM, it is presently believed by some that these cells are of the same lineage as CLL cells. See Roitt, *Essential Immunology*, 375. As a borderline entity, the well-known disorder did not fit all classifications. When presenting the "European concept," Lennert had this to say about the disease: "The macroglobulinemia (lymphoid myeloma) could not yet be localized in our classification. Cytologically in macroglobulinemia different types of cells are present. . . . We consider it most suitable to group this disease to the 'progressive hyperplasias' according to Robb-Smith (1947, 1964)" (Lennert, "Classification of Malignant," 104–5). In Lennert's 1973 scheme Waldenström's macroglobulinemia lost its status as an unclassifiable "nosological entity" and became a mere "symptom." See Lennert, Stein, and Kaiserling, "Cytological and Functional Criteria for the Classification of Malignant Lymphomata."

173. Preud'homme and Seligmann, "Surface Bound Immunoglobulins."

174. Lennert, "Classification of Malignant,"103.

175. Lennert, "Preface," v.

176. Lennert, "Classification of Malignant,"104.

177. Taylor, "Changing Concepts in the Classification of Lymphoma."

178. Lennert and his coworkers proposed "functional criteria" for the diagnosis and classification of lymphomas. These criteria would allow correlation of pathological cells with normal cells by demonstrating the persistence of a normal cell function in the pathological state. See Lennert, Stein, and Kaiserling, "Cytological and Functional Criteria." It should be noted that the addition of functional criteria did not initially make the classification functional. This was a later transformation. As Robb-Smith, Tearloch, and Taylor point out, "It [the Kiel classification] does not claim to be 'functional,' but recognition of immunoglobulin synthesis, as an indication of B-cell derivation, is important in its taxonomy; however the Kiel classification proper, as against Lennert's (1978) modifications, did not accept the terms B- and T-cell in its nomenclature" (Robb-Smith, Tearloch, and Taylor, *Lymph Node Biopsy*, 252).

179. From an immunological point of view (Hansen and Good, "Malignant Disease of the Lymphoid System in Immunological Perspective") the two classifications are the same. From a pathologist's view (Berard et al., "Discussion II: Roundtable Discussion of Histopathologic Classification") they are different.

180. While we cannot go into details here, this is an important point, because both the Kiel and the Lukes-Collins classifications are uncritically presented as the first example of immunology-based classifications. Not quite so! See Sreenan and Tubbs, "The Influence of Immunology."

181. Lennert, Stein, and Kaiserling, "Cytological and Functional Criteria," 29. It was not possible to culture cells from lymphomas and show that the "histiocytes" are B cells until 1978. See A. L. Epstein, "The Cell Culture, Heterotransplantation and Biological Characterization of the Human Malignant Lymphomas."

182. For the table, see Lukes and Collins, "Approaches to the Classification of the Lymphomata," 24. As Lukes and Collins had pointed out in a publication the previous year, "On the basis of our clinical morphological correlation studies, the majority of FCC (follicular center cells) lymphomas can be correlated to the stages in B cell (FCC) transformation" (Lukes and Collins, "Immunologic Characterization of Human Malignant Lymphomas," 1492).

183. Cottier, Turk, and Sobin, "A Proposal for a Standardized System of Reporting Human Lymph Node Morphology in Relation to Immunological Function."

184. Robb-Smith, Tearloch, and Taylor, *Lymph Node Biopsy*, 271.

185. Nancy Lee Harris et al., "A Revised European-American Classification of Lymphoid Neoplasms."

186. Nancy Lee Harris et al., "The World Health Organization Classification of Neoplastic Diseases of the Hematopoietic and Lymphoid Tissues."

187. Interview with Keith Miller, London, 5 May 1999.

188. Coons et al., "The Demonstration of Pneumococcal Antigen in Tissues by the Use of Fluorescent Antibody." See also Coons, "The Beginnings of Immunofluorescence;" Coons, "Introduction: The Development of Immunohistochemistry."

189. Graham and Karnovsky, "The Early Stages of Absorption of Injected Horseradish Peroxidase in the Proximal Tubules of Mouse Kidney;" Nakane and Pierce, "Enzyme-Labelled Antibodies: Preparation and Application for the Localization of Antigen"; Avrameas and Uriel, "Méthode de marquage d'antigènes et d'anticops avec des enzymes et son application en immunodiffusion." For additional details concerning these methods, see Sternberger, *Immunocytochemistry*.

190. Sternberger et al., "The Unlabeled Antibody Enzyme Method of Immunohistochemistry;" Heitzmann and Richards, "Use of the Avidin-Biotin Complex for Specific Staining of Biological Membranes in Electron Microscopy."

191. Cordell et al., "Immunoenzymatic Labeling;" Erber, Pinching, and Mason, "Immunocytochemical Detection of T and B Cell Populations in Routine Blood Smears."

192. Brandtzaeg, "The Increasing Power," 51.

193. For an overview of these possibilities and the corresponding literature, see Sreenan and Tubbs, "The Influence of Immunology," 575–6.

194. See James R. Wright, "The Development of the Frozen Section Technique."

195. Interview with Keith Miller, London, 5 May 1999.

196. Davey, Elghetany, and Kurec, "Immunophenotyping of Hematologic Neoplasms in Paraffin-Embedded Tissue Sections," S18.

197. Taylor, "Immunocytochemical Methods in the Study of Lymphoma and Related Conditions," 507. This problem was not confined to IPT. As the Pathology Ad Hoc Working Group explained to the National Cancer Institute at the end of the 1970s, the procedures used for morphology blocked clinical research initiatives in a variety of ways: "Almost all pathological diagnosis of cancer is made on formalin-fixed paraffin-embedded and hematoxylin and eosin–stained slides. The first thing the pathologist does after examining the tissue is to fix it in formalin. This makes it impossible to do tissue culture, electron microscopy, histochemistry, enzymatology, hormone determinations, electrophoresis, autoradiography, and high pressure liquid chromatography" ("More Oncopathology Research Asked, Development Workshop Approved," 4).

198. The Berlin and Oslo events are recalled in Brandtzaeg, "The Increasing Power," 59.

199. Not all pathologists felt this way. Some felt immunofluorescence techniques were more sensitive than (enzyme-based) immunohistochemical techniques, particularly in the detection of immunoglobulin in B-cell lymphomas. See Warnke et al., "A Study of Lymphoproliferative Diseases Comparing Immunofluorescence with Immunohistochemistry," 67. And, according to Brandtzaeg, "frozen tissue sections remain the gold standard for the reliable detection of many cell surface markers and a variety of tissue antigens based on immunostaining with [monoclonal antibodies]" (Brandtzaeg, "The Increasing Power," 63).

200. Taylor, "Immunohistologial Approach," 195. As Taylor pointed out, just because there was immunoglobulin in the cytoplasm didn't necessarily qualify a cell as a B lymphocyte capable of secreting lymphocytes. It was, however, the most plausible explanation. "It must be noted that the simple demonstration of a substance within a cell is not necessarily evidence of its in situ synthesis, but in the absence of other explanations for its presence (such as phagocytosis or absorption by specific receptors) this provides a tenable working hypothesis" (Taylor, "Immunocytochemical Methods," 499). This "working hypothesis" was, moreover, widely accepted. German researchers studying intracanial lymphomas concluded on the basis of immunoperoxidase examination that "In all cases intracellular immunoglobulins were demonstrable in tumor cells and in a majority of the tumors these were monoclonal. Thus, all malignant lymphomas proved to be of B cell origin with demonstrable cytoplasmic immunoglobulin production." (Houthoff et al., "Intracranial Malignant Lymphomas. A Morphologic and Immunocytologic Study of Twenty Cases," 203.) Note that, pace the previous quotation, the staining pattern could be either monoclonal (either one light chain or one heavy chain) or polyclonal. If the staining was monoclonal, then there was no reason to believe that the cell in question was in the process of ingesting antibodies rather than producing them, for, if ingested, antibodies would, by definition, have been polyclonal (containing different heavy and light chains).

201. Indeed, this was the case in Taylor's view: "Immunoperoxidase studies strongly suggest that lymphomas corresponding to four normal cell types, namely the small lymphocytes, follicle center cell, immunoblast, and plasma cell, are all variants of a single cell type, the B lymphocyte, not four completely distinct cell types as previously supposed (i.e., chronic lymphocytic leukemia, small lymphocytic lymphoma, follicle center cell lymphoma, immunoblastic sarcoma and multiple myeloma share a common origin from the B lymphocyte series)" (Taylor, "Immunohistologial Approach," 195).

202. For example: "Even more striking is the observation that in many cases of follicle center cell lymphoma and immunoblastic sarcoma, many of the cells shown to contain monoclonal immunoglobulin are indistinguishable morphologically from normal reactive plasma cells. This serves to emphasize the morphological diversity of the neoplastic cells occurring within a single neoplasm, and questions the tacit assumption, inherent in most histological classifications, that the different morphological forms of lymphoma are completely distinct from one another" (Taylor, "Immunohistological Approach," 195).

203. Mason, "Summary: Philadelphia Stories," unpublished text presented to the Society for Applied Immunohistochemistry, 2 June 1997. Many thanks to Dr. Mason for sending us a copy of his text.

204. The name was a tribute to three scientists who played a key role in the development of electrophoresis and the ultracentrifuge: Kai O. Pedersen (KOP), Arne Tiselius (AT), and The Svedberg (TS).

205. Haughland, cited in Brandtzaeg, "The Increasing Power," 55–6.

206. Centers for Disease Control, "Guidelines for the Performance of CD4+ T-Cell Determinations in Persons with Human Immunodeficiency Virus Infection."

Chapter 8

1. A major (Neo-Marxist) school of contemporary French political economy has called their approach "théorie de la régulation." Members of this school explicitly reject the identification of their approach with the study of increased state intervention through "réglementation"; see Boyer, *La théorie de la régulation*, 30–1.

2. Canguilhem, "Régulation," 1. Our translation of: "L'ajustement, conformément à quelque règle ou norme, d'une pluralité de mouvements ou d'actes et de leurs effets ou produits que leur diversité ou leur succession rend d'abord étrangers les uns aux autres".

3. For instance, according to the CDC, "[as IPT] has moved from research laboratories to clinical laboratories, the need for standardization has increased" (Centers for Disease Control, "Guidelines for the Performance of CD4+ T-Cell Determinations in Persons with Human Immunodeficiency Virus Infection").

4. For other exceptions to the one-way model, see Reines, "On the Locus of Medical Discovery," and Sinding, *Le clinicien et le chercheur.*

5. For a pathologist's view of the "mechanics of operating an immunophenotyping laboratory," see Foucar, Chen, and Crago, "Organization and Operation of a Flow Cytometric Immunophenotyping Laboratory." For a technician's description of a "clinical" flow laboratory, see Oakley, "Bravely Entering the New World of Flow Cytometry."

6. For example: "So by suggesting these [IPT procedures] in a document like this [clinical-laboratory guidelines], this will be accepted in the framework of the United States in the clinical laboratories at least, and now many research laboratories as well are beginning to take this as a document that will have some use" (interview with Alan Landay, Chicago, 21 November 1991).

7. As one respondent put it, "we want to set [standards and guidelines] based on real practice that can be instituted into a regular lab that grinds out a lot of data, not just the Olympian lab that might do this on an occasional basis" (interview with Alan Landay, Chicago, 21 November 1991).

8. Reiser, *Medicine and the Reign of Technology*, 184–9. For a more recent, although rather cursory examination of these issues, see also Rosenfeld, *Four Centuries of Clinical Chemistry*, esp. 466–8 and 503–14. For a history of the regulation of the clinical laboratory in general, see also Derman and Dorsey, "The Pathology of Regulation," and Kingham, "History of FDA Regulation of Clinical Research."

9. To speak of quality control is somewhat of a misnomer as the process is predicated on the regulation of quantities. On the distinction between internal quality control and external quality assessment, see England, "Internal Quality Control and Calibration"; Lewis, "External Quality Assessment in Europe." On the American situation, see Koepke, "The College of American Pathologists Survey Programme." See also National Committee for Clinical Laboratory Standards, *Clinical Applications of Flow Cytometry: Quality Assurance and Immunophenotyping of Peripheral Blood Lymphocytes. Tentative Guideline*, 3.

10. World Health Organization, *External Quality Assessment of Health Laboratories.* For an editorial comment on the WHO report, see "Quality of Performance in Pathology Laboratories," 599.

11. See, e.g., O'Connell, "Metrology"; Schaffer, "Late Victorian Metrology and Its Instrumentation." Another example is provided by the field of thermometry, where direct measurement has been impossible. As Herbert Arthur Klein points out, "The first widely used temperature scales—Fahrenheit, Réaumur and Celsius—provided degrees of various sizes for comparing one temperature with another. But none of them permits measurements in magnitudes proportional to the average atomic and molecular kinetic energies of the substances in question. Only a thermodynamic scale can do this." Moreover, since such a scale has yet to be forthcoming, even today, temperature cannot be measured directly. Herbert Arthur Klein, *The Science of Measurement*, 322.

12. Kidd and Vogt, "Report of the Workshop on the Evaluation of T-Cell Subsets during HIV Infection and AIDS," 4.

13. Interview with Francis F. Mandy, Ottawa, 16 December 1994.

14. As pointed out many years ago by Canguilhem, "The normal is the effect obtained by the execution of the normative project, it is the norm exhibited in the fact". Canguilhem, *The Normal and the Pathological*, 243.

15. Lewis, "Standardization and Harmonization of the Blood Count."

16. Ibid., 10.

17. Ibid., 10.

18. Ibid., 10.

19. Ibid., 10.

20. Ibid., 11. The hemocytometer counting chamber is an instrument for measuring the number of blood cells in a sample, and the Romanowsky stain is a mixture of cytological dyes.

21. Ibid., 12–13.

22. Things are becoming more complex. According to a 2000 European Union's In Vitro Diagnostics Directive, it is no longer enough to demonstrate that a given in vitro diagnostic device has been designed and manufactured in such a way that it can achieve the required accuracy, sensitivity, specificity, and so on. In addition, manufacturers must demonstrate the traceability of values assigned to calibrators and control materials: "Traceability means that a calibrator value is systematically derived from a higher-order reference material or reference method through an unbroken chain of comparisons. In other words, the value-assignment scheme must start with the highest available reference method or reference material—ideally . . . a World Health Organization (WHO) standard, or another certified reference material. Accuracy is transferred from these primary reference materials or methods, through secondary or intermediate reference materials and methods, to the product calibrators and, ultimately, to the measurement of patients' specimens." In what looks like an epistemological fight between relativists and realists, while "U.S. laboratories accept differences among methods as inevitable and compensate with method-specific reference ranges, their European counterparts have refused to abandon the pursuit of analytical truth." See Powers, "Traceability of Assay Calibrators."

23. As for Asia, Tatsumi et al. ("Standardization in Flow Cytometry") complain that, in Japan, regulatory work lags behind that in Western countries. Japanese quality-control surveys have revealed the existence of "differences in data . . . among instruments and laboratories." In an unintentional flight of Foucaultian oratory, the authors argue that the way to minimize those differences is through the establishment of "nation-wide surveillance."

24. Lewis, "External Quality Assessment in Europe," 55.

25. Ibid.

26. Goguel, "Interlaboratory Trials;" Goguel et al., "Interlaboratory Quality Assessment of Lymphocyte Phenotyping."

27. Lewis, "External Quality Assessment in Europe," 55–6.

28. Lewis and Burgess, "Quality Control in Haematology."

29. Ibid., 256.

30. The information on the UK NEQAS is based on the following documents: UK NEQAS, *Report and Directory*, 3rd ed. (March 1998); UK NEQAS for Leucocyte Immunophenotyping, *Handbook and Report*, 2nd ed. (n.d.); David Barnett, interview, Sheffield, U.K., 24 April 1999. For a criticism of exclusive reliance on EQA schemes, see "How to Ensure Quality," 196.

31. Aboulker and Swart, "Preliminary Analysis of the Concorde Trial," 889–90.

32. The four schemes concerned only fresh blood samples; a separate histopathology UK NEQAS dealt with histopathological, formalin-fixed samples such as those used in the diagnosis of lymphomas.

33. Of the participants, 153 were located in the United Kingdom, 32 in France, 25 in Italy and Sweden, 24 in Switzerland, 12 in Australia, and 11 in Ireland, with the remaining being located in 27 other countries (European, African, Middle Eastern, South and North American, and Asian).

34. See., e.g., General Haematology Task Force of BCSH, "Immunophenotyping in the Diagnosis of Acute Leukaemias."

35. Interview with David Barnett, Sheffield, U.K., 24 April 1999.

36. These de facto guidelines thus have an even stronger feedback on the establishment of the official ones when the same person participates in both activities. For instance, David Barnett was a member of the committee drafting guidelines for CD34 IPT.

37. On SIHON, see van't Veer et al., "Quality Assessment of Immunological Marker Analysis and the Immunological Diagnosis in Leukaemia and Lymphoma"; van't Veer and Gratama, "Quality Assessment for Immunophenotyping of Leukaemias and Lymphomas"; Kluin-Nelemans et al., "Pitfalls in the Immunophenotyping of Leukaemia and Leukaemic Lymphomas"; Gratama, Bolhuis, and van 't Veer, "Quality Control of Flow Cytometric Immunophenotyping of Haematological Malignancies."

38. Gratama, Bolhuis, and van't Veer, "Quality Control of Flow Cytometric," 155.

39. Kluin-Nelemans et al. "Pitfalls in the Immunophenotyping of Leukaemia," 697.

40. See Martini et al., *First European Quality Control of Cellular Phenotyping by Flow Cytometry.*

41. Martini and D'Hautcourt, "Contrôle de qualité Franco-Belge des phénotypages cellulaires analysés en cytométrie en flux."

42. Martini et al., *First European Quality Control,* 15.

43. Ibid., 60. Even though the study documented the different makes of flow cytometers in use, for the purposes of the study all machines were considered equal. In terms of market share, the "big three" (Becton Dickinson, Coulter, Ortho) controlled the market.

44. Ibid., 25. A recent survey of external quality-control programs in the United States has typed hospital laboratories using IPT into "general," "university," "military," and "other." See Koepke, "Survey of Quality Assurance/Quality Control Practices for CD4+ Lymphocyte Counting."

45. Martini et al., *First European Quality Control,* 55–6.

46. EQALM has asked for recognition from a motley of relevant European scientific associations, including the Forum for European Societies of Clinical Chemistry (FESCC); the European Confederation of Laboratory Medicine (ECLM); the International Council for Standardisation in Haematology, European Division; the European branch of World Association of Societies in Pathology (WASP); the European Society of Clinical Microbiology and Infectious Diseases; the European Federation of Immunology Societies; the European Conference for External Quality Assessment Organisations (ECEQAO); and the Nordic Committee for External Quality Assurance Programmes in Laboratory Medicine (NQLM).

47. "Standardization of flow cytometry assays for clinical cell analysis" (project reference: BMH4972611); information posted on the European Union Website: http://dbs.cordis.lu (information updated on 2000-07-04).

48. Koepke, "The College of American Pathologists Survey Programme."

49. For example, a recent interlaboratory study out of Brigham and Women's Hospital in Boston found that "Of the 24 patients in this survey, 14 had CD4-count results with enough variation to have led to conflicting treatment recommendations; three of the 24 patients fulfilled the revised Centers for Disease Control and Prevention case definition on the basis of results from some but not all laboratories" (Sax et al., "Potential Clinical Implications of Interlaboratory Variability in CD4+ T-Lymphocyte Counts of Patients Infected with Human Immunodeficiency Virus," 1121).

50. Belgium, for example, requires patients to have less than 100 CD4+ cells/mm^3 to be eligible for triple therapy. See D'Hautcourt, "Contrôle de qualité," 87.

51. Interview with Alan Landay, Chicago, 21 November 1991.

52. Paxton et al., "Results of the Flow Cytometry ACTG Quality Control Program."

53. Interview with Alan Landay, Chicago, 21 November 1991.

54. See Wagner, "The College of American Pathologists."

55. "As these [IPT] and other flow cytometric assays leave the research laboratory and become integrated into the mainstream of diagnostic pathology, the performance of proper quality control for these assays becomes crucial not only for optimal patient care, but also to fulfill the requirements for reimbursement by third-party carriers" (McCoy, Carey, and Krause, "Quality Control in Flow Cytometry for Diagnostic Pathology I," 27).

56. Nicholson, "Quality Control in Immunophenotyping," 7.

57. National Committee for Clinical Laboratory Standards, *Clinical Applications of Flow Cytometry: Quality Assurance and Immunophenotyping of Peripheral Blood Lymphocytes. Tentative Guideline.* As noted by McCoy and colleagues, "Because of

controversies concerning the optimum anticoagulant, method of specimen preparation, and data analysis, flow cytometry quality control programs are still evolving. With a careful dissection of each aspect of flow cytometric analysis, a consensus on these matters should eventually be reached. The subcommittee on flow cytometry for the National Committee for Clinical Laboratory Standards is providing a leadership role in this endeavor" (McCoy, Carey, and Krause. "Quality Control in Flow Cytometry for Diagnostic Pathology I," 37).

58. See National Committee for Clinical Laboratory Standards [NCCLS], *Clinical Applications of Flow Cytometry: Immunophenotyping of Leukemic Cells; Proposed Guideline*; NCCLS, *Clinical Applications of Flow Cytometry: Immunophenotyping of Leukemic Cells; Approved Guideline*; NCCLS, *Methods for Reticulocyte Counting.*

59. For a review of the problems associated with CD4+ counts and clinical trials, see Fei, Paxton, and Chen, "Difficulties in Precise Quantitation of CD4+ T-Lymphocytes for Clinical Trials."

60. According to a survey carried out by the CDC, of 270 laboratories canvassed, 158 were hospital laboratories of which 71 were privately owned (Centers for Disease Control, *Model Performance Evaluation Program,* 3).

61. Although it originated in the United States, because of the worldwide diffusion of flow cytometry instrumentation produced in that country, the effects of the movement have been anything but local. For instance, the basic units of analysis for a recent Italian quality-control study are inevitably Becton Dickinson and Coulter; see Danesi, Spanò, and Altavista, "Quality Control Study of the Italian Group of Cytometry on Flow Cytometry Cellular DNA Content Measurements."

62. Parker et al., "Leukocyte Immunophenotyping by Flow Cytometry in a Multisite Study," 188.

63. Marti et al., "Normal Human Blood Density Gradient Lymphocyte Subset Analysis."

64. Ibid., 50.

65. Waxdal et al., "Interlaboratory Survey of Lymphocyte Immunophenotyping," 345.

66. Ibid., 353.

67. Ibid., 346.

68. Ibid., 354.

69. Interview with Francis F. Mandy, Ottawa, 16 December 1994. The interviewee noted that when the flow cytometer and the hematology instrument sit side by side in the same laboratory so that you can run the same sample on both instruments within six hours, results are quite comparable. Problems arise when, as is often the case in the United States, CD4 counts are performed by

large reference laboratories that, in order to profit from economies of scale, concentrate flow in one city and hematology in another.

70. Waxdal et al., "Interlaboratory Survey," 354.

71. Becton Dickinson, *Normal Values*, 11.

72. National Committee for Clinical Laboratory Standards, *Clinical Applications of Flow Cytometry: Quality Assurance and Immunophenotyping of Peripheral Blood Lymphocytes. Tentative Guideline*, 61. Some companies now sell flow cytometers that work with finite volumes of blood and thus give absolute numbers. Referred to as volumetric capillary cytometry (VCC), the new equipment has "consolidated the process to a single platform," although a recent study found that on samples containing less than 200 CD4+ cells/mm^3, "VCC variability was higher than the flow cytometry and hematology variability" (O'Gorman et al., "Inter- and Intra-institutional Evaluation of Automated Volumetric Capillary Cytometry," 173).

73. Homburger et al., "Assessment of Interlaboratory Variability of Immunophenotyping."

74. It should be pointed out that CAP has since undertaken the certification of clinical flow laboratories and that, in addition to on-site visits by CAP inspectors, one of the certification requirements is participation in a recognized proficiency program (interview with Alan Landay, Chicago, 21 November 1991).

75. Homburger et al., "Assessment of Interlaboratory Variability of Immunophenotyping," 48.

76. Ibid., 47.

77. Ibid., 48.

78. Gerber, "Centers for Disease Control Programs in Flow Cytometric Immunophenotyping."

79. The Model Performance Evaluation Program for T-Lymphocyte Immunophenotyping is still regularly performed twice a year at the time of this writing and the results, as well as the analysis of the results, are posted on the CDC Website.

80. National Committee for Clinical Laboratory Standards, *Clinical Applications of Flow Cytometry: Quality Assurance and Immunophenotyping of Peripheral Blood Lymphocytes. Tentative Guideline*, 1.

81. Keeping the number 400 in mind, the Walter Reed group offers an interesting example of how contingent this figure can be. For example, in addition to flow cytometry, one can obtain CD4 percentages using a standard hematology analyzer. However, unlike flow cytometers, the numbers generated by hematology analyzers tend to vary according to the anticoagulant used and the storage time. A study conducted at the Walter Reed Army Institute of Research concluded that, using a hematology analyzer, "[t]he CD4 absolute count was

increased by as much as 236 cells/mm^3 48 h after collection" (Rentas, Perfetto, and Rickman, "The Effect of Anticoagulant and Room Temperature Storage on Lymphocyte Markers").

82. Rickman et al., "Department of Army Lymphocyte Immunophenotyping Quality Assurance Program," 85.

83. Statistical Graphics Inc. of Denver, Colo. furnished software for the statistical analysis. See Rickman et al., "Department of Army Lymphocyte Immunophenotyping," 88.

84. Ibid., 88, table 1.

85. Rickman, Monical, and Waxdal, "Improved Precision in the Enumeration of Absolute Numbers of Lymphocyte Phenotypes," 54–5.

86. Rickman et al., "Department of Army Lymphocyte Immunophenotyping," 95.

87. Coulter Electronics Inc., "Interlaboratory Quality Assurance Program."

88. Muirhead, "Establishment of Quality Control Procedures in Clinical Flow Cytometry," 9.

89. As pointed out by the authors of an Italian nationwide quality-control trial on lymphocyte IPT, their "study design proved valid and suitable for a large-scale evaluation of both instrument performance and cytometer operators' skill" (Brando and Sommaruga, "Nationwide Quality Control Trial on Lymphocyte Immunophenotyping," 294). For a review of the factors involved in quality control in IPT, see McCarthy and Fetterhoff, "Issues for Quality Assurance in Clinical Flow Cytometry."

90. The following passage is largely based on an interview with Francis F. Mandy, Ottawa, 16 December 1994.

91. It should be noted that, insofar as the laboratories are aware that they are being monitored, they will usually use extra care in analyzing the test samples. In other words, monitored activities are not necessarily representative of everyday operations.

92. D'Hautcourt, "Contôle de qualité," 91.

93. The absence of external norms has not prevented the onset of sanctions. For example, using the NCCLS guidelines as a base, the AIDS section of the National Institute of Allergy and Infectious Diseases (NIAID) has defined performance criteria to discipline and punish laboratories participating in their obligatory Flow Cytometry Quality Assessment Program. "An unsatisfactory level of performance is defined as 33% of a laboratory's CD4 analyses with residual values greater than or equal to ±5% and with deviates greater than or equal to 2. The residual value is a laboratory's CD4 value minus the median of all participating laboratories. The deviate is the residual divided by the interquartile

range (IQR). The IQR is three-quarters of the difference between the 25th and 75th percentiles of all participating laboratories" (Kagan and Mayall, "Introduction to the NIAID Guideline for Flow Cytometric Immunophenotyping," 709). Contingent upon quarterly assessments, a laboratory's status may move from "certified" to "provisionally certified" and further on down the road to "probationary" and "suspended." Late reports receive, in addition to a knuckle-rapping written notification, a penalty "equivalent to one unsatisfactory sample" (ibid., 710).

94. IHCs are different from so-called analyte-specific reagents (ASRs) which are, so to speak, the active ingredients (antibodies, receptor proteins, nucleic acid sequences, etc.) entering into the production of IHCs by manufacturers of in vitro diagnostic products or by specialized laboratories producing their own "homebrewed" assays. For a discussion of the regulation of ASRs by the FDA, see Gibbs, "ASRs: FDA Issues Final Rule."

95. Ricki, "New Antibody Classification May Restrict Research."

96. Graziano, "FDA Panel Recommends Class II for IHC Reagents," 1, 45; Stone, "Companies Fear FDA Rule on Antibodies," 494.

97. For reasons that are too long to detail here, the CAP intervention was restricted to antibodies used in vitro on tissue sections. It thus does not concern directly flow cytometric (or serological) reagents. However, the relevance of this episode for practices, such as flow cytometry, resorting to similar or the same antibody reagents has not escaped observers in the field.

98. Ricki, "New Antibody Classification May Restrict Research."

99. This does not mean that biological stains have not been subject to complex regulatory interventions. The Biological Stain Commission was founded in 1944 to address this issue and has acted since as a certifying agency and repository for batches of stains. It has been argued that it is precisely the success of this voluntary certification program that led the FDA to classify these products in the class I category. See Taylor, "An Exaltation of Experts," 233.

100. Graziano, "FDA Panel Recommends Class II for IHC Reagents," 45.

101. Takes and Graham, "Letter to *Science*," 619–20.

102. Takes, "Letter to *Cap Today*," 6–7.

103. Gibbs, "Regulations and Standards: "FDA Makes a Better Rule for IHC's"; Graziano, "Final Chapter Inked in IHC Saga."

104. Hutt, "A History of Government Regulation of Adulteration and Misbranding of Medical Devices."

105. Kahan, "The Evolution of FDA Regulation of New Medical Device Technology and Product Applications." For a general review of the broader issues involved, see Estrin, *The Medical Device Industry*.

106. Stelzer and Grimauld, "Reimbursement for Clinical Flow Cytometry Testing."

107. See, e.g., Shapin and Schaffer, *Leviathan and the Air Pump*, on the use of anomalous suspension to calibrate the earliest vacuum pumps.

108. One comparison is between the antibody that is used to stain the cells with a similar antibody from the same class in order to eliminate nonspecific staining. This comparison is termed an "isotype control" and opinion varies on its utility. See Sreenen et al., "The Use of Isotypic Control Antibodies in the Analysis of CD3+ and CD3+, CD4+ Lymphocyte Subsets in Flow Cytometry."

109. From, e.g., Flow Cytometry Standards Corp.

110. QC3 from Flow Cytometry Standards Corp. or Cytotrol from Coulter or, in an interesting turn by which biological material assumes some of the qualities of nonbiological material, chicken erythrocytes. A veritable cellular menagerie can be mobilized to this effect; see, e.g., Pierrez and Ronot, "Use of Diploid and Triploid Trout Erythrocytes as Internal Standards in Flow Cytometry."

111. Vogt et al., "Model System Evaluating Fluorescein-Labeled Microbeads," 301.

112. Ibid.

113. National Committee for Clinical Laboratory Standards, *Clinical Applications of Flow Cytometry: Quality Assurance and Immunophenotyping of Peripheral Blood Lymphocytes. Tentative Guideline*, 31.

114. Vogt et al., "Model System Evaluating Fluorescein-Labeled Microbeads." Similarly, Vogt et al., in "Interlaboratory Study of Cellular Fluorescence Intensity Measurements," claim that "[u]ncharacterized differences in the operating conditions of flow cytometers can influence cellular [fluorescence intensity] measurements, but consistent results can be obtained if a stained cellular calibrator [fluoresceinated calf thymocyte nuclei (Fluorotrol)], is analyzed in addition to the proper microbead standards."

115. Other systems are available. Quickcal, e.g., offers a mix of beads "which match the fluorescence spectra of the labeled cells." The claim is that "[n]ow comparisons of fluorescent cell intensities may be made directly from histograms obtained from different instruments under different operating conditions" (Schwartz et al., "Quickcal Plus: An Automated System to Determine the Fluorescence Intensity of Labeled Cells in MESF Units," 136).

116. Becton Dickinson, *Normal Values*. McCoy and Overton, in "Quality Control in Flow Cytometry for Diagnostic Pathology: II", after noting that "[i]mmunophenotyping, as many other clinical assays, is interpreted only in the context of reference values obtained from healthy control individuals," pointed out that "[w]hile the use of these reference values, or ranges, has been commonplace in the clinical flow cytometry laboratory for well over a decade, there has been little consensus in standardizing how these values should be obtained, analyzed, or expressed."

117. Giorgi, Kesson, and Chou, "Immunodeficiency and Infectious Diseases," 174.

118. Marti et al., "CD20 and CD5 Expression in B-Chronic Lymphocytic Leukemia," 481.

119. Statland and Winkel, "Physiological Variability of Leukocytes in Healthy Subjects."

120. A short section entitled "Race" in a clinical monograph on "normal values" by Becton Dickinson (*Normal Values*) reads as follows: "All the individuals in this study were [white]. Preliminary studies using this system with patients of other races confirm earlier observations, which suggest that [Asian] individuals have relatively more NK cells and, therefore, studies with such populations will require that appropriate reference ranges are determined separately." The text refers to an earlier paper by Prince et al., "Influence of Racial Background on the Distribution of T-Cell Subsets." More recent articles on the topic are Senju et al., "Two-Color Immunofluorescence and Flow Cytometric Analysis of Peripheral Blood Lymphocyte Subsets in Caucasian and Japanese Healthy Subjects;" and Mili et al., "The Associations of Race, Cigarette Smoking, and Smoking Cessation to Measures of the Immune System in Middle-Aged Men." In spite of the dubious claim in this latter study, namely that "[t]he associations between race and immunologic status are important because they reflect the effect of race on the immune system and therefore the variation of immune measures within each race category" (ibid., 187), all the clinicians we interviewed pointed out that the limited diagnostic significance of the supposed differences has drastically curtailed the number of studies devoted to this topic. The term "biological variables," however, does not necessarily refer to a macroconstruct such as "race." For instance, an interviewee pointed out that "what we are learning is that only about half of the variables can be attributed to the instrument, the operator, the technical component. The other half is biological variation, that is, has to do with the patient and how the blood was taken, the hour of the day, what the patient ate, what the patient drank, what the patient smoked" (interview with Francis F. Mandy, Ottawa, 15 December 1994). The search, however, continues. See Kam et al., "Lymphocyte Subpopulation Reference Ranges for Monitoring Human Immunodeficiency Virus–Infected Chinese Adults"; Reichert et al., "Lymphocyte Subset Reference Ranges in Adult Caucasians." A report from Thailand carried out by Becton Dickinson and local researchers claimed that not only is there a significant difference between white and Thai CD4+ counts but that the count placed "the lower limit of normal for Thai males within approximately 2% of the US CDC surveillance definition of AIDS," thus suggesting that standard Western values for staging and monitoring HIV disease were not appropriate. See Webster et al., "Lymphocyte Immunophenotype Reference Ranges in Healthy Thai Adults," 427.

121. Hensleigh, Waters, and Herzenberg, "Human T Lymphocyte Differentiation Antigens: Effects of Blood Sample Storage on Leu Antibody Binding"; Loken, Meiners, and Terstappen, "Comparison of Sample Preparation Techniques for Flow Cytometric Analysis of Immunofluorescence," 53.

122. Carter et al., "Flow Cytometric Analysis of Whole Blood Lysis, Three Anticoagulants, and Five Cell Preparations."

123. In a letter to us (5 May 1995), Dr. Gerald E. Marti explained that the study was carried out "because at the time that the NCCLS guidelines were being written no such study existed." He also insisted that the study did uncover one difference ("FACS Lyse consistently produced a smaller signal on the forward light scatter") and that he "did not conceive of that series of experiments as a consumer report. Nonetheless I can understand how you might perceive it that way."

123. National Committee for Clinical Laboratory Standards, *Clinical Applications of Flow Cytometry: Quality Assurance and Immunophenotyping of Peripheral Blood Lymphocytes. Tentative Guideline.*

125. Ibid., 71.

126. "Consensus guidelines for immunophenotyping of peripheral blood lymphocytes recommend evaluation of a specimen collected from a healthy individual, prepared using the laboratory's standard protocol. . . . [However] [o]ther types of quality control specimens are also increasingly available commercially (e.g., cryopreserved mononuclear cells, stabilized whole blood specimens). The value of such materials is that they provide a more constant reference point than do 'normal' specimens from different individuals" (Muirhead, "Establishment of Quality Control Procedures in Clinical Flow Cytometry," 9).

127. Loken et al., *Establishing Optimal Lymphocyte Gates for Immunophenotyping Using Leucogate.*

128. Coulter Cytometry, *Optimizing Cytometry Systems for Measurement of Biologic Samples.* These are mononuclear cells. As far as blood cells are concerned, D. Barnett in Britain has recently produced a stabilized form of blood marketed by Ortho under the ominous-sounding name ABSOLUTECONTROL. See Barnett et al., "Evaluation of a Novel Stable Whole Blood Quality Control Material for Lymphocyte Subset Analysis."

129. 29 November 1994—Louisiana State University, New Orleans.

130. 29 November 1999—Stanford University, Stanford, Calif. The "skills" expected from competent operators have changed over time and with the switch from the laboratory to the clinic. As a contributor to a flow cytometry electronic bulletin board explained in September 1995, "I began to learn flow more than 15 years ago. I started the hard way on old FACS I's and II's steering beams through small holes, replacing fuses and proteus wheels in power supplies so lasers would run, tracking down leaks in tubing to obtain stable dropoffs for sorts, clearing clogs in nozzles and holders, and aligning mirrored quartz flow cells. Then when we became proficient at flow cytometry in the research setting, the daring and wise hematopathologists who foresaw the powerful tool flow would be in the clinical lab came to us with their stained samples for us to count

their T and B cells. This was about 10 years ago. For the last 5 years we have readily and graciously incorporated the [quality-control] standards and protocols and the many samples generated for proficiency testing into our daily routine even though we had been recording and plotting the channels where bead standards have fallen for years. Today we frantically rush to keep familiar with all aspects of computer technology from selecting hardware platforms, TCP/IP protocols, networking products, and getting on the world wide web. All so we are not left behind the big research laboratories and can deal with the huge amount of data flow cytometry produces." 1 September 1995—University of Massachusetts, Worcester.

131. 30 November 1994—Centenary Institute of Cancer Medicine & Cell Biology, Newtown, NSW, Australia.

132. 2 December 1994—Memorial Sloan-Kemering Cancer Center, New York.

133. 23 February 1995—University of Midingan, Ann Arbor.

134. 24 February 1995—Wayne State University, Detroit, Mich.

135. Here is how the professional in charge of a Canadian regulatory facility described how he learned to use the machine: "So the way it works is that the instrument is purchased, the instrument is delivered. Some technical people come with the instrument to unpack it and tune it and run it for you and you sort of learn the most rudimentary operation from the technical people who actually set up the instrument so before they leave you know how to set it up, you know what not to do, the basic do's and don'ts, but just very fundamentals. Then you tinker with the instrument for a few weeks and either you mess it up and you just give up and you say well they'll train me anyway and you give up at that point or you are lucky and you can bring it back alive and get some preliminary data out of it and then you go off for training for a week and the way most people negotiate it, certainly on the Canadian sites, we included training of two individuals per site and not necessarily at the same time. So, most of these sites sent off someone for training within the first month of the instrument being on site. And then, we usually send someone who also had the capacity to train others" (interview with Francis F. Mandy, Ottawa, 16 December 1994).

136. Electronic bulletin boards constitute a virtual user group, to which researchers and technicians can and do resort with a wide range of questions ranging from such "practical" issues as to what homemade or commercial washing solution should be utilized to avoid the clogging and deterioration of the viewing orifice, to such "decisive" issues as what methods, protocols, and antibody reagents should be used to measure a given cell population, or which statistical algorithm will allow for the interpretation of unclear results. On setting up a flow cytometry user group, see Sorensen, "Starting a Flow Cytometry User Group," 52–3.

137. Zito, "American Society of Clinical Pathologists Cytometry Qualification," 60.

138. In the case of flow cytometry, because the evaluation was based on a technique, it was called a qualification, rather than a certification (ibid., 61). This aspect of the evaluation was somewhat controversial and led in August 1995 to a lively discussion on a flow cytometry electronic bulletin board. A contributor pointed out that the ASCP qualification was "not a true certification process and means very little to many in the field (i.e., as a lab director, this does not by itself indicate to me any significant degree of expertise or experience)." The criticism had a dual target: the "narrowness" of the technology involved and of the theoretical knowledge expected from candidates. After admitting that "some detractors have put forth the argument that [the ASCP is] merely 'certifying' a particular technology, which the ASCP does not wish to do," and after also admitting that the qualification "does address a relatively (in the minds of some) narrow aspect of clinical laboratory science," a champion of the ASCP approach noted that while the organization did indeed think that "theoretical 'book knowledge' is no substitute for hands-on clinical experience," it also maintained that the cytometry "qualification does address theoretical knowledge, but in a more practical fashion."

139. Ibid., 61. To be eligible for the examination, candidates must hold a previous ASCP certification or a relevant university degree and a variable amount of hands-on experience in the field.

140. Nicholson, "Quality Control in Immunophenotyping," 11.

141. According to an informant, the variability among instruments found in a survey by CAP was due, in part, to the fact that one manufacturer's model was of a "black-boxed" variety, whereas another manufacturer's model was a research instrument with much built-in flexibility, that, when located in "some of the worst laboratories," was "badly set up." According to the same informant, the second manufacturer learned the lesson, "and the next generation instrument had a lot less knob on it" (interview with Francis F. Mandy, Ottawa, 16 December 1994).

142. Interview with Gerald E. Marti, Bethesda, Md., 15 February 1995.

143. Bessis and Brecher, *Unclassifiable Leukemias,* 79.

144. Organized by the New York Academy of Sciences, the proceedings were published in Landay et al., *Clinical Flow Cytometry.*

145. See Dubois, "The Use of Slides in Biomedical Speeches," and "'And the Last Slide, Please,' Regulatory Language Function at Biomedical Meetings."

146. We are here also confronted with the fact that the role of immunophenotypic imagery seems to go beyond the "technical" role attributed to diagrams. As pictures, they entail judgments that are not reducible to statistical probabilities. Indeed, one could go as far as to argue that they play a "mythological" function (in the sense of Barthes, *Mythologies,* 191–247), insofar as their role as a visual representation of data relative to cell populations is subsumed under their role as persuasive exemplar of competently performed work, and thus of

competent performers. The demonstrative/persuasive power of flow cytometric imagery is captured in an advertisement for ReproMan, a flow cytometry software package from a company called TrueFacts Software: "Do you need . . . a three dimensional plot that will inform (and impress) the most critical audience? . . . Tap the power of persuasion in flow cytometry. . . ."

147. See, e.g., Gnanadesikan, *Methods for Statistical Data Analysis of Multivariate Observations*; Hartigan, *Clustering Algorithms*.

148. For a distinction, from a scientist's point of view, between intrinsic and extrinsic parameters in flow cytometry, see Shapiro, *Practical Flow Cytometry*. 3rd ed., 1–3. See also n. 171.

149. We are nonetheless aware that this distinction between the two forms of IPT cannot be taken for granted. Some observers have tended to emphasize it, thus promoting flow cytometry as a radical innovation in itself (see, e.g., Loken and Herzenberg, "Analysis of Cell Populations with a Fluorescence-Activated Cell Sorter," 163), while others, in an effort to familiarize readers with an esoteric technology, have tended to play it down (e.g., Givan, *Flow Cytometry*, 90). Distinctions can be based on multiple arguments and evolve over time. For instance, writing in 1975, Loken and Herzenberg claimed that flow cytometry eliminated the subjectivity involved in classifying cells as fluorescent or nonfluorescent under a microscope and that flow cytometry produced quantitative rather than qualitative results. Speed (Fortun, "Projecting Speed Genomics") and the sheer quantity of cells examined are "obvious" differences/advantages ascribed to flow cytometric equipment over traditional fluorescence microscopy: a flow cytometer analyzes thousands of cells per second. Although the resulting analysis is "low resolution compared to imaging of cells," this implies a gain in terms of statistical sample; see Haynes, "Principles of Flow Cytometry." The fact remains that the distinction is relevant to participants.

150. See, e.g., Blume, *Insight and Industry*.

151. See, e.g., Dumit, "Objective Brains, Prejudicial Images."

152. Similarly, equipment based on the use of tracers (thermography, scintillography) provides reconstituted views of the inside of the body, and does not lead to measurement, counting, and control. We are grateful to Daniel Jacobi for pointing this out to us. It should be added that biomedical instruments can be divided into "meters"—instruments for the production of measurements, such as thermometers, sphygomanometers, and so on—and "scopes"—instruments for the production of images, such as microscopes, endoscopes, and so on. While the traces produced by "meters" can be contrasted with the events made available by "scopes," the relevant issue here is that a flow cytometer produces (quantitative) imagery, thus collapsing meters and scopes. As we will see below, flow cytometric imagery can acquire iconic qualities that stress its "scope" characteristics, or can be reduced to statistical tables, thus enhancing its "meter" characteristics. It is precisely this essential tension that makes for a sociologically interesting piece of equipment.

153. Foucault, *This Is Not a Pipe.* Of some relevance here is Umberto Eco's, discussion, (in *A Theory of Semiotics,* 250) of "invention as code-making." The latter is defined as "a semiotic mode of production in which something is mapped from something else which was not defined and analyzed before the act of mapping took place. We are witnessing a case in which a significant convention is posited at the very moment in which both the functives of the correlation are invented."

154. See, e.g., Sun, *Color Atlas/Text of Flow Cytometric Analysis of Hematologic Neoplasms.*

155. Star, "Triangulating Clinical and Basic Research."

156. Sun, in *Color Atlas,* 1, complains that "[t]he major limitations of [flow cytometry], at this stage, are the high cost of the instrument, the special skill required to operate it, and the lack of a morphologic record to correlate with markers."

157. As noted by a Dutch biomedical scientist quoted in chapter 4. Another researcher complained that things had gone so far that morphological information was now routinely disregarded: "I spend a lot of time looking at these cells under the microscope . . . that's not a fashionable thing to talk about, you don't talk about a microscope unless you have 100,000 dollars of digital image stuff; if you are still using your eye, God forbid! . . . This is a real problem in flow cytometry: the majority of flow cytometrists have never seen a lymphocyte" (interview with Gerald E. Marti, Bethesda, Md., 15 February 1995). Attempts to automate (see below) lead even further away from the optical domain and convey us to a mathematically defined space that is often contrasted with biologically relevant observations. For example:

> I think it was hard for biologists to really be comfortable with [data synthesis on visual displays]. I think it's hard for a lot of people to be comfortable with it. The people who are comfortable with it . . . were mathematicians, physicists and engineers who are quite comfortable taking data and making a graph out of it and understanding what the graph is saying. That wasn't as true for biologists.
>
> I mean [biologists] have very simple graphs, like histograms. In fact, a lot of biologists or medical doctors, when they do clinical studies, hire a statistician to go through their data and get the number out with the right confidence levels. And they just use those numbers. They don't really understand where they're coming from, or what the limitations are. That's not their training, and they feel they only need to have a, not an intimate knowledge of it, but sort of a superficial knowledge (interview with Martin Bigos, Stanford University, 17 February 1993).

158. See Wood, *The Power of Maps,* 4–6.

159. Field notes, 29 November 1994. On artifacts and shop talk, see Lynch, *Art and Artefact in Laboratory Science*; see also Rasmussen, "Facts, Artifacts, and Mesosomes."

160. A limited survey of the evolution of published IPT imagery, confined to the *Journal of Immunology* and a sample of 100 articles over a ten-year period (1982–92), clearly points in the direction of an increasing "entrenchment" of the translation from dots into cell populations. Given the limitation of the sample, no truly quantitative result can be reported; however, some interesting trends can be identified. We found, first of all, that there are fewer and less explicit references—in the text or in the figure captions—to technical details. By "technical details" we refer both to the instrumental setup leading to image production and to the data analysis techniques constitutive of the image, for instance, the basis for drawing contours in contour plots. This confirms the previously mentioned trend, made explicit in figure 7.6, concerning the "backgrounding" of IPT as a laboratory technique. Obviously, authors increasingly take for granted that readers will immediately recognize the illustrations as flow cytometric and will thus be able to make sense of their various aspects without the help of explicit instructions. More interesting still, the technique has been subordinated to the platform on which it functions. Mention of flow cytometry in, say, the caption of an illustration, is often replaced by terms such as "expression of surface markers," "phenotypic analysis," and so on. In other words, mention of the technique is replaced by reference to the function of the technique. Similarly, one finds evident changes in diagrams illustrating the presence and statistical distribution of subpopulations. While axis labels of early plots referred to the signal being recorded, i.e., fluorescence intensity, more recent axis labels mention surface markers. The external identification now points directly to measurement targets and not to the measurements themselves: traces become equated with what they are presumed to be traces of, and the intervening translations are assumed to be unproblematic. Last but not least, since the fluorescence signal is equated with the expression of a surface marker, the clusters on the diagram become cell populations as defined by surface markers, and no longer data points.

161. Hacking, *Representing and Intervening.* It could be objected that the term *representation* has two distinct meanings, the first denoting various inscriptions such as diagrams, graphs, microphotographs, and so on, and the second denoting abstract scientific theories or even logical arguments about those theories. If one accepts this distinction, our argument would seem to apply only to the former. Insofar, however, as scientific theories cannot be divorced from practice, this objection is groundless. Moreover, the representation/practice dichotomy in itself is insufficient. There are good reasons for this: while representations are indeed the product of intervention, the latter, in turn, are grounded in representations. We intervene not in nature, but on representations of nature be they samples, specimens, events, or images thereof.

162. Kidd and Vogt, "Report of the Workshop on the Evaluation of T-Cell Subsets during HIV Infection and AIDS," 6. On the "art and science" trope in immunology, see Cambrosio and Keating, "'Going Monoclonal.'"

163. Originally, gating was hardware-based and thus generally restricted to cursor-defined quadrilaterals; the shift from hardware to software has diversified the gating options.

164. This was not always the case. Early flow cytometric equipment, such as that constructed in Herzenberg's Stanford University laboratory, used the "conventional technology at the time," namely analog oscilloscopes (interview with Martin Bigos, Stanford University, 17 February 1993). They served both for the handling of the apparatus and for data representation in published articles; indeed, the first published images of histograms and dot plots were real-time Polaroid pictures of analog oscilloscope screens (see figure 4.5). Oscilloscopes, however, provided only limited data analysis capacity and, precisely because of those limitations, the FACS was conceived not simply as a measurement instrument but, first and foremost, as a sorting instrument. The sorted cells could become the object of further, more traditional biological manipulations, producing results that, while predicated on the initial sorting procedure, did not necessarily borrow the representational conventions associated with the latter. The introduction of increasingly powerful computers and of sophisticated software not only multiplied the range of available displays, it also introduced a separation between real-time handling of the flow cytometer and data analysis. Measurements made by the apparatus could be stored (in "list mode") on the hard disk and various data analysis procedures performed offline. This led to the development of more advanced forms of data representation such as contour plots.

165. Shapiro, *Practical Flow Cytometry*, 3rd ed., 5.

166. Software such as the one just mentioned is not a one-step innovation but, rather, the outcome of a longer process. Given the complex operations involved in gating, one may wonder whether flow cytometrists speak of raw data. Talk of raw data can easily be found in both articles and shoptalk. Kidd and Vogt, for instance, note when discussing gating that "[i]deally, the *raw data* from sample analysis would be accumulated with completely 'open' gates and stored in 'list mode' files, where it could be played back if necessary under different gating constraints" (Kidd and Vogt, "Report of the Workshop," 6; our emphasis). Similarly, Vogt et al. in "Model System Evaluating Fluorescein-Labeled Microbeads," 301, in discussing calibration, vaunt the merits of internal calibrators that "remain a permanent part of the *raw data* for each analysis" (our emphasis). Similar mentions of "raw data" can be found in shoptalk. Take, for instance, the following exchange that took place during a presentation by the head of a new academic flow cytometry unit to fellow researchers. The speaker had been discussing at length the various transformations (compensation, gating, and so on) that data displays undergo as part of a typical flow cytometric experiment. One of the participants asked, "You showed that the final image is the result of many manipulations. How do raw data look?" Referring to a previous slide of uncompensated, ungated data, the speaker answered: "I showed the raw data at the beginning. They look messy!" (field notes, 19 November 1994). Judging from the above examples, flow cytometrists attach a commonsense meaning to the term "raw data." They use it to refer to data generated by the equipment previous to any manipulation of the data display; in other words, they refer to the measurements stored in list mode on a hard disk as "raw data." However, in doing so they gloss over the manipulations that make the production of those

"raw data" possible in the first place. Certain operations spoil the rawness of data, while others do not. Thus, the question, "How do raw data look?," while implying a belief in the existence of original data as a basis for experimental inquiry, translates a certain puzzlement as to precisely how "raw" (or cooked) flow cytometric data are. The point, in other words, is that the distinction between "raw data" and "manipulated data" does not provide for two clearly defined, mutually exclusive domains; rather, technical manipulations result in thresholds of rawness. Below a consensual, though in principle questionable, threshold, data count as raw.

167. Articles claiming that accepted, routine gating approaches lead to erroneous results are to be found in the literature: see, e.g., Krömer and Grossmüller, "Light Scatter Based Lymphocyte Gate," for the case of T cells, and Lagaay et al., "Gating of the So-Called 'Lymphocytic' Cell Population," for the case of natural killer cells.

168. A technician described to us how researchers in his unit would often have him retrieve and manipulate stored data in order to produce a particularly good diagram for publication. And a researcher pointed out that textbook images are the result of the operator's fiddling with the machine. The final result looks very different from what shows up first on the screen: "When I first found that out, I became suspicious of everybody else's" (field notes, 19 November 1994). Similarly, as another researcher told us: ". . . there are often only minimal explanations [in published articles] as to how the data was obtained, whether samples were gated, and the 'significance' of a result by comparison to controls. Illustrations of flow cytometric data (dot-plots, histograms, etc.) are rarely explained, as it is assumed the reader is familiar with this data presentation. Dot-plots from anything other than laser printers often reproduce badly, and tricks like thresholding out, gating, etc. are not always mentioned . . . multiparameter cubes, hexagons etc. . . . are sometimes used to 'represent' multiparameter data, but . . . usually only serve to confuse. Contour plots and 3-D plots are fraught with difficulties. Depending upon where the contour is drawn (and the spacing), data can be presented or eliminated as desired" (John Lawry, University of Sheffield, letter to the authors, 19 September 1994).

169. We wrote to the editors of twenty-nine journals routinely publishing flow cytometric images, asking whether the journal had specific guidelines concerning flow cytometric imagery. We received twelve replies, all claiming that no specific guidelines had been developed other than the vague requirement that figures "must be clear and legible." Editors, in most replies, shifted the responsibility to referees. Yet, both from interviews with researchers and from a letter we sent to a sample of about fifty researchers, we learned that referees seldom, if ever, comment on the quality or relevance of the illustrations of submitted manuscripts.

170. According to a March 1998 discussion on the flow cytometry electronic bulletin board. On a contrary note, some participants in the discussion maintain that formal guidelines will be of little help in this matter.

171. Rolf Loertscher, letter to the authors, 1 November 1994. Similar difficulties are experienced with histograms. Some of the issues involved in quantitating histograms are discussed in Agrawal, Agrawal, and Mantyjarvi, "Flow Cytometric Quantitation of C-myc and P53 Proteins"; and Sladek and Jacobberger, "Flow Cytometric Titration of Retroviral Expression Vectors."

172. Givan, *Flow Cytometry*, 93; see also Dean, "Helpful Hints in Flow Cytometry and Sorting."

173. As put by Givan, *Flow Cytometry*, 73: "A serious concern . . . is that the superficial simplicity of the instruments may lull users into a false sense of security about the ease of interpretation of the results; the basis for this concern is particularly clear in the medical community, where clinicians have been conditioned to expect that laboratory reports will contain unambiguous numbers and may not be accustomed to the need for an intellectual framework in which to interpret those numbers." As far as this issue was concerned, the NCCLS was obviously trying to steer a middle course between full automation and the idiosyncrasies of local operators, taking into account the existence of different gating approaches and of conflicting goals, as well as the additional difficulties presented by abnormal samples. This attitude has been summarized by Givan (*Flow Cytometry*, 97) as one of aiming at objectivity while being aware of the necessity of subjective compromise.

174. See, e.g., National Committee for Clinical Laboratory Standards, *Clinical Applications of Flow Cytometry: Quality Assurance and Immunophenotyping of Peripheral Blood Lymphocytes. Tentative Guideline*, 29–31.

175. See, e.g., Young, "Proof without Prejudice"; and Murphy, "Automated Identification of Subpopulations." These attempts have always been fraught with ambiguity. For instance, the author of an early method for the statistical analysis of histogram data ended his article with a "cautionary note," saying that while his test provided "an objective mechanism for possibly distinguishing one population from another," it did not and could not "prove that the difference [was] biologic and substantive as opposed to, say, an artifact of the stain or the flow methodology" (Young, "Proof without Prejudice," 936). Some authors have been quite adamant about the fact that, while "the most sophisticated mathematical model is biologically useless if it is inconsistent with known biological principles," the "ultimate objective" was the "quantitative description of biological systems" (Gray and Dean, "Display and Analysis of Flow Cytometric Data," 536).

176. Routine clinical situations are characterized by the presence of a norm (e.g., a "normal blood picture") and by a predefined set of relevant entities. Software can thus be more easily devised for the automatic performance of a particular task and, in turn, this kind of automation is seen as an important condition for the widespread use of flow cytometry in clinical settings (see, e.g., Ault, "Between the Idea and the Reality Falls the Shadow"). Examples of this kind of software include SimulSET for lymphocyte gating and subset analysis, and Retic-COUN for the enumeration of reticulocytes. Interestingly enough, this software is labeled "for in-vitro diagnostic use," while other kinds of software

(such as LYSIS II and PAINT-A-GATE) only qualify for the label "for research use only" (the software mentioned in this note is commercialized by Becton Dickinson; flow cytometric software is also available from other manufacturers of flow cytometers, such as Coulter, and from third-party suppliers such as Verity House and Phoenix Flow Systems).

177. Calvelli et al., "Guideline for Flow Cytometric Immunophenotyping."

178. See, e.g., Givan, *Flow Cytometry*, 93–7; Loken et al., *Establishing Optimal Lymphocyte.*

179. While light scatter maintains a link with fluorescence microscopy, immunofluorescence-based gating implies a redefinition of the immune cells in flow cytometric, phenotypic terms. This move, as we have previously seen, can be controversial for morphologically oriented researchers. Accordingly, forward and side scatter are termed "intrinsic parameters," whereas those parameters measured and visualized through the use of antibody "probes" are termed "extrinsic parameters." See Shapiro, *Practical Flow Cytometry*, 3rd ed., 2, for a list of parameters, measurement methods, and probes.

180. See, e.g., Murphy, "Automated Identification of Subpopulations in Flow Cytometric List Mode Data Using Cluster Analysis"; Reinhold C. Mann, "On Multiparameter Data Analysis in Flow Cytometry"; Kosugi et al., "An Interactive Multivariate Analysis of FCM Data."

181. Sychra et al., "Dimensionality Reducing Displays in Cell Image Analysis," 747–8.

182. Bellman, cited in Reinhold C. Mann, "On Multiparameter Data Analysis in Flow Cytometry," 184.

183. Ibid. One can overcome this problem by attempting to "reduce" multi-dimensional data to two- or three-dimensional graphic displays. Alternatively, imagery can be discarded and replaced by mathematical calculations. In practice, one finds a mix of these two options. For instance, the author of a cluster analysis method for the automated identification of subpopulations pointed out that the validation of statistically obtained clusters should be sought in the visual inspection of clusters in two-parameter displays (Murphy, "Automated Identification," 308). Similarly, after describing his method for "dimensionality reduction," Mann cautioned that "visual inspection of the results and validation of the clusters obtained are an absolute necessity in order to assure results that are biologically meaningful" (Reinhold C. Mann, "On Multiparameter Data," 189). It is interesting to note that visual inspection does not mean here the inspection of biological material, but of the cells as represented in a geometrical-statistical space. It is biology within Cartesian coordinates. The importance of visual displays over their reduction to numbers has been stressed by other scientists: "Images in flow cytometry are the heart, are the guts, the spirit, the essence. I mean the numbers are important, I don't want to diminish the importance of the numbers, but everywhere you look around here [pointing to various dot and contour plots on posters hanging from the office walls], we spend a great deal

of our time looking at patterns and then only afterwards do we want to know what the number is" (interview with Gerald E. Marti, Bethesda, Md., 15 February 1995). Imagery has thus not been eliminated. One should not, however, forget that, in these approaches, gating is reduced to mathematical "at once" operations. "[D]iscriminant functions" and "Boolean expressions" replace the moving of cursors or the drawing of polygons. A commercial embodiment of this trend is Becton Dickinson's Attractors software, a system of "dynamic gates," whereby the oval-shaped Attractor is "a cluster-seeking object that automatically tracks user-defined populations." According to its developers, Attractors will "quickly [make] obsolete existing software approaches, relegating them to their true function as automatic file readers" (undated Attractors brochure).

184. Kidd and Vogt, "Report of the Workshop on the Evaluation of T-Cell Subsets during HIV Infection and AIDS."

185. Centers for Disease Control and Prevention, "1997 Revised Guidelines for Performing CD4+ T-Cell Determinations," 17 (fig. 2) and 18 (fig. 3).

186. Sun, *Color Atlas*, 1

187. See, e.g., Duque, "Flow Cytometric Analysis of Lymphomas and Acute Leukemias."

188. Interview with Carleton Stewart, Bethesda, Md., 17 November 1995.

Chapter 9

1. See Temkin, "The Scientific Approach to Disease."

2. Interview with a Dr. Raul C. Braylan, Bethesda, Md., 18 November 1995.

3. Dagognet, *Le catalogue de la vie*, 162.

4. Ibid., 20–1.

5. Béné et al., "Proposals for the Immunological Classification of Acute Leukemias."

6. Rothe and Schmitz, "Consensus Protocol for the Flow Cytometric Immunophenotyping of Hematopoietic Malignancies."

7. First MIC Cooperative Study Group, "Morphologic, Immunologic, and Cytogenetic (MIC) Working Classification of Acute Lymphoblastic Leukemia"; Second MIC Cooperative Study Group, "Morphologic, Immunologic, and Cytogenetic (MIC) Working Classification of the Acute Myeloid Leukaemias."

8. Bennett, "World Health Organization Classification of the Acute Leukemias and Myelodysplastic Syndrome."

9. Béné et al., "Proposals for the Immunological Classification of Acute Leukemias," 1785.

10. Paietta, "Proposals for the Immunological Classification of Acute Leukemias."

11. Ibid., 2148.

12. From this point of view, according to GEIL, immunology lies somewhere between cytology/morphology (high number of successful studies) and cytogenetics (high number of unsuccessful karyotypic studies); see Béné et al., "Immunologic Analysis of a Thousand Cases of Acute Leukemia."

13. This latter approach allows each hospital team to retain full ownership of the data provided to the group, a device aimed at decreasing fears of cannibalization by leading centers while ensuring access on request to locally archived, complementary clinical data, without which immunological information would be meaningless.

14. In fact, it appears that differences can still be observed among certain reagents belonging to the cluster but produced by different suppliers; see Béné et al., "Immunologic Analysis;" field notes, Bethesda Consensus Conference.

15. Interview with Marie-Christine Béné and Gilbert Faure, Nancy, France, 13 February 1997.

16. See Keating and Cambrosio, "From Screening to Clinical Research."

17. Although reference laboratories were designated for morphology and cytogenetics, the work in these cases was essentially a review of what had been done in local laboratories. The immunophenotype, on the other hand, was initially established by the reference laboratory itself.

18. Since then, E-1485 has persisted as an appendix to the ECOG clinical protocol.

19. See Bettelheim et al., "Expression of a Myeloid Marker on TdT-positive Acute Lymphocytic Leukemic Cells."

20. Wiernik went on to become the director of ECOG. See Peter H. Wiernik, "Curriculum Vitae," *National Archives II* (USA), RG 443, Research Grant Files.

21. Interview with Elisabeth Paietta, New York, 30 May 1999.

22. For a discussion of the different kinds of objectivities that have characterized the evolution of clinical trial design, see Marks, *The Progress of Experiments.*

23. See ibid. for a discussion of the tension between statisticians and clinicians.

24. Paietta, Anderson, and Wiernik, "A New Approach to Analyzing the Utility of Immunophenotyping for Predicting Clinical Outcome in Acute Leukemia," 1. The authors offer the following example: "An example would be the newly defined leukemia subtype of immature acute monocytic leukemia (AMOL) which is characterized by limited CD14 expression antigen expression and associated with poor prognosis, inferior to that of mature AMOL with CD14

expression by the majority of blast cells. This clinically significant segregation of AMOL into immature and mature emerged only through the retrospective determination of the prognostically significant cutoff point for CD14 which was found to lie at 58%, much higher than any arbitrary prognostic expression level ever chosen for analysis of this antigen before, suggesting considerable differentiating ability within the immature AMOL population" (ibid., 2).

25. Bennett, "World Health Organization Classification of the Acute Leukemias and Myelodysplastic Syndrome."

26. See Nancy Lee Harris et al., "A Revised European-American Classification of Lymphoid Neoplasms."

27. Dehner, "Here We Go Again"; Meijer et al., "The Revised European-American Lymphoma (REAL) Classification of Non-Hodgkin's Lymphoma"; Schwarze, "Amerika, du sollst es besser haben"; Mason and Gatter, "Not Another Lymphoma Classification!"

28. Rosenberg, "Classification of Lymphoid Neoplasms [editorial]."

29. Note, in this respect, the pragmatic attitude of the ILSG: "It is necessary to split before meaningful lumping can occur. If several morphologically, immunologically, and genetically distinct neoplasms prove to respond identically to currently available treatment, they can be lumped for the purpose of clinical treatment selection. However, if new forms of treatment become available . . . it will be important to recognize and study each disease separately" (Nancy Lee Harris et al., "A Revised European-American Classification," 1384).

30. Nancy Lee Harris, Jaffe, and Stein, "Response [Letter]."

31. Nancy Lee Harris, "A Practical Approach to the Pathology of Lymphoid Neoplasms," 111.

32. The club was created by Karl Lennert in 1973 as a vehicle for the Kiel classification.

33. Lennert and Stein, "Personal Points of View on the Kiel Classification," 35–6.

34. O'Conor and Sobin, "Conclusions of the First Session: Correlations between Current Morphologic Categorizations," 126.

35. Dorfman objected to this system: "The term 'prolymphocytic' in the WHO classification makes use of a designation familiar to hematologists from their examinations of Romanovsky-stained preparations, but not to pathologists working with histologic sections stained with hematoxylin and eosin" (Dorfman, "Pathology of the Non-Hodgkin's Lymphomas," 948–9).

36. Kaplan, "Introduction," vii–viii; quoted in Berard and Hutchison, "The Problem of Classifying Lymphomas," S4.

37. Entitled the "Invitational Workshop for the Planning of Retrospective and Prospective Studies to Delineate Optimal Classification of the Non-Hodgkin's

Lymphomas," the meeting was held in Warrenton, Va., 4–5 September 1975. See Mathé, "Workshop for the Classification of Non-Hodgkin's Lymphoma."

38. Ibid.

39. More precisely, the experts visited four participating institutions and classified slides according to their own system without any clinical information. They were then given three pieces of clinical information (age, sex, site of biopsy) and allowed to revise their diagnosis (which they did only 2.4% of the time). Then the experienced pathologists (without any special knowledge of any of the systems) visited the four institutions and classified the same slides. Herein is what they were allowed to know about the six systems.

40. Non-Hodgkin's Lymphoma Pathologic Classification Project, "National Cancer Institute Sponsored Study of Classifications of Non-Hodgkin's Lymphomas," 2121.

41. Ibid., 2122. According to NCI researchers, in clinical protocols only the categories "high grade" and "low grade" were used. See Fornace and Jaffe, "Pathology of Malignant Lymphomas," 712.

42. Lennert, "Commentary on Working Formulation of Non-Hodgkin's Lymphomas," 2133.

43. Lukes, "Commentary on Working Formulation of Non-Hodgkin's Lymphomas," 2134.

44. Rappaport, "Commentary on Working Formulation of Non-Hodgkin's Lymphomas," 2134.

45. Jaffe, "Predictability of Immunologic Phenotype by Morphologic Criteria in Diffuse Aggressive Non-Hodgkin's Lymphomas," 46. The opposite, however, was not true. IPT carried out on frozen tissue section could be easily integrated into the working formulation. See, e.g., Tubbs et al., "Immunohistologic Cellular Phenotypes of Lymphoproliferative Disorders," 207.

46. Lymphomas in patients that underwent multiple biopsies could be diffuse in one lymph node and nodular in another; see Fisher et al., "Natural History of Malignant Lymphomas with Divergent Histologies at Staging Evaluation." Patients that began with a nodular pattern, often (37% in one NIH study) progressed to diffuse; see Hubbard et al., "Histologic Progression in Non-Hodgkin's Lymphoma."

47. Grogan et al., "Immunologic Approaches to the Classification of Non-Hodgkin's Lymphomas," 31.

48. Ibid.

49. Ibid., 32.

50. See Shimoyama et al., "Final Results of Cooperative Study of VEPA"; Coiffier et al., "T-Cell Lymphomas"; Lippman et al., "The Prognostic Significance of the Immunophenotype in Diffuse Large-Cell Lymphoma."

51. Cossman et al., "Low-grade Lymphomas," 120.

52. Mtasiwa et al., "Immunophenotype, Histopathology and Clinical Stage," 100.

53. Simon et al., "The Non-Hodgkin's Lymphoma Pathologic Classification Project," 939.

54. Nancy Lee Harris, "Lymphoma 1987," 1.

55. Ibid., 21.

56. Hiddemann et al., "Lymphoma Classification," 4086. This did not prevent other groups, for instance, the European Organization for Research and Treatment of Cancer (EORTC), from coming up with yet other classificatory proposals; see, e.g., Russell-Jones, "Primary Cutaneous B-Cell Lymphoma."

57. Nancy Lee Harris et al., "The World Health Organization Classification of Hematological Malignancies," 193.

58. A subsequent WHO classification project included members of the ISLG and is considered "a slightly modified REAL classification." See, Pileri et al., "From the R.E.A.L. Classification to the Upcoming WHO Scheme," 609.

59. Koeppen and Vardiman, "New Entities, Issues and Controversies in the Classification of Malignant Lymphoma," 421.

60. De Wolf-Peeters and Pittaluga, "Further Considerations on the Revised European-American Lymphoma Classification," 366.

61. The Southwest Oncology Group (SWOG) and the Non-Hodgkin's Classification (NHL) Project set out to test the REAL classification in 1996. "The analyses conducted by the SWOG Lymphoma Committee and the NHL Classification Project have demonstrated that the REAL classification does define 'real' clinical entities [as opposed to merely biological ones] that can be diagnosed by expert hematopathologists" (Fisher, Miller, and Grogan, "New REAL Clinical Entities").

62. The sites included nine different clinical centers (Omaha, Vancouver, Capetown, London, Bellizona/Locarno, Lyon, Hong Kong, Würzburg, Göttingen). Cytogenetic and molecular genetic data were also used when available. "In each case, the expert was then presented with the immunophenotypic profile, along with any available cytogenetic and molecular genetic data, and the immunostains and/or flow cytometry report" (Armitage and Weisenburger, "New Approach to Classifying Non-Hodgkin's Lymphomas," 2781; data originally reported in the Non-Hodgkin's Lymphoma Pathologic Classification Project, "A Clinical Evaluation of the International Lymphoma Study Group Classification of Non-Hodgkin's Lymphoma").

63. Following classification, the ILSG calculated survival times that allowed them to stratify patients into four prognostic groups. The survival time also allowed them to make comparisons with the International Prognostic Index; see the Non-Hodgkin's Lymphoma Pathologic Classification Project (1997). Yet

another part of the study showed that non-Hodgkin's lymphoma subtypes differed by geographic location. Although this had been known, especially with regard to the T-cell lymphomas, the existence of a single international classification made possible findings that before could have been attributed to differing diagnostic practices and classification systems; see Anderson, Armitage, and Weisenburger, "Epidemiology of the Non-Hodgkin's Lymphomas."

64. Fisher, Miller, and Grogan, "New REAL Clinical Entities," 55.

65. We say "closely monitored" because the REAL classification was used as an occasion to redefine the relations between pathologists and clinicians; for instance, one finds in the literature statements like the following: "The previous anachronism of basing therapy on opinions of non-specialist pathologists, without appropriate review, is unwise. Furthermore, treatment by lone practitioners, or even single-specialty groups that lack the discipline to analyse their findings critically and regularly report their updated results, can no longer be considered standard of practice and should be discouraged" (Jacobs, "Lymphoma—Histopathology in Changing Clinical Perspective," 135). An overview of findings for common lymphoma types, targeting the clinician, contained the following sentence: "Since patients will be given these diagnoses by pathologists, it is important that clinicians be knowledgeable with regard to their clinical characteristics" (Armitage and Weisenburger, "New Approach to Classifying Non-Hodgkin's Lymphomas," 2780).

66. Nancy Lee Harris et al. "The World Health Organization Classification of Hemafologic Malignancies," 193.

67. Nancy Lee Harris et al., "The World Health Organization Classification." This article was published under the same title in the following four journals: *Annals of Oncology* (1999); *Histopathology* (2000); *Journal of Clinical Oncology* (1999); *Modern Pathology* (2000). The International Prognostic Index is the result of yet another cooperative endeavor designed to standardize ways of predicting the risk of disease recurrence and overall survival; it uses a scoring system that takes into account factors such as stage of disease, general health, and number of sites affected other than lymph nodes; the index is used to make therapeutic decisions concerning conventional vs. more aggressive therapies; see International Non-Hodgkin's Lymphoma Prognostic Factors Project, "A Predictive Model for Aggressive Non-Hodgkin's Lymphoma."

68. Hacking, "The Self-Vindication of the Laboratory Sciences."

69. See, e.g., Asch and Lowe, "The Consensus Development Program"; Jacoby, "Consensus Development at NIH." For an international comparative overview of consensus conferences, see Giraud and Jolly, *Le consensus en médecine.*

70. Battista and Hodge, "The Development of Health Care Technology Assessment."

71. Borowitz et al., "U.S.-Canadian Consensus Recommendations on the Immunophenotypic Analysis of Hematologic Neoplasia by Flow Cytometry."

72. Davis et al., "U.S.-Canadian Consensus Recommendations on the Immunophenotypic Analysis of Hematologic Neoplasia by Flow Cytometry."

73. Stewart et al., "U.S.-Canadian Consensus Recommendations on the Immunophenotypic Analysis of Hematologic Neoplasia by Flow Cytometry."

74. Borowitz et al., 'U.S.-Canadian Consensus Recommendations."

75. Stelzer et al., "U.S.-Canadian Consensus Recommendations on the Immunophenotypic Analysis of Hematologic Neoplasia by Flow Cytometry."

76. Braylan et al., "U.S.-Canadian Consensus Recommendations on the Immunophenotypic Analysis of Hematologic Neoplasia by Flow Cytometry."

77. See, e.g., Hill and Goodale, "The Delphi Predictions of Pathology Chairmen."

78. The following statements are derived not from the published consensus statements but, rather, from our field notes of the actual discussions during the conference.

79. M2, M3, etc. are subcategories of the myeloid leukemias as defined in the FAB classification. It was generally recognized that this was not the case with all FAB categories. There were some categories that apparently only IPT could display, leading to yet another problem: "So far, flow is confirmatory; what should be done when it is at odds with morphology? Won't an increased use of flow make new diseases? M7 used to be rare. With flow it is common. Flow is the only way to get M0 or M7" (fieldnotes, Bethesdol Consensus conference, 17 November 1995).

Chapter 10

1. Calvino, *Invisible Cities.*

2. Cambrosio and Keating, *Exquisite Specificity.*

3. Herzenberg, De Rosa, and Herzenberg, "Monoclonal Antibodies and the FACS."

4. On the notion of the trading zone, see Galison, *Image and Logic.*

5. In Foucault's sense of "a decidedly heterogeneous set of discourses, institutions, architectural arrangements, regulatory decisions, laws, administrative decisions, scientific statements, philosophical, moral, philanthropic propositions, in short, the said and the unsaid. . . . The 'dispositif' itself is the network that can be established between these elements." See Foucault, "Le jeu de Michel Foucault," 299 (our translation).

6. See Vinck, *Du laboratoire aux réseaux.*

7. See, e.g., Latour, *Science in Action*; Callon, *La science et ses réseaux.*

8. See also Cambrosio and Keating, "Monoclonal Antibodies: From Local to Extended Networks."

9. Reiser, *Medicine and the Reign of Technology.*

10. Howell, *Technology in the Hospital.*

11. Wailoo, *Drawing Blood.*

12. Wailoo examines many specific examples of technologies, but his theoretical account of these heterogeneous events is constructed in terms of the technology vs. medicine trope.

13. For a recent list of proposed taxonomies, as well as related considerations concerning the administration of clinical research, see Heinig et al., "The Changing Landscape for Clinical Research."

14. A similar criticism has been made, in the sociology of (medical) professions, with regard to early attempts to account for professions in terms of traits. On this, see, e.g., Abbot, *The System of Professions.*

15. De Chadarevian and Kamminga, *Molecularizing Biology and Medicine.*

16. Star and Ruhleder, "Steps Toward an Ecology of Infrastructure."

17. Fujimura, *Crafting Science,* 16–17.

18. A similar critique is to be found in Gaudillière, "Oncogenes as Metaphors for Human Cancer," and in Morange, "From the Regulatory Vision of Cancer to the Oncogene Paradigm," 1.

19. Rheinberger, *Toward a History of Epistemic Things.*

20. Ibid., 133–42.

21. Knorr-Cetina, *Epistemic Cultures.*

22. What holds together and separates science and technology is not how they are produced. More precisely, rather than an economy of the production of epistemic things, we suggest that the regulation of those things determines which unprecedented differences produced within an experimental system attain significance or acquire the status of an epistemic thing. Without an economy of regulation, it is impossible to tell which differences produced by an experimental system are significant and which are trivial.

23. Rheinberger, *Toward a History of Epistemic Things,* 176–86.

24. See, for example, Alizadeh et al., "Distinct Types of Diffuse Large B-Cell Lymphoma Identified by Gene Expression Profiling"; Ramaswamy et al., "Multiclass Cancer Diagnosis Using Tumor Gene Expression Signatures;" Lakhani and Ashworth, "Microarray and Histopathological Analysis of Tumors."

25. For clinical trials, see *The Progress of Experiments*; for epidemiology, see Fagot-Largeault, *Les causes de la mort*; for clinical medicine, see Aronowitz, *Making Sense of Illness.*

26. Daston and Galison, "The Image of Objectivity"; see also Daston, "Objectivity and the Escape from Perspective."

27. See, e.g., Nelson and Winter, *An Evolutionary Theory of Economic Change,* 134.

28. On the "heterogeneity of medical practices," see Kerleau, "L'hétérogénéité des pratiques médicales."

29. On "styles of reasoning," see Hacking, "Statistical Language, Statistical Truth and Statistical Reason."

References

Abbas, Abul K., Andrew H. Lichtman, and Jordan S. Pober. *Cellular and Molecular Immunology*. Philadelphia: Saunders, 1991.

Abbot, Andrew. *The System of Professions: An Essay on the Division of Expert Labor*. Chicago: University of Chicago Press, 1988.

Aboulker, Jean-Pierre, and A. M. Swart. "Preliminary Analysis of the Concorde Trial." *Lancet* 341 (3 April 1993), 889–90.

Ackerknecht, Erwin H. *Rudolf Virchow: Doctor, Statesman, Anthropologist*. Madison: University of Wisconsin Press, 1953.

Adams, Annmarie. *Architecture in the Family Way. Doctors, Houses, and Women, 1870–1900*. Montreal: McGill-Queen's, 1996.

Agrawal, Reitus S., Yash P. Agrawal, and Rauno A. Mantyjarvi. "Flow Cytometric Quantitation of C-myc and P53 Proteins in Bovine Papillomavirus Type 1–Transformed Primary Mouse Fibroblasts." *Cytometry* 17 (1994), 237–45.

Ahrens, Edward H. *The Crisis in Clinical Research: Overcoming Institutional Obstacles*. New York: Oxford University Press, 1992.

Aiuti, Fernando, Vincenzo Lacava, Massimo Fiorilli, and Maria Vera Ciarla. "Lymphocyte Surface Markers in Lymphoproliferative Diseases." *Acta Haematalogica* 50 (1973), 275–83.

Algeo, David. "Developing a Safe Way of Screening." *Denver Post* (9 June 1996), 2D.

Alizadeh, Ash A., Michael B. Eisen, R. Eric Davis, Chi Ma, Izidore S. Lossos, Andreas Rosenwald, Jennifer C. Boldrick, Hajeer Sabet, Truc Tran, Xin Yu, John I. Powell, Liming Young, Gerald E. Marti, Troy Moore, James Hudson Jr., Lisheng Lu, David B. Lewis, Robert Tibshirani, Gavin Sherlock, Wing C. Chan, Timothy C. Greiner, Dennis D. Weisenburger, James O. Armitage, Roger Warnke, Ronald Levy, Wyndham Wilson, Michael R. Grever, John C. Byrd, David Batstein, Patrick O. Brown, and Louis M. Staudt. "Distinct Types of Diffuse Large B-cell Lymphoma Identified by Gene Expression Profiling." *Nature* 403 (2000), 503–11.

Alvey, P. L., and M. F. Greaves. "A Computer Program for Interpreting Immunophenotypic Data as an Aid to the Diagnosis of Leukemia." *Leukemia* 1 (1987), 527–40.

Amsterdamska, Olga. "Chemistry in the Clinic: The Research Career of Donald Dexter Van Slyke." In *Molecularizing Biology and Medicine: New Practices and Alliances, 1910–1970*, ed. Soraya de Chadarevian and Harmke Kamminga, 47–82. Amsterdam: Harwood, 1998.

Amsterdamska, Olga. "Stabilizing Instability: The Controversy over Cyclogenic Theories of Bacterial Variation during the Interwar Period." *Journal of the History of Biology* 24 (1991), 191–222.

Anderson, Carl, and John J. Bartholdi. "Centralized versus Decentralized Control in Manufacturing: Lessons From Social Insects." In *Complexity and Complex Systems in Industry*, ed. I. P. McCarthy and T. Rakotobe-Joel, 92–105. Warwick, UK: University of Warwick Press, 2000.

Anderson, James R., James O. Armitage, and Dennis D. Weisenburger. "Epidemiology of the Non-Hodgkin's Lymphomas: Distribution of the Major Subtypes Differ by Geographic Locations. Non-Hodgkin's Lymphoma Classification Project." *Annals of Oncology* 9 (1998), 717–20.

Ansell, Phillip R. J. "Hybridoma Technology: A View from the Patent Arena." *Immunology Today* 21 (2000), 357–8.

Antabi, Elizabeth, and David Fishlock, *Biotechnology: Strategies for Life.* Cambridge, MA: MIT Press, 1986.

"Antibodies Rescue 10 Grafts from Rejection." *McGraw-Hill's Biotechnology Newswatch,* 7 (September 1984), 3.

Architecture et conception hospitalière. Paris: Institut Français d'Architecture; Direction des Hôpitaux; Ministère des Affaires Sociales et de la Solidarité Nationale; Secrétariat d'Etat chargé de la Santé, 1985.

L'architecture hospitalière au XIXe siècle. L'exemple parisien. Les dossiers du Musée d'Orsay 27, Paris: Éditions de la Réunion des Musées Nationaux, 1988.

Armed Forces Institute of Pathology. *Annual Report.* Washington, DC: U.S. Armed Forces Institute of Pathology, 1954.

Armed Forces Institute of Pathology. *Annual Report,* Washington, DC: U.S. Armed Forces Institute of Pathology, 1957.

Armitage, James O., and Dennis D. Weisenburger. "New Approach to Classifying Non-Hodgkin's Lymphomas: Clinical Features of the Major Histologic Subtypes." *Journal of Clinical Oncology* 16 (1998), 2780–95.

Aronowitz, Robert A. *Making Sense of Illness. Science, Society and Disease.* Cambridge, UK: Cambridge University Press, 1998.

Asch, S. M., and C. U. Lowe. "The Consensus Development Program: Theory, Process, and Critique." *Knowledge: Creation, Diffusion, Utilization* 5 (1984), 369–85.

Asgmore, Malcom. *The Reflexive Thesis: Wrighting Sociology of Scientific Knowledge.* Chicago: University of Chicago Press, 1989.

Atkinson, Paul. *Medical Talk and Medical Work.* London: Sage, 1995.

Ault, Kenneth A. "Between the Idea and the Reality Falls the Shadow: Clinical Flow Cytometry Comes of Age?" *Cytometry* Supplement 3 (1988), 2–6.

Austoker, Joan. *A History of the Imperial Cancer Research Fund, 1902–1986.* Oxford: Oxford University Press, 1988.

"Automation: What to Measure and Why." Special double issue of *Blood Cells* 6 (2–3) (1980).

L'automatisme en hématologie. Special issue of *Nouvelle Revue Française d'Hématologie* 20, no. 2 (1978).

"Availability of Flow Cytometric Immunophenotyping of Lymphocytes to Hospital Patients—United States, 1990." In Centers for Disease Control and Prevention, *Reports on HIV/AIDS 1992.* Atlanta: U.S. Department of Health and Human Services, 1993, 109–11 [reprinted from *MMWR. Morbidity and Mortality Weekly Report* 41 (21 August 1992), 608–10.

Avrameas, S., and J. Uriel. "Méthode de marquage d'antigènes et d'anticops avec des enzymes et son application en immunodiffusion." *Comptes Rendus Hebdomadaires des Séances de l'Académie des Sciences D: Sciences naturelles.* Paris, 262 (1966), 2543–5.

Bach, J. F., G. Biozzi, M. F. Greaves, I. McConnell, H. S. Micklem, E. Möller, and O. B. Zaalberg. "Summary of Round-Table Discussion on the Technical Aspects of the Rosette Test." *Transplantation Proceedings* 4 (1972), 335–7.

Baehr, R. V., H. D. Volk, P. Reinke, P. Falck, and H. Wolff. "An Immune Monitoring Program for Controlling Immunosuppressive Therapy." *Transplantation Proceedings* 21 (1989), 1189–91.

Baffert, Sandrine, Stéphane Jouveshomme, Emmanuel Charpentier, A. Souag, D. Tiah, M.-C. Vacher-Lavenu, and E. Fery-Lemonnier. "Évaluation médicale et économique d'un système d'analyse des frottis cervico-utérines (FCU) assistée par ordinateur." Poster presented at the 2nd French Health Economists Conference, Paris, 1–2 February 2001.

Bahr, G. F., and E. H. Zeitler. "Distribution of Erythrocyte Volumes [letter]." *Blood* 23 (1964), 402–4.

Baker, M. A., K. Ramachandar, and R. N. Taub. "Specificity of Heteroantisera to Human Acute Leukemia–Associated Antigens." *Journal of Clinical Investigation* 54 (1974), 1273–8.

Banda-Gamboa, Hugo, Ian Ricketts, Alistair Cairns, Kudair Hussein, James H. Tucker, and Nasseem Hussain. "Automation in Cervical Cytology: An Overview." *Analytical Cellular Pathology* 4 (1992), 25–48.

Barley, Stephen R. "Technology, Power, and the Social Organization of Work: Towards a Pragmatic Theory of Skilling and Deskilling." *Research in the Sociology of Organization* 6 (1988), 33–80.

Barnett, D., V. Granger, P. Mayr, I. Storie, G. A. Wilson, and J. T. Reilley. "Evaluation of a Novel Stable Whole Blood Quality Control Material for Lymphocyte Subset Analysis: Results from the UK NEQAS Immune Monitoring Scheme." *Cytometry* 26 (1996), 216–22.

Barnhart, Clarence L., Sol Steinmetz, and Robert K. Barnhart. *The Barnhart Dictionary of New English Since 1963.* Bronxville, NY: Barnhart/Harper & Row, 1973.

Barthes, Roland. *Mythologies.* Paris: Seuil, 1957.

Bartholdi, M. "A High-Sensitivity Flow Chamber." In Los Alamos Scientific Laboratory of the University of California, *Progress Report. Biomedical and Environmental Research Program of the LASL Health Division, Progress Report, January–December 1977.* LA-7254-PR, Los Alamos, NM, 1977, 165.

Bartholdi, M., and G. S. Salzman. "A Light-Scattering Flow, Photometer." In Los Alamos Scientific Laboratory of the University of California, *Progress Report. Biomedical and Environmental Research Program of the LASL Health Division, January–December 1978.* LA-8023-PR, Los Alamos, NM, 1978, 98–9.

Baszanger, Isabelle, and Nicolas Dodier. "Totalisation et altérité dans l'enquête ethnographique." *Revue française de sociologie* 38 (1997), 37–66.

Battista, Renaldo N., and Matthew J. Hodge. "The Development of Health Care Technology Assessment. An International Perspective." *International Journal of Technology Assessment in Health Care* 11 (1995), 287–300.

"Battle Continues in Ortho v Becton Dickinson Patent Case." *BioEngineering News* (15 January 1985), 1–2.

Becton Dickinson. *Normal Values: Definition of a Reference Range for Lymphocyte Subsets of Healthy Adults.* Clinical Monograph no. 1. San José, CA: Becton Dickinson Immunocytometry Systems, 1991.

Benaroyo, Lazare. "La renaissance de la pensée biologique de Rudolf Virchow dans l'oeuvre de Ludwig Aschoff." *Revue d'histoire des sciences* 50 (1997), 447–60.

Béné, M. C., L. Boumsell, J. P. Vannier, R. Garand, E. Solary, G. Faure, A. Bernard, and the members of the French Groupe d'Étude Immunologique des Leucémies (GEIL). "Immunologic Analysis of a Thousand Cases of Acute Leukemia." *Nouvelle revue française d'hématologie* 31 (1989), 133–6.

Béné, M. C., G. L. Castoldi, W. Knapp, W. D. Ludwig, E. Matutes, A. Orfao, and M. B. van't Veer. "Proposals for the Immunological Classification of Acute

Leukemias. European Group for the Immunological Characterization of Leukemias (EGIL)." *Leukemia* 9 (1995), 1783–6.

Bennett, John M. "World Health Organization Classification of the Acute Leukemias and Myelodysplastic Syndrome." *International Journal of Hematology* 72 (2000), 131–3.

Bennett, John M., Daniel Catovsky, M. T. Daniel, Georges Flandrin, D. A. Galton, H. R. Gralnick, and Claude Sultan. "Proposed Revised Criteria for the Classification of Acute Myeloid Leukemia. A Report of the French-American-British Cooperative Group." *Annals of Internal Medicine* 103 (1985), 620–5.

Bennett, John M., Daniel Catovsky, M. T. Daniel, Georges Flandrin, D. A. G. Galton, H. R. Gralnick, and Claude Sultan. "Proposals for the Classification of the Acute Leukaemias (French-American-British (FAB) Co-operative Group)." *British Journal of Haematology* 33 (1976), 451–8.

Berard, Costan W., and R. E. Hutchison. "The Problem of Classifying Lymphomas: An Orderly Prescription for Progress." *Annals of Oncology* 8 (Suppl. 2) (1997), S3–S9.

Berard, Costan W., E. Jaffe, R. J. Lukes, H. Rappaport, and R. Dorfman. "Discussion II: Roundtable Discussion of Histopathologic Classification." *Cancer Treatment Reports* 61 (1977), 1037–58.

Berg, Marc. "Practices of Reading and Writing: The Constitutive Role of the Patient Record in Medical Work." *Sociology of Health & Illness* 18 (1996), 499–524.

Bergeron, Michèle, F. Lacroix, Tracy Minkus, C. Chabot, S. Phaneuf, R. Somorjai, and F. Mandy. "Comparison of Single Versus Double Platform Absolute Count Determination of T-Cell Subsets by Flow Cytometry." *International Conference on AIDS* (Vancouver, Canada, July 7–12 1996), abstract no. Th.A.4008, 255.

Berlin, R. D., J. M. Oliver, T. E. Ukena, and H. H. Yin. "The Cell Surface." *New England Journal of Medicine* 292 (1975), 515–20.

Bernard, Alain, Laurence Boumsell, Jean Dausset, Cesar Milstein, and Stuart F. Schlossman, eds. *Leucocyte Typing. Human Leucocyte Differentiation Antigens Detected by Monoclonal Antibodies.* Berlin: Springer-Verlag, 1984.

Bernard, Alain, L. Boumsell, E. L. Reinherz, L. M. Nadler, J. Ritz, H. Coppin, Y. Richard, F. Valensi, J. Dausset, G. Flandrin, J. Lemerle, and S. F. Schlossman. "Cell Surface Characterization of Malignant T Cells from Lymphoblastic Lymphoma Using Monoclonal Antibodies: Evidence for Phenotypic Differences between Malignant T Cells from Patients with Acute Lymphoblastic Leukemia and Lymphoblastic Lymphoma." *Blood* 57 (1981), 1105–10.

Bernard, Claude. *Introduction à l'étude de la médecine expérimentale.* Paris: Garnier-Flammarion, 1966 [1865].

Bernard, Jean. "Summing Up." *Blood Cells* 6 (1980), 499–500.

Bernard, Jean, and Marcel Bessis. "The Impact of Automation on the Future of Hematology." *Blood Cells* 6 (1980), 115–7.

Bessis, Marcel, and George Brecher, eds. *Unclassifiable Leukemias.* New York: Springer-Verlag, 1975.

Bettelheim, P., E. Paietta, O. Majdic, H. Gadner, J. D. Schwarzmeier, and W. Knapp. "Expression of a Myeloid Marker on TdT-positive Acute Lymphocytic Leukemic Cells: Evidence by Double Fluorescence Staining." *Blood* 60 (1982), 1392–6.

Bibel, Debra Jan. *Milestones in Immunology: A Historical Exploration.* Madison, WI: Science Tech Publishers, 1988.

Binet, Jacques-Louis. *Les architectes de la médecine.* Besançon, France: Les Éditions de l'Imprimeur, 1996.

Biozzi G., C. Stiffel, D. Mouton, Y. Bouthillier, and C. Decreusefond. "Morphology and Differentiation of Rosette-Forming Cells during the Immune Response." *Transplantation Proceedings* 4 (1972), 339–43.

Block, Sharon E. *Acute Leukemias.* Study no. 42. Waltham, MA: Pharmacor, Onkos/Decision Resources, 2000.

Block, Sharon E., and Lucy J. Sannes. *Therapeutic and Diagnostic Monoclonal Antibodies for Cancer.* Study no. 40. Waltham, MA: Decision Resources, 1999.

Blume, Stuart S. *Insight and Industry. On the Dynamics of Technological Change in Medicine.* Cambridge, MA: MIT Press, 1992.

Blustein, Bonnie Ellen. "Medicine as Biology: Neurospychiatry at the University of Chicago." *Perspectives on Science* 1 (1993), 416–44.

Bogdanich, Walt. "False Negative." *Wall Street Journal* (2 February 1987), 1.

Bogdanich, Walt. "Lax Laboratories." *Wall Street Journal* (2 November 1987), 1.

Boltanski, Luc. *L'amour et la justice comme compétences.* Paris: Métailié, 1990.

Boltanski, Luc, and Laurent Thévenot. *De la justification. Les économies de la grandeur.* Paris: Gallimard, 1991.

Bonah, Christian. "Pathological Anatomy versus Pathological Physiology: A Franco-German Dispute Over a 'Province for Pathology.'" In *Pathology in the 19th and 20th Centuries. The Relation Between Theory and Practice,* ed. Cay-Ruediger Pruell, 31–53. Sheffield, UK: European Association for the History of Medicine and Health Publications, 1998.

Bonner, William A., Richard G. Sweet, and Henry R. Hulett. *Particle Sorting Method and Apparatus.* U.S Patent no. 3826364, 1974.

Booth, Christopher C. "Clinical Research." In *Companion Encyclopedia of the History of Medicine,* vol. 1, ed. William F. Bynum and Roy Porter, 205–29. London: Routledge, 1993.

Borella, Luis, and Luisa Sen. "T- and B-Lymphocytes in Untreated Acute Lymphocytic Leukemia." *Cancer* 34 (1974) 646–54.

Borella, Luis, and Luisa Sen. "T Cell Surface Markers on Lymphoblasts from Acute Lymphocytic Leukemia." *Journal of Immunology* 3 (1973), 1257–60.

Borowitz, Michael J., Robert Bray, Randy Gascoyne, Steven Melnick, John W. Parker, Louis Picker, and Maryalise Stetler-Stevenson. "U.S.-Canadian Consensus Recommendations on the Immunophenotypic Analysis of Hematologic Neoplasia by Flow Cytometry: Data Analysis and Interpretation." *Cytometry* 30 (1997), 236–44.

Bostrom, R. G., and W. G. Holcomb. "CYDAC: A Digital Scanning Cytophotometer." *IEEE International Convention Record* pt. 9 (1963), 110–9.

Boumsell, L., A. Bernard, E. L. Reinherz, L. M. Nadler, J. Ritz, H. Coppin, Y. Richard, L. Dubertret, F. Valensi, L. Degos, J. Lemerle, G. Flandrin, J. Dausset, and S. F. Schlossman. "Surface Antigens on Malignant Sézary and T-CLL Cells Correspond to Those of Mature T Cells." *Blood* 57 (1981), 526–30.

Bourret, Pascale, and François Eisinger. "Guidelines of 'Good Practices' in Cancer Genetic Clinics: Regulatory Tools for Practices and/or Coordination Tools for Actors?" Presented at the 1998 Annual Meeting of the Society for Social Studies of Science, Halifax, Nova Scotia, 28 October–1 November, 1998.

Bowker, Geoffrey C., and Susan Leigh Star. *Sorting Things Out. Classification and Its Consequences.* Cambridge, MA: MIT Press, 1999.

Bowler, F. "Review: Translational Research: Bench to Bedside and Back Again." *Gray Laboratory Annual Report, Cancer Research Campaign* (1993), 12–24.

Boyer, Robert. *La théorie de la régulation: une analyse critique.* Paris: La Découverte, 1987.

Boyse, Edward A. "The Invitation to Surveillance." In *Immune Surveillance: Proceedings of an International Conference Held at Brook Lodge, Augusta, Michigan, May 11–13, 1970,* ed. Richard T. Smith and Maurice Landy, 7–21. New York: Academic Press, 1970.

Boyse, Edward A., and Lloyd J. Old. "Some Aspects of Normal and Abnormal Cell Surface Genetics." *Annual Review of Genetics* 3 (1969), 269–90.

Boyse, Edward A., Lloyd J. Old, Elisabeth Stockert, and Naoya Shigeno. "Genetic Origin of Tumor Antigens." *Cancer Research* 28 (1968), 1280–7.

Boyse, Edward A., M. Miyazawa, T. Aoki, and Lloyd J. Old, "Ly-A and Ly-B: Two Systems of Lymphocyte Isoantigens in the Mouse." *Proceedings of the Royal Society of London. Series B. Biological Sciences* 170 (1968), 175–93.

Boyse, Edward A., Elisabeth Stockert, and Lloyd J. Old. "Modification of the Antigenic Structure of the Cell Membrane by Thymus-Leukemia (TL) Antigen." *Proceedings of the National Academy of Sciences U.S.A.* 58 (1967), 954–7.

Bracegirdle, Brian. *A History of Microtechnique.* Ithaca, NY: Cornell University Press, 1978.

Brando, B., G. Civati, G. Busnach, M. L. Broggi, L. S. Belli, C. Brunati, M. Seveso, E. Sommaruga, and L. Minetti. "The Leu-2+7+ Cell Subset as a Marker of Immune Activation in Renal Transplant Recipients." *Transplantation Proceedings* 19 (1987), 1611–2.

Brando, Bruno, and Elisabetta Sommaruga. "Nationwide Quality Control Trial on Lymphocyte Immunophenotyping and Flow Cytometer Performance in Italy." *Cytometry* 14 (1993), 294–306.

Brandt, Allan M., and David Charles Sloane. "Of Beds and Benches: Building the Modern American Hospital." In *The Architecture of Science,* ed. Peter Galison and Emily Thompson, 281–305. Cambridge, MA: MIT Press, 1999.

Brandtzaeg, Per. "The Increasing Power of Immunohistochemistry and Immunocytochemistry." *Journal of Immunological Methods* 216 (1998), 49–67.

Braverman, Harry. *Labor and Monopoly Capital. The Degradation of Work in the Twentieth Century.* New York and London: Monthly Review Press, 1974.

Braylan, Raul C., Susan K. Atwater, Lawrence Diamond, Joseph M. Hassett, Margaret Johnson, Pamela G. Kidd, Catherine Leith, and Doyen Nguyen. "U.S.-Canadian Consensus Recommendations on the Immunophenotypic Analysis of Hematologic Neoplasia by Flow Cytometry: Data Reporting." *Cytometry* 30 (1997), 245–84.

Bréchot, Christian, "Les enjeux pour l'INSERM." *INSERM Actualités.* 181 (Suppl.) (January–February 2002), 1–4.

Brent, Leslie. *A History of Transplantation Immunology.* New York: Academic Press, 1997.

Bresnahan, Timothy F., and Shane Greenstein. "Technological Competition and the Structure of the Computer Industry." *Journal of Industrial Economics* 47 (1999), 1–40.

"Bridging the Gap." *Bio-medical Engineering* 1 (1965), 3.

Brodwin, Paul E., ed. *Biotechnology and Culture: Bodies, Anxieties, Ethics.* Bloomington, IN: Indiana University Press, 2000.

Brouet, Jean-Claude. "Marqueurs immunologiques des leucémies." *Actualités immunologiques* 15 (1981), 299–307.

Brouet, Jean-Claude, Jean-Louis Preud'homme, Georges Flandrin, Françoise Valensi, Marie-Thèrese Daniel, and Maxime Seligmann. "Classification immunologique des leucémies aiguës lymphoblastiques. Corrélations cliniques et morphologiques." In *Actualités hématologiques, dixième série,* 148–55. Paris: Masson, 1976.

Brouet, Jean-Claude, Françoise Valensi, M. T. Daniel, Georges Flandrin, Jean-Louis Preud'homme, and Maxime Seligmann. "Immunological Classification of Acute Lymphoblastic Leukemias: Evaluation of Its Clinical Significance in a Hundred Patients." *British Journal of Haematology* 3 (1976), 319–28.

Brown, Geoffrey, and Melvyn F. Greaves. "Cell Surface Markers for Human T and B Lymphocytes." *European Journal of Immunology* 4 (1974), 302–10.

Brown, Geoffrey, David Capellaro, and Melvyn Greaves. "Leukemia-Associated Antigens in Man." *Journal of the National Cancer Institute* 55 (1975), 1281–9.

Brown, Geoffrey, Melvyn F. Greaves, T. A. Lister, N. Rapson, and M. Papamichael. "Expression of Human T and B Lymphocyte Cell-Surface Markers on Leukaemic Cells." *Lancet* 2 (1883) (1974), 753–5.

Brown, Geoffrey, Nancy Hogg, and Melvyn Greaves. "Candidate Leukemia-Specific Antigen in Man." *Nature* 258 (1975), 454–6.

Bucher, Rue. "Pathology: A Study of Social Movements within a Profession." *Social Problems* 10 (1962), 40–51.

Bucher, Rue, and Anselm Strauss. "Professions in Process." *American Journal of Sociology* 66 (1961), 325–34.

Bud, Robert. *The Uses of Life. A History of Biotechnology.* Cambridge, UK: Cambridge University Press, 1993.

Burton, Robert C. "Lymphocyte Monitoring in Renal Transplantation." *Transplantation Proceedings* 16 (1984), 983–7.

Bury, Michael R. "Social Constructionism and the Development of Medical Sociology." *Sociology of Health & Illness* 8 (1986), 137–69.

Bury, Michael R. "Social Constructionism and Medical Sociology: A Rejoinder to Nicolson and McLaughlin." *Sociology of Health & Illness* 9 (1987), 439–41.

Büttner, Johannes. "Clinical Chemistry: A Professional Field for Physicians and Natural Scientists in Europe." *European Journal of Clinical Chemistry and Clinical Biochemistry* 29 (1991), 3–12.

Büttner, Johannes, and Christa Habrich. *Roots of Clinical Chemistry. A Guide through the Historical Exhibition.* Darmstadt, Germany: GIT-Verlag, 1987.

Cain, A. J. "Thomas Sydenam, John Ray, and Some Contemporaries on Species." *Archives of Natural History* 26 (1999), 55–83.

Calder, Nigel. "Immunology: Research at Mill Hill Institute." *Science* 157 (1967), 177–9.

Callendar, G. R. "Tumors and Tumor-like Conditions of the Lymphocyte, the Myelocyte, the Erythrocyte and the Reticulum Cell." *American Journal of Pathology* 10 (1943), 443–65.

Callon, Michel. "Is Science a Public Good?" *Science, Technology, and Human Values* 19 (1994), 395–424.

Callon, Michel, ed. *La science et ses réseaux. Genèse et circulation des faits scientifiques.* Paris: La Découverte, 1989.

Callon, Michel, and John Law. "On the Construction of Sociotechnical Networks: Content and Context Revisited." *Knowledge and Society: Studies in the Sociology of Science Past and Present* 8 (1989), 57–86.

Calvelli, Theresa, Thomas N. Denny, Helene Paxton, Rebecca Gelman, and Jonathan Kagan. "Guideline for Flow Cytometric Immunophenotyping: A Report from the National Institute of Allergy and Infectious Diseases, Division of AIDS." *Cytometry* 14 (1993), 702–15.

Calvino, Italo. *Invisible Cities,* trans. William Weaver. New York: Harcourt Brace Jovanovich, 1974.

Cambrosio, Alberto, and Peter Keating. *Exquisite Specificity. The Monoclonal Antibody Revolution.* New York: Oxford University Press, 1995.

Cambrosio, Alberto, and Peter Keating. "'Going Monoclonal': Art, Science and Magic in the Day-to-Day Use of Hybridoma Technology." *Social Problems* 35 (1988), 244–60.

Cambrosio, Alberto, and Peter Keating. "A Matter of FACS: Constituting Novel Entities in Immunology." *Medical Anthropology Quarterly* 6 (1992), 362–84.

Cambrosio, Alberto, and Peter Keating. "Monoclonal Antibodies: From Local to Extended Networks." In *Private Science: Biotechnology and the Rise of the Molecular Sciences,* ed. Arnold Thackray, 165–81. Philadelphia: University of Pennsylvania Press, 1998.

Cambrosio, Alberto, Peter Keating, and Ronald D. Guttmann. "New Medical Technologies and Clinical Practice: A Survey of Lymphocyte Subset Monitoring." *Clinical Transplantation* 8 (1994), 532–40.

Cambrosio, Alberto, Camille Limoges, and Denyse Pronovost. "Representing Biotechnology: An Ethnography of Quebec Science Policy." *Social Studies of Science* 20 (1990), 195–227.

Cambrosio, Alberto, Peter Keating, and Andrei Mogoutov. "Mapping Collaborative Work and Innovation in Biomedicine: A Computer-Assisted Analysis of Antibody Reagent Workshops." *Social Studies of Science* (forthcoming).

Cameron, Charles S. *Cytology—Best Early Detector of Cancer,* Public Affairs Pamphlet no. 252A. Washington, DC: American Cancer Society, 1966.

Campana, Dario, and George Janossy, "Leukemia Diagnosis and Testing of Complement-Fixing Antibodies for Bone Marrow Purging in Acute Lymphoid Leukemia." *Blood* 68 (1986), 1264–71.

Campana Dario, and C. H. Pui. "Detection of Minimal Residual Disease in Acute Leukemia: Methodologic Advances and Clinical Significance." *Blood* 85 (1995), 1416–34.

Campana Dario, E. Coustan-Smith, and George Janossy. "The Immunologic Detection of Minimal Residual Disease in Acute Leukemia." *Blood* 76 (1990), 163–71.

Canguilhem, Georges. "Régulation." *Encyclopaedia Universalis*, vol. 14, 1–3. Paris: Encyclopaedia Universalis, 1980.

Canguilhem, Georges. *The Normal and the Pathological*, trans. Cardyn R. Fawcett *Le normal et le pathologique.* Paris: Presses Universitaires de France, 1972. New York: Zone Books, 1989. Originally published as.

Canguilhem, Georges. "Le statut épistémologique de la médecine." *History and Philosophy of the Life Sciences* 10 (Suppl.) (1988), 15–29.

Cantor, Harvey, and Richard Asofsky. "Synergy among Lymphoid Cells Mediating the Graft-versus-Host Response II. Synergy in Graft-versus-Host Reactions Produced by Balb/C Lymphoid Cells of Differing Anatomic Origin." *Journal of Experimental Medicine* 131 (1970), 235–46.

Cantor, Harvey, and Edward A. Boyse. "Functional Subclasses of T Lymphocytes Bearing Different Ly Antigens. I. The Generation of Functionally Distinct T-Cell Subclasses Is a Differentiative Process Independent of Antigen." *Journal of Experimental Medicine* 141 (1975), 1376–89.

Cantor, Harvey, and Edward A. Boyse. "Functional Subclasses of T Lymphocytes Bearing Different Ly Antigens. II. Cooperation between Subclasses of Ly+ Cells in the Generation of Killer Activity." *Journal of Experimental Medicine* 141 (1975), 1390–9.

Cantor, Harvey, Richard Asofsky, and Normal Talal. "Synergy among Lymphoid Cells Mediating the Graft-versus-Host Response I. Synergy in Graft-versus-Host Reactions Produced by Cells from NZB/BL Mice." *Journal of Experimental Medicine* 131 (1970), 223–34.

Cantor, Harvey, Elizabeth Simpson, Vicki L. Sato, C. Garrison Fathman, and Leonard A. Herzenberg. "Characterization of Subpopulations of T Lymphocytes I. Separation and Functional Studies of Peripheral T-Cells Binding Different Amounts of Anti-Thy 1.2 (Theta) Antibody Using a Fluorescence-Activated Cell Sorter (FACS)." *Cellular Immunology* 15 (1975), 180–96.

Carter, Patricia H., Sandra Resto-Ruiz, Glenelle C. Washington, Steve Ethridge, Alessio Palini, Robert Vogt, Myron Waxdal, Thomas Fleisher, Philip D. Noguchi, and Gerald E. Marti. "Flow Cytometric Analysis of Whole Blood Lysis, Three Anticoagulants, and Five Cell Preparations." *Cytometry* 13 (1992), 68–74.

Casper, Monica J., and Adele E. Clarke. "Making the Pap Smear into the 'Right Tool' for the Job: Cervical Cancer Screening in the USA, circa 1940–95." *Social Studies of Science* 28 (1998), 255–90.

Caspersson, Torbjörn O. "History of the Development of Cytophotometry from 1935 to Present." *Analytical and Quantitative Cytology and Histology* 9 (1987), 2–6.

Catovsky, Daniel. "Ph1-Positive Acute Leukaemia and Chronic Granulocytic Leukaemia: One or Two Diseases?" *British Journal of Haematology* 42 (1979), 493–8.

Catovsky, Daniel, S. Pittman, M. O'Brien, M. Cherchi, C. Costello, R. Foa, H. E. Pearce, A. V. Hoffbrand, George Janossy, K. Ganeshaguru, and Melvyn F. Greaves. "Multiparameter Studies in Lymphoid Leukemias." *American Journal of Clinical Pathology* 72 (1979), 736–45.

Cazaubiel, M. "Une nécessité: le plateau technique de biologie." *Techniques Hospitalières* 566 (1992), 39–44.

CDC/HIV/AIDS Prevention. *Meeting on the Expansion of the AIDS Surveillance Case Definition. September 2, 1992.* HIV/OAD/9–92/027. Atlanta: Centers for Disease Control, 1992.

Cecil, Russell L. *A Text-Book of Medicine.* Philadelphia: Saunders, 1930.

Centers for Disease Control. "Guidelines for the Performance of CD4+ T-Cell Determinations in Persons with Human Immunodeficiency Virus Infection." *MMWR. Mortality and Morbidity Weekly Report* 41 (RR-8), 1992, 1–17.

Centers for Disease Control. *Model Performance Evaluation Program. Testing for T-Lymphocyte Immunophenotyping by Flow Cytometry.* Atlanta: U.S. Department of Health and Human Services, Public Health Service, 1991.

Centers for Disease Control and Prevention. "1997 Revised Guidelines for Performing CD4+ T-Cell Determinations in Persons Infected with Human Immunodeficiency Virus (HIV)." *MMWR. Mortality and Morbidity Weekly Report* 46 (RR-2), 1997, 1–29.

Centre National de la Recherche Scientifique. *Trésor de la langue française,* vol. 13. Paris: Gallimard, 1988.

Chabner, Bruce A., Anthony L. Boral, and Patrik Multani. "Translational Research: Walking the Bridge between Idea and Cure. Seventeenth Bruce F. Cain Memorial Award Lecture." *Cancer Research* 58 (1998), 4211–6.

Chang, Sophie W., Mitchell H. Kate, and Sandra R. Hernandez. "The New AIDS Case Definition. Implications for San Francisco." *JAMA* 267 (1992), 973–75.

Chatenoud, L., N. Chkoff, H. Kreis, and J. F. Bach. "Correlation between Immunoregulatory T-Cell Imbalances and Renal Allograft Outcome." *Transplantation Proceedings* 15 (1983), 1184–5.

Chess, Leonard, and Stuart F. Schlossman. "Anti-Immunoglobulin Columns and the Separation of T, B and Null Cells." In *In-vitro Methods in Cell-Mediated and*

Tumor Immunity, ed. Barry R. Bloom and John R. David, 255–61. New York: Academic Press, 1976.

Chess, Leonard, and Stuart F. Schlossman. "Methods for the Separation of Unique Human Lymphocyte Subpopulations." In *Manual of Clinical Immunology*, ed. Noel R. Rose and Herman Friedman, 77–80. Washington, DC: American Society for Microbiology, 1976.

Chessels, Judith M., R. M. Hardisty, N. T. Rapson, and Melvyn F. Greaves. "Acute Lymphoblastic Leukaemia in Children: Classification and Prognosis." *Lancet*, 24 and 31 December (1977), 1307–9.

Christakis, Nicholas A. *Death Foretold: Prophecy and Prognosis in Medical Care.* Chicago: University of Chicago Press, 1999.

Ciborra, Claudio U. "The Platform Organization: Recombining Strategies, Structures and Surprises." *Organizational Science* 7 (1996), 103–18.

Cioran, Emile M. *Syllogismes de l'amertume.* Paris: Gallimard, 1952.

Claman, Henry N., Edward A. Chaperon, and R. Fraser Triplett. "Thymus-Marrow Cell Combinations. Synergism in Antibody Production." *Proceedings of the Society for Experimental Biology and Medicine* 122 (1966), 1167–71.

Clark, William R. *The Double-Edged Sword of Immunity: At War Within.* Oxford: Oxford University Press, 1995.

Clarke, Adele E. *Disciplining Reproduction. Modernity, American Life Sciences, and the Problems of Sex.* Berkeley: University of California Press, 1998.

Clarke, Adele E. "A Social Worlds Research Adventure: The Case of Reproductive Science." In *Theories of Science in Society*, ed. Susan E. Correns and Thomas F. Gieryn, 15–42. Bloomington: Indiana University Press, 1990.

Clarke, Adele E., and Monica J. Casper. "From Simple Technology to Complex Arena: Classification of Pap Smears, 1917–90." *Medical Anthropology Quarterly* 10 (1996), 601–23.

Clarke, Adele E., and Joan H. Fujimura, eds. *The Right Tools for the Job: At Work in Twentieth-Century Life Sciences.* Princeton, NJ: Princeton University Press, 1992.

Cline, Martin J. *The White Cell.* Cambridge, MA: Harvard University Press, 1975.

"Clinical Immunology: Report on the Joint Meeting of the Antibody Club and the Dutch Society of Immunology, Leiden, 13 June 1970." *British Journal of Hospital Medicine* (October 1970), 467–70.

Cobbold, Steve, and Su Metcalfe. "Monoclonal Antibodies That Define Canine Homologues of Human CD Antigens: Summary of the First International Canine Leukocyte Antigen Workshop (CLAW)." *Tissue Antigens* 43 (1994), 137–54.

Coiffier, Bertrand, Françoise Berger, Paul-André Bryon, and Jean-Pierre Magaud. "T-Cell Lymphomas: Immunologic, Histologic, Clinical and Therapeutic Analysis of 63 Cases." *Journal of Clinical Oncology* 6 (1988), 1584–9.

Cole, Rufus. "Hospital and Laboratory." *Science* 61 (1927), 545–52.

Coleman, C. Norman, and Jay R. Harris. "Current Scientific Issues Related to Clinical Radiation Oncology." *Radiation Research* 150 (1998), 125–33.

Collard, Patrick. *The Development of Microbiology.* Cambridge, UK: Cambridge University Press, 1976.

Collen, Morris F., Leonard Rubin, and Lou S. Davis. "Computers in Multiphasic Screening." In *Computers in Biomedical Research,* vol. 1, ed. Ralph W. Stacy and Bruce Waxman, chap. 14. New York: Academic Press, 1965.

Collen, Morris F., Leonard Rubin, Jerzy Neyman, George B. Danzig, Robert M. Baer, and A. B. Siegelaub. "Automated Multiphasic Screening and Diagnosis." *American Journal of Public Health* 54 (1964), 742–50.

Collins, Harry M. *Artificial Experts: Social Knowledge and Intelligent Machines.* Cambridge, MA: MIT Press, 1990.

Collins, Harry. "Hubert L. Dreyfus, Forms of Life, and a Simple Test for Machine Intelligence." *Social Studies of Science* 22 (1992), 726–39.

Collins, Harry, and Martin Kusch. *The Shape of Actions: What Humans and Machines Can Do.* Cambridge, MA: MIT Press, 1998.

Colvin, R. B., A. B. Cosimi, R. C. Burton, F. L. Delmonico, G. Jaffers, R. H. Rubin, N. E. Tolkoff-Rubin, J. V. Giorgi, R. T. McCluskey, and P. S. Russel. "Circulating T-Cell Subsets in 72 Human Renal Allograft Recipients: The OKT4+/OKT8+ Cell Ratio Correlates with Reversibility of Graft Injury and Glomerulopathy." *Transplantation Proceedings* 15 (1983), 1166–9.

Commission on Chronic Illness. *Chronic Illness in the United States,* vol. 1. Cambridge, MA: Harvard University Press, 1956.

Committee for Scientific and Technological Policy. *Biotechnology and Government Policies.* Paris: Organisation for Economic Co-operation and Development, 1981.

Conein, Bernard, Nicolas Dodier, and Laurent Thévenot, eds. *Les objets dans l'action. De la maison au laboratoire. Raisons Pratiques* 4. Paris: Éditions de l'École des Hautes Études en Sciences Sociales, 1993.

"Conference on Tumor Specific Antigens [conference proceedings]." *Cancer Research* 28 (1968), 1275–459.

Cook, Harold J. "The New Philosophy and Medicine in Seventeenth-Century England." In *Reappraisals of the Scientific Revolution,* ed. David C. Lindberg and Robert S. Westman, 397–436. Cambridge, UK: Cambridge University Press, 1990.

Coon, John S., Alan L. Landay, and Ronald S. Weinstein. "Flow Cytometric Analysis of Paraffin-Embedded Tumors: Implications for Diagnostic Pathology." *Human Pathology* 17 (1986), 435–7.

Coons, Albert H. "The Beginnings of Immunofluorescence." *Journal of Immunology* 87 (1961), 499–503.

Coons, Albert. H. "Fluorescent Antibodies as Histochemical Tools." *FASEB Journal* 10 (1951), 558–9.

Coons, Albert H. "Introduction: The Development of Immunohistochemistry." *Annals of the New York Academy of Sciences* 177 (1971), 5–9.

Coons, Albert H., H. J. Creech, and R. N. Jones. "Immunological Properties of an Antibody Containing a Fluorescent Group." *Proceedings of the Society for Experimental Biology and Medicine* 47 (1941), 200–2.

Coons, Albert H., H. J. Creech, R. N. Jones, and E. Berliner. "The Demonstration of Pneumococcal Antigen in Tissues by the Use of Fluorescent Antibody." *Journal of Immunology* 45 (1942), 159–70.

Cooper, Max D., Daniel Y. Perey, Raymond D. Peterson, Ann E. Gabrielsen, and Robert A. Good. "The Two-Component Concept of the Lymphoid System." In *Immunologic Deficiencies in Man, Birth Defects. Original Article Series (4)*, ed. Daniel Bergsma and Robert A. Good, 7–16. New York: National Foundation, 1968.

Cordell, Jacqueline L., Brunangelo Falini, Wendy N. Erber, Anna K. Ghosh, Zainalabideen Abdulaziz, Stuart MacDonald, Karen A. Pulford, Harald Stein, and David Y. Mason. "Immunoenzymatic Labeling of Monoclonal Antibodies Using Immune Complexes of Alkaline Phosphatase and Monoclonal Anti-Alkalilne Phosphatase (APAAP Complexes)." *Journal of Histochemistry and Cytochemistry* 32 (1984), 219–29.

Cosimi, A. Benedict, Robert B. Colvin, Robert C. Burton, Robert H. Rubin, Gideon Goldstein, Patrick C. Kung, W. Peter Hansen, Francis L. Delmonico, and Paul S. Russell. "Use of Monoclonal Antibodies to T-Cell Subsets for Immunologic Monitoring and Treatment in Recipients of Renal Allografts." *New England Journal of Medicine* 305 (1981), 308–14.

Cossman, Jeffrey, Leonard M. Neckers, Su Ming Hsu, Dan Longo, and Elaine S. Jaffe. "Low-grade Lymphomas. Expression of Developmentally Regulated B-Cell Antigens." *American Journal of Pathology* 115 (1984), 117–24.

Cottier, H., J. Turk, and L. Sobin. "A Proposal for a Standardized System of Reporting Human Lymph Node Morphology in Relation to Immunological Function." *Bulletin of the World Health Organization* 47 (1972), 375–408.

"Coulter Corp. Is Sued by Stanford University on Patent Violation." *Wall Street Journal* (4 June 1986), 1.

Coulter Cytometry. *Optimizing Cytometry Systems for Measurement of Biologic Samples.* Hialeah, FL: Coulter Cytometry Technical Monograph, 1990.

Coulter Electronics Inc. "Interlaboratory Quality Assurance Program." *U.S. Patent* no. 4, 858, 154 (1989).

Coulter, Wallace H. "High Speed Automatic Blood Cell Counter and Size Analyzer." *Proceedings of the National Electronics Conference* 12 (1956), 1034–40.

Courtney, W. B., A. W. Hilberg, S. C. Ingraham, R. F. Kaiser, J. C. Pruitt, and M. M. Bouser. "Field Trial of the Cytoanalyzer; 1, 184 Specimens Analyzed." *Journal of the National Cancer Institute* 24 (1960), 1167–79.

Craigie, William Alexander. *A Dictionary of American English on Historical Principles.* Chicago: University of Chicago Press, 1940.

Crespin, Renaud, and Pierre Lascoumes. "Régulation de la carrière d'un instrument de santé. Les parcours de l'usage du test du VIH dans l'emploi en France et aux États-Unis." *Sociologie du travail* 42 (2000), 133–57.

Crosland-Taylor, P. J. "A Device for Counting Small Particles Suspended in a Fluid through a Tube." *Nature* 171 (1953), 37–8.

Cunningham, Andrew, and Perry Williams, eds. *The Laboratory Revolution in Medicine.* Cambridge, UK: Cambridge University Press, 1992.

Dagognet, François. *Le catalogue de la vie.* Paris: Presses Universitaires de France, 1970.

Dagognet, François. "La nature de la pensée médicale (II). Point de vue de Dagognet." *Le Concours médical* (22 October 1966), 6281–5.

Dagognet, François. "Le normal et le pathologique: Prolégomènes." *Prospective et santé* 40 (1986–7), 7–10.

Danesi, D. T., M. Spanò, and P. Altavista. "Quality Control Study of the Italian Group of Cytometry on Flow Cytometry Cellular DNA Content Measurements." *Cytometry* 14 (1993), 576–83.

Danielli, J. F., and H. Davson. *The Permeability of Natural Membranes.* London: University Press, 1952.

Daston, Lorraine. "Objectivity and the Escape from Perspective." *Social Studies of Science* 22 (1992), 597–618.

Daston, Lorraine, ed. *Biographies of Scientific Objects.* Chicago: University of Chicago Press, 2000.

Daston, Lorraine, and Peter Galison. "The Image of Objectivity." *Representations* 40 (fall 1992), 81–128.

Dausset, Jean. *Clin d'œil à la vie. La grande aventure HLA.* Paris: Odile Jacob, 1998.

Davey, Frederick R., M. Tarek Elghetany, and Anthony S. Kurec. "Immunophenotyping of Hematologic Neoplasms in Paraffin-Embedded Tissue Sections." *American Journal of Clinical Pathology* 93 (Suppl. 1) (1990) S17–S26.

David, Paul A. "Path Dependence and Varieties of Learning in the Evolution of Technological Practice." In *Technological Innovation as an Evolutionary Process,* ed. John Ziman, 118–33. Cambridge, UK: Cambridge University Press, 2000.

David, Paul A. "Clio and the Economics of QWERTY." *American Economic Review* 75 (1985), 332–7.

Davis, Bruce H., Kathy Foucar, Wlodek Szczarkowski, Edward Ball, Tom Witzig, Kenneth A. Foon, Denise Wells, Pat Kotylo, Rebecca Johnson, Curtis Hanson, and David Bessman. "U.S.-Canadian Consensus Recommendations on the Immunophenotypic Analysis of Hematologic Neoplasia by Flow Cytometry: Medical Indications." *Cytometry* 30 (1997), 249–63.

Dean, Phillip N. "Helpful Hints in Flow Cytometry and Sorting." *Cytometry* 6 (1985), 62–4.

Dean, Philip N. "Membership Profile of the International Society for Analytical Cytology." *Cytometry* 15 (1994), 185–8.

Debru, Claude. *Philosophie de l'inconnu: le vivant et la recherche.* Paris: Presses Universitaires de France, 1998.

De Chadarevian, Soraya, and Harmke Kamminga, eds. *Molecularizing Biology and Medicine: New Practices and Alliances, 1910s–1970s.* Amsterdam: Harwood Academic Publishers, 1998.

Dehner, Louis P. "Here We Go Again: A New Classification of Malignant Lymphomas. A Viewpoint from the Trenches." *American Journal of Clinical Pathology* 103 (1995), 539–40.

Delaporte, François, and Patrice Pinell. *Histoire des myopathies.* Paris: Payot, 1998.

"Deposit Case before CAFC." *BioEngineering News* (13 May 1985), 1.

Derman, Herbert, and Dennis B. Dorsey. "The Pathology of Regulation." *Clinics in Laboratory Medicine* 11 (1991), 793–802.

Deschamps, Jacques. "Paris: L'Hôpital Saint-Louis." *Revue de la Société Française d'Histoire des Hôpitaux* no. 89 (1998), 25–7.

Desowitz, Robert S. *The Thorn in the Starfish: The Immune System and How It Works.* New York: Norton, 1987.

Devilder, R. "Une nouvelle logistique pour les laboratoires hospitaliers." *Techniques Hospitalières* 613 (1997), 31–42.

DeVita, Vincent T., Jr., and Samuel Hellman. "Hodgkin's Disease and the Non-Hodgkin's Lymphomas." In *Cancer: Principles and Practice of Oncology,* ed. Vincent

T. DeVita Jr., Samuel Hellman, and S. Rosenberg, 1331–1401. Philadelphia: Lippincott, 1982.

DeVita, Vincent T., Jr., Henry Rappaport, and Emil Frei. "Announcement of Formation of the Lymphoma Task Force and Pathology Reference Center." *Cancer* 22 (1968), 1087–8.

Dewhurst, Kenneth, ed. *Dr. Thomas Sydenham (1624–1689). His Life and Writings.* Berkeley: University of California Press, 1968.

De Wolf-Peeters, C., and S. Pittaluga. "Further Considerations on the Revised European-American Lymphoma Classification." *Current Opinion in Oncology* 8 (1996), 366–70.

Deyoung, H. Garrett. "Many Factors Must Be Weighed in Decision to Purchase Antibodies." *The Scientist* 10 (September 1996), 18.

D'Hautcourt, Jean-Luc. "Contrôle de qualité: revue de l'offre et des résultats." In *Immunologie de l'infection à VIH,* 87–95. Paris: Glyphe & Biotem, 1997.

Dick, Fred R., J. O. Armitage, and C. P. Burns. "Diagnostic Concurrence in the Subclassification of ALL Using FAB Criteria." *Cancer* 49 (1982), 916–20.

Dill, Ken A. "Strengthening Biomedicine's Roots." *Nature* 400 (22 July 1999), 309–10.

Dittrich, W., and W. Göhde. "Impulsfluorometrie bei Einzelzellen in Suspensionen." *Zeitschrift für Naturforschung* 24B (1969), 360–1.

Dodier, Nicolas, and Janine Barbot. "Le temps des tensions épistémiques. Le développement des essais thérapeutiques dans le cadre du sida." *Revue française de sociologie* 41 (2000), 79–118.

Doljanski, F. "A New Look at the Cell Surface." *Israeli Journal of Medical Science* 9 (1973), 251–7.

Dorfman, Ronald F. "Pathology of the Non-Hodgkin's Lymphomas: New Classifications." *Cancer Treatment Reports* 61 (6) (1977), 945–51.

Dorland, William Alexander Newman. *The American Illustrated Medical Dictionary.* Philadelphia: Saunders, 1923.

Downey, Hal, ed. *Handbook of Hematology,* vol. 3. New York: P. B. Hoeber, 1938.

Drexler, H. G., and J. Minowada. "History and Classification of Human Leukemia-Lymphoma Cell Lines." *Leukemia and Lymphoma* 31 (1998), 305–16.

Dreyfus, Hubert L. "Response to Collins' *Artificial Experts.*" *Social Studies of Science* 22 (1992), 717–26.

Dubois, Betty Lou. "'And the Last Slide, Please,' Regulatory Language Function at Biomedical Meetings." *World Language English* 1 (1982), 263–8.

Dubois, Betty Lou. "The Use of Slides in Biomedical Speeches." *The ESP Journal* 1 (1980), 45–50.

Dubuisson, Sophie, and Antoine Hennion. *Le design: l'objet dans l'usage. La relation objet-usage-usager dans le travail de trois agences de design.* Paris: Presses de l'École des Mines, 1996.

Duchesneau, François. "La philosophie médicale de Sydenham." *Dialogue* 9 (1970), 54–68.

Dumit, Joseph. "Objective Brains, Prejudicial Images." *Science in Context* 12 (1999), 173–201.

Duque, Ricardo E. "Flow Cytometric Analysis of Lymphomas and Acute Leukemias." *Annals of the New York Academy of Sciences* 677 (1993), 309–25.

Duval, Georges. "L'Hôpital moderne: 1920–1980." *Monuments Historiques* 114 (April–May 1981), 59–64.

Eco, Umberto. *A Theory of Semiotics.* Bloomington: Indiana University Press, 1979.

Engel, Eloise, and Arnold S. Lott. *Man in Flight. Biomedical Achievements in Aerospace.* Annapolis, MD: Leeward, 1979.

England, John M. "Internal Quality Control and Calibration." In *Automation and Quality Assurance in Haematology*, ed. R. M. Rowan and John M. England, 3–17. Oxford: Blackwell, 1986.

Engleman, Edgar C., Claudia Benike, Barbara Osborne, and Richard Goldsby. "Functional Characteristics of Human T-Cell Subpopulations Distinguished by a Monoclonal Antibody." *Proceedings of the National Academy of Sciences U.S.A.* 77 (1980), 1607–11.

Epstein, A. L. "The Cell Culture, Heterotransplantation and Biological Characterization of the Human Malignant Lymphomas." *Dissertation Abstracts International* (B) 40 (1979), 36.

Epstein, Steven. "Activism, Drug Regulation, and the Politics of Therapeutic Evaluation in the AIDS Era: A Case Study of ddC and the 'Surrogate Markers' Debate." *Social Studies of Science* 27 (1997), 691–726.

Epstein, Steven. *Impure Science. AIDS, Activism, and the Politics of Knowledge.* Berkeley: University of California Press, 1996.

Erber, W. N., L. C. Mynheer, and D. Y. Mason. "APAAP Labelling of Blood and Bone Marrow Samples for Immunophenotyping Leukaemia." *Lancet* 1, 8484 (April 1986), 761–5.

Erber, W. N., A. J. Pinching, and D. Y. Mason. "Immunocytochemical Detection of T and B Cell Populations in Routine Blood Smears." *Lancet* 1, 8385 (May 1984), 1042–6.

Erickson, Cyrus C., Bennett E. Everett Jr., Edward E. Siegler, Frank Whitacre, John Stirling, John E. Dunn, L. M. Graves, and Douglas H. Sprunt. "Preliminary Report of 20,000 Women Studied by the Vaginal Smear Technic in a General Population Cancer Screening Project." *Proceedings of the American Association for Cancer Research,* 1 (April 1953), 14.

Escobar, Mario R. "Oncogenic Viruses." In *The Pathobiology of Neoplasia,* ed. Alphonse E. Sirica, 81–109. New York: Plenum Press, 1989.

Estrin, Norman F., ed. *The Medical Device Industry: Science, Technology and Regulation in a Competitive Environment.* New York: Marcel Dekker, 1990.

Evans, Robert L., Jacqueline M. Breard, Herbert Lazarus, Stuart F. Schlossman, and Leonard Chess. "Detection, Isolation and Functional Characterization of Two Human T-Cell Subclasses Bearing Unique Differentiation Antigens." *Journal of Experimental Medicine* 145 (1977), 221–33.

Evans, Robert L., Herbert Lazarus, Ann C. Penta, and Stuart F. Schlossman. "Two Functionally Distinct Subpopulations of Human T Cells That Collaborate in the Generation of Cytotoxic Cells Responsible for Cell-mediated Lympholysis." *Journal of Immunology* 120 (1978), 1423–8.

Faber, Knud. *Nosography in Modern International Medicine.* New York: Hoeber, 1923.

Fagot-Largeault, Anne. *Les causes de la mort. Histoire naturelle et facteurs de risque.* Paris: Vrin, 1989.

Farber, S., R. Toch, E. M. Sears, and D. Pinkel. "Advances in Chemotherapy of Cancer in Man." *Advances in Cancer Research* 4 (1956), 1–71.

Fausto, Nelson. "What's in a Name? The American Society for Investigative Pathology." *American Journal of Pathology* 142 (1993), 1.

Feinstein, Alvan R. "The Crisis in Clinical Research." *Bulletin of the History of Medicine* 69 (1995), 288–91.

Fei, David T. W., Helene Paxton, and Anthony B. Chen. "Difficulties in Precise Quantitation of CD4+ T-Lymphocytes for Clinical Trials: A Review." *Biologicals* 21 (1993), 221–31.

First MIC Cooperative Study Group. "Morphologic, Immunologic, and Cytogenetic (MIC) Working Classification of Acute Lymphoblastic Leukemias." *Cancer Genetics and Cytogenetics* 23 (1986), 189–97.

Fisher, Richard I., R. B. Jones, V. T. De Vita Jr., R. M. Simon, A. J. Garvin, C. W. Berard, and R. C. Young. "Natural History of Malignant Lymphomas with Divergent Histologies at Staging Evaluation." *Cancer* 47 (1981), 2022–5.

Fisher, Richard I., Thomas P. Miller, and Thomas M. Grogan. "New REAL Clinical Entities." *Cancer Journal from Scientific American* 4 (Suppl. 2) (1998), S5–12.

Fleisher, Thomas A. "Introduction to Diagnostic Laboratory Immunology." In *Primer on Allergic and Immunologic Diseases, 4th ed. JAMA*, 278, 22 (1997), 1823–34.

Flexner, Stuart Berg, ed. *Random House Unabridged Dictionary*. 2nd edn. New York: Random House, 1993 [1982].

Fortanier, Cécile, Louis-André Gérard-Varet, and Jean-Paul Moatti. "Un cas de recherche et développement dans le champ biomédical: les thérapies cellulaires." In *Dix ans d'avancées en économie de la santé. Actes des XIXes Journées des économistes de la santé française*, ed. Jean-Claude Sailly and Thérèse Lebrun, 289–304. Montrouge, France: J. Libbey Eurotext, 1997.

Ford, W. I. "The Lymphocyte—Its Transformation from a Frustrating Enigma to a Model of Cellular Function." In *Blood: Pure and Eloquent*, ed. M. M. Wintrobe, 457–507. New York: McGraw-Hill, 1980.

Fornace Albert J., Jr., and Elaine S. Jaffe. "Pathology of Malignant Lymphomas." In *Neoplastic Diseases of the Blood*, vol. 2, ed. Peter H. Wiernik, George P. Canellos, Robert A. Kyle, and Charles A. Schiffer, 707–36. New York: Churchill Livingston, 1985.

Forsum, U., K. Claesson, L. Frödin, A. Parra-Karlson, L. Klareskog, B. Odlind, B. Stenkvist, and G. Tufveson. "Methods for Monitoring T-Lymphocyte Subsets in Renal Allografts." *Transplantation Proceedings* 15 (1983), 1179–81.

Fortun, Michael. "Projecting Speed Genomics." In *Practices of Human Genetics: International and Interdisciplinary Perspectives* (Sociology of the Sciences Yearbook), ed. Michael Fortun and Everett Mendelsohn, 25–48. Dordrecht, Netherlands: Kluwer, 1999.

Fosdick, Raymond B. *The Rockefeller Foundation. A Review for 1947*. New York: Rockefeller Archives Center, 1947.

Foucar, K., I. M. Chen, and S. Crago. "Organization and Operation of a Flow Cytometric Immunophenotyping Laboratory." *Seminars in Diagnostic Pathology* 6 (1989), 13–36.

Foucault, Michel. *The Birth of the Clinic: An Archeology of Medical Perception*. New York: Vintage Books, 1975.

Foucault, Michel. "Le jeu de Michel Foucault." In *Dits et écrits*, vol. 2, 298–329. Paris: Quarto Gallimard, 2001.

Foucault, Michel. "Pierre Boulez: L'écran traversé." In *Dits et écrits*, vol. 2, 1038–41. Paris: Quarto Gallimard, 2001.

Foucault, Michel. *This Is Not a Pipe*. Berkeley: University of California Press, 1983.

Foucault, Michel, Blandine Barret Kriegel, Anne Thalamy, François Beguin, and Bruno Fortier. *Les machines à guérir. Aux origines de l'hôpital moderne*. Brussels and Liège: Pierre Mardaga, 1979.

Fowkes, F. G. R. "Containing the Use of Diagnostic Tests." *British Medical Journal* 290 (1985), 488–90.

Fox, Jeffrey L. "Encroaching on Research Freedom." *Science* 224 (1994), 584–6.

"Frei, Freireich Share One GM Award." *The Cancer Letter* 9 (24) (1983), 5.

Freireich, Emil J., and Noreen A. Lemak. *Milestones in Leukemia Research and Therapy.* Baltimore: Johns Hopkins University Press, 1991.

Friedman, Henry S., Sandra H. Bigner, and Darrell D. Bigner. "Cyclophosphamide Therapy of Medulloblastoma: From the Laboratory to the Clinic and Back Again (and Again and Again)." *Journal of Neuro-Oncology* 24 (1995), 103–8.

Fröland, S. S. "Binding of Sheep Erythrocytes to Human Lymphocytes. A Probable Marker of T Lymphocytes." *Scandinavian Journal of Immunology* 1 (1972), 269–80.

Fujimura, Joan H. "The Molecular Biological Cancer Research Bandwagon: Where Social Worlds Meet." *Social Problems* 35 (1988), 261–83.

Fujimura, Joan H. *Crafting Science: A Sociohistory of the Quest for the Genetics of Cancer.* Cambridge, MA: Harvard University Press, 1996.

Fujimura, Joan H. "Crafting Science: Standardized Packages, Boundary Objects, and 'Translations.'" In *Science as Practice and Culture,* ed. Andrew Pickering, 169–211. Chicago: University of Chicago Press, 1992.

Fulginiti, Vincent A., William E. Hathaway, David S. Pearlman, Will R. Blackburn, C. W. Reiquam, John H. Githens, Henry N. Claman, and C. Henry Kempe. "Dissociation of Delayed-Hypersensitivity and Antibody Synthesizing Capacities in Man. Report of Two Sibships with Thymic Dysplasia, Lymphoid Tissue Depletion and Normal Immunoglobulins." *Lancet* 2, no. 7453 (July 1966), 5–8.

Fulwyler, Mack J. "An Electronic Particle Separator with Potential Biological Applications." In Los Alamos Scientific Laboratory of the University of California, *Biological and Medical Research Groups (H-4) of the Health Division. Annual Report July 1964 through June 1965.* LA-3432-MS, 114–8, Los Alamos, NM, 1965.

Fulwyler, Mack J. "Electronic Separation of Biological Cells by Volume." *Science* 150 (1965), 910–1.

Fulwyler, Mack J. *Electronic Volume Analysis and Volume Fractionation Applied to Mammalian Cells.* PhD thesis, University of Colorado, Boulder, 1967.

Fulwyler, Mack J. "Further Development of the Cell Separator." In Los Alamos Scientific Laboratory of the University of California, *Biological and Medical Research Groups (H-4) of the Health Division. Annual Report July 1965 through June 1966.* LA-3610-MS, 222–4, Los Alamos, NM, 1966.

Fulwyler, Mack J. *Particle Separator.* U.S. Patent no. 3.380.584, 1968.

Gajewska, Muriel. "Sida: la trithérapie entre la vie et la mort." *Le Monde* (2 November 1996), 11.

Galison, Peter. *Image and Logic. A Material Culture of Microphysics.* Chicago: University of Chicago Press, 1997.

Gallagher, Richard B., Jean Gilder, G. J. V. Nossal, and Gaetano Salvatore. *Immunology: The Making of a Modern Science.* New York: Academic Press, 1995.

Galton, D. A. G., and H. E. M. Kay. *U.K. Leukaemia Clinical Trials for Children and Adults.* London: Leukaemia Research Fund, 1978.

Garrett, Laurie. *The Coming Plague: Newly Emerging Diseases in a World out of Balance.* New York: Farrar, Straus and Giroux, 1994.

Gatter, K. C., C. Alcock, A. Heryet, and D. Y. Mason, "Clinical Importance of Analysing Malignant Tumours of Uncertain Origin with Immunohistological Techniques." *Lancet* 1, no. 8441 (June 1985), 1302–5.

Gaudillière, Jean-Paul. "Biochimistes et biomédecine dans l'après-guerre: deux itinéraires entre laboratoire et hôpital." *Sciences sociales et santé* 10 (1992), 107–47.

Gaudillière, Jean-Paul. "Les biochimistes français entre légitimité médicale et légitimité biologique, 1930–1960." In *Les sciences biologiques et médicales en France, 1920–1950,* ed. Claude Debru, Jean Gayon, and Jean-François Picard, 265–82. Paris: CNRS, 1994.

Gaudillière, Jean-Paul. *Inventer la biomédecine. La France, l'Amérique et la production des savoirs du vivant après 1945.* Paris: La Découverte, 2002.

Gaudillière, Jean-Paul. "Oncogenes as Metaphors for Human Cancer: Articulating Laboratory Practices and Medical Demands." In *Medicine and Change. Historical and Sociological Studies of Medical Innovation,* ed. Ilana Löwy, 212–48. Montrouge France: John Libbey Eurotext, 1993.

Gay, Tim. "How 'Team Learning' Raises Customer Service Levels." *Health Industry Today* 59 (1996), 9.

Geiger, Robert L. "Science and the University." In *Science in the Twentieth Century,* ed. John Krige and Dominique Pestre, 159–74. Amsterdam: Harwood Academic, 1997.

General Haematology Task Force of BCSH [British Society for Haematology]. "Immunophenotyping in the Diagnosis of Acute Leukemias." *Journal of Clinical Pathology* 47 (1994), 777–81.

Gerber, A. Russel. "Centers for Disease Control Programs in Flow Cytometric Immunophenotyping." *Annals of the New York Academy of Sciences* 677 (1993), 40–2.

Gershon, Richard K., and K. Kondo. "Cell Interactions in the Induction of Tolerance: The Role of Thymic Lymphocytes." *Immunology* 18 (1970), 723–37.

Gerstein, Marc S. "From Machine Bureaucracies to Networked Organizations: An Architectural Journey." In *Organizational Architecture. Designs for Changing Organizations*, ed. David A. Nadler, Marc S. Gerstein, and Robert B. Shaw, 11–38. San Francisco: Jossey-Bass, 1992.

Gibbs, Jeffrey N. "ASRs:FDA Issues Final Rule." *IVD Technology Magazine* (January 1998).

Gibbs, Jeffrey N. "Regulations and Standards: FDA Makes a Better Rule for IHC's." *IVD Technology Magazine* (September 1998).

Gilbert, Pierre. *Dictionnaire des mots nouveaux*. Paris: Hachette, 1971.

Giorgi, Janis V., Hui-Ling Cheng, Joseph B. Margolick, Kenneth D. Bauer, John Ferbas, Myron Waxdal, Ingrid Schmid, Lance E. Hultin, Anne L. Jackson, Larry Park, Jeremy M. G. Taylor, and the Multicenter AIDS Cohort Study Group. "Quality Control in the Flow Cytometric Measurement of T-Lymphocyte Subsets: The Multicenter AIDS Cohort Study Experience." *Clinical Immunology and Immunopathology* 55 (1990), 173–86.

Giorgi, Janis V., Alison M. Kesson, and Cheng-Cheng Chou. "Immunodeficiency and Infectious Diseases." In *Manual of Clinical Laboratory Immunology*, ed. Noel R. Rose, Everly Conway de Macario, John L. Fahey, Herman Friedman, and Gerald M. Penn, 174–81. Washington, DC: American Society for Microbiology, 1992.

Giraud, Alexandra, and Dominique Jolly. *Le consensus en médecine. Analyse et bilan des conférences de consensus dans le monde*. Paris: Doin, 1991.

Givan, Alice Longobardi. *Flow Cytometry: First Principles*. New York: Wiley-Liss, 1992.

Glick, B., T. S. Chang, and R. G. Jaap. "The Bursa of Fabricius and Antibody Production." *Poultry Science* 35 (1956), 224–5.

Gnanadesikan, Ram. *Methods for Statistical Data Analysis of Multivariate Observations*. New York: John Wiley & Sons, 1977.

Goguel, Alain F. "Interlaboratory Trials: Surveys in France." In *Quality Control in Haematology: Symposium of the International Committee for Standardization in Haematology*, ed. Shirley Mitchell Lewis and Johannes Ferdinand Coster, 69–78. London: Academic Press, 1975.

Goguel, Alain F., K. Crainic, A. Ducailar, and M. Ouin. "Interlaboratory Quality Assessment of Lymphocyte Phenotyping. Etalonorme 1990–1992 Surveys." *Biology of the Cell* 78 (1993), 79–84.

Göhde, Wolfgang. *Zellzyklusanalysen mit dem Impulscytophotometer: Der Einfluss chemischer und physikalischer Noxen auf die Proliferationskinetik von Tumorzellen*. Habilitationsschrift des Fachbereichs Vorklinische und Theoretische Medizinischen Fakultät, Westfälischen Wilhelms-Universität, Münster, Germany, 1973.

Göhde, Wolfgang, Johannes Schumann, and Th. Büchner, eds. *Pulse-Cytophotometry: Application in Cancer Research and Hematology with Special Reference to Cell Kinetics. 2d International Symposium on Pulse-Cytophotometry—Münster 1976.* Ghent, Belgium: European Press, 1976.

Goldin, Grace, and John D. Thompson. *The Hospital: A Social and Architectural History.* New Haven, CT: Yale University Press, 1975.

Gomez, E., J. F. San Miguel, M. Gonzalez, A. Orfao, M. C. Canizo, J. M. Moraleda, and A. Lopez Borrasca. "The Value of the Immunological Subtypes and Individual Markers Compared to Classical Parameters in the Prognosis of Acute Lymphoblastic Leukemia." *Hematological Oncology* 9 (1991), 33–42.

Good, Robert A. "Experiments of Nature in Immunobiology." *New England Journal of Medicine* 279 (1968), 1344–5.

Good, Robert A. "Lymphocyte Surface Markers [editorial]." *New England Journal of Medicine* 287 (1972), 305–6.

Good, Robert A. "The Minnesota Scene: A Crucial Portal of Entry to Modern Cellular Immunology." In *The Immunologic Revolution. Facts and Witnesses,* ed. Andor Szentuvanyi and Herman Friedman, 105–68. Boca Raton, FL: CRC Press, 1994.

Good, Robert A. "Runestones in Immunology: Inscriptions to Journeys of Discovery and Analysis." *Journal of Immunology* 117 (1976), 1413–28.

Goodhart, James F. "The Passing of Morbid Anatomy." *Lancet* (26 October 1912), 1129–33.

Gordon, Deborah R. "Tenacious Assumptions in Western Medicine." In *Biomedicine Examined,* ed. Margaret M. Lock and Deborah R. Gordon, 19–56. Dordrecht, Netherlands: Kluwer, 1988.

Gorer, Peter A. "Further Studies on Antigenic Differences in Mouse Erythrocytes." *Journal of Pathological Bacteriology* 44 (1937), 691–7.

Gosselin, Roger. "Probing into Task Interdependencies: The Case of Physicians in a Teaching Hospital." *Journal of Management Studies* 22 (1985), 466–97.

Gouget, Bernard, Christophe Bielle, Maurice Le Mandat, and Josy Pollet. "La dynamique de la biologie au sein du plateau technique hospitalier." *Gestions Hospitalières* no. 337 (June–July 1994), 453–8.

Gouvernement du Québec. *À l'heure des biotechnologies. Programme d'intervention pour le développement de la recherche en biotechnologies au Québec. Phase I: 1982–1987.* Québec City: Secrétariat au développement scientifique, 1982.

Government of Canada. *Biotechnology: A Development Plan for Canada. Report of the Task Force on Biotechnology.* Ottawa: Ministry of Supply and Services, 1981.

Gowans, J. L. "The Mysterious Lymphocyte." In *Immunology: The Making of a Modern Science*, ed. Richard B. Gallagher, Jean Gilder, G. J. V. Nossal, and Gaetano Salvatore, 65–74. New York: Academic Press, 1995.

Grace, James T. "Discussion of the Paper." *Annals of the New York Academy of Sciences* 73 (1958), 651.

Grady, Denise. "Going Overboard on Medical Tests." *Time* (25 April 1988), 54–5.

Graham, Richard C., and Morris J. Karnovsky. "The Early Stages of Absorption of Injected Horseradish Peroxidase in the Proximal Tubules of Mouse Kidney: Ultrastructural Cytochemistry by a New Technique." *Journal of Histochemistry and Cytochemistry* 14 (1966), 291–302.

Gralnick, Harvey R., D. A. G. Galton, Daniel Catovsky, Claude Sultan, and John M. Bennet. "Classification of Acute Leukemia (NIH Conference)." *Annals of Internal Medicine* 87 (1977), 740–53.

Gratama, Jan Willem. *Immunological Studies in Allogeneic Marrow Grafting.* PhD thesis, University of Leiden, Netherlands, 1986.

Gratama, Jan Willem, R. L. H. Bolhuis, and M. B. van't Veer. "Quality Control of Flow Cytometric Immunophenotyping of Haematological Malignancies." *Clinical and Laboratory Haematology* 21 (1999), 155–60.

Gray, J. W., and P. N. Dean. "Display and Analysis of Flow Cytometric Data." *Annual Review of Biophysics and Bioengineering* 9 (1980), 509–39.

Graziano, Carl. "FDA Panel Recommends Class II for IHC Reagents." *CAP Today* 8 (December 1994), 1, 45.

Graziano, Carl. "Final Chapter Inked in IHC Saga." *CAP Today* 12 (July 1998), 1, 28, 32.

Greaves, Melvyn F. *Biology of Acute Lymphoblastic Leukaemia.* London: Leukemia Research Fund, 1981.

Greaves, Melvyn F. "Clinical Applications of Cell Surface Markers." *Progress in Hematology* 9 (1975), 255–303.

Greaves, Melvyn F. "The Expression of Immunoglobulin Determinants on the Surface of Antigen-Binding Lymphoid Cells in Mice. I. An Analysis of Light and Heavy Chain Restrictions on Individual Cells." *European Journal of Immunology* 1 (1971), 186–94.

Greaves, Melvyn F. "The Expression of Immunoglobulin Determinants on the Surface of Antigen-Binding Lymphoid Cells in Mice. II. Allotypes of the Ig-1 Locus." *European Journal of Immunology* 1 (1971), 195–201.

Greaves, Melvyn F. "An Immunological Window on Leukemia." *Immunology* Supplement 2 (1989), 56–63.

Greaves, Melvyn F. "Molecular Phenotypes: A New Perspective on Diagnosis and Classification of Leukemias." In *Topics in Paediatrics 1. Haematology and Oncology*, ed. P. H. Morris-Jones, 36–50. Tunbridge Wells, UK: Pitman Medical, 1979.

Greaves, Melvyn F. "Recent Progress in the Immunological Characterization of Leukemic Cells." *Blut: Zeitschrift für die Gesamte Blutforschung* 34 (1977), 349–56.

Greaves, Melvyn F. "Regulation of Cell-Surface Structures in Malignancy, Differentiation and Proliferation." *Biochemical Society Transactions* (1984), 532–3.

Greaves, Melvyn F. "Subtypes of Acute Lymphoblastic Leukemia: Implications for the Pathogenesis and Epidemiology of Leukemia." In *Pathogenesis of Leukemias and Lymphomas: Environmental Influences*, vol. 27, ed. I. T. Magrath, G. T. O'Connor, and B. Ramot, 129–39. New York: Raven Press, 1984.

Greaves, Melvyn F. "'Target' Cells, Cellular Phenotypes, and Lineage Fidelity in Human Leukaemia." *Journal of Cellular Physiology* 1 (Suppl.) (1982), 113–15.

Greaves, Melvyn F., and N. M. Hogg. "Inhibition of Rosette Formation by Antisera to Cell Surface Determinants: An Approach to the Antigen Receptor Problem." *Transplantation Proceedings* 4 (1972), 351–6.

Greaves, Melvyn F., and E. Möller. "Studies on Antigen-Binding Cells. I: The Origin of Reactive Cells." *Cellular Immunology* 1 (1970), 372–85.

Greaves, Melvyn F., G. Brown, and A. Hayward. "A Panel of Markers for Human Lymphocyte Subpopulations: Applications to Disease." In *The Role of Immunological Factors in Infectious, Allergic and Autoimmune Processes (Proceedings of the 8th Miles Immunopathology Symposium)*, ed. Roland F. Beers, Jr. and Edward Basset, 265–80. New York: Raven Press, 1976.

Greaves, Melvyn F., L. C. Chan, A. J. Furley, S. M. Watt, and H. V. Molgaard. "Lineage Promiscuity in Hemopoietic Differentiation and Leukemia." *Blood* 67 (1986), 1–11.

Greaves Melvyn F., Domenico Delia, Fay Katz, Claudio Schneider, Robert Sutherland, and Roland Newman. "Biological Diversity of Acute Lymphoblastic Leukemia." In *Leukemia Research: Advances in Cell Biology and Treatment*, ed. Sharon B. Murphy and John R. Gilbert, 97–116. New York: Elsevier, 1983.

Greaves, Melvyn F., Domenico Delia, Jean Robinson, Robert Sutherland, and Roland Newman. "Exploitation of Monoclonal Antibodies: A 'Who's Who' of Haematopoietic Malignancy." *Blood Cells* 7 (1981), 257–80.

Greaves, Melvyn F., George Janossy, and Micheal Doenhoff. "Selective Triggering of Human T and B Lymphocytes in Vitro by Polyclonal Mitogens." *Journal of Experimental Medicine* 140 (1) (1974), 1–18.

Greaves, Melvyn F., George Janossy, Julien Peto, and Humphrey Kay. "Immunologically Defined Subclasses of Acute Lymphocytic Leukaemia in Children:

Their Relationship to Presentation Features and Prognosis." *British Journal of Haematology* 48 (1981), 179–97.

Greaves, Melvyn F., S. M. Pegram, and L. C. Chan. "Collaborative Group Study of the Epidemiology of Acute Lymphoblastic Leukaemia Subtypes: Background and First Report." *Leukemia Research* 9 (1985), 715–33.

Grey, Howard M., Enrique Rabellino, and Bernard Priofsky. "Immunoglobulins on the Surface of Lymphocytes IV. Distribution in Hypogammaglobulinemia, Cellular Immune Deficiency and Chronic Lymphatic Leukemia." *Journal of Clinical Investigation* 50 (1971), 2368–75.

Grogan, Thomas M., Catherine M. Spier, Lynne C. Richter, and Catherine S. Rangel. "Immunologic Approaches to the Classification of Non-Hodgkin's Lymphomas." In *Immunologic Approaches to the Classification and Management of Lymphomas and Leukemias,* ed. John M. Bennett and Kenneth A. Foon, 31–147. Dordrecht, Netherlands: Kluwer, 1988.

Grohs, Dawn H. "Impact of Automated Technology on the Cervical Cytologic Smear. A Comparison of Cost." *Acta Cytologica* 42 (1998), 165–70.

Gross, U., F. Thomas, C. Matthews, P. Cunningham, and T. Ritter. "In Vivo–in Vitro Correlates of Human Rejection Using Flow Cytometry with Two-Color Fluorescence on Peripheral Blood Mononuclear Cells." *Transplantation Proceedings* 19 (1987), 1609–10.

Gruhier, Fabien. "La machine à explorer le cancer." *Le nouvel observateur* (20 April 1984).

Grunze, Heinz, and Arthur I. Spriggs, *History of Clinical Cytology: A Selection of Documents.* Darmstadt: E. Giebeler, 1980.

Gunz, Frederick W. "The Dread Leukemias and the Lymphomas: Their Nature and Their Prospects." In *Blood, Pure and Eloquent: A Story of Discovery, of People, and of Ideas,* ed. Maxwell M. Wintrobe, 511–46. New York: McGraw-Hill, 1980.

Guralnik, David Bernard, ed. *Webster's New World Dictionary of the American Language,* 2nd college ed. New York: World Pub., 1970.

Guttmann, Ronald D. "The Graft Survival Curve: Ideology and Rhetoric." *Transplantation Proceedings* 24 (1992), 2407–10.

Guttmann, Ronald D., and R. S. Poulsen. "Fluorescence Activated Cell Sorter Analysis of Lymphocyte Subsets after Renal Transplantation." *Transplantation Proceedings* 15 (1983), 1160–2.

Haanen, C. A. M., T. K. A. Eskes, H. F. P. Hillen, and J. M. C. Wessels, eds. *First International Symposium on Pulse-Cytophotometry.* Ghent, Belgium: European Press Medikon, 1975.

Hacking, Ian. *Representing and Intervening: Introductory Topics in the Philosophy of Natural Science.* Cambridge, UK: Cambridge University Press, 1983.

Hacking, Ian. "The Self-Vindication of the Laboratory Sciences." In *Science as Practice and Culture,* ed. Andrew Pickering, 29–64. Chicago: University of Chicago Press, 1992.

Hacking, Ian. *The Social Construction of What?* Cambridge, MA: Harvard University Press, 1999.

Hacking, Ian. "Statistical Language, Statistical Truth and Statistical Reason: The Self-Authentication of a Style of Scientific Reasoning." In *The Social Dimensions of Science,* ed. Ernan McMullin, 130–57. Notre Dame, IN: University of Notre Dame Press, 1992.

Hagenmuller, Jean-Baptiste. "Projet du plateau technique et enjeux de la gestion des ressources humaines." *Technologie et santé* no. 16 (July 1996), 11–25.

Halicka, H. D., K. Seiter, E. J. Feldman, F. Traganos, A. Mittelman, T. Ahmed, and Z. Darzynkiewicz. "Cell Cycle Specificity of Apoptosis during Treatment of Leukemias." *Apoptosis* 2 (1997), 25–39.

Hall, Stephen S. *A Commotion in the Blood: Life, Death and the Immune System.* New York: Henry Holt, 1997.

Hannaway, Caroline, and Ann La Berge, eds. *Constructing Paris Medicine.* Amsterdam and Atlanta: Rodopi, 1998.

Hansen, J. A., and R. A. Good. "Malignant Disease of the Lymphoid System in Immunological Perspective." *Human Pathology* 5 (1974), 567–99.

Harden, Victoria A. *Inventing the NIH: Federal Biomedical Research Policy, 1887–1937.* Baltimore: Johns Hopkins University Press, 1986.

Harlow, F. H., and M. A. Van Dilla. "Flow of Particles through a Coulter Aperture: Hydrodynamic Considerations." In Los Alamos Scientific Laboratory of the University of California, *Biological and Medical Research Groups (H-4) of the Health Division. Annual Report July 1964 through June 1965.* LA-3432-MS, Los Alamos, NM, 1965, 107–13.

Harris, Nancy Lee. "Lymphoma 1987: An Interim Approach to Diagnosis and Classification." *Pathology Annual* 22 (1987), 1–68.

Harris, Nancy Lee. "A Practical Approach to the Pathology of Lymphoid Neoplasms: A Revised European-American Classification from the International Lymphoma Study Group." *Important Advances in Oncology* (1995), 111–40.

Harris, Nancy Lee, Elaine S. Jaffe, Jacques Diebold, Georges Flandrin, H. Konrad Muller-Hermelink, James Vardiman, T. Andrew Lister, and Clara D. Bloomfield. "The World Health Organization Classification of Neoplastic Diseases of the Hematopoietic and Lymphoid Tissues. Report of the Clinical Advisory Committee Meeting, Airlie House, Virginia, November, 1997." *Annals of Oncology* 10 (1999), 1419–32.

Harris, Nancy Lee, Elaine S. Jaffe, Jacques Diebold, Georges Flandrin, H. Konrad Muller-Hermelink, James Vardiman, T. Andrew Lister, and Clara D.

Bloomfield. "World Health Organization Classification of Neoplastic Diseases of the Hematopoietic and Lymphoid Tissues: Report of the Clinical Advisory Committee Meeting—Airlie House, Virginia, November 1997." *Journal of Clinical Oncology* 17 (1999), 3835–49.

Harris, Nancy Lee, Elaine S. Jaffe, Jacques Diebold, Georges Flandrin, H. Konrad Muller-Hermelink, James Vardiman, T. Andrew Lister, and Clara D. Bloomfield. "The World Health Organization Classification of Hematological Malignancies. Report of the Clinical Advisory Committee Meeting, Airlie House, Virginia, November 1997." *Modern Pathology* 13 (2000), 193–207.

Harris, Nancy Lee, Elaine S. Jaffe, Jacques Diebold, Georges Flandrin, H. Konrad Muller-Hermelink, James Vardiman, T. Andrew Lister, and Clara D. Bloomfield. "The World Health Organization Classification of Neoplastic Diseases of the Haematopoietic and Lymphoid Tissues: Report of the Clinical Advisory Committee Meeting, Airlie House, Virginia, November 1997." *Histopathology* 36 (2000), 69–86.

Harris, Nancy Lee, Elaine S. Jaffe, and Harald Stein. "Response [letter]." *Blood* 85 (1995), 857–60.

Harris, Nancy Lee, Elaine S. Jaffe, Harald Stein, Peter M. Banks, John K. C. Chan, Michael L. Cleary, Georges Delsol, Christine De Wolf-Peeters, Brunangelo Falini, Kevin C. Gatter, Thomas M. Grogan, Peter G. Isaacson, Daniel M. Knowles, David Y. Mason, Hans-Konrad Muller-Hermelink, Stefano A. Pileri, Miguel A. Piris, Elisabeth Ralfkiaer, and Roger A. Warnke. "A Revised European-American Classification of Lymphoid Neoplasms: A Proposal from the International Lymphoma Study Group." *Blood* 84 (1994), 1361–92.

Harris, R. "Leukemia Antigens and Immunity in Man." *Nature* 241 (1973), 95–100.

Hartigan, John A. *Clustering Algorithms.* New York: John Wiley & Sons, 1975.

Hatchuel, Armand. "Les axiomatiques de la production: éléments pour comprendre les mutations industrielles." In *La performance économique en entreprise,* ed. Jacques-Henri Jacot and Jean-Pierre Micaelli, 35–53. Paris: Hermes, 1996.

Hatchuel, Armand, and Benoît Weil. *Experts in Organizations: A Knowledge-Based Perspective on Organizational Change.* Berlin and New York: Walter de Gruyter, 1995.

Hayes, J. M., R. Valenzuela, A. C. Nowick, D. R. Steinmuller, and G. Williams. "Correlation between Two-Color Flow Cytometry Quantitation of Activated T-Cells and Acute Allograft Rejection." *Transplantation Proceedings* 19 (1987), 1605–8.

Haynes, John L. "Principles of Flow Cytometry." *Cytometry* Supplement 3 (1988), 7–17.

Head, David R., L. Cerezo, R. A. Savage, C. M. Craven, J. N. Bickers, R. Hartsack, T. A. Hosty, J. H. Saiki, H. E. Wilson, and F. S. Morrison.

"Reproducibility of the FAB Classification of Acute Leukemia: The Southwest Oncology Group Experience." *American Journal of Hematology* 18 (1985), 47–57.

Hedley David W. "Flow Cytometry Using Paraffin-Embedded Tissue: Five Years On." *Cytometry* 10 (1989), 229–41.

Hedley, David W., Michael L. Friedlander, Ian W. Taylor, Catherine A. Rugg, and Elizabeth A. Musgrove. "DNA Flow Cytometry of Paraffin-Embedded Tissue." *Cytometry* 5 (1984), 660.

Hedley, David W., Michael L. Friedlander, Ian W. Taylor, Catherine A. Rugg, and Elizabeth A. Musgrove. "Method for Analysis of Cellular DNA Content of Paraffin-Embedded Pathological Material Using Flow Cytometry." *Journal of Histochemistry and Cytochemistry* 31 (1983), 1333–5.

Heinig, Stephen J., Andrew S. W. Quon, Roger E. Meyer, and David Korn. "The Changing Landscape for Clinical Research." *Academic Medicine* 74 (1999), 726–45.

Heitzmann, H., and Frederick M. Richards. "Use of the Avidin-Biotin Complex for Specific Staining of Biological Membranes in Electron Microscopy." *Proceedings of the National Academy of Sciences U.S.A.* 71 (1974), 3537–41.

Hensleigh, Paul A., Virginia Bryan Waters, and Leonard A. Herzenberg. "Human T Lymphocyte Differentiation Antigens: Effects of Blood Sample Storage on Leu Antibody Binding." *Cytometry* 31 (1983), 453–5.

Herman, Chester J., and Bill Bunnag. "Goals of the Cytology Automation Program of the National Cancer Institute." *Journal of Histochemistry and Cytochemistry* 24 (1976), 2–5.

Herzenberg, Leonore A., Stephen C. De Rosa, and Leonard A. Herzenberg. "Monoclonal Antibodies and the FACS: Complementary Tools for Immunobiology and Medicine." *Immunology Today* 21 (2000), 383–90.

Herzenberg, Leonard A., Richard G. Sweet, and Leonore A. Herzenberg. "Fluorescence-Activated Cell Sorting." *Scientific American* 234 (March 1976), 108–17.

Hewlitt, Richard G., and Francis Duncan. *A History of the United States Atomic Energy Commission.* Vol. 2, *Atomic Shield, 1947–1952.* University Park: Pennsylvania State University Press, 1969.

Hiddemann, Wolgang, Dan L. Longo, Bertrand Coiffier, Richard I. Fisher, Fernando Cabanillas, Franco Cavalli, Lee M. Nadler, Vincent T. De Vita, T. Andrew Lister, and James O. Armitage. "Lymphoma Classification—The Gap between Biology and Clinical Management Is Closing." *Blood* 88 (1996), 4085–9.

Hill, Rolla B., and Fairfield Goodale. "The Delphi Predictions of Pathology Chairmen: A Six-Year Retrospective View." *Journal of Medical Education* 56 (1981), 537–46.

Hillen, Harry Frans Peter, J. M. C. Wessels, and Clemens Antonius Maria Haanen. *Cell Proliferation Patterns in Acute Leukemia Monitored by Pulse-Cytophotometry*. Ghent, Belgium: European Press Medikon, 1975.

Homburger, Henry A., Wendy Rosenstock, Helene Paxton, Mary L. Paton, and Alan L. Landay. "Assessment of Interlaboratory Variability of Immunophenotyping: Results of the College of American Pathologists Flow Cytometry Survey." *Annals of the New York Academy of Sciences* 667 (1993), 43–9.

Houthoff, H. J., S. Poppema, E. J. Ebels, and J. D. Elema. "Intracranial Malignant Lymphomas. A Morphologic and Immunocytologic Study of Twenty Cases." *Acta Neuropathologica (Berlin)* 44 (1978), 203–10.

"How to Ensure Quality [editorial]." *Lancet* (24 July 1982), 196.

Howell, Joel D. *Technology in the Hospital. Transforming Patient Care in the Early Twentieth Century*. Baltimore: Johns Hopkins University Press, 1995.

Hubbard S. M., B. A. Chabner, V. T. DeVita Jr., R. Simon, C. W. Berard, R. B. Jones, A. J. Garvin, G. P. Canellos, C. K. Osborne, and R. C. Young. "Histologic Progression in Non-Hodgkin's Lymphoma." *Blood* 59 (1982), 258–64.

Hughes, Jonathan. "The 'Matchbox on a Muffin': The Design of Hospitals in the Early NHS." *Medical History* 44 (2000), 21–56.

Hulett, Henry R., William A. Bonner, Richard G. Sweet, and Leonard A. Herzenberg. "Development and Application of a Rapid Cell Sorter." *Clinical Chemistry* 19 (1973), 813–16.

Humphrey, J. H. "The Growth of Immunology." *The Biologist* 27 (1980), 13–17.

Hunter, Kathryn Montgomery. *Doctor's Stories. The Narrative Structure of Medical Knowledge*. Princeton, NJ: Princeton University Press, 1991.

Hutt, Peter Barton. "A History of Government Regulation of Adulteration and Misbranding of Medical Devices." *Food Drug Cosmetic Law Journal* 44 (1989), 99–117.

"Identification, Enumeration, and Isolation of B and T Lymphocytes from Human Peripheral Blood. Special Technical Report." *Scandinavian Journal of Immunology* 3 (1974), 521–32.

International Academy of Cytology. "Specifications for Automated Cytodiagnostic Systems Proposed by the International Academy of Cytology." *Analytical and Quantitative Cytology* 6 (1984), 146.

International Non-Hodgkin's Lymphoma Prognostic Factors Project. "A Predictive Model for Aggressive Non-Hodgkin's Lymphoma." *New England Journal of Medicine* 329 (September 1993), 987–94.

"Introduction." In Los Alamos Scientific Laboratory of the University of California, *Biological and Medical Research Groups (H-4) of the Health Division. Semi-*

annual Report. January through June. LAMS-2627, Los Alamos, NM, 1961, 9–14.

Jacobs, P. "Lymphoma—Histopathology in Changing Clinical Perspective. Non-Hodgkin's Lymphoma Classification Project." *South African Medical Journal* 90 (2000), 135–41.

Jacoby, Itzhak. "Consensus Development at NIH: What Went Wrong?" *Risk. Issues in Health and Safety* 4 (1993), 133–42.

Jaffe, Elaine S. "Predictability of Immunologic Phenotype by Morphologic Criteria in Diffuse Aggressive Non-Hodgkin's Lymphomas." *American Journal of Clinical Pathology* 77 (1982), 46–9.

James, Paul, and Tony Noakes. *Hospital Architecture.* Essex, UK: Longman, 1994.

Jamous, Haroun. *Sociologie de la décision. La réforme des études médicales et des structures hospitalières.* Paris: Éditions du Centre National de la Recherche Scientifique, 1969.

Jamous, Haroun, and B. Peloille. "Professions or Self-Perpetuating Systems? Changes in the French University-Hospital System." In *Professions and Professionalization,* ed. J. A. Jackson, 109–52. Cambridge, UK: Cambridge University Press, 1970.

Janossy, George. *Polyclonal Activation of Murine and Human T and B Lymphocytes.* PhD thesis, University of London, 1974.

Janossy, George, and Melvyn F. Greaves. "Lymphocyte Activation 1: Response of T and B Lymphocytes to Phytomitogens." *Clinical and Experimental Immunology* 9 (1971), 483–98.

Janossy, George, I. Jani, and W. Göhde. "Affordable CD4 (+) T-Cell Counts on 'Single Platform' Flow Cytometers I. Primary CD4 Gating." *British Journal of Haematology* 111 (2000), 1198–208.

Janossy, George, M. M. Roberts, D. Capellaro, Melvyn F. Greaves, and G. E. Francis. "Use of the Fluorescence Activated Cell Sorter in Human Leukaemia." In *Immunofluorescence and Related Staining Techniques,* ed. W. Knapp, K. Holubar, and G. Wick, 111–22. Elsevier/North-Holland, 1978.

Janossy, George, Roger K. Woodruff, Ann Paxton, Melvyn F. Greaves, David Capellaro, Barbara Kirk, Elizabeth M. Innes, O. B. Eden, Daniel Catovsky, and A. Victor Hoffbrand. "Membrane Marker and Cell Separation Studies in Ph^1-positive Leukemia." *Blood* 51 (1978), 861–77.

Joly, Robert. *Hippocrate médecin grec.* Paris: Gallimard, 1964.

Jouanna, Jacques. *Hippocrate.* Paris: Fayard, 1992.

Julius, Michael H., T. Masuda, and L. A. Herzenberg. "Demonstration That Antigen-Binding Cells Are Precursors of Antibody-Producing Cells after Purification with a Fluorescence-Activated Cell Sorter." *Proceedings of the National Academy of Sciences U.S.A.* 69 (1972), 1934–8.

Julius, Michael H., Elizabeth Simpson, and Leonard A. Herzenberg. "A Rapid Method for the Isolation of Functional Thymus-Derived Murine Lymphocytes." *European Journal of Immunology* 3 (1973), 645–9.

Julius Michael H., Richard G. Sweet, C. Garrison Fathman, and Leonard A. Herzenberg. "Fluorescence-Activated Cell Sorting and Its Applications." In *Mammalian Cells: Probes and Problems. Proceedings of the First Los Alamos Life Sciences Symposium Held at Los Alamos, New Mexico, October 17–19, 1973,* ed. C. R. Richmond, Donald F. Petersen, Paul F. Mullaney, and E. C. Anderson, 107–24. Oak Ridge, TN: Technical Information Center, Office of Public Affairs, U.S. Energy Research and Development Administration, 1975.

Kadens, Darien. *Sales of in Vitro Diagnostic Products to 2004.* Study no. 08. Waltham, MA: Decision Resources, 2000.

Kagan, Jonathan M., and Brian H. Mayall. "Introduction to the NIAID Guideline for Flow Cytometric Immunophenotyping." *Cytometry* 14 (1993), 701–11.

Kahan, Jonathan S. "The Evolution of FDA Regulation of New Medical Device Technology and Product Applications." *Food Drug Cosmetic Law Journal* 41 (1989), 207–14.

Kajita, Akira. "Rudolf Virchow and His Successors." In *History of Pathology,* ed. Teizo Ogawa, 163–84. Osaka, Japan: Taniguchi Foundation, 1983.

Kam, Kai Man, Wai Lin Leung, Mei Yee Kwok, Mi Yim Hung, Shui Shan Lee, and Wai Ping Mak. "Lymphocyte Subpopulation Reference Ranges for Monitoring Human Immunodeficiency Virus–Infected Chinese Adults." *Clinical and Diagnostic Laboratory Immunology* 3 (1993), 326–30.

Kamentsky, Louis A. "Photoelectric Particle Separator Using Time Delay," U.S. Patent no. 3, 560, 754 (1971).

Kamentsky, Louis A., and Myron R. Melamed, "Instrumentation for Automated Examinations of Cellular Specimens." *Proceedings of the Institute of Electrical and Electronic Engineers,* special issue on technology and health services, 57 (November 1969), 2007–16.

Kamentsky, Louis A., and Myron R. Melamed. "Spectrophotometric Cell Sorter," *Science* 156 (1967), 1364–5.

Kamentsky, Louis A., Herbert Derman, and Myron R. Melamed. "Ultraviolet Absorption in Epidermoid Cancer Cells." *Science* 142 (1964), 1580–3.

Kamentsky, Louis A., Myron R. Melamed, and Herbert Derman. "Spectrophotometer: New Instrument for Ultrarapid Cell Analysis." *Science* 150 (1965), 630–1.

Kaplan, Henry S. "Introduction." *British Journal of Cancer* 31 (Suppl. 2) (1975), vii–viii.

Kaufert, Patricia A. "Screening the Body: The Pap Smear and the Mammogram." In *Living and Working with the New Medical Technologies. Intersections of Inquiry,* ed.

Margaret Lock, Allan Young, and Alberto Cambrosio, 165–83. Cambridge, UK: Cambridge University Press, 2000.

Keating, Peter, and Alberto Cambrosio. "From Screening to Clinical Research: The Cure of Leukemia and the Early Development of the Cooperative Oncology Groups: 1955–1966." *Bulletin of the History of Medicine* 76 (2002), 299–334.

Keating, Peter, and Alberto Cambrosio. "Interlaboratory Life: Regulating Flow Cytometry." In *The Invisible Industrialist: Manufacturers and the Construction of Scientific Knowledge,* ed. Jean-Paul Gaudillière and Ilana Löwy, 250–95. London: Macmillan, 1997.

Keating, Peter, Camille Limoges, and Alberto Cambrosio. "The Automated Laboratory: The Generation and Replication of Work in Molecular Genetics." In *The Practices of Human Genetics,* ed. Michael Fortun and Everett Mendelsohn, 125–42. Dordrecht, Netherlands: Kluwer, 1999.

Keel, Othmar. "La pathologie tissulaire de John Hunter." *Gesnerus* 37 (1980), 47–61.

Keel, Othmar. *La généalogie de l'histopathologie, une révision déchirante: Philippe Pinel, lecteur discret de J.-C. Smyth (1741–1821)* Paris: Vrin, 1979.

Keene, Nancy. *Childhood Leukemia: A Guide for Families, Friends and Caregivers.* Sebastopol, CA: O'Reilly and Associates, 1997.

Kenney, Martin. *Biotechnology: the University-Industry Complex.* New Haven, CT: Yale University Press, 1986.

Kerleau, Monique. "L'hétérogénéité des pratiques médicales, enjeu des politiques de maîtrise des dépenses de santé." *Sciences Sociales et Santé* 16 (4) (1998), 5–32.

Kerman, R. H., C. T. Van Buren, and W. Payne. "Monitoring of T-Cell Subsets in Renal Allograft Recipients." *Transplantation Proceedings* 15 (1983), 1170–2.

Kersey, J. H., and T. W. LeBien. "What Happened to Lineage- and Leukemia-Specific Antigens? Implications for the Therapeutic Use of Monoclonal Antibodies." In *Leucocyte Typing,* ed. A. Bernard, L. Boumsell, J. Dausset, C. Milstein, and F. Schlossmann, 651–6. New York: Springer-Verlag, 1984.

Kidd, Pamela G., and Robert F. Vogt, Jr. "Report of the Workshop on the Evaluation of T-Cell Subsets during HIV Infection and AIDS." *Clinical Immunology and Immunopathology* 52 (1989), 3–9.

Kingham, Richard F. "History of FDA Regulation of Clinical Research." *Drug Information Journal* 22 (1988), 151–5.

Kisielow, P., J. A. Hirst, H. Shiku, P. C. L. Beverley, M. K. Hoffman, E. A. Boyse, and H. F. Oettgen. "Ly Antigens as Markers for Functionally Distinct Subpopulations of Thymus-Derived Lymphocytes of the Mouse." *Nature* 253 (1975), 219–20.

Klein, Eva, Trond Eskeland, Masaharu Inque, Roberto Strom, and Bo Johansson. "Surface Immunoglobulin-Moieties on Lymphoid Cells." *Experimental Cell Research* 62 (1970), 133–48.

Klein, Herbert Arthur. *The Science of Measurement. A Historical Survey.* New York: Dover, 1988 [1974].

Klein, J. B. "Immune Monitoring in the Monoclonal Era." *Clinical Transplantation* 2 (1988), 177–9.

Klein, Jan. "Seeds of Time: Fifty Years Ago Peter A. Gorer Discovered the H-2 Complex." *Immunogenetics* 24 (1986), 331–8.

Kling, James. "Flow Cytometry: It's Not Just for Immunologists Anymore." *The Scientist* 11 (June 1997), 14.

Kluin-Nelemans, J. C., E. R. van Wering, M. B. van't Veer, C. E. van der Schoot, H. J. Adriaansen, F. J. van der Burgh, and J. W. Gratama. "Pitfalls in the Immunophenotyping of Leukaemia and Leukaemic Lymphomas: Survey of 9 Years of Quality Control in the Netherlands. Dutch Cooperative Study Group on Immunophenotyping of Haematological Malignancies (SIHON)." *British Journal of Haematology* 95 (1996), 692–9.

Knapp, W., P. Rieber, B. Dörken, R. E. Schmidt, H. Stein, and A. E. vondem Borne. "Towards a Better Definition of Human Leucocyte Surface Molecules." *Immunology Today* 10 (1989), 253–8.

Knorr-Cetina, Karin. *Epistemic Cultures. How the Sciences Make Knowledge.* Cambridge, MA: Harvard University Press, 1999.

Koepke, John A. "The College of American Pathologists Survey Programme." In *Automation and Quality Assurance in Haematology*, ed. R. M. Rowan and John M. England 62–83. Oxford: Blackwell, 1986.

Koepke, John A. "Survey of Quality Assurance/Quality Control Practices for CD4+ Lymophocyte Counting." *Cytometry* 26 (1996), 178–80.

Koeppen, Harmut, and James W. Vardiman. "New Entities, Issues and Controversies in the Classification of Malignant Lymphoma." *Seminars in Oncology* 25 (1998), 421–34.

Kohen, Elli. "In Memoriam: Bo Thorell, a Pioneer of Blood Cell Microspectrofluorometry. A Forerunner of Living Cell Biochemistry and Pathology." *Nouvelle Revue Française d'Hématologie* 26 (1984), 53–5.

Kohler, Robert E. "The Enzyme Theory and the Origins of Biochemistry." *Isis* 64 (1973), 181–96.

Kohler, Robert E. *From Medical Chemistry to Biochemistry. The Making of a Biomedical Discipline.* Cambridge, UK: Cambridge University Press, 1982.

Koo, Gloria C., Christopher W. Stackpole, Edward A. Boyse, Ulrich Hämmerling, and Michael P. Lardis. "Topographical Location of H-Y Antigen on Mouse Spermatozoa by Immunoelectronmicroscopy." *Proceedings of the National Academy of Sciences U.S.A* 70 (1973), 1502–5.

Koss, Leopold G. "Analytical and Quantitative Cytology: A Historical Perspective." *Analytical and Quantitative Cytology* 4 (1982), 251–6.

Koss, Leopold G. "The Papanicolaou Test for Cervical Cancer Detection: A Triumph and a Tragedy." *JAMA* 261 (3 February 1989), 737–43.

Kosugi, Yukio, Ryuichi Sato, Shigeru Genka, Nobuyuki Shitara, and Kintomo Takakura. "An Interactive Multivariate Analysis of FCM Data." *Cytometry* 9 (1988), 405–8.

Kroker, Kenton. *From Reflex to Rhythm: Sleep, Dreaming, and the Discovery of Rapid Eye Movement, 1870–1960.* PhD thesis, University of Toronto, 2000.

Krömer, Elisabeth, and Friedrich Grossmüller. "Light Scatter Based Lymphocyte Gate. Helpful Tool or Source of Error?." *Cytometry* 15 (1994), 87–9.

Krumm, Rebecca. "Flow Cytometry Expanding in Clinical and Research Labs." *The Scientist* 8 (1994), 17–8.

Kubitschek, H. E. "Apertures for Coulter Counters." *Review of Scientific Instruments* 35 (1964), 1598–9.

Kuhn, Thomas S. "Second Thoughts on Paradigms." In *The Essential Tension*, Thomas S. Kuhn, 293–319. Chicago: University of Chicago Press, 1977.

Kung, Patrick C., Gideon Goldstein, Ellis L. Reinherz, and Stuart F. Schlossman. "Monoclonal Antibodies Defining Distinctive Human T Cell Surface Antigens." *Science* 206 (1979), 347–9.

Kung, Patrick C., John C. Long, Ronald P. McCaffrey, Robert L. Ratliff, Thomas A. Harrison, and David Baltimore. "Terminal Deoxynucleotidyl Transferase in the Diagnosis of Leukemia and Malignant Lymphoma." *American Journal of Medicine* 64 (1978), 788–94.

Kunkel, H. G. "Surface Markers of Human Lymphocytes." *Johns Hopkins Medical Journal* 137 (1975) 216–23.

Laedlein-Greilsammer, Denis. "Place de l'Anatomo-Cyto-Pathologie dans le plateau technique hospitalier." *Technologie et santé* no. 26 (July 1996), 48–50.

Laerum, Ole D., and Tore Farsund. "Clinical Applications of Flow Cytometry: A Review." *Cytometry* 2 (1981), 1–13.

Laerum, Ole D., Tore Lindmo, and E. Thorud. *Flow Cytometry IV: Proceedings of the IVth International Symposium on Flow Cytometry (Pulse Cytophotometry)—Voss, June 4–8, 1979.* Bergen, Norway: Universitetsforlaget, 1980.

Lagaay, A. M., C. B. Bosman, M. Van den Keur, G. J. Lightart, H. R. E. Schuit, H. J. Tanke, and W. Hijmans. "Gating of the So-Called 'Lymphocytic' Cell Population for the Quantification of Natural Killer Cells (CD16+) by Flow Cytometry Causes Loss of CD16 Positive Cells." *Journal of Immunological Methods* 133 (1990), 235–44.

Lajtha, L. G. *Stem Cells: Properties and Malfunctions.* London: Leukemia Research Fund, 1982.

Lakhani, Sunil R., and Alan Ashworth. "Microarray and Histopathological Analysis of Tumors: The Future and the Past?" *Nature Reviews Cancer* 1 (2001), 151–7.

Landay, Alan L., Kenneth A. Ault, Kenneth D. Bauer, and Peter S. Rabinovitch, eds. *Clinical Flow Cytometry. Annals of the New York Academy of Sciences,* 677. New York: New York Academy of Sciences, 1993.

Laszlo, John. *The Cure of Childhood Leukemia: Into the Age of Miracles.* New Brunswick, NJ: Rutgers University Press, 1995.

Latour, Bruno. "Give Me a Laboratory and I Will Raise the World." In *Science Observed,* ed. Karin D. Knorr-Cetina and Michael Mulkay, 141–70. Beverly Hills, CA: Sage, 1983.

Latour, Bruno. "The 'Pédofil' of Boa Vista: A Photo-Philosophical Montage." *Common Knowledge* 4 (1995), 142–87.

Latour, Bruno. *Science in Action. How to Follow Scientists and Engineers through Society.* Cambridge, MA: Harvard University Press, 1987.

Lawrence, Christopher. "Clinical Research." In *Science in the Twentieth Century,* ed. John Krige and Dominique Pestre, 439–59. Amsterdam: Harwood Academic, 1997.

Lay, Wlatraut H, Nalson F. Mendes, Celso Bianco, and Victor Nussenzweig. "Binding of Sheep Red Blood Cells to a Large Population of Human Lymphocytes." *Nature* 230 (1971), 531–2.

Ledbetter, Jeffrey A., James W. Goding, Tokuhisa Takeshi, and Leonard A. Herzenberg. "Murine T Cell Differentiation Antigens Detected by Monoclonal Antibodies." In *Monoclonal Antibodies: Hybridomas, a New Dimension in Biological Analyses,* ed. Roger H. Kennett, Thomas Joseph McKearn, and Kathleen B. Bechtol, 235–49. New York: Plenum Press, 1980.

Leif, S. B., R. C. Leif, and R. Auer. "The EPICS C Analyzer: An Ergonomically Designed Flow Cytometer Computer System." *Analytical and Quantitative Cytology and Histology* 7 (1985), 187–91.

Lennert, Karl. "Classification of Malignant Lymphomas (European Concept)." In *Progress in Lymphology. Proceedings of the International Symposium on Lymphology, Zurich, Switzerland, July 19–23, 1966,* ed. Alois Rüttimann, 103–09. Stuttgart: Georg Thieme Verlag, 1967.

Lennert, Karl. "Commentary on Working Formulation of Non-Hodgkin's Lymphomas." *Cancer* 49 (May 1982), 2133.

Lennert, Karl. "Preface." In *Electron Microscopic Atlas of Lymph Node Cytology and Pathology*, ed. Yoshitaka Mori and Karl Lennert, i–ii. Berlin: Springer-Verlag, 1969.

Lennert, Karl, and H. Stein. "Personal Points of View on the Kiel Classification." In *Lymphoid Neoplasias I: Classification, Categorization and Natural History*, ed. Georges Mathé, Maxime Seligmann, and Maurice Tubiana, 31–7. Berlin: Springer-Verlag, 1978.

Lennert, Karl, H. Stein, and E. Kaiserling. "Cytological and Functional Criteria for the Classification of Malignant Lymphomata." *British Journal of Cancer* (Proceedings of the First International Symposium on the Non-Hodgkin's Lymphomata; London, 1973) 31 (Suppl. 2) (1975), 29–43.

Lenoir, Timothy. "Science for the Clinic: Science Policy and the Formation of Carl Ludwig's Institute in Leipzig." In *The Investigative Enterprise: Experimental Physiology in Nineteenth-Century Medicine*, ed. William Coleman and Frederic L. Holmes, 139–78. Berkeley: University of California Press, 1988.

Lenoir, Timothy, and Marguerite Hays. "The Manhattan Project for Biomedicine." In *Controlling Our Destinies. Historical, Philosophical, Ethical, and Theological Perspectives on the Human Genome Project*, ed. Philip R. Sloan, 29–62. South Bend, IN: University of Notre Dame Press, 2000.

Lesec, Guy. "Exercice en anatomocytopathologie dans le cadre de la loi sur la biologie de 1975. Paris, 28 octobre 1994." *Bulletin d'information et de liason du syndicat des médecins anatomo-cyto-pathologistes Français* no. 43 (1995), 10–12.

Levinthal, Elliott, L. Hundley, and Joshua Lederberg. "Multivator. A Biochemical Laboratory for Martian Experiments." In *Life Sciences and Space Research II*, ed. Marcel Florkin and A. Dollfus, 112–23. Amsterdam: North-Holland, 1964.

Lewis, S. Mitchell. "External Quality Assessment in Europe." In *Automation and Quality Assurance in Haematology*, ed. R. M. Rowan and John M. England, 18–61. Oxford: Blackwell, 1986.

Lewis, S. Mitchell. "Standardization and Harmonization of the Blood Count: The Role of International Committee for Standardization in Haematology (ICSH)." *European Journal of Haematology Supplement* 45 (Suppl. 53) (1990), 9–13.

Lewis, S. Mitchell, and B. J. Burgess. "Quality Control in Haematology: Report of Interlaboratory Trials in Britain." *British Medical Journal* 4 (1969), 253–6.

Linder, James. "Automation in Cytopathology." *American Journal of Clinical Pathology* 98 (Suppl. 1) (1992), S47–S51.

Lippman, S. M., T. P. Miller, C. M. Spier, D. J. Slymen, and T. M. Grogan. "The Prognostic Significance of the Immunotype in Diffuse Large-Cell Lymphoma. A Comparative Study of the T-Cell and B-Cell Phenotype." *Blood* 72 (1988), 436–41.

Loken, Michael R., and Leonard A. Herzenberg. "Analysis of Cell Populations with a Fluorescence-Activated Cell Sorter." *Annals of the New York Academy of Sciences* 254 (1975), 163–71.

Loken, Michael R., Jeanne M. Brosnan, Kenneth A. Ault, and Bruce Allen Bach. *Establishing Optimal Lymphocyte Gates for Immunophenotyping Using LeucoGATE*, Monograph no. 2. San José, CA: Becton Dickinson Immunocytometry Systems, n.d., c. 1990.

Loken, Michael R., H. Meiners, and M. L. Terstappen. "Comparison of Sample Preparation Techniques for Flow Cytometric Analysis of Immunofluorescence." *Cytometry* Supplement 2 (1988), 53.

Lopez, Manuel, Thomas Fleisher, and Richard deShazo. "Use and Interpretation of Diagnostic Immunologic Laboratory Tests." *Primer on Allergic and Immunologic Diseases*, 3rd ed. *JAMA* 268, 20 (1992), 2970–90.

Los Alamos Scientific Laboratory, *Annual Report of the Biomedical and Environmental Research Program of the LASL Health Division. January through December 1973.* LA-5633-PR. Los Alamos, NM, 1974.

Los Alamos Scientific Laboratory. *Biological and Medical Research Group (H-4) of the Health Division—Semiannual Report July through December 1959.* LAMS-2445. Los Alamos, NM, 1960.

Los Alamos Scientific Laboratory. *Health Division Annual Report 1949.* LA-1072. Los Alamos, NM, 1950.

Löwy, Ilana. *Between Bench and Bedside. Science, Healing, and Interleukin-2 in a Cancer Ward.* Cambridge, MA: Harvard University Press, 1996.

Löwy, Ilana. "The Impact of Medical Practice on Biomedical Research: The Case of Human Leucocyte Antigens Studies." *Minerva* 25 (1987), 171–200.

Löwy, Ilana. "Tissue Groups and Cadaver Kidney Sharing: Socio-cultural Aspects of a Medical Controversy." *International Journal of Technology Assessment in Health Care* 2 (1986), 195–218.

Löwy, Ilana. "Trustworthy Knowledge and Desperate Patients: Clinical Tests for New Drugs from Cancer to AIDS." In *Living and Working with the New Medical Technologies. Intersections of Inquiry*, ed. Margaret Lock, Allan Young, and Alberto Cambrosio, 49–81. Cambridge, UK: Cambridge University Press, 2000.

Löwy, Ilana. "Variances in Meaning of Discovery Accounts: The Case of Contemporary Biology." *Historical Studies in the Physical and Biological Sciences* 21 (1990), 87–121.

Löwy, Ilana, and Jean-Paul Gaudillière. "Disciplining Cancer: Mice and the Practice of Genetic Purity." In *The Invisible Industrialist: Manufactures and the*

Production of Scientific Knowledge, ed. Jean-Paul Gaudillière and Ilana Löwy, 209–49. London: Macmillan, 1998.

Lucio, A. Parreira, M. W. van den Beemd, E. G. van Lochem, E. R. van Wering, E. Baars, A. Porwit-MacDonald, E. Bjorklund, G. Gaipa, A. Biondi, A. Orfao, G. Janossy, J. J. M. van Dongen, and J. F. San Miguel. "Flow Cytometric Analysis of Normal B Cell Differentiation: A Frame of Reference for the Detection of Minimal Residual Disease in Precursor-B-ALL." *Leukemia* 13 (1999), 419–27.

Lukes, Robert. "Commentary on Working Formulation of Non-Hodgkin's Lymphomas." *Cancer* 49 (May 1982), 2133.

Lukes, Robert J. "A Review of the American Concept of Malignant Lymphoma." In *Progress in Lymphology. Proceedings of the International Symposium on Lymphology, Zurich, Switzerland, July 19–23, 1966*, ed. Alois Rüttimann, 109–19. Stuttgart: Georg Thieme Verlag, 1967.

Lukes, Robert J., and Robert D. Collins. "Approaches to the Classification of the Lymphomata." *British Journal of Cancer* 3 (Suppl. 2) (1975), 1–28.

Lukes, Robert J., and Robert D. Collins, "Immunologic Characterization of Human Malignant Lymphomas." *Cancer* 34 (1974), 1488–1503.

Lushbaugh, C. C. "A Rejoinder." *Blood* 23 (1964), 404–5.

Lushbaugh, C. C., and D. B. Hale. "Clinical Applications of Whole Body Scintillometry. III. Whole Body Retention of Iodine^{131} as a Method of Studying Thyroid Function in Man." In Los Alamos Scientific Laboratory, Biological and Medical Research Group (H-4) of the Health Division. *Semiannual Report*, July through December, 1959, 361–75.

Lushbaugh, C. C., and D. B. Hale. "Iodine^{131} Retention in Normal and Starved Rats." In Los Alamos Scientific Laboratory, Biological and Medical Research Group (H-4) of the Health Division. *Semiannual Report*, July through December, 1959, 375–83.

Lushbaugh, C. C., N. J. Basmann, and H. Israel. "Electronically Determined Erythrocyte Volumes. III. Further Observations on the Skewed Population Profile." In University of California, Los Alamos Scientific Laboratory, Biological and Medical Research Group (H-4) of the Health Division. *Annual Report*, November 1962, 198–202.

Lushbaugh, C. C., J. A. Maddy, and N. J. Bamann. "Electronic Measurement of Cellular Volumes I. Calibration of the Apparatus." *Blood* 20 (1962), 233–9.

Lushbaugh, C. C., J. A. Maddy, and N. J. Bamann. "Electronic Measurement of Cellular Volumes II. Frequency Distribution of Erythrocyte Volumes." *Blood* 20 (1962), 241–8.

Lutz, Dieter, ed. *Pulse-Cytophotometry. 3rd International Symposium on Pulse-Cytophotometry—Vienna, Austria 1978*. Ghent, Belgium: European Press, 1978.

Lynch, Michael. *Art and Artefact in Laboratory Science. A Study of Shop Work and Shop Talk in a Research Laboratory*. London: Routledge and Kegan Paul, 1985.

Lynch, Michael. "The Discursive Production of Uncertainty. The OJ Simpson 'Dream Team' and the Sociology of Knowledge Machine." *Social Studies of Science* 28 (1998), 829–68.

Lynch, Michael. "The Externalized Retina: Selection and Mathematization in the Visual Documentation of Objects in the Life Sciences." In *Representation in Scientific Practice*, ed. Michael Lynch and Steve Woolgar, 153–86. Cambridge, MA: MIT Press, 1990.

Lynch, Michael. *Scientific Practice and Ordinary Action Ethnomethodology and Social Studies of Science*. Cambridge, UK: Cambridge University Press, 1993.

Lynch, Michael. "Technical Work and Critical Inquiry: Investigations in a Scientific Laboratory." *Social Studies of Science* 12 (1982), 499–533.

Mackenzie, Ian F. C., and Terry Potter. "Murine Lymphocyte Surface Antigens." *Advances in Immunology* 27 (1979), 179–337.

Madec, Y. "La biologie hospitalière. Regards sur une fabuleuse et irrésistible ascension." *Techniques Hospitalières* 613 (1997), 23–30.

Maillard, Christian. *Histoire de l'hôpital de 1940 à nos jours. Comment la santé est devenue une affaire d'État*. Paris: Dunod, 1986.

Majno, Guido, and Isabelle Joris. *Cells, Tissues and Disease: Principles of General Pathology*. Oxford: Blackwell, 1996.

Mann, D. L., G. N. Rogentine, R. Halterman, and B. Leventhal. "Detection of an Antigen Associated with Acute Leukemia." *Science* 174 (1971), 1136–7.

Mann, Reinhold C. "On Multiparameter Data Analysis in Flow Cytometry." *Cytometry* 8 (1987), 184–9.

Mant, David, and Godfrey Fowler. "Mass Screening: Theory and Ethics." *British Medical Journal* 300 (1990), 916–8.

Marks, Harry M. *The Progress of Experiments: Science and Therapeutic Reform in the United States, 1900–1990*. Cambridge, UK: Cambridge University Press, 1997.

Marti, Gerald E., G. Faguet, P. Bertin, J. Agee, G. Washington, S. Ruiz, P. Carter, V. Zenger, R. Vogt, and P. Noguchi. "CD20 and CD5 Expression in B-Chronic Lymphocytic Leukemia." *Annals of the New York Academy of Sciences* 651 (1992), 480–3.

Marti, Gerald E., L. Magruder, K. Patrick, M. Vail, W. Schuette, R. Keller, K. Muirhead, P. Horan, and H. R. Gralnick. "Normal Human Blood Density Gradient Lymphocyte Subset Analysis: I. An Interlaboratory Flow Cytometric Comparison of 85 Normal Adults." *American Journal of Hematology* 20 (1985), 41–52.

Martini, E., J. L. D'Haucourt, B. Brando, J. Lawry, J. E. O'Connor, and F. Sansonetty. *First European Quality Control of Cellular Phenotyping by Flow Cytometry.* Paris: Frison-Roche, 1990.

Martini, E., and J. L. D'Haucourt. "Contrôle de qualité Franco-Belge des phénotypages cellulaires analysés en cytométrie en flux." *Annales du contrôle de qualité national.* Paris: Laboratoire National de la Santé, 1989.

Mason, David Y. "HLDA Workshops: Past and Present." Unpublished document, c. 1997.

Mason, David Y., and K. C. Gatter. "Not Another Lymphoma Classification!" *British Journal of Haematology* 90 (1995), 493–7.

Mason, David Y., and Clive R. Taylor. "The Distribution of Muramidase (Lysozyme) in Human Tissues." *Journal of Clinical Pathology* 28 (1975), 124–32.

Mason, David Y., and Clive R. Taylor. "Staining of the A Antigen Human Erythrocytes." *Journal of Clinical Pathology* 28 (1975), 594–5.

Mason, David Y., Caroline Farrell, and Clive R. Taylor. "The Detection of Intracellular Antigens in Human Leucocytes by Immunoperoxidase Staining." *British Journal of Haematology* 31 (1975), 361–70.

Mason David Y., Sylvaine Labaume, and Jean-Louis Preud'homme. "The Detection of Membrane and Cytoplasmic Immunoglobulins in Human Leucocytes by Immunoperoxidase Staining. *Clinical and Experimental Immunology* 29 (1977), 413–21.

Mathé, Georges. "Workshop for the Classification of Non-Hodgkin's Lymphoma." *Biomedicine* 22 (1975), 466–7.

Mathé, Georges, D. Dantchev, P. Pouillart, and I. Florentin. "De l'hématologie *avec* à l'hématologie *sans* microscope." *Nouvelle Presse Médicale* 1 (1972), 3135–40.

Maurice, John. "Immunology Powerhouse in the Marseilles Hills." *Science* 260 (18 June 1993), 1750.

Mayall, B. H. "Technical Tutorial—A New Feature." *Cytometry* 8 (1987), 247.

Mazumdar, Pauline M. H. *Immunology 1930–1980: Essays in the History of Immunology.* Toronto: Wall and Thompson, 1989.

McCaffrey Ronald, Thomas A. Harrison, Patrick C. Kung, Robertson Parkman, Allen E. Silverstone, and David Baltimore. "Terminal Deoxynucleotidyl Transferase in Normal and Neoplastic Hematopoietic Cells." *Hämatologie und Bluttransfusion* 19 (1976), 503–13.

McCarthy, Robert C., and Terry J. Fetterhoff. "Issues for Quality Assurance in Clinical Flow Cytometry." *Archives of Pathology and Laboratory Medicine* 113 (1989), 658–66.

McCoy, J. Phillip, Jr., and W. Roy Overton. "Quality Control in Flow Cytometry for Diagnostic Pathology: II. A Conspectus of Reference Ranges for Lymphocyte Immunophenotyping." *Cytometry* 18 (1994), 129–39.

McCoy, J. P., Jr., John L. Carey, and John R. Krause. "Quality Control in Flow Cytometry for Diagnostic Pathology I. Cell Surface Phenotyping and General Laboratory Procedures." *American Journal of Clinical Pathology* 93 (4 Suppl. 1) (1990), S27–37.

McGough, Kevin J., and Daniel P. Burke. "The End of Monoclonal Patents?" *Biotechnology* 10 (1992), 1082–3.

McGraw-Hill Dictionary of Scientific and Technical Terms, 5th ed., New York: McGraw-Hill, 1994.

Meijer, C. J., P. van der Valk, P. C. de Bruin, and R. Willemze. "The Revised European-American Lymphoma (REAL) Classification of Non-Hodgkin's Lymphoma: A Missed Opportunity?" *Blood* 85 (1995), 1971–2.

Meijer, G. A., J. A. M. Beliën, P. J. van Dienst, and J. P. A. Baak. "Image Analysis in Clinical Pathology." *Journal of Clinical Pathology* 50 (1997), 365–70.

Melamed, Myron R., and Louis A. Kamentsky. "An Assessment of the Potential Role of Automatic Devices in Cytology Screening." *Obstetrical and Gynecological Survey* 24 (1969), 914–26.

Melamed, Myron R., Paul F. Mullaney, and Howard M. Shapiro. "An Historical Review of the Development of Flow Cytometers and Sorters." In *Flow Cytometry and Sorting,* 2nd ed., ed. Myron R. Melamed, Tore Lindmo, and Mortimer L. Mendelsohn, 1–9. New York: Wiley-Liss, 1990.

Mendelsohn, Mortimer L. "Introduction." In *Automation of Cytogenetics, Asilomar Workshop, Nov. 30–Dec. 2, 1975,* ed. Mortimer L. Mendelsohn, 1–2. Springfield, VA: National Technical Information Service, 1976.

Mendelsohn, Mortimer L., and Brian H. Mayall. "Chromosome Identification by Image Analysis and Quantitative Cytochemistry." In *Human Chromosome Methodology.* 2nd ed., ed. Jorge J. Yunis, 311–46. New York: Academic Press, 1974.

Mendelsohn, Mortimer L., T. J. Conway, D. A. Hungerford, Wilfred A. Kolman, Benson H. Perry, and Judith M. S. Prewitt. "Computer-Oriented Analysis of Human Chromosomes I. Photometric Estimation of DNA Content." *Cytogenetics* 5 (1966), 223–42.

Mendelsohn, Mortimer L., Wilfred A. Kolman, and R. C. Bostrum. "Initial Approaches to the Computer Analysis of Cytophotometric Fields." *Annals of the New York Academy of Sciences* 115 (1964), 998–1009.

Mendelsohn, Mortimer L., Wilfred A. Kolman, Benson Perry, and Judith M. S. Prewitt. "Morphological Analysis of Cells and Chromosomes by Digital Computer." *Methods of Information in Medicine* 4 (1965), 163–7.

Mendelsohn, Mortimer L., Brian H. Mayall, and Judith M. S. Prewitt. "Approaches to the Automation of Chromosome Analysis." In *Image Processing in Biological Science,* ed. Diane M. Ramsay, 119–36. Berkeley: University of California Press, 1969.

Ménoret, Marie. *Le temps du cancer.* Paris: CNRS Éditions, 1999.

Merriam-Webster's Collegiate Dictionary, 10th ed., Springfield, MA: Merriam-Webster, 1993.

Métézeau, Philippe, and Marie-Hélène Ratinaud. "Flow Cytometry: Technical Description and Some Applications in France." *Biology of the Cell* 58 (1986), 103–12.

Métézeau, Philippe, and Marie-Hélène Ratinaud. "L'implantation et l'environnement de la cytométrie en flux." *Spectra Biologie* 90/4 (1990), 25–6.

Metz, Lance E., and Ivan M. Viest. *The First 75 Years: A History of the Engineering Foundation.* New York: Engineering Foundation, 1991.

Metzgar, R. S., T. Mohanakumar, and D. S. Miller. "Antigens Specific for Human Lymphocytic and Myeloid Leukemia Cells: Detection by Nonhuman Primate Antiserum." *Science* 178 (1972), 986–8.

Michel, Huguette. *L'informatique dans les laboratoires centraux d'hématologie de l'Assistance publique.* Mémoire de maîtrise de sciences et techniques de gestion des organisations sanitaires et sociales: Gestion Hospitalière, Université de Paris-Dauphine, 1983.

Mili, Fatima, W. Dana Flanders, John R. Boring, J. Lee Annest, and Frank Destefano. "The Associations of Race, Cigarette Smoking, and Smoking Cessation to Measures of the Immune System in Middle-Aged Men." *Clinical Immunology and Immunopathology* 59 (1991), 187–200.

Miller, J. A. F. P. "The Discovery of Thymus Function." In *Immunology: The Making of a Modern Science,* ed. Richard B. Gallagher, Jean Gilder, G. J. V. Nossal, and Gaetano Salvatore, 75–84. New York: Academic Press, 1995.

Milstein, César. "Introductory Remarks." In *Leucocyte Typing. Human Leucocyte Differentiation Antigens Detected by Monoclonal Antibodies. Specification-Classification-Nomenclature,* ed. Alain Bernard, Laurence Boumsell, Jean Dausset, César Milstein, and Stuart F. Schlossman, 3–8. Berlin: Springer Verlag, 1984.

Milstein, César. "What Next?" In *Leucocyte Typing IV. White Cell Differentiation Antigens,* ed. W. Knapp, B. Dörken, W. R. Gilks, E. P. Rieber, R. E. Schmidt, H. Stein, and A. E. G. Von dem Borne, 1–5. Oxford: Oxford University Press, 1989.

Milstein, César. "With the Benefit of Hindsight," *Immunology Today* 21 (2000), 359–63.

Mishler, Elliot George. *The Discourse of Medicine: Dialectics of Medical Interviews.* Norwood, NJ: Ablex, 1984.

Missmahl, H. P. "Fluoreszenzmikroskopie." In *100 Jahre Histochemie in Deutschland,* ed. W. Sandritter, 63–79. Stuttgart: Schattauer Verlag, 1964.

Mitchell, G. F., and J. F. Miller. "Cell to Cell Interaction in the Immune Response. II. The Source of Hemolysin-Forming Cells in Irradiated Mice Given Bone Marrow and Thymus or Thoracic Duct Lymphocytes." *Journal of Experimental Medicine* 128 (1968), 821–37.

Mohanakumar, T., R. S. Metzgar, and D. S. Miller. "Human Leukemia Cell Antigens: Serologic Characterization with Xenoantisera." *Journal of the National Cancer Institute* 52 (1974), 1435–44.

Möller, G. "Citation Classic Commentary on the *Journal of Experimental Medicine* 114: 415–34, 1962." *Current Contents/Life Sciences* 27, (2 July 1984): 20.

Morange, Michel. "From the Regulatory Vision of Cancer to the Oncogene Paradigm, 1975–1985." *Journal of the History of Biology* 30 (1997), 1–29.

"More Oncopathology Research Asked, Development Workshop Approved." *The Cancer Letter* 4 (1978), 4.

Morris, P. J., N. P. Carter, P. R. Cullen, J. F. Thompson, and R. F. Wood. "Role of T-Cell-Subset Monitoring in Renal Allograft Recipients." *New England Journal of Medicine* 306 (1982), 110–1.

Morse, Herbert C., III, "Genetic Nomenclature for Loci Controlling Surface Antigens of Mouse Hemopoietic Cells." *Journal of Immunology* 149 (1992), 3129–34.

Moulin, Anne Marie. *Le dernier langage de la médecine. Histoire de l'immunologie de Pasteur au Sida.* Paris: Presses Universitaires de France, 1991.

Moulin, Anne Marie. "The Immune System: A Key Concept for the History of Immunology." *History and Philosophy of the Life Sciences* 11 (1989), 221–36.

Moulin, Anne Marie. "Un objet scientifique à la charnière des sciences biologiques et sociales: le système immunitaire." *Historia, Ciencias, Saude-Manguinhos* 3 (2) (1996), 300–18.

Mtasiwa, Deodatus M., Nobutaka Imamura, Yasuo Takimoto, Kosuke Okada, Koji Nanba, Hideki Asaoku, and Atsushi Kuramoto. "Immunophenotype, Histopathology and Clinical Stage: Their Predictive Value in the Prognosis of Non-Hodgkin's Lymphomas." *Hiroshima Journal of Medical Science* 39 (1990), 95–100.

Muirhead, Katherine A. "Establishment of Quality Control Procedures in Clinical Flow Cytometry." *Annals of the New York Academy of Sciences* 677 (1993), 1–20.

Mullaney, Paul F., D. E. Burger, and G. C. Salzman. "An Instrument for Static Light-Scattering Measurements on Individual Cells." In Los Alamos Scientific Laboratory of the University of California, *Progress Report. Biomedical and Envi-*

ronmental Research Program of the LASL Health Division, January–December 1977. LA-7254-PR, 168–9. Los Alamos, NM, 1978.

Mullaney, Paul F., J. A. Steinkamp, G. C. Salzman, J. M. Crowell, Z. V. Svitra, and J. C. Martin. *Automated Cancer-Cell Sorting and Analysis: Progress Report, December 1, 1977–May 31, 1978* LA-7412-PR. Los Alamos, NM: Los Alamos Scientific Laboratory, 1978.

Mullaney, Paul F., J. A. Steinkamp, G. C. Salzman, Z. V. Zvitra, J. M. Crowell, J. C. Martin, K. M. Hansen, M. J. Skogen-Hagenson, R. D. Hiebert, and F. C. Genter. *Automated Cancer-Cell Sorting and Analysis: Progress Report, June 1–November 30, 1977.* LA-7076-PR. Los Alamos, NM: Los Alamos Scientific Laboratory, 1978.

Müller, Johannes. *On the Finer Structure and the Forms of Morbid Tumors* (*Über den feinern Bau und die Formen der krankhaften Geschwülste.* Berlin, 1938). In *Johannes Müller and the Nineteenth-Century Origins of Tumor Cell Theory,* ed. Lelland Joseph Rather, Patricia Rather, and John B. Frerichs, 56–150. Canton, MA: Science History Publications, 1986.

Murken, Axel Hinrich. *Vom Armenhospital zum Grossklinikum. Die Geschichte des Krankenhauses vom 18. Jahrhundert bis zur Gegenwart.* Cologne: DuMont Buchverlag, 1988.

Murphy, Robert F. "Automated Identification of Subpopulations in Flow Cytometric List Mode Data Using Cluster Analysis." *Cytometry* 6 (1985), 302–9.

Myers, Greg. *Writing Biology. Texts in the Social Construction of Scientific Knowledge.* Madison: University of Wisconsin Press, 1982.

Nadel, Elie M. "Computer Analysis of Cytophotometric Fields by CYDAC and Its Historical Evolution from the Cytoanalyzer." *Acta Cytologica* 9 (1965), 203–6.

Nakane, P. K., and G. B. Pierce. "Enzyme-Labelled Antibodies: Preparation and Application for the Localization of Antigen." *Journal of Histochemistry and Cytochemistry* 14 (1967), 929–31.

Narin, Francis, and Elliot Noma. "Is Technology Becoming Science?" *Scientometrics* 7 (1985), 369–81.

National Cancer Institute. *Digest of Scientific Recommendations for the National Cancer Program Plan.* U.S. Dept. of Health, Education, and Welfare publication no. (NIH) 74–570. Bethesda, MD: National Institutes of Health, 1973.

National Committee for Clinical Laboratory Standards [NCCLS]. *Clinical Applications of Flow Cytometry: Immunophenotyping of Leukemic Cells; Approved Guideline.* Document H43-A. Villanova, PA: NCCLS, 1998.

National Committee for Clinical Laboratory Standards [NCCLS]. *Clinical Applications of Flow Cytometry: Immunophenotyping of Leukemic Cells; Proposed Guideline.* Document H43-P. Villanova, PA: NCCLS, 1993.

National Committee for Clinical Laboratory Standards [NCCLS]. *Clinical Applications of Flow Cytometry: Quality Assurance and Immunophenotyping of Peripheral Blood Lymphocytes. Tentative Guideline.* Document H42-T. Villanova, PA: NCCLS, 1992.

National Committee for Clinical Laboratory Standards [NCCLS]. *Methods for Reticulocyte Counting (Flow Cytometry and Supravital Dyes); Approved Guideline.* Document H44-A. Villanova, PA: NCCLS, 1997.

Nelson, Richard R., and Sidney G. Winter. *An Evolutionary Theory of Economic Change.* Cambridge, MA: Harvard University Press, 1982.

Nenning, P., and H. Bourcevet. "Zum Rechtsschutz monoklonaler Antikörper." *Die Pharmazie* 45 (1990), 525–7.

Nicholas, Robin, and Davis Nicholas. *Immunology: An Information Profile.* London: Mansell, 1985.

Nicholson, J. K. "Quality Control in Immunophenotyping: US Efforts to Establish Common Methodology and Their Impact. American Society for Histocompatibility and Immunogenetics." *European Journal of Histochemistry* 38 (Suppl. 1) (1994), 7–12.

Nicolson, Malcom, and Cathleen McLaughlin. "Social Constructionism and Medical Sociology: A Reply to M. R. Bury." *Sociology of Health & Illness* 9 (1987), 107–26.

"Nomenclature for Clusters of Differentiation (CD) of Antigens Defined on Human Leukocyte Populations." *Bulletin of the World Health Organization* 62 (1984), 809–15.

Non-Hodgkin's Lymphoma Pathologic Classification Project. "A Clinical Evaluation of the International Lymphoma Study Group Classification of Non-Hodgkin's Lymphoma." *Blood* 89 (1997), 3909–18.

Non-Hodgkin's Lymphoma Pathologic Classification Project. "National Cancer Institute Sponsored Study of Classifications of Non-Hodgkin's Lymphomas. Summary and Description of a Working Formulation for Clinical Usage." *Cancer* 49 (May 1982), 2112–35.

Nossal, G. J. V. "Triumphs and Trials of Immunology in the 1980s." *Immunology Today* 9 (1988), 286–91.

"Note on Nomenclature." *Nature* 325 (1987), 660.

Nukaga, Yoshio, and Alberto Cambrosio, "Medical Pedigrees and the Visual Production of Family Disease in Canadian and Japanese Genetic Counselling Practices." In *The Sociology of Medical Science and Technology*, ed. Mary Ann Elston, 29–55. London: Blackwell, 1997.

Oakley, Therese. "Bravely Entering the New World of Flow Cytometry." *Medical Laboratory Observer* 24 (1992), 42–4.

Oboler, Silvya K., and F. Marc LaForce. "The Periodic Physical Examination in Asymptomatic Adults." *Annals of Internal Medicine* 110 (1989), 214–26.

O'Connell, Joseph. "Metrology: The Creation of Universality by the Circulation of Particulars." *Social Studies of Science* 23 (1993), 129–73.

O'Conor, Gregory T., and L. H. Sobin. "Conclusions of the First Session: Correlations between Current Morphologic Categorizations." In *Lymphoid Neoplasias I: Classification, Categorization, and Natural History*, ed. Georges Mathé, Maxime Seligmann, and Maurice Tubiana, 126–8. Berlin: Springer-Verlag, 1978.

O'Gorman, Maurice R., Rebecca Gelman, Site Investigators, and the NIAID New CD4 Technologies Focus Group. "Inter and Intrainstitutional Evaluation of Automated Volumetric Capillary Cytometry for the Quantitation of CD4- and CD8-positive T Lymphocytes in the Peripheral Blood of Persons Infected with Human Immunodeficiency Virus." *Clinical and Diagnostic Laboratory Immunology* 4 (1997), 173–9.

Office of Technology Assessment. *Commercial Biotechnology: An International Analysis.* Washington, DC: U.S. Government Printing Office, 1984.

Oi, Vernon T., Alexander N. Glazer, and Luber Stryer. "Fluorescent Phycobiliprotein Conjugates for Analyses of Cells and Molecules." *Journal of Cell Biology* 93 (1982), 981–6.

Old, Lloyd J. "Cancer Immunology: The Search for Specificity." *National Cancer Institute Monographs* 60 (1982), 193–209.

Old, Lloyd J., and Edward A. Boyse. "Current Enigmas in Cancer Research." *The Harvey Lectures* 67 (1973), 273–315.

Old, Lloyd J., Edward A. Boyse, and Elisabeth Stockert. "Antigenic Properties of Experimental Leukemias. I. Serological Studies in Vitro with Spontaneous and Radiation Leukemias." *Journal of the National Cancer Institute* 31 (1963): 977–86.

Orfao, A., G. Schmitz, B. Brando, A. Ruiz-Arguelles, G. Basso, R. Braylan, G. Rothe, F. Lacombe, F. Lanza, S. Papa, P. Lucio, and J. F. San Miguel. "Clinically Useful Information Provided by the Flow Cytometric Immunophenotyping of Hematological Malignancies: Current Status and Future Directions." *Clinical Chemistry* 45 (1999), 1708–17.

Orsi, Fabienne. *Droits de propriété intellectuelle et marches financiers dans les nouvelles relations science/industrie. Le cas de la recherche sur le génome humain.* PhD thesis, Université de la Méditerranée (Aix-Marseille II), 2001.

Osmond, Denis H. "Classification and Staging of HIV Disease." In *The AIDS Knowledge Base*, ed. Philip T. Cohen, Merle A. Sande, and Paul A. Volberding. Boston: Little, Brown, 1994, 1.1, 1–15.

OTA, [Office of Technology Assessment]. *The CDC's Case Definition of AIDS: Implications of the Proposed Revisions.* Document OTA-BP-H-89. Springfield, VA: National Technical Information Service, June 1992.

Oxford English Dictionary. Oxford: Clarendon Press, 1970.

Oxford English Dictionary. 2nd ed. Prepared by John A. Simpson and Edmund S.C. Weiner. Oxford: Clarendon Press, 1989.

Paietta, Elisabeth. "Proposals for the Immunological Classification of Acute Leukemias." *Leukemia* 9 (1995), 2147–57.

Paietta, Elisabeth, J. Anderson, Peter H. Wiernik, and Eastern Cooperative Oncology Group. "A New Approach to Analyzing the Utility of Immunophenotyping for Predicting Clinical Outcome in Acute Leukemia." *Leukemia* 10 (1996), 1–4.

Pallez, Gabriel. "Une politique architecturale pour l'Assistance publique." *Monuments Historiques* 114 (April–May 1981), 2–7.

Pambianchi, Wayne. "Biotechnology Marketing Strategies: Case Studies from the Monoclonal Antibody Field." *Genetic Engineering News* (July–August 1983), 6, 34.

Panem, Sandra. *The Interferon Crusade.* Washington, DC: Brookings Institution, 1984.

Parker, John W., Bernard Adelsberg, Stanley P. Azen, Donna Boone, Mary Ann Fletcher, George F. Gjerset, Joseph Hassett, Joseph Kaplan, Joyce C. Niland, Tamara Odom-Maryon, Evan A. Operskalski, Harry Prince, Diane Scott, Daniel P. Stites, James W. Mosley, and the Transfusion Safety Study Group (USC). "Leucocyte Immunophenotyping by Flow Cytometry in a Multisite Study: Standardization, Quality Control, and Normal Values in the Transfusion Safety Study." *Clinical Immunology and Immunopathology* 55 (1990), 187–220.

Parks, David R., Leonore A. Herzenberg, and Leonard A. Herzenberg. "Flow Cytometry and Fluorescence-activated Cell Sorting." In *Fundamental Immunology,* 2nd edn., ed. William E. Paul, 781–802. New York: Raven Press, 1989.

Paxton, Helene, Pamela Kidd, Alan Landay, Janis Giorgi, Neal Flomenberg, Edward Walker, Fred Valentine, John Fahey, and Rebecca Gelman. "Results of the Flow Cytometry ACTG Quality Control Program: Analysis and Findings." *Clinical Immunology and Immunopathology* 52 (1989), 68–84.

Pegrum, G. D. "Leukaemic Antigens." *British Journal of Haematology* 24 (1973), 1–6.

Pelissolo, J. C. *La biotechnologie, demain? Rapport au Premier Ministre.* Paris: Délégation générale à la recherche scientifique et technique, 1980.

Perkins, Mary L., J. Michael Odell, and Rita M. Braziel. "Introduction to Leukemia and the Acute Leukemias." In *Clinical Hematology and Fundamentals of Hemostasis,* 3rd edn. ed. Denise M. Harmening, 294–332. Philadelphia: Davis, 1997.

Pernis, Benvenuto, Luciani Forni, and Luisa Amante. "Immunoglobulins as Cell Receptors." *Annals of the New York Academy of Sciences* 190 (1971), 420–31.

Perutz, Max F. "Fundamental Research in Molecular Biology: Relevance to Medicine." *Nature* 262 (1976), 449–53.

Petersdorf, Robert G. "The Evolution of Departments of Medicine." *New England Journal of Medicine* 303 (1980), 489–96.

"Physician-Scientists Receive $7.5 Million in Awards." *Focus (U.S. Burroughs Wellcome Fund)* (spring 2000), 1, 7–8.

Picard, Jean-François. "De la médecine expérimentale (1865) à l'INSERM (1964)." In *Les sciences biologiques et médicales en France, 1920–1950,* ed. Claude Debru, Jean Gayon, and Jean-François Picard, 329–44. Paris: CNRS, 1994.

Picard, Jean-François. "Poussée scientifique ou demande des médecins? La recherche médicale en France de l'Institut national d'hygiène à l'INSERM." *Sciences Sociales et Santé* 10 (1992), 47–106.

Pickering, Andrew. *The Mangle of Practice: Time, Agency, and Science.* Chicago: University of Chicago Press, 1995.

Pierrez, José, and Xavier Ronot. "Use of Diploid and Triploid Trout Erythrocytes as Internal Standards in Flow Cytometry." *Cytometry* 12 (1991), 275–8.

Pileri, Stefano A., Marina Milani, Giulio Fraternali-Orcioni, and Elena Sabattini. "From the R.E.A.L. Classification to the Upcoming WHO Scheme: A Step Towards Universal Categorization of Lymphoma Entities?" *Annals of Oncology* 9 (1998), 607–12.

Piller, Gordon J. *The History and Presentation of Leukaemia: 1845–1960.* Doctoral thesis, Open University, U.K., 1992.

Piller, Gordon J. "John Hughes Bennett and the Discovery of Leukaemia." *Proceedings of the Royal College of Physicians of Edinburgh.* 27 (Suppl. 3) (1997), 1–11.

Piller, Gordon J. *Rays of Hope. The Story of the Leukaemia Research Fund.* London: Leukaemia Research Fund, 1994.

Pinch, Trevor. "Towards an Analysis of Scientific Observation: The Externality and Evidential Significance of Observational Reports in Science." *Social Studies of Science* 15 (1985), 3–36.

Pinkel, Donald. "Curing Children of Leukemia." *Cancer* 59 (1987), 1683–91.

Pinkus, G. S., J. L. Pinkus, E. Langhoff, F. Matsumura, S. Yamashiro, G. Mosialos, and J. W. Said. "Fascin, a Sensitive New Marker for Reed-Sternberg Cells of Hodgkin's Disease: Evidence for a Dendritic or B Cell Variation?" *American Journal of Pathology* 150 (1997), 543–62.

Pitts, John A. *The Human Factor. Biomedicine in the Manned Space Program to 1980.* Washington, DC: National Aeronautics and Space Administration, 1985.

Plant, David W., Niels J. Reimers, and Norton D. Zinder, eds. *Patenting Life Forms. Banbury Report 10.* Cold Spring Harbor, NY: Cold Spring Harbor Laboratory, 1982.

"Le plateau technique hospitalier: points de vue et expériences." *Technologie et santé* no. 26 (July 1996).

Podolsky, Scott H., and Alfred I. Tauber. *The Generation of Diversity: Clonal Selection Theory and the Rise of Molecular Immunology.* Cambridge, MA: Harvard University Press, 1997.

Pollak, Michael. "Peptide Growth Factors and Breast Cancer Treatment: Recent Translational Research." *Recent Results in Cancer Research* 140 (1996), 43–9.

Porter, Roy. "The Enemy Within." *The New Republic* (20 April 1998), 38–40.

"The Possible Rele of Immunology in Cancer [conference proceedings]." *Cancer Research* 21 (1961), 1167–325.

Powers, Donald M. "Traceability of Assay Calibrators: The EU's IVD Directive Raises the Bar." *IVD Technology Magazine* (Web edition, July 2000).

Prehn, Richmond T. "Tumor-Specific Antigens of Putatively Nonviral Tumors." *Cancer Research* 28 (1968), 1326–30.

Preud'homme, Jean-Louis. "Lymphocyte Markers: Diagnostic Help or Costly Vogue?" *Diagnostic Immunology* 2 (1984), 242–8.

Preud'homme, Jean-Louis, and Maxime Seligmann. "Critical Evaluation of B and T Cell Markers in Man." *Rheumatology* 6 (1975), 178–89.

Preud'homme, Jean-Louis, and Maxime Seligmann. "Immunoglobulins on the Surface of Lymphoid Cells in Waldenström's Macroglobulinemia." *Journal of Clinical Investigation* 51 (1972), 701–5.

Preud'homme, Jean-Louis, and Maxime Seligmann. "Surface Bound Immunoglobulins as a Cell Marker in Human Lymphoproliferative Diseases." *Blood* 40 (1972), 777–94.

Price, B. J., V. H. Kollman, and G. C. Salzman. "Classification of Microalgal Species." In Los Alamos Scientific Laboratory of the University of California, *Progress Report. Biomedical and Environmental Research Program of the LASL Health Division, January–December 1976.* LA-6898-PR, Los Alamos, NM, 1977, 125–7.

Prince, Harry E., Karim Hirji, Lilian S. Waldbeser, Susan Plaeger-Marshall, Steven Kleinman, and Lewis L. Lanier. "Influence of Racial Background on the Distribution of T-Cell Subsets and Leu 11-positive Lymphocytes in Healthy Blood Donors." *Diagnostic Immunology* 3 (1985), 33–7.

Prior, Lindsay. "The Architecture of the Hospital: A Study of Spatial Organization and Medical Knowledge." *The British Journal of Sociology* 39 (1988), 86–113.

Prior, Lindsay. "The Local Space of Medical Discourse. Disease, Illness and Hospital Architecture." In *The Social Construction of Illness. Illness and Medical*

Knowledge in Past and Present, ed. Jens Lachmund and Gunnar Stollberg, 67–84. Stuttgart: Franz Steiner Verlag, 1992.

Proctor, Robert N. *Cancer Wars. How Politics Shapes What We Know and Don't Know about Cancer.* New York: Basic Books, 1995.

Proffitt, Michael, ed. *Oxford English Dictionary Additions Series*, vol. 3. Oxford: Clarendon Press, 1997.

Purdy, William C., and Robert S. Melville. "The Manpower Crisis in Clinical Chemistry." *Analytical Chemistry* 42 (12) (1970), 32A–38A.

"Quality of Performance in Pathology Laboratories." *Lancet* (14 March 1981), 599.

Rabellino, Enrique, Sonia Colon, Howard M. Grey, and Emil R. Unanue. "Immunoglobulins on the Surface of Lymphocytes I. Distribution and Quantitation," *Journal of Experimental Medicine* 133 (1971), 156–67.

Rabinow, Paul. *French DNA. Trouble in Purgatory.* Chicago: University of Chicago Press, 1999.

Raff, Martin C. "Cell-Surface Immunology." *Scientific American* 234 (May 1976), 30–9.

Raff, Martin C. "Citation Classic Commentary on *Immunology* 19: 637–50, 1970." *Current Contents/Life Sciences* 27 (July 2) (1984), 21.

Raff, Martin C. "Selective Removal of Lymphocyte Populations." In *Immunologic Intervention: Proceedings of an International Conference Held at Brook Lodge, Augusta, Michigan, April 26–28, 1971*, ed. Jonathan W. Uhr and Maurice Landy, 53–104. New York: Academic Press, 1971.

Raff, Martin C. "Surface Antigenic Markers for Distinguishing T and B Lymphocytes in Mice." *Transplantation Reviews* 6 (1971), 52–80.

Raff, Martin C. "Theta Isoantigen as a Marker of Thymus-Derived Lymphocytes in Mice." *Nature* 224 (1969), 378–9.

Raff, Martin C. "Two Distinct Populations of Peripheral Lymphocytes in Mice Distinguishable by Immunofluorescence." *Immunology* 19 (1970), 637–50.

Raff, Martin C., and Harvey Cantor. "Subpopulations of Thymus Cells and Thymus-Derived Lymphocytes." In *Progress in Immunology*, ed. Bernard Amos, 83–93. New York: Academic Press, 1971.

Raff, Martin C., M. Sternberg, and R. B. Taylor. "Immunoglobulin Determinants in the Surface of Mouse Lymphoid Cells." *Nature* 225 (1970), 553–4.

Rall, J. E. "Epilogue." In *NIH: An Account of Research in Its Laboratories and Clinics*, ed. De Witt Stetten Jr. and William T. Carrigan, 527–8. New York: Academic Press, 1984.

Ramaswamy, Seidhar, Pablo Tamayo, Ryan Rifkin, Sayan Mukherjee, Chen-Hsiang Yeang, Michael Angela Christine Ladd, Michael Reich, Era Latulippe, Jill Pi Mesirov, Tomaso Poggio, William Gerald Massimoloda, Eric S. Lander, and Todd R. Golub. "Multiclass Cancer Diagnosis Using Tumor Gene Expression Signatures." *Proceedings of the National Academy of Sciences U.S.A.* 98 (2001), 15149–54.

Rappaport, Henry. "Commentary on Working Formulation of Non-Hodgkin's Lymphomas." *Cancer* 49 (May 1982), 2134.

Rappaport, Henry. "Tumors of the Hematopoietic System." In *Atlas of Tumor Pathology*, sec. 3, fasc. 8, Washington, DC: U.S. Armed Forces Institute of Pathology, 1966.

Rasmussen, Nicolas. "Facts, Artifacts, and Mesosomes: Practicing Epistemology with the Electron Microscope." *Studies in History and Philosophy of Science* 24 (1993), 227–65.

Rather, Lelland Joseph. "Johannes Müller, Theodor Schwann, Mathias Schleiden, Jacob Henle and the Nature of Plant and Animal Cells." In *Johannes Müller and the Nineteenth-Century Origins of Tumor Cell Theory*, ed. Lelland Joseph Rather, Patricia Rather, and John B. Frerichs, 1–55. Canton, MA: Science History Publications, 1986.

Rather, Lelland Joseph. "The Place of Virchow in Medical Thought." In *Cellular Pathology as Based upon Physiological and Pathological Histology*, Rudolf Virchow, v–xxvii trans. Frank Chance. New York: Dover, 1971.

Ratinaud, Marie-Hélène, and Philippe Métézeau. "Cytomètres en flux: implantation en France et description des appareils commercialisés." *Spectra Biologie* 95/4 (1995), 34–9.

Reichert, T., M. DeBruyere, V. Deneys, T. Totterman, P. Lydyard, F. Yuksel, H. Chapel, D. Jewell, L. Van Hove, J. Linden, and L. Buchner. "Lymphocyte Subset Reference Ranges in Adult Caucasians." *Clinical Immunology and Immunopathology* 60 (1991), 190–208.

Reif, Arnold E. "The Discovery of Thy-1 and Its Development." In *Cell Surface Antigen Thy-1. Immunology, Neurology, and Therapeutic Applications*, ed. Arnold E. Reif and Michael Schlesinger, 3–45. New York: Marcel Dekker, 1989.

Reif, Arnold E., and Joan M. V. Allen. "Specificity of Isoantisera against Leukemic and Thymic Lymphocytes." *Nature* 200 (1963), 1332–3.

Reines, Brandon P. "On the Locus of Medical Discovery." *Journal of Medicine and Philosophy* 16 (1991), 183–209.

Reinherz, Ellis L., Patrick C. Kung, Gideon Goldstein, and Stuart F. Schlossman. "A Monoclonal Antibody with Selective Reactivity with Functionally Mature Human Thymocytes and All Peripheral Human T Cells." *Journal of Immunology.* 123 (1979), 1312–7.

Reinherz, Ellis L., Patrick C. Kung, Gideon Goldstein, and Stuart F. Schlossman. "Separation of Functional Subsets of Human T Cells by a Monoclonal Antibody." *Proceedings of the National Academy of Sciences U.S.A.* 76 (1979), 4061–5.

Reiser, Stanley Joel. *Medicine and the Reign of Technology*. Cambridge, UK: Cambridge University Press, 1981 [1978].

Rentas, F., S. P. Perfetto, and W. J. Rickman. "The Effect of Anticoagulant and Room Temperature Storage on Lymphocyte Markers." *Clinical Applications of Cytometry. Abstracts*, 7th Annual Meeting, Charleston, SC., 1992.

Rettig, Richard A. *Cancer Crusade: The Story of the National Cancer Act of 1971*. Princeton, NJ: Princeton University Press, 1977.

Rey, Alain, ed. *Dictionnaire historique de la langue française*. Paris: Dictionnaires Le Robert, 1992–8.

Rheinberger, Hans-Jörg. "Beyond Nature and Culture: Modes of Reasoning in the Age of Molecular Biology and Medicine." In *Living and Working with the New Medical Technologies*, ed. Margaret Lock, Allan Young, and Alberto Cambrosio, 19–30. Cambridge, UK: Cambridge University Press, 2000.

Rheinberger, Hans-Jörg. *Toward a History of Epistemic Things. Synthesizing Proteins in the Test Tube*. Stanford, CA: Stanford University Press, 1997.

Rhoads, C. P. "The Sword and the Ploughshare." *Journal of Mount Sinai Hospital* 13 (1946), 299–309.

Ricki, Lewis. "New Antibody Classification May Restrict Research." *Genetic Engineering News* 14 (1994), 1, 16, 32.

Rickman, William J., Christine Monical, and Myron J. Waxdal. "Improved Precision in the Enumeration of Absolute Numbers of Lymphocyte Phenotypes with Long-Term Monthly Proficiency Testing." *Annals of the New York Academy of Sciences* 677 (1993), 53–8.

Rickman, William J., Myron J. Waxdal, Christine Monical, James D. Damato, and Donald S. Burke. "Department of Army Lymphocyte Immunophenotyping Quality Assurance Program." *Clinical Immunology and Immunopathology* 52 (1989), 85–95.

Ritz, Jerome, John M. Pesando, Jean Notis-McConarty, Herbert Lazarus, and Stuart F. Schlossman. "A Monoclonal Antibody to Human Acute Lymphoblastic Leukemia Antigen." *Nature* 238 (1980), 583–5.

Robb-Smith, Alastair Hamish Tearloch, and Clive R. Taylor. *Lymph Node Biopsy: A Diagnostic Atlas*. London: Harvey Miller and Oxford University Press, 1981.

Robert, Paul. *Dictionnaire alphabétique et analogique de la langue française*. Paris: Société du Nouveau Littré, 1962.

Roitt, Ivan M. *Essential Immunology*, 8th ed. Oxford: Blackwell, 1994.

Roitt, Ivan M., Jonathan Brostoff, and David K. Male. *Immunology*, 2nd ed. Edinburgh: Churchill Livingstone, 1989.

Roitt, Ivan M., Melvyn F. Greaves, G. Torrigiani, and J. Brostoff. "The Cellular Basis of Immunological Responses. A Synthesis of Some Current Views." *Lancet* (16 August 1969), 367–71.

Rosenberg, Saul A. "Classification of Lymphoid Neoplasms [editorial]." *Blood* 84 (1994), 1359–60.

Rosenfeld, Louis. *Four Centuries of Clinical Chemistry*. Amsterdam: Gordon and Breach, 1999.

Rosnay, Joël de. *Biotechnologies et bioindustries*. Paris: Seuil—La documentation française, 1979.

Ross, Walter S. *Crusade: The Official History of the American Cancer Society*. New York: Arbor House, 1987.

Rössle, Robert. "Eröffnungsansprache." *Verhandlungen der Deutschen Pathologischen Gesellschaft* 25 (1930), 1–10.

Rothe, G., and G. Schmitz, for the Working Group on Flow Cytometry and Image Analysis. "Consensus Protocol for the Flow Cytometric Immunophenotyping of Hematopoietic Malignancies." *Leukemia* 10 (1996), 877–95.

Rothstein, William G. *American Medical Schools and the Practice of Medicine: A History*. New York: Oxford University Press, 1987.

Rotman, Boris, and Ben W. Papermaster. "Membrane Properties of Living Mammalian Cells as Studied by Enzymatic Hydrolysis of Fluorogenic Esters." *Proceedings of the National Academy of Sciences U.S.A.* 55 (1966), 134–41.

Roussel, Martine. *Une nouvelle fonction à l'étude: coordonnateur du plateau médico-technique*. Rapport de stage auprès de M. Joubert, coordonnateur du plateau médico-technique de l'hôpital Saint-Louis de l'A.P.-H.P. Paris, June 1995.

Rousselet, F., A. Legrand, P. Chappuis, and F. Thuillier. Dimanches biologiques de Lariboisière, 1960–1990: 30 ans de biologie clinique et de formation permanente. Paris: CNB, 1990.

Royal Society. *Biotechnology: Report of a Joint Working Party*. London: Her Majesty's Stationery Office, 1980.

Rubin, Martin, and Per Lous. *Education and Training for Clinical Chemistry*. Lancaster, UK: MTP Press, 1977.

Rushefsky, Mark E. *Making Cancer Policy*. Albany: State University of New York Press, 1986.

Russell-Jones, R. "Primary Cutaneous B-Cell Lymphoma: How Useful Is the New European Organization for Research and Treatment of Cancer (EORTC) Classification?" *British Journal of Dermatology* 139 (1998), 945–9.

Ryder, Robert W., and Roy D. Mugerwa. "The Clinical Definition and Diagnosis of AIDS in African Adults." In *AIDS in Africa,* ed. Max Essex, Souleymane Mboup, Phyllis J. Kanki, and Mbowa R. Kalengayi, 269–81. New York: Raven Press, 1994.

Saalmuller, A., T. Pauly, B. Aasted, K. T. Jensen, D. H. Sachs, S. Arn, W. C. Davis, Y. H. Park, K. McCullough, A. Summerfield, M. Murtaugh, M. S. Pampusch, K. D. Burger, J. Laber, J. Nielsen, M. D. Pescovitz, C. Stokes, K. Haverson, P. Boyd, and J. K. Lunney. "Overview of the Second International Workshop to Define Swine Cluster of Differentiation (CD) Antigens." *Veterinary Immunology and Immunopathology* 60 (1998), 207–28.

Salmon, Sidney E., and Maxime Seligmann. "B-Cell Neoplasia in Man." *Lancet* 23 November (1974), 1230–3.

Salzman, Gary C. "Light Scattering Analysis of Single Cells." In *Cell Analysis,* vol. 1, ed. Nicholas Catsimpoolas, 111–43. New York: Plenum Press, 1982.

Salzman, Gary C., J. M. Crowell, J. C. Martin, J. A. Steinkamp, P. F. Mullaney, M. T. Butler, J. H. Jet, and C. A. Goad. "Development of Flow-Systems Instrumentation for Rapid Cell Analysis and Sorting." In Los Alamos Scientific Laboratory of the University of California, *Annual Report of the Biomedical and Environmental Research Program of the LASL Health Division, January through December 1974.* LA-5883-PR, Los Alamos, NM, 1975, 104–8.

Salzman Gary C., J. M. Crowell, J. C. Martin, T. T. Trujillo, A. Romero, P. F. Mullaney, and P. M. LaBauve. "Cell Classification by Laser Light Scattering: Identification and Separation of Unstained Leukocytes." *Acta Cytologica* 19 (1975), 374–7.

Samet, Jonathan M. "Concepts of Time in Clinical Research." *Annals of Internal Medicine* 132 (2000), 37–44.

Sandritter, W., Bertha L. Lobel, and G. Kiefer. "Photometric Cytodiagnosis of Vaginal Smears." *Journal of the National Cancer Institute* 32 (1964), 1221–8.

Sannes, Lucy J. *Sales of in Vitro Diagnostic Products to 2001.* Study no. 01. Waltham, MA: Decision Resources, 1998.

Sannes, Lucy J. *Sales of in Vitro Diagnostic Products to 2002.* Study no. 09. Waltham, MA: Decision Resources, 1998.

Sannes, Lucy J. *Sales of in Vitro Diagnostic Products to 2003.* Study no. 04. Waltham, MA: Decision Resources, 1999.

Sax, Paul E., Stephen L. Boswell, M. Guthro-White, and Martin S. Hirsch. "Potential Clinical Implications of Interlaboratory Variability in CD4+ T-Lymphocyte Counts of Patients Infected with Human Immunodeficiency Virus." *Clinical Infectious Disease* 21 (1995), 1121–5.

"Scanning the Issue." *Proceedings of the Institute of Electrical and Electronic Engineers* 57, special issue on technology and health services, (November 1969), 1799.

Schaffer, Simon. "Late Victorian Metrology and Its Instrumentation: A Manufactory of Ohms." In *Invisible Connections. Instruments, Institutions, and Science*, ed. Robert Bud and Susan E. Cozzens, 23–55. Bellingham, WA: SPIE Optical Engineering Press, 1992.

Schechter, Alan N. "The Crisis in Clinical Research: Endangering the Half-Century National Institutes of Health Consensus." *JAMA* 280 (1998), 1440–2.

Schechter, Alan N. "Medicine and Biology Are More Than Biomedicine." *Nature* 401 (30 September 1999), 424.

Schena, Mark, Renu A. Heller, Thomas P. Theriault, Ken Konrad, Eric Lachenmeier, and Ronald W. Davis. "Microarrays: Biotechnology's Discovery Platform for Functional Genomics." *Trends in Biotechnology* 16 (1998), 301–6.

Schlesinger, Michael. "Antigens of the Thymus." *Progress in Allergy* 16 (1972), 214–99.

Schlesinger, Michael, and I. Yron. "Antigenic Changes in Lymph-Node Cells after Administration of Antiserum to Thymus Cells." *Science* 164 (1969), 1412–3.

Schneider, V. "The Bethesda System: The European Perspective." In *Recent Results in Cancer Research.* Vol. 113, *Current Status of Diagnostic Cytology*, ed. Peter Pfitzer and Ekkehard Grundmann, 113–15. Berlin: Springer-Verlag, 1993.

Schwartz, Abe, A. Dorn Hetzel, Jr., Emma Fernandez-Repollet, and Robert F. Vogt. "Quickal Plus: An Automated System to Determine the Fluorescence Intensity of Labeled Cells in MESF Units." *Cytometry* Supplement 5 (1991), 136.

Schwarze, E. W. "Amerika, du sollst es besser haben. Zur Diskussion um eine aktuelle Lymphom-Klassification." *Pathologe* 16 (1995), 241–4.

Scott, Mitchell G. "Monoclonal Antibodies: Approaching Adolescence in Diagnostic Immunoassays." *Trends in Biotechnology* 3 (1985), 170–5.

Second MIC Cooperative Study Group. "Morphologic, Immunologic, and Cytogenetic (MIC) Working Classification of the Acute Myeloid Leukaemias." *British Journal of Haematology* 68 (1988), 487–94.

Seligmann, Maxime, Jean-Claude Brouet, and Jean-Louis Preud'Homme. "The Immunological Diagnosis of Human Leukemias and Lymphomas: An Overview." In *Immunological Diagnosis of Leukemias and Lymphomas*, ed. Stefan Thierfelder, Hans Rodt, and Eckhard Thiel, 1–16. Berlin: Springer-Verlag, 1977.

Seligmann, Maxime. *Lymphocyte Membrane Markers in Human Leukaemias and Lymphomas*, London: Leukaemia Research Fund, 1976.

Senju, Masahiro, Kazuya Makiyama, Kohei Hara, Frank Hulstaert, James N.

Lowder, and Derek P. Jewell. "Two-Color Immunofluorescence and Flow Cytometric Analysis of Peripheral Blood Lymphocyte Subsets in Caucasian and Japanese Healthy Subjects." *Japanese Journal of Medicine* 30 (1991), 509–15.

Shapin, Steven, and Simon Schaffer. *Leviathan and the Air Pump: Hobbes, Boyle, and the Experimental Life.* Princeton, NJ: Princeton University Press, 1985.

Shapiro, Carl, and Hal R. Varian. *Information Rules. A Strategic Guide to the Network Economy.* Boston: Harvard Business School Press, 1998.

Shapiro, Howard M. *Practical Flow Cytometry.* New York: Allan R. Liss, 1985.

Shapiro, Howard M. *Practical Flow Cytometry,* 2nd ed., New York: Allan R. Liss, 1988.

Shapiro, Howard M. *Practical Flow Cytometry,* 3rd ed., New York: Wiley-Liss, 1994.

Shaw, Stephen, "Characterization of Human Leukocyte Differentiation Antigens." *Immunology Today* 8 (1987), 1–3.

Shevach, Ethan, Ira Green, and Leonard Ellman "Heterologous Antiserum to Thymus-Derived Cells in the Guinea-Pig." *Nature New Biology* 235 (1972), 19–21.

Shevach, Ethan M., Ronald Heberman, Michael M. Frank, and Ira Green. "Receptors for Complement and Immunoglobulin on Human Leukemic Cells and Human Lymphoblastoid Cell Lines." *Journal of Clinical Investigation* 51 (1972), 1933–8.

Shi, Shan-Rong, Richard J. Cote, and Clive R. Taylor. "Antigen Retrieval Immunohistochemistry: Past, Present, and Future." *Journal of Histochemistry and Cytochemistry* 45 (1997), 327–43.

Shiku, H., P. Kisielow, M. A. Bean, T. Takahashi, E. A. Boyse, H. F. Oettgen, and L. J. Old. "Expression of T-Cell Differentiation Antigens on Effector Cells in Cell-Mediated Cytotoxicity in Vitro." *Journal of Experimental Medicine* 141 (1975), 227–41.

Shimoyama, M., K. Yunoki, M. Ichimaru, K. Ota, and M. Ogawa. "Final Results of Cooperative Study of VEPA (Vincristine, Cyclophosphamide, Prednisone and Adriamycin) Therapy in Advanced Adult Non-Hodgkin's Lymphoma. Relation Between T- and B-Cell Phenotype and Response." *Japanese Journal of Clinical Oncology* 12 (1982), 227–38.

Shorter, Edward. *The Health Century.* New York: Doubleday, 1987.

Shryock, Richard H. *American Medical Research: Past and Present.* London: Oxford University Press, 1947.

Silverman, David. *Communication and Medical Practice. Social Relations in the Clinic.* London: Sage, 1987.

Silverstein, Arthur M. *A History of Immunology.* New York: Academic Press, 1989.

Silverstein, Arthur M., and Thomas Söderqvist. "The Structure and Dynamics of Immunology, 1951–1972: A Prosopographical Study of International Meetings." *Cellular Immunology* 158 (1994), 1–28.

Simon, Claude. *Le jardin des plantes.* Paris: Les Éditions de Minuit, 1977.

Simon, Richard, Sylvain Durrleman, Richard T. Hoppe, Gianni Bonadonna, Clara D. Bloomfield, Richard A. Rudders, Bruce D. Cheson, and Costan W. Berard. "The Non-Hodgkin's Lymphoma Pathologic Classification Project: Long-Term Follow-up of 1153 Patients with Non-Hodgkin's Lymphomas." *Annals of Internal Medicine* 109 (1988), 939–45.

Sinding, Christiane. "Basic Science and Clinical Research. The Development of the Concept of Organ Resistance to a Hormone." *Journal of the History of Medicine and Allied Sciences* 45 (1990), 198–232.

Sinding, Christiane. *Le clinicien et le chercheur. Des grandes maladies de carence à la médecine moléculaire, 1880–1980.* Paris: Presses Universitaires de France, 1991.

Singer, S. J. "The Molecular Organization of Biological Membranes." In *Structure and Function of Biological Membranes,* ed. L. I. Rothfield, 145–223. Academic Press: New York, 1971.

Singer, S. J., and Garth L. Nicolson. "The Fluid Mosaic Model of the Structure of Cell Membranes." *Science* 175 (1972), 720–31.

Singleton, Vicky, and Mike Michael. "Actor-Networks and Ambivalence: General Practitioners in the UK Cervical Screening Programme." *Social Studies of Science* 23 (1993), 227–64.

Sladek, T. L., and J. W. Jacobberger. "Flow Cytometric Titration of Retroviral Expression Vectors: Comparison of Methods for Analysis of Immunofluorescence Histograms Derived from Cells Expressing Low Antigen Levels." *Cytometry* 14 (1993), 23–31.

Smit, B. J. " 'Translational Research,' the 'Linker Laboratory' or a Paradigm Shift in Cancer Care?" *South African Medical Journal* 86 (1996), 388.

Smith, Barbara Herrnstein. *Belief and Resistance: Dynamics of Contemporary Intellectual Controversy.* Cambridge, MA: Harvard University Press, 1997.

Smith, W. J., J. F. Burdick, and G. M. Williams. "Immunologic Monitoring of Renal Transplant Recipients." *Transplantation Proceedings* 15 (1983), 1182–3.

Sorensen, L. Lee. "Starting a Flow Cytometry User Group." *Medical Laboratory Observer* (June 1994), 52–3.

Sournia, Jean-Charles. *Histoire du diagnostic en médecine.* Paris: Éditions de Santé, 1995.

Sournia, Jean-Charles. "La place actuelle de la biologie dans la pratique médicale et dans les dépenses de santé." *Bulletin de l'Académie Nationale de Médecine* 165 (1981), 213–19.

Southam, Chester M. "Application of Immunology to Clinical Cancer: Past Attempts and Future Possibilities." *Cancer Research* 21 (1961), 1302–16.

Southam, Chester M., and Alice E. Moore. "Induced Immunity to Cancer Cell Homografts in Man." *Annals of the New York Academy of Sciences* 73 (1958), 635–51.

Spicker, Stuart F. "An Introduction to the Medical Epistemology of Georges Canguilhem: Moving beyond Michel Foucault." *Journal of Medicine and Philosophy* 12 (1987), 397–411.

Sprenger, E., W. Sandritter, N. Bohm, D. Wagner, M. Hilgarth, and M. Schaden. "Flow-through-Cytophotometry—A Step towards Automated Cytology?" *Acta Cytologica,* 16 (1972), 297–303.

Springer, Timothy. "Adhesion Receptors of the Immune System." *Nature* 346 (1990), 425–34.

Sreenan, Joseph J., and Raymond R. Tubbs. "The Influence of Immunology and Genetics on Lymphoma Classification: A Historical Perspective." *Cancer Investigation* 14 (1996), 572–88.

Sreenan, Joseph J., Abdelghani Tbakhi, Mark G. Edinger, and Raymond R. Tubbs. "The Use of Isotypic Control Antibodies in the Analysis of CD3+ and CD3+, CD4+ Lymphocyte Subsets in Flow Cytometry. Are They Really Necessary?" *Archives of Pathology and Laboratory Medicine* 121 (1997), 118–21.

Stamatakis, Konstantinos. *Immunotech: conception, création et démarrage d'une société de biotechnologie.* Paris: DEA thesis, Université Paris VII, 1996.

Star, Susan Leigh. "Triangulating Clinical and Basic Research: British Localizationists, 1870–1906." *History of Science* 24 (1986), 29–48.

Star, Susan Leigh, and James Griesemer. "Institutional Ecology, 'Translations' and Boundary Objects. Amateurs and Professionals in Berkeley's Museum of Vertebrate Zoology, 1907–1939." *Social Studies of Science* 19 (1989), 387–420.

Star, Susan Leigh, and Karen Ruhleder. "Steps Toward an Ecology of Infrastructure: Design and Access for Large Information Space." *Information Systems Research* 7 (1996), 111–34.

Statland, Bernard E., and P. Winkel. "Physiological Variability of Leukocytes in Healthy Subjects." In *Differential Leukocyte Counting,* ed. John A. Koepke, 23–38. Skokie, IL: College of American Pathologists, 1978.

Stedman, Thomas Lathrop. *Medical Dictionary: A Vocabulary of Medicine and Its Allied Sciences, with Pronunciations and Derivations.* 21st ed. Baltimore: Williams & Wilkins, 1966.

Steinkamp, John A. "Flow Cytometry." *Review of Scientific Instruments* 55 (1984), 1375–1400.

Stelzer, Gregory T., and Dennis L. Grimaud. "Reimbursement for Clinical Flow Cytometry Testing." *Annals of the New York Academy of Sciences* 677 (1993), 21–7.

Stelzer, Gregory T., Gerald E. Marti, Anne Hurley, J. Phillip McCoy Jr., E. J. Lovett, and Abe Schwartz. "U.S.-Canadian Consensus Recommendations on the Immunophenotypic Analysis of Hematologic Neoplasia by Flow Cytometry: Standardization and Validation of Laboratory Procedures." *Cytometry* 30 (1997), 214–30.

Sternberger, Ludwig A. *Immunocytochemistry.* Englewood, NJ: Prentice-Hall, 1974.

Sternberger, Ludwig A., Paul H. Hardy Jr., John J. Cuculis, and Howard G. Meyer. "The Unlabeled Antibody Enzyme Method of Immunohistochemistry: Preparation and Properties of Soluble Antigen-Antibody Complex (Horseradish Peroxidase–Antihorseradish Peroxidase) and Its Use in Identification of Spirochetes." *Journal of Histochemistry and Cytochemistry* 18 (1970), 315–33.

Stewart, Carleton C., Frederick G. Behm, John L. Carey, Joanne Cornbleet, Ricardo E. Duque, S. David Hudnall, Paul E. Hurtubise, Mike Loken, Raymond R. Tubbs, and Susan Wormsley. "U.S.-Canadian Consensus Recommendations on the Immunophenotypic Analysis of Hematologic Neoplasia by Flow Cytometry: Selection of Antibody Combinations." *Cytometry* 30 (1997), 231–5.

Stillwell, Craig R. "Thymectomy as an Experimental System in Immunology." *Journal of the History of Biology* 27 (1994), 379–401.

Stoker, Michael. "Limits to Oncology." *Nature* 254 (1975), 547–8.

Stoker, Michael. "New Medicine and New Biology." *British Medical Journal* 281 (1980), 1678–82.

Stone, Richard. "Companies Fear FDA Rule on Antibodies." *Science* 268 (1995), 494.

Strauss, Anselm. "A Social World Perspective." *Studies in Symbolic Interaction* 1 (1978), 119–28.

Strauss, Anselm. "Social Worlds and Their Segmentation Processes." *Studies in Symbolic Interaction* 5 (1984), 123–39.

Studer, Kenneth E., and Daryl E. Chubin. *The Cancer Mission: Social Contexts of Biomedical Research.* Beverly Hills, CA: Sage, 1980.

Sun, Tsieh. *Color Atlas/Text of Flow Cytometric Analysis of Hematologic Neoplasms.* New York: Igaku-Shoin, 1993.

Swann, John P. *Academic Scientists and the Pharmaceutical Industry: Cooperative Research in Twentieth Century America.* Baltimore: Johns Hopkins University Press, 1988.

Swazey, Judith P., and Karen Reeds, eds. *Today's Medicine, Tomorrow's Science. Essays on Paths of Discovery in the Biomedical Sciences.* U.S. Dept. of Health, Education, and Welfare (DHEW) publication no. (NIH) 78–244. Washington, DC: DHEW, 1978.

Sweet, Richard G. "High Frequency Recording with Electrostatiscally Deflected Ink Jets." *Review of Scientific Instruments* 36 (1965), 131–6.

Sychra, Jaroslav J., Peter H. Bartels, Marluce Bibbo, and George L. Wied. "Dimensionality Reducing Displays in Cell Image Analysis." *Acta Cytologica* 21 (1977), 747–52.

Takes, Peter. "Letter to CAP Today." *CAP Today* 8 (December 1994), 6–7.

Takes, Peter A., and Delores Graham. "Letter to *Science*." *Science* 269 (1995), 619–20.

Tanke, Hans J. *Cytochemical Staining of DNA and RNA for Analytical Cytology: Development of Methods for Image and Flow Cytometry and Their Diagnostic Application.* PhD thesis, University of Leiden, Netherlands, 1982.

Tatsumi, N., S. Kitahashi, H. Kubota, I. Tsuda, Y. Yasui, K. Tanaka, and H. Kondo. "Standardization in Flow Cytometry" (in Japanese). *Rinsho Byori. Japanese Journal of Clinical Pathology* 41 (9) (1993), 982–9.

Taylor, Clive R. "An Exaltation of Experts: Concerted Efforts in the Standardization of Immunochemistry." *Applied Immunohistochemistry* 1 (1993), 232–43.

Taylor, Clive R. "Changing Concepts in the Classification of Lymphoma." In *Malignant Lymphoproliferative Diseases*, ed. J. G. van den Tweel, C. R. Taylor, and F. T. Bosman, 175–84. The Hague: Leiden University Press, 1980.

Taylor, Clive R. *Hodgkin's Disease and the Lymphomas*, vol. 1. Montreal: Eden Press, 1976.

Taylor, Clive R. *Hodgkin's Disease and the Lymphomas*, vol. 4. Montreal: Eden Press, 1980.

Taylor, Clive R. "Immunocytochemical Methods in the Study of Lymphoma and Related Conditions." *Journal of Histochemistry and Cytochemistry* 26 (1978), 496–512.

Taylor, Clive R. "Immunohistologial Approach to Tumor Diagnosis." *Oncology* 35 (1978), 189–97.

Taylor, Clive R. *An Immunohistological Study of Human and Murine Lymphomata.* PhD thesis, Oxford University, 1974.

Taylor, Clive R., and D. Y. Mason. "The Immunohistological Detection of Intracellular Immunoglobulin in Formalin-Paraffin Sections from Multiple Myeloma and Related Conditions Using the Immunoperoxidase Technique." *Clinical and Experimental Immunology* 18 (1974), 417–29.

Temkin, Oswei. "The Scientific Approach to Disease: Specific Entity and Individual Sickness." In *The Double Face of Janus and Other Essays in the History of Medicine*, Owsei Temkin, 441–55. Baltimore: Johns Hopkins University Press, 1977.

Temkin, Owsei. "The Scientific Approach to Disease: Specific Entity and Individual Sickness." In *Scientific Change: Historical Studies in the Intellectual, Social and*

Technical Conditions for Scientific Discovery and Technical Invention, from Antiquity to the Present. Symposium on the History of Science, University of Oxford, 9–15 July 1961, ed. Alistair Cameron Crombie, 629–47. London: Heinemann Educational, 1963.

Terstappen, L. W., and M. R. Loken, "Five-Dimensional Flow Cytometry as a New Approach for Blood and Bone Marrow Differentials." *Cytometry* 9 (1988), 548–56.

Terstappen, L. W., S. Konemann, M. Safford, M. R. Loken, K. Zurlutter, T. Buchner, W. Hiddemann, and B. Wormann. "Flow Cytometric Characterization of Acute Myeloid Leukemia. Part I. Significance of Light Scattering Properties." *Leukemia* 5 (1991), 315–21.

Terstappen, L. W., M. Safford, S. Konemann, M. R. Loken, K. Zurlutter, T. Buchner, W. Hiddemann, and B. Wormann. "Flow Cytometric Characterization of Acute Myeloid Leukemia. Part II. Phenotypic Heterogeneity at Diagnosis." *Leukemia* 6 (1992), 70–80.

Thévenot, Laurent. "Les investissements de forme." In *Les conventions économiques. Cahiers du centre d'études de l'emploi* 29, Paris: Presses Universitaires de France, 1985, 21–71.

Thévenot, Laurent. "Rules and Implements: Investments in Forms." *Social Science Information* 23 (1984), 1–45.

Thomas, Lewis. *Aspects of Biomedical Science Policy.* Washington, DC: National Academy of Sciences, Institute of Medicine 1972.

Thomas, Lewis. *The Youngest Science: Notes of a Medicine-Watcher.* New York: The Viking Press, 1983.

Thomson, Arthur Landsborough. *Half a Century of Medical Research.* Vol. 1, *Origins and Policy of the Medical Research Council.* London: Her Majesty's Stationery Office, 1973.

Thomson, Arthur Landsborough. *Half a Century of Medical Research.* Vol. 2, *The Programmes of the Medical Research Council.* London: Her Majesty's Stationery Office, 1975.

Tillemans, G. "The Netherlands AIDS Platforms: From National Policy-Making to Local and Regional Implementation." *International Conference on AIDS* (San Francisco, June 20–23, 1990), abstract no. F.D.885, 303.

Tolles, W. E. "The Cytoanalyzer: An Example of Physics in Medical Research." *Transactions of the New York Academy of Sciences* 17 (1954), 250–6.

Tolles, W. E., and R. C. Bostrom. "Automatic Screening of Cytologic Smears for Cancer: Instrumentation." *Annals of the New York Academy of Sciences* 63 (1955), 1211–18.

Tomes, Nancy. *The Gospel of Germs. Men, Women, and the Microbe in American Life.* Cambridge, MA: Harvard University Press, 1998.

Toner, Robin. "Who Gets What Slice of the President's First Federal Budget Pie." *The New York Times* (10 April 2001).

Tubbs, Raymond R., A. Fishleder, R. A. Weiss, R. A. Savage, B. A. Sebek, and J. K. Weick. "Immunohistologic Cellular Phenotypes of Lymphoproliferative Disorders. Comprehensive Evaluation of 564 Cases Including 257 Non-Hodgkin's Lymphomas Classified by the International Working Formulation." *American Journal of Pathology* 113 (November 1983), 207–21.

Tuchman, Arleen M. "From the Lecture to the Laboratory: The Institutionalization of Scientific Medicine at the University of Heidelberg." In *The Investigative Enterprise: Experimental Physiology in Nineteenth-Century Medicine,* ed. William Coleman and Frederic L. Holmes, 65–99. Berkeley: University of California Press, 1988.

Tucker, J., and B. Stenkvist. "Whatever Happened to Cervical Cytology Automation?" *Analytical Cellular Pathology* 2 (1990), 259–66.

Ungeleider, Richard S. "Introduction to the Conference on Cell Markers in Acute Leukemia." *Cancer Research* 41 (1981), 4751.

Upbin, Bruce. "What Have You Invented for Me Lately?" *Forbes* 158 (14) (16 December 1996), 330–4.

Urist, Marshall R. "Phoenix of Physiology and Medicine: Franklin Chambers McLean." *Perspectives in Biology and Medicine* 19 (1975), 41–6.

U.S. Department of Commerce, International Trade Administration. *High Technology Industries: Profiles and Outlooks: Biotechnology.* Washington, DC: U.S. Government Printing Office, July 1984.

Valet, Günter. "Analytical Cellular Pathology and Biology: Presence and Future." *Analytical Cellular Pathology* 18 (1999), 3.

Valet, Günter. "Cytometry, a Biomedical Key Discipline." Unpublished document, n.d., c. 1998.

Van Dilla, Marvin A., and E. C. Anderson. "Personnel Monitoring with Large Liquid Scintillation Counters." *Armed Forces Medical Journal* 11 (1960), 526–34.

Van Dilla, Marvin A., Paul F. Mullaney, and Jeff R. Coulter. "The Fluorescent Cell Photometer: A New Method for the Rapid Measurement of Biological Cells Stained with Fluorescent Dyes." In *Annual Report (July 1966–June 1967) of the Biological and Medical Research Group (H-4) of the Health Division of the Los Alamos Scientific Laboratory,* 100–5.

Van Dilla, Marvin A., T. T. Trujillo, Paul F. Mullaney, and Jeff R. Coulter. "Cell

Microfluorometry: A Method for Rapid Fluorescence Measurement." *Science* 163 (1969), 1213–4.

Van Dongen, Jacques J. M., and Henk J. Adriaansen. "Immunobiology of Leukemia." In *Leukemia*, 6th edn, ed. Edward S. Henderson, T. Andrew Lister, and Mel F. Greaves, 83–130. Philadelphia: Saunders, 1996.

Van Es, Adrian. *Immunological and Clinical Factors Influencing Rejection of Human Renal Allografts: A Single Center Study*. PhD thesis: University of Leiden, Netherlands, 1984.

Van't Veer, M. B., and J. W. Gratama. "Quality Assessment for Immunophenotyping of Leukaemias and Lymphomas: the Dutch Experience. The SIHON Study Group." *Leukaemia and Lymphoma* 13 (Suppl. 1) (1994), 77–9.

Van't Veer, M. B., J. C. Kluin-Nelemans, C. E. van der Schoot, W. L. van Putten, H. J. Adriaansen, and E. R. van Wering, on behalf of the Dutch Cooperative Study Group on Immunophenotyping of Leukaemia and Lymphomas (SIHON). "Quality Assessment of Immunological Marker Analysis and the Immunological Diagnosis in Leukaemia and Lymphoma: a Multi-Centre Study." *British Journal of Haematology* 80 (1992), 458–65.

Vayena, Eftychia. *Cancer Detectors: An International History of the Pap Test and Cervical Cancer Screening, 1928–1970*. PhD thesis, University of Minnesota, Minneapolis, 1999.

Veggeberg, Scott. "Immunology: Highlights from a Hot Biological Field." *The Scientist* 7 (1993), 14–15.

Verderber, Stephen, and David J. Fine. *Healthcare Architecture in an Era of Radical Transformation*. New Haven, CT: Yale University Press, 2000.

Videbaek, Aage. "Do Malignant Lymphomas Represent Varying Differentiation of the Same Growth?" *Acta Haematologica* 2 (1949), 201–12.

Vinck, Dominique. *Du laboratoire aux réseaux. Le travail scientifique en mutation*. Luxembourg City: Office des Publications Officielles des Communautés Européennes, 1992.

Virchow, Rudolf Ludwig Karl. *Cellular Pathology, as Based upon Physiological and Pathological Histology*. New York: Dover, 1971.

Virchow, Rudolf Ludwig Karl. *Disease, Life, and Man: Selected Essays*, trans. Lelland J. Rather. Stanford, CA: Stanford University Press, 1958.

Viza, D., D. A. L. Davies, and R. Harris. "Solubilization and Partial Purification of Human Leukemic Specific Antigens." *Nature* 227 (1970), 1249–51.

Vogel, Karl M. "The Leukemias." In *Nelson Loose-Leaf Living Medicine: Diseases of Blood, Circulatory System, and Kidney*, ed. George R. Minot and Roger I. Lee, 66–90. New York: Thomas Nelson & Sons, 1920.

Vogt, Robert F. Jr., G. David Cross, L. Omar Henderson, and Donald L. Phillips.

"Model System Evaluating Fluorescein-Labeled Microbeads as Internal Standards to Calibrate Fluorescence Intensity on Flow Cytometers." *Cytometry* 10 (1989), 294–302.

Vogt, Robert F. Jr., G. David Cross, Donald L. Phillips, L. Omar Henderson, and W. H. Hannon. "Interlaboratory Study of Cellular Fluorescence Intensity Measurements with Fluorescein-Labeled Microbead Standards." *Cytometry* 12 (1991), 525–36.

Wagner, Loyd R. "The College of American Pathologists, 1946–1996: Laboratory Standards." *Archives of Pathology and Laboratory Medicine* 121 (1996), 536–41.

Wailoo, Keith. *Drawing Blood. Technology and Disease Identity in Twentieth-Century America.* Baltimore: Johns Hopkins University Press, 1997.

Warnke, Roger, Marilyn Pederson, Christopher Williams, and Ronald Levy. "A Study of Lymphoproliferative Diseases Comparing Immunofluorescence with Immunohistochemistry." *American Journal of Clinical Pathology* 70 (1978), 867–75.

Watson, Jim. "From the President: The State of the Society." ISAC E-News (ISAC Website), Summer 1999.

Waxdal, Myron J., Christine Monical, T. A. Fleisher, and Gerald E. Marti. "Interlaboratory Survey of Lymphocyte Immunophenotyping." *Pathology and Immunopathology Research* 7 (1988), 345–56.

Webster, H. Kyle, Kovit Pattanapanyasat, Praphan Phanupak, Chantapong Wasi, Choedchai Cheunchitra, Lupe Ybarra, and Leonard Buchner. "Lymphocyte Immunophenotype Reference Ranges in Healthy Thai Adults: Implications for Management of HIV/AIDS in Thailand." *Southeast Asian Journal of Tropical Medicine and Public Health* 27 (1996), 418–29.

Webster's Third New International Dictionary of the English Language, vol. 2. Chicago: Encyclopaedia Britannica, 1971.

Weissmann, Gerald. "Cell Biology and Medicine." *Hospital Practice* (October 1976), 15–16.

Weisz, George. "The Emergence of Medical Specialization in the Nineteenth Century." *Bulletin of the History of Medicine* 77 (2003), forthcoming.

Weisz, George. "Medical Directories and Medical Specialization in France, Britain and the United States." *Bulletin of the History of Medicine*, 71 (1997), 23–68.

Weisz, George. "Regulating Specialties in France during the First Half of the Twentieth Century." *Social History of Medicine*, 15 (2002), 457–80

Whittaker, M. H., and Cheryl L. Willman. "A Practical Guide to the Use of Molecular Genetic Techniques in the Diagnosis of Lymphoid Malignancies." In *Molecular Diagnostics in Pathology*, ed. Cecilia M. Fenoglio-Preiser and Cheryl L. Willman, 123–48. Baltimore: Williams & Wilkins, 1991.

Wied, George L. "Automated Cell Screening—A Practical Reality or a Daydream?" In *Cytology Automation*, Proceedings of the Second Tenovus Symposium, Cardiff, 24–5 October 1968, ed. David Maclean Demetrius Evans, 43–7. Edinburgh: E. & S. Livingstone, 1970.

Wied, George L. "History of Clinical Cytology and Outlook for the Future." In *Compendium on Diagnostic Cytology*, 7th edn, ed. George L. Wied, Catherine M. Keebler, Leopold G. Koss, Stanley F. Patten, and Dorothy L. Rosenthal, 1–21. Chicago: Tutorials of Cytology, 1992.

Williams, Simon J., and Gillian A. Bendelow. "'Recalcitrant Bodies'? Children, Cancer and the Transgression of Corporeal Boundaries." *Health* 4 (2000), 51–71.

Wilmanns, W., K. Wilms, and M. F. Rajewsky. "Biochemische Grundlagen der Behandlung von Leukosen." In *Leukämie*, ed. Rudolf Gross and Jurgen van de Loo 459–77. Berlin and New York: Springer-Verlag,1972.

Wilson, David. *Body and Antibody. A Report on the New Immunology*. New York: Knopf, 1972.

Wilson, J. M. G., and G. Jungner. *Principles and Practice of Screening for Disease*. Geneva: World Health Organization, 1968.

Wintrobe, Maxwell M. *Hematology: The Blossoming of a Science*. Philadelphia: Lea & Febiger, 1985.

Wofsy, Leon, Paolo Truffa-Bachi, and David Naor. "Chemical Approaches to the Cell Receptor Problem." *Annals of the New York Academy of Sciences* 190 (1971), 432–42.

Wood, Denis. *The Power of Maps*. New York: Guilford, 1992.

Woodruff, H. Boyd, and Brinton M. Miller. "Patenting of Hybridomas and Genetically Engineered Microorganisms." *In Vitro* 17 (1981), 1078–80.

Wooldridge, Dean E. *Biomedical Science and Its Administration. A Study of the National Institutes of Health*. Washington, DC: U.S. Government Printing Office, 1965.

Woolgar, Steve, and Dorothy Pawluch. "Ontological Gerrymandering: The Anatomy of Social Problems Explanations." *Social Problems* 32 (1985), 214–27.

World Health Organization, *External Quality Assessment of Health Laboratories*. Euro Reports and Studies 38. Copenhagen: WHO Regional Office for Europe, 1981.

Wright, James R. "The Development of the Frozen Section Technique, the Evolution of Surgical Biopsy, and the Origins of Surgical Pathology." *Bulletin of the History of Medicine* 59 (1985), 295–326.

Wright, Susan. "Recombinant DNA Technology and Its Social Transformations: 1972–1982." *Osiris* 2nd ser. 2 (1986), 303–60.

Wybran, Joseph, Martin C. Carr, and H. Hugh Fudenberg. "The Human Rosette-

Forming Cell as a Marker of a Population of Thymus-Derived Cells." *Journal of Clinical Investigation* 51 (1972), 2537–43.

Ye, K., K.-C. Koch, B. D. Clark, and C. A. Dinarello. "Interleukin-1 Down-regulates Gene and Surface Expression of Interleukin-1 Receptor Type I by Destabilizing Its mRNA whereas Interleukin-2 Increases Its Expression," *Immunology* 75 (1992), 427–34.

Yorkton Securities Inc. "Valuation." In *Canadian Life Sciences Handbook.* Toronto: BioCatalyst Yorkton Inc., February 1997.

Young, Ian T. "Proof without Prejudice: Use of the Komolgorov-Smirnov Test for the Analysis of Histograms from Flow Systems and Other Sources." *Journal of Histochemistry and Cytochemistry* 25 (1977), 935–41.

Ziegler-Heitbrock, H. W. L., and R. J. Ulevitch. "CD14: Cell Surface Receptor and Differentiation Marker." *Immunology Today* 14 (March 1993), 121–5.

Zito, Denise R. "American Society of Clinical Pathologists Cytometry Qualification." *Cytometry* 18 (1994), 60–1.

Zola, Heddy. "The CD Nomenclature. A Brief Historical Summary of the CD Nomenclature, Why It Exists and How CDs Are Defined." *Journal of Biological Regulators and Homeostatic Agents* 13 (1999), 226–8.

Zuckerman, Steven H. *Cancer Research. A Report by Lord Zuckerman.* London: Her Majesty's Stationery Office, 1972.

Zuckerman, Steven H., and Steven D. Douglas. "The Lymphocyte Plasma Membrane: Markers, Receptors, and Determinants." *Pathobiology Annual* 6 (1976), 119–62.

Index